Stone's Plastic Surgery Facts and Figures

Stone's Plastic Surgery Facts and Figures

Tor Wo Chiu

Resident Specialist, Division of Plastic Reconstructive and Aesthetic Surgery, Prince of Wales Hospital, Hong Kong

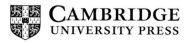

CAMBRIDGE UNIVERSITY PRESS
Cambridge, New York, Melbourne, Madrid, Cape Town,
Singapore, São Paulo, Delhi, Tokyo, Mexico City

Cambridge University Press
The Edinburgh Building, Cambridge CB2 8RU, UK

Published in the United States of America by Cambridge University Press, New York

www.cambridge.org
Information on this title: www.cambridge.org/9780521139786

First edition published 2000
Second edition published 2006
Third edition published 2011

Printed in the United Kingdom at the University Press, Cambridge

A catalogue record for this publication is available from the British Library

Library of Congress Cataloguing in Publication data
Chiu, Tor Wo.
Stone's plastic surgery facts and figures. – 3rd ed. / Tor Wo Chiu.
   p. ; cm.
Plastic surgery facts and figures
Rev. ed. of: Plastic surgery / Christopher Stone. 2nd ed. 2006. Includes index.
ISBN 978-0-521-13978-6 (Hardback)
1. Surgery, Plastic. I. Stone, Christopher (Christopher A.) Plastic surgery. II. Title. III. Title: Plastic surgery
facts and figures. [DNLM: 1. Reconstructive Surgical Procedures. 2. Wounds and Injuries – surgery. WO 600]
RD118.S76   2011
617.9′5–dc22

2011004248

ISBN 978-0-521-13978-6 Hardback

In memory of my loving father.

Contents

Abbreviations

18 FDG–PET	18F-Fluorodeoxyglucose–positron emission tomography	CO	Carbon monoxide
5-FU	5-Fluorouracil	COHb	Carboxyhaemoglobin
ADM	Abductor digiti minimi	CPO	Cleft palate alone
ADSC	Adipose derived stem cells	CRPS	Complex regional pain syndrome
AER	Apical ectodermal ridge	CTA	Computed tomography angiography
AIS	Androgen-insensitivity syndrome	CTS	Carpal tunnel syndrome
ALM	Acral lentiginous melanoma	DCIA	Deep circumflex iliac artery
ALT	Anterolateral thigh	DCIS	Ductal carcinoma *in situ*
AMA	American Medical Association	DD	Dupuytren's disease
ANA	Antinuclear antibody	DFSP	Dermatofibrosarcoma protruberans
APL	Abductor pollicis longus	DIC	Disseminated intravascular coagulation
APR	Abdominoperineal resection	DIEA	Deep inferior epigastric artery
ASA	American Society of Anesthesiologists	DIEP	Deep inferior epigastric perforator
ASD	Atrial septal defect	DIPJ	Distal interphalangeal joint
ASIS	Anterosuperior iliac spine	DISI	Dorsal intercalated segment instability
AVM	Arteriovenous malformation	DP	Distal phalanx
AVN	Avascular necrosis	DRUJ	Distal radioulnar joint
BAD	British Association of Dermatologists	DVT	Deep venous thrombosis
BCC	Basal cell carcinoma	ECRB	Extensor carpi radialis brevis
BCS	Breast conservation surgery	ECRL	Extensor carpi radialis longus
BEAM	Bulbar elongation anastomotic meatoplasty	EDC	Extensor digitorum communis
bFGF	Basic fibroblast growth factor	EDM	Extensor digiti minimi
BMP	Bone morphogenetic protein	EGF	Epidermal growth factor
BRBNS	Blue rubber bleb nevus syndrome	EI	Extensor indicis
BSA	Body surface area/burn surface area	ELND	Elective lymph node dissection
BXO	Balanitis xerotica obliterans	EPB	Extensor pollicis brevis
CAH	Congenital adrenal hyperplasia	ePTFE	Expanded polytetrafluoroethylene (Gore-Tex)
CEA	Cultured epithelial autograft	ESR	Erythrocyte sedimentation rate
CFNG	Cross facial nerve graft	EUA	Examination under anaesthesia
CGRP	Calcitonin growth-related peptide	FCR	Flexor carpi radialis
CL	Cleft lip	FCU	Flexor carpi ulnaris
CL/P	Cleft lip with or without cleft palate	FDM	Flexor digiti minimi
CMCJ	Carpometacarpal joint	FDP	Flexor digitorum profundus
CMN	Congenital melanocytic naevi	FDS	Flexor digitorum superficialis
		FGF	Fibroblast growth factor
		FHL	Flexor hallucis longus

FPL	Flexor pollicis longus	NICE	National Institute for Health and Clinical Excellence
FTSG	Full thickness skin graft	NPWT	Negative pressure wound therapy
GAG	Glycosaminoglycan	NRSTS	Non-rhabdomyosarcoma soft tissue sarcoma
GM-CSF	Granulocyte macrophage colony-stimulating factor	NSAID	Non-steroidal anti-inflammatory drug
GRAP	Glandular reconstruction and prepucioplasty	OA	Osteoarthritis
HBO	Hyperbaric oxygen	OPG	Orthopantomogram
HBV	Hepatitis B virus	ORIF	Open reduction and internal fixation
HCV	Hepatitis C virus	ORL	Oblique retinacular ligament
HLA	Human leucocyte antigen	PDGF	Platelet-derived growth factor
HPV	Human papilloma virus	PDL	Pulsed-dye laser
HSV	Herpes simplex virus	PDT	Photodynamic therapy
ICP	Intracranial pressure	PE	Pulmonary embolism
IDDM	Insulin-dependent diabetes mellitus	PET	Positron emission tomography
IFN	Interferon	PIPJ	Proximal interphalangeal joint
IGAP	Inferior gluteal artery perforator	PLLA	Poly-L-lactic acid
IGF	Insulin-like growth factor	PM	Pectoralis major
IMA	Internal mammary artery	POP	Plaster of Paris
IMF	Intermaxillary fixation	PP	Proximal phalanx
IMRT	Intensity modulated radiotherapy	PRP	Platelet-rich plasma
IPJ	Interphalangeal joint	PSA	Pleomorphic salivary adenoma
IPL	Intense pulsed light	PSIS	Posterior superior iliac spine
ILP	Isolated limb perfusion	PWS	Port wine stain, plagiocephaly without synostosis
KTP	Potassium titanyl phosphate		
LASER	Light amplification by stimulated emission of radiation	PZ	Progress zone
		QSRL	Q-switched ruby laser
LCIS	Lobular carcinoma *in situ*	RA	Rheumatoid arthritis
LDH	Lactate dehydrogenase	RF	Rheumatoid factor
LMM	Lentigo maligna melanoma	RFF	Radial forearm flap
LND	Lymph node dissection	RL	Ringer's lactate
MAGPI	Meatoplasty and glanuloplasty	RT-PCR	Reverse transcriptase–polymerase chain reaction
MCPJ	Metacarpophalangeal joint		
MESS	Mangled extremity severity score	SAL	Suction-assisted liposuction
MFH	Malignant fibrous histiocytoma	SAN	Spinal accessory nerve
MM	Malignant melanoma	SCC	Squamous cell carcinoma
MMP	Matrix metalloproteinase	SIEA	Superficial inferior epigastric artery
MRA	Magnetic resonance angiography	SGAP	Superior gluteal artery perforator
MRSA	Methicillin resistant *Staphylococcus aureus*	SLAC	Scapholunate advanced collapse
		SLD	Scapholunate dissociation
MSH	Melanocyte-stimulating hormone	SLNB	Sentinel lymph node biopsy
NAI	Non-accidental injury	SMAS	Superficial musculo-aponeurotic system
NCS	Nerve conduction study		
Nd:YAG	Neodymium:yttrium aluminium garnet	SNAC	Scaphoid non-union advanced collapse
		SSD	Silver sulphadiazine
NGF	Nerve growth factor	SSG	Split skin graft

SSKI	Saturated solution of potassium iodide	TRAM	Transverse rectus abdominis muscle
SSM	Skin-sparing mastectomy	TXA2	Thromboxane A2
SSM	Superficial spreading melanoma	UAL	Ultrasound-assisted liposuction
STS	Soft tissue sarcomas	UCL	Ulnar collateral ligament
TAP	Thoracodorsal artery perforator	VAC*	Vacuum-assisted closure
TAR	Thrombocytopaenia, absent radius	VASER	Vibration amplification of sound energy at resonance
TCA	Trichloroacetic acid		
TCS	Treacher Collins syndrome	VEGF	Vascular endothelial growth factor
TENS	Transcutaneous electrical nerve stimulation	VISI	Volar intercalated segment instability
TFCC	Triangular fibrocartilage complex	VPI	Velopharyngeal incompetence
TFG	Transforming growth factor	VRAM	Vertical rectus abdominis muscle
TFL	Tensor fascia lata	VSD	Ventricular septal defect
TNF	Tumour necrosis factor-α TNF-α	vWF	von Willebrand factor
TNM	Tumour-node-metastasis	WLE	Wide local excision
TNP	Topical negative pressure	XP	Xeroderma pigmentosum
TPN	Total parenteral nutrition	ZPA	Zone of polarizing activity

Foreword

We live and practice in revolutionary times: never before have there been such rapid advances in knowledge and technology. Our training systems have evolved rapidly in response to political and commercial forces and patient expectations. Against this background, the third edition of Stone's Plastic Surgery Facts and Figures is a timely innovation. The original books were excellent but the third edition is a major improvement with article summaries, avoidance of repetitions and a strong classification.

The many drivers to surgical training include evidence based treatment, which in turn requires an understanding of molecular and cellular biology. Treatment is now becoming strongly influenced by guidelines and protocols and the trainee must be familiar with such systems of classification when selecting appropriate treatments and attending MDTs.

This book provides an excellent framework covering the curriculum for plastic surgery training in the UK. It is an ideal reference source and a checklist for patient-based discussions. Key points are highlighted and knowledge is nicely classified. It will not be the sole source for learning, but it provides an excellent classification of all the points needed for examination revision or the general knowledge required to undertake safe practice.

D A McGrouther MD, MSc, FRCS F Med Sci
Professor of Plastic & Reconstructive Surgery,
The University of Manchester February 2011

Preface

I remember buying the first edition of Plastic Surgery Facts. I was not alone in appreciating its easy to read format and the fact that it was born out of the author's revision notes made it all the more useful for those of us studying for our own Exit examinations in Plastic Surgery.

Since the second edition was published, Plastic Surgery training in the UK has undergone a major overhaul and the Intercollegiate Surgical Curriculum Programme has provided detailed guidance on what is expected of trainees. The material in the new edition has been arranged to follow the syllabus as closely as possible; the chapter layout is based on the Key Topics. Obviously, discussion of everything on the syllabus is not possible in a book of this size, nor is this intended to be the scope of this book.

There was a great deal of information in the previous editions; this edition has focused on altering the layout and presenting the material in a more organized manner, to improve clarity. Of course, the material has been updated to include new material including the AJCC 2009 Staging for Melanoma and propranolol therapy for haemangiomas, for example. The article summaries were a favourite feature of the book and have been retained and updated. Every reference has been rechecked and reviewed; the full reference now given in a more standard format – first author, journal, year, volume and page numbers. Finally there are now line drawings that should make understanding certain topics much easier.

Last but not least, I would like to acknowledge the contribution of Dr Dai Q. A. Nguyen, Welsh Center of Burns and Plastic Surgery, Morriston Hospital.

Wound care

A. Wounds and wound healing

I. Wound healing and tissue transplantation

Adult wound healing

Wound repair proceeds through several stages that overlap:

- Inflammation (coagulation, inflammation).
- Proliferation (re-epithelialization, fibroplasia).
- Remodelling (maturation).

Inflammatory phase (days 0–6)

Coagulation/haemostasis – after wounding, bleeding occurs and haemostatic cascades are activated leading to the formation of a thrombin–platelet plug (clot), adherent to type II collagen exposed by endothelial disruption. This platelet clot is a source of:

- Growth factors – **platelet-derived growth factor** (PDGF), transforming growth factor alpha and beta (TGF-α and –β).
- Inflammatory vasoactive and chemotactic cytokines.
- Fibrinogen, fibronectin, thrombospondin and von Willebrand factor.

Subsequent formation of a **fibrin–thrombin mesh** traps more platelets to continue the cycle. After an initial period of vasoconstriction there is active vasodilatation due to the inflammatory mediators (histamine, kinins, complement).

Inflammation – activation of mast cells (release histamine) and influx of **neutrophils** (production of inflammatory mediators and cytokines), **macrophages** (remove debris, release TGF-β) and **T-lymphocytes** (recruit and activate fibroblasts), conversion of differentiated keratinocytes to immature cells that migrate over the wound surface. There is initial vasoconstriction of injured vessels followed by vasodilatation (and increased permeability) due to histamine and other vasoactive substances.

- Within **12 hours** of wounding, cells appear in the wound – **neutrophils** and **monocytes** are attracted by chemotaxins including fibrin degradation products, complement proteins, leukotrienes, TGF-β and PDGF.
- Translocation of marginating neutrophils (24–48 hours) through capillary endothelium and basement membrane is facilitated by secretion of collagenase. Unless there is a continuing inflammatory stimulus, the neutrophil response and population declines after a few days, whereupon debris is removed by macrophages.
- **Macrophages** are attracted to the wound (48–96 hours) where they synthesize and release further **cytokines and growth factors**; they are **vital to wound healing**.
- Dermal **fibroblasts** migrate into the wound by forming cell–matrix contacts with matrix

proteins such as fibronectin, vitronectin and fibrinogen.

- **T-lymphocytes** migrate into wounds following the influx of macrophages (5–7 days) and persist for up to 1 week – a reduced response may lead to poorer wound healing. Their primary role seems to be to mediate in **fibroblast recruitment** and activation.

Proliferative phase (4 days to 3 weeks)

Re-epithelialization begins within hours of wounding with **migration** of marginal keratinocytes over the matrix but beneath the forming eschar. There is a phenotypic conversion of differentiated keratinocytes into non-polarized cells expressing basal cytokeratins similar to cultured cells; increased mobility comes from dissolution of anchoring junctions and reorganization of the cortical actin cytoskeleton to form lamellipodia. Cells stop migrating when they form a contiguous layer due to **contact inhibition**. Restitution of the basement membrane then induces the cells to adopt their previous morphology and form anchoring junctions with fibronectin.

- **Epidermal growth factor** (EGF) mRNA levels increase rapidly after wounding to promote re-epithelialization. Abnormalities of EGF expression are thought to impair wound healing whilst glucocorticoids suppress EGF expression in cutaneous wounds but have less effect on EGF receptor levels.
- **Melanocyte growth-stimulating activity**, or growth-related gene (MGSA/GRO), is normally expressed by suprabasal, differentiated keratinocytes and is up-regulated in regenerating human epithelium. It is a ligand for the type B IL-8 receptor which is also up-regulated in proliferating keratinocytes (as well as dermal fibroblasts, macrophages and smooth muscle), suggesting that this cytokine may act as an autocrine or paracrine factor-mediating cutaneous wound repair.
- **Insulin-like growth factor-1** (IGF) and IGF-binding protein-1 have been demonstrated to act synergistically to accelerate the healing of adult skin wounds.

Fibroplasia – there is an influx of fibroblasts over the fibronectin scaffold; they are activated by PDGF and TGF-β. These cells synthesize type III collagen, which with ongoing neovascularization forms granulation tissue. Wound **tensile strength** increases during this fibroblastic phase.

- **Activin** is strongly expressed in wound skin. Overexpression in transgenic mice improves wound healing and enhances scar formation; activin A has been implicated in stimulating formation of granulation tissue whilst activin B mRNA has been localized to hyperproliferative epithelium at the wound edge.
- Secretion of glycosaminoglycans (hyaluronic acid, chondroitin sulphate, dermatan sulphate), which become hydrated to form an amorphous **ground substance** within which fibrillar collagen is deposited.
- Zinc, vitamins A (retinoids) and C are also required for normal collagen synthesis.

Angiogenesis – induced by *vascular endothelial growth factor* (VEGF).

Remodelling phase (3 weeks to 18 months)

The extracellular matrix appears to modulate fibroblast activity through changes in composition during healing. When fibronectin initially predominates, fibroblasts actively synthesize hyaluronic acid and collagen, but in a maturing wound, when the amount of collagen reaches a certain, abundant level, fibroblast proliferation and collagen production ceases irrespective of any stimulation by TGF-β. At this point, usually ~10 days, the wound becomes a relatively acellular scar.

- Residual fibroblasts mature into **myofibroblasts** and form cell–matrix and cell–cell contacts that **contract** the wound (scar contracture). Type III collagen is gradually replaced by **type I collagen** by the activity of metallomatrix proteins released by macrophages, keratinocytes and fibroblasts, slowly returning to normal type I : III ratio of 3 : 1. Collagen is initially disorganized but then becomes **lamellar** (and aligned along lines of stress) by the activity of fibroblasts and collagenases with permanent cross-links.
- The abundant capillaries regress.
- Peak wound tensile strength is achieved at ~60 days and is a maximum of ~80% of unwounded skin strength.

Factors affecting wound healing

Discussions generally divide these into patient factors and wound factors. Most factors impairing wound healing may be attributed to a lowering of the oxygen concentration in the wound including radiotherapy and diabetes. An oxygen tension of more than 40 mmHg augments **fibroblastic activity** and is required for the hydroxylation of proline and lysine residues to form **cross linkages** in the collagen α-chain. Oxygen also facilitates **cell-mediated killing** of pathogens in the wound.

Wound infection causes a prolonged inflammatory phase; reduced oxygen tension affects fibroplasia, causes collagen lysis and inefficient keratinocyte migration.

- Tissue expansion – increased rate and strength of healing.
- Low serum protein – prolonged inflammatory phase and impaired fibroplasia.
- Increased ambient temperature (30 °C) – accelerated wound healing.

Patient factors

- Age – there is a reduction in the cellular multiplication and production rate with age. The tensile strength and wound closure rates also decrease with age – the stages of wound healing are protracted.
- Nutrition – malnutrition is associated with impairment of fibroblast function and reduced wound tensile strength.
  ○ Vitamin C – essential for hydroxylation of collagen.
  ○ Vitamin E – antioxidant actions that neutralize lipid peroxidation (and thus cell damage) caused by ionizing radiation, for example.
  ○ Minerals – many are cofactors in collagen production, e.g. zinc influences re-epithelialization and collagen deposition.
- Systemic illness – many impair oxygen delivery and collagen synthesis (fibroblasts are oxygen-sensitive and collagen production is reduced if PaO_2 is below 40 mmHg). Examples include anaemia and pulmonary disease.
  ○ Smoking (multifactorial – the nicotine in one single cigarette causes vasoconstriction that lasts 90 minutes, cyanide impairs oxidative enzymes whilst carbon monoxide impairs the oxygen-carrying capacity of haemoglobin). Stopping will improve:
    – Carbon monoxide (12 hours).
    – Free radicals (1 week).
    – Nicotine effects (10 days).
  ○ Diabetes – multiple factors. These patients are prone to infection, whilst vascular disease reduces oxygenation and neuropathy increases vulnerability to ischaemia.
- Drugs.
  ○ Steroids – anti-inflammatory actions affect wound healing in many ways including macrophage and fibroblast function, reduced angiogenesis and contracture. Vitamin A is usually said to reverse steroid effects and increases collagen synthesis.
  ○ Non-steroidal anti-inflammatory drugs (NSAIDs) – almost halve collagen synthesis in some studies, which is related to the reduction in prostaglandins.
  ○ Chemotherapy – e.g. cyclophosphamide is anti-inflammatory and methotrexate potentiates infections.
- Genetic conditions e.g. Ehlers–Danlos/cutis hyperelastica, progeria etc.

Wound factors

- Infection – this prolongs the inflammatory phase. Endotoxins reduce tissue oxygenation, stimulate phagocytosis and release of collagenases and radicals that may damage normal tissue.
- Oedema – reduces tissue perfusion.
- Denervation – prone to ulceration (also increased collagenases).
- Radiation – endarteritis obliterans.

Collagen

Collagen forms about one-third of the total protein in the human body. The aminoacids hydroxyproline and hydroxylysine are important components of (pro)collagen; deficiencies of vitamin C and iron inhibit their hydroxylation.

- Procollagen – three polypeptide chains as triple helix form tropocollagen.
- Tropocollagen units form collagen filaments.
- Filaments form fibrils, which form fibres.

There are at least 16 different types of collagen.

- Type I – most common and predominates in bone, tendon and skin.
- Type II – hyaline cartilage, cornea.
- Type III – immature scar, blood vessels, bowel, uterus.
- Type IV – basement membrane.
- Type V – fetal and placental tissue.

Dystrophic epidermolysis bullosa is associated with mutations of collagen VII, which form anchoring fibril-specific proteins.

Contraction versus contracture

Contraction is a physiological process which is part of wound repair, whilst contracture is a pathological process which may be related to undesirable healing, fibrosis and tissue damage, which causes shortening, distortion, deformity and limitation of movement.

Myofibroblasts are the source of contraction in wounds; they are found dispersed throughout granulating wounds and appear on the third day, peaking on the tenth day. They are specialized fibroblasts with contractile myofilaments and cellular adhesion structures and their action leads to contraction of the entire wound bed.

Adjuncts to healing

- **Negative wound pressure** – the exact mechanism of action is unclear but negative pressure may help by reducing oedema and interstitial pressure, improving tissue oxygenation and removing inflammatory exudate/mediators and bacteria. See also VAC®.
- **Hyperbaric oxygen** – increases oxygen delivery to wounds. It may be useful in selected wounds e.g. ischaemic (acute arterial insufficiency, crush injuries), radionecrosis, gas gangrene and diabetic ulcers (Medicare covers its use if there are 'no measurable signs of healing for at least 30 days of standard wound therapy').
- **Growth factors** – use is mostly experimental. Recombinant PDGF B-chain (becaplermin) marketed as Regranex, the only agent shown to be efficacious in double-blind studies. It has FDA approval, however, there is a warning that there is an increased cancer mortality in patients who used three or more tubes.
- **Laser biostimulation**.
- **Ultrasound** – results equivocal.

Debridement

Debridement of necrotic, non-viable tissue is an important part of wound management.

- Non-selective – mechanical e.g.
  - Scrubbing.
  - Wet-to-dry dressings.
  - **Hydrogen peroxide** (usually 3%) – this is highly reactive and a source of reactive oxygen species. When applied to tissues it bubbles due to the reaction with tissue catalase releasing water and oxygen; Staphylococci tend to be catalase positive whilst Streptococci do not have catalase and are thus said to be more susceptible to peroxide. It is commonly used as a wound antiseptic and whilst in vitro it shows broad activity, the few studies on its clinical efficacy generally show that it is relatively ineffective in reducing bacterial count but does appear not to delay wound healing. The AMA (Roderheaver GT. In Krasner D, Kane D (eds). *Chronic Wound Care: A Clinical Source Book for Healthcare Professionals*, 2nd Edn. 1997;97–108) suggested that the effervescence may have some mechanical benefit in loosening debris and necrotic tissue in a wound.
  - Pulsed lavage systems, Versajet®.
- Selective debridement.
  - Sharp/surgical.
  - **Enzymatic** – selectively digest dead tissue/ slough e.g. Iruxol Mono® which is a collagenase, clostridiopeptidase A, but takes several days. Others include Debridase (bromelain, derived from pineapple stems) which seems to work quicker (Rosenberg L. *Burns* 2004;**30**:843–850).
    - Autolytic – the combination of moist dressings e.g. hydrocolloids and endogenous enzymes can lead to the breakdown of necrotic tissue.
  - Biological – maggots of certain species, e.g. *Lucilia sericata*, can cause benign myiasis – i.e. the larvae only eat dead tissue. They also have antimicrobial action and promote healing to a certain extent.

Fetal wound healing

Rowlatt U. *Virchows Archiv* 1979;**381**:353–361. This was the first report of scar-free healing in humans.

The term fetal wound healing is used to describe the regenerative process that occurs with minimal or no scar formation; it only occurs in the skin and bone of the fetus, but not nerve or muscle i.e. it is organ specific. The exact reasons for this are unclear though some have postulated on the significance of various findings including:

- Environment: fetal wounds are rich in hyaluronic acid and fibronectin.
- Wounds are conspicuous by an absence of inflammation and angiogenesis; healing is largely controlled by fibroblasts rather than macrophages.
- Reduced levels of TGF-β, PDGF, bFGF.
- Type III collagen is deposited in a more organized manner close to normal structure.
- Tenascin is a modulator of cell growth and migration in fetal wounds.

Bone

Bone is composed of 25% organic material (mostly type I collagen), 60% mineral (mainly hydroxyapatite) and 5% trace elements.

- Endochondral bone – laid down as cartilage first, usually at an epiphysis, followed by ossification. This occurs in long bones.
- Membranous bone – osteoid is laid down directly by osteoblasts without a cartilaginous stage – this occurs in facial bones.
- Cortical – concentric lamellae around a Haversian canal.
- Cancellous – made up of lamellar bone but in loosely woven spicules/trabeculae. It is not the same as immature/woven bone.

Fracture healing

There are four phases similar to wound healing described above:

- **Haemorrhage, inflammation and proliferation** (1–7 days) – activation of clotting cascade to form a fibrin coagulum between the bone ends which is invaded by neutrophils, then by macrophages and fibroblasts to form granulation tissue.
- **Soft callus stage** (3–4 days) – capillaries from the periosteum invade the fibrin clot. Undifferentiated periosteal mesenchymal cells differentiate to become chondrocytes that form a cartilaginous external or **bridging callus** (its extent increases when there is movement of the bone ends) with further differentiation of chondrocytes into osteoblasts with **endochondral ossification** of callus to form woven bone (hard callus stage about 3 weeks after injury).

- **Remodelling** (years) of woven bone to mature lamellar bone, orientated along lines of stress.

Primary cortical union/bone healing occurs when bone ends are anatomically reduced and there is rigid fixation (also for membranous bone or for vascularized bone flaps). Bone regeneration occurs from within the opposed Haversian canals with little or no external callus reaction; it takes about 6 weeks i.e. typically longer than secondary bone healing described above (for fractures that are not rigidly fixed or have a small gap).

Bone reconstruction

A good blood supply and stability of the bony ends is essential for healing. Blood supply:

- Nutrient artery which enters medulla and usually supplies the inner two-thirds of the cortex.
- Periosteal artery which supplies the outer third of the cortex.
- Metaphyseal, apophyseal (at tendon/ligament attachments) and epiphyseal.

Healing of bone grafts

- **Osteoinduction** – pluripotential cells in the recipient site (pericytes) are 'induced' to become bone cells; this is controlled by bone morphogenic proteins.
- **Osteoconduction** – bone graft acts as scaffold for the ingrowth of cells and capillaries. Old bone is reabsorbed and new bone deposited i.e. 'creeping substitution'.
- **Osteointegration** – new bone formation by surviving cells within vascularized bone graft.

Vascularized bone grafts i.e. bone flaps are recommended for defects larger than 5–6 cm. It can take over a year for stable union. Distraction osteogenesis can be used for defects > 10 cm.

Factors affecting healing of bone grafts

- Patient factors e.g. age, nutrition, immunosuppression, diabetes, obesity, drugs.
- Bone graft factors.
  - Intrinsic properties – there is usually less resorption if the periosteum is intact and in membranous bone. Preparation, i.e. fresh or treated, will make a difference.
  - Placement – orthotopic (graft placed in position normally occupied by bone) grafts are less prone to resorption whilst heterotopic

Table 1.1. The characteristics of types of bone grafts related to their healing and strength over time.

	Vascularized bone	Cortical graft	Cancellous bone
Osteoinduction	+/−	+/−	++
Osteoconduction	+	+	++++
Osteoprogenitor cells	++	−	+++
Immediate strength	+++	+++	−
6-month strength	+++	+++	++
12-month strength	+++	+++	+++

(in position not normally occupied by bone) are more prone to resorption.

○ Recipient site – irradiation, infected or scarred.
○ Fixation.
○ Mechanical stress – physiological loading speeds up union and creeping substitution.

Tendon healing e.g. in the hand

Tendons consist of a dense network of spiralling collagen fibres that are predominantly type I; there is some type III collagen and a small amount of elastin. They are relatively acellular but do contain tenocytes, fibroblasts and synoviocytes.

● The endotenon holds tendon fascicles together and supports the sparse vessels and nerves; it is continuous with perimysium and periosteum.
● The epitenon is a vascular, cellular outer layer of a tendon which runs through a synovial sheath (zones 1 and 2) whilst in zones 3 and beyond, where there is no tendon sheath, the outer vascular layer is called 'paratenon'.

The blood supply in zones 1 and 2 comes via mesenteries ('mesotenons') called the vinculae – long and short, that enter the dorsal surface of the tendons from the transverse digital arteries at the level of the cruciate pulleys.

Synovial fluid also contributes to nutrition via imbibition and is the more important source in the hand; in the forearm, tendon nutrition is derived from vessels in the paratenon.

Tendon healing occurs by analogous processes of inflammation, fibroplasia and remodelling:

● Intrinsic healing by cells within the tendon itself.
● Extrinsic healing by cells recruited from synovial sheaths and surrounding tissues forming adhesions.

Studies have demonstrated that the strength and rate of healing are maximal in a tendon that is moving and stressed. A repaired tendon is weakest during period of collagen lysis at about day 14.

Cytokines, growth factors and plastic surgery
Rumalla VK. *Plast Reconstr Surg* 2001; **108**: 719–733.

Cytokines

Cytokines are proteins required for cell defence that are secreted predominantly by immune cells. They mediate in protective and reparative processes and also regulate cell growth and maturation.

Tumour necrosis factor-α

Tumour necrosis factor-α (TNFα) is released by macrophages/monocytes when stimulated by interaction with pathogens, tumour cells and toxins. It appears at wound sites after 12 hours of wounding and peaks at 72 hours.

● Mediates in chemotaxis of inflammatory cells.
● Up-regulation of cellular adhesion molecules at neutrophil target cell sites e.g. vascular endothelium (margination).
● Other effects include haemostasis, increased vascular permeability and collagen synthesis (although may impair wound healing if persists at high levels beyond natural peak and excess TNFα is associated with multi-system organ failure).

Interleukin-1

Interleukin-1 (IL-1) is produced by macrophages/monocytes and keratinocytes at wound sites and is detectable at wound sites after 24 hours, peaking around day 2 then rapidly declining.

● Neutrophil activation and chemotaxis.
● Increased collagen synthesis and keratinocyte maturation.
● High levels at chronic non-healing wound sites.

Interleukin-2

Interleukin-2 (IL-2) is produced by T lymphocytes.

- Sustains the post-injury inflammatory response via T-cell activation.
- Promotes fibroblast infiltration at wound sites.

Interleukin-6

Interleukin-6 (IL-6) is released by macrophages/monocytes, polymorphs and fibroblasts and is detectable at wound sites within 12 hours (as polymorphs arrive) and persists for up to a week.

- Promotes stem cell growth, B- and T-cell activation and mediates in hepatic acute phase protein synthesis (involved in the immune response).
- Stimulates fibroblast proliferation.
- High IL-6 increases scarring and high systemic IL-6 levels have been described as a marker of wound extent/severity (e.g. major burns) and a poor prognostic indicator.
- Low IL-6 in elderly patients with impaired wound healing and at scar-less fetal wound sites.

Interleukin-8

Interleukin-8 (IL-8) is released by macrophages and fibroblasts at wound sites.

- Neutrophil chemotaxis, adhesion (via up-regulated expression of endothelial cell adhesion molecules) and activation.
- Promotes keratinocyte maturation and migration.
- High levels in patients with psoriasis and low levels at fetal wound sites.

Interferon γ

Interferon γ is produced by T-cells and macrophages.

- Macrophage and polymorph activation.
- Mediates in wound remodelling; reduces wound contraction.
- Possible role for decreasing scar hypertrophy but may decrease wound strength.
- Anti-inflammatory cytokine.

Interleukin-4

Interleukin-4 (IL-4) is produced by T-cells, mast cells and B-lymphocytes.

- Promotes B-cell proliferation and IgE mediated immunity and inhibits the release of pro-inflammatory cytokines by macrophages.
- Promotes fibroblast proliferation and collagen synthesis at wound sites.
- High levels are found in patients with scleroderma.

Interleukin-10

Interleukin-10 (IL-10) is produced by macrophages and T-cells.

- Inhibits production of pro-inflammatory cytokines at acute wound sites.
- If persistent at high levels at chronic wound sites, e.g. venous ulcers, it contributes to impairment of the wound healing response.

Growth factors

Growth factors are polypeptides whose primary role is in regulation of cell growth and maturation.

Platelet-derived growth factor

Platelet-derived growth factor (PDGF) is released from α granules within platelets and by macrophages.

- Recruitment and activation of immune cells and fibroblasts in the early post-injury phase.
- Later stimulates the production of collagen and glycosaminoglycans; reduced levels are found in non-healing wounds.
- Three isomers of PDGF (2 polypeptide chains 'A' and 'B'):
  - AA: elevated at acute wound sites.
  - BB: most useful clinically, used for chronic and diabetic ulcers (Regranex®).
  - AB.

Transforming growth factor β

Transforming growth factor β (TGF-β) is released by macrophages, platelets and fibroblasts.

- Fibroblast maturation, collagen and proteoglycan synthesis.
- Inhibition of proteases.
- There are three isomers: TGF-β1, TGF-β2 and TGF-β3.
  - TGF-β1 and TGF-β2 associated with hypertrophic and keloid scarring, and neutralizing antibodies decrease scarring at rat wound sites (Shah M. *J Cell Sci* 1994;**107**:1137–1157).
  - Low TGF-β at fetal wound sites.
  - TGF-β3 shown to decrease scarring.
  - Ratio of TGF-β1 and TGF-β2: TGF-β3 determines nature of scar.

Fibroblast growth factor

Fibroblast growth factor (FGF) is released from fibroblasts and endothelial cells.

- Regulates angiogenesis and keratinocyte migration at wound sites.
- Two main forms: acidic FGF (aFGF or FGF-1) and basic FGF (bFGF or FGF-2) that binds to the same receptors as aFGF but is ten times more potent.
  - Eight other isoforms complete the family: FGF-7 and FGF-10 known as keratinocyte growth factor (KGF) 1 and 2. KGF-1 is low in diabetics and steroid immunosuppression; recombinant KGF shown to improve re-epithelialization at wound sites.
- Application of exogenous bFGF to wound sites accelerates re-epithelialization.

Epidermal growth factor

Epidermal growth factor (EGF) is released from keratinocytes.

- EGF promotes epithelialization.
- Promotes collagenase release from fibroblasts (remodelling).
- Inhibits wound contraction at fetal wound sites.

Vascular endothelial growth factor

Vascular endothelial growth factor (VEGF) is released mainly from keratinocytes, also macrophages and fibroblasts.

- Promotes angiogenesis at wound sites.
- Mediates in the formation of granulation tissue.

Insulin-like growth factor

At wound sites, insulin-like growth factor (IGF) is released by macrophages, neutrophils and fibroblasts; levels rise to a peak within 24 hours of wounding and persist for several weeks.

- Promotes fibroblast and keratinocyte proliferation, with possible role in angiogenesis.
- Two isoforms: IGF-1 and IGF-2.
- Low IGF levels are observed in diabetic and steroid-suppressed wounds.

Immunology

Major histocompatability antigens (called human leucocyte antigens – HLA, in humans).

- Type 1 – all nucleated cells and platelets.
- Type 2 – antigen-presenting cells: Langerhans cells, macrophages and lymphocytes.

Sequence

- Antigen-presenting cells present alloantigen to T-cells and express IL-1.
- IL-1 causes T-helper (CD4+) to produce IL-2.
- IL-2 causes clonal expansion of T-helper cells and B-lymphocytes.
- IL-2 also activates Tc-cells and NK cells (cellular immunity).
- B lymphocytes mediate antibody-mediated cell lysis (humoral immunity).

Allograft rejection

- Acute rejection occurs after 7–10 days, due to T-cell infiltrate (cellular immunity). It may be delayed in immunocompromised patients until the immunodeficient state has passed, e.g. recovery from a burn or stopping immunosuppressant drugs.
- Late rejection is due to antibody-mediated cell lysis (humoral immunity).
- Hyperacute rejection is due to preformed antibodies and the rejection response begins immediately.

Graft versus host reaction occurs when allograft containing lymphoid tissue reacts against an immunocompromised host.

Immunosuppressant drugs

- Cyclosporin blocks IL-2 which blocks clonal expansion of Tc-cells.
- Azathioprine inhibits T-cell-mediated rejection by preventing cell division.
- Prednisolone blocks the generation and release of T-cells.

Biomaterials

These are materials used to replace or augment tissues in the human body and can be classified as:

- Autograft – living tissue from host.
- Isograft – from a genetically identical twin.
- Allograft – tissue from same species.
- Xenograft – tissue from different species.
- Alloplast – derived from synthetic material.

The biological reactions to a foreign body include:

- Immediate inflammation with early rejection.
- Delayed rejection.

- Fibrous encapsulation.
- Incomplete encapsulation with continuing cellular reaction.
- Slow resorption.
- Incorporation.

Cultured epithelial autograft

A cultured epithelial autograft (CEA) begins with a full-thickness skin biopsy of several square centimetres taken from the patient for culturing. After 3 weeks' preparation time, there are enough cells to cover a $1.8\,m^2$ sheet five cells thick. The overall take is 80% under favourable conditions, though late loss can occur. The new skin separates easily from underlying dermis – these bullae contain high levels of thromboxane A2 (TXA2) and prostaglandin E2 (PGE2) suggesting on going inflammation.

- Cultured cells can be delivered as a sheet or as a suspension, which takes less time (cells are less mature) and less ligand-specific integrins/adhesion molecules are expressed facilitating graft take. CEA cell suspension may be used in combination with widely meshed split skin graft (SSG; e.g. 'sandwich' graft). It may also be used to speed up donor site re-epithelialization.
- A variant (mixed cell culture – ReCell®) is said to reduce pigmentary problems.

Bone grafts and cartilage grafts

Bone autografts

- Can be incorporated without host reaction, and is relatively resistant to infection.
- Donor site morbidity is a problem, as is the variable resorption rate in the graft – cortical grafts maintain their volume better than cancellous.

Cartilage autografts

- Relatively easy harvest and less donor site morbidity; infection and resorption is rare but may calcify.
- Has a tendency to warp and quantities are quite limited (septum, rib, conchal).

Allografts

These generally do not contain living cells due to processing to reduce antigenicity, though bone allograft may have osteoconductive and osteoinductive properties. They are **incorporated** into host tissues providing a structural framework for ingrowth of host tissues.

- Their advantages include a plentiful supply, a donor site is not required and operation time is usually reduced.
- Disadvantages include a potential for infection/disease transmission, and variable amount of resorption.

Examples include:

- Lyophilized fascia (dura mater, fascia lata) – risk of Creutzfeldt–Jakob disease (CJD) transmission in the former. Typically there is a 10% resorption rate.
- Homologous cartilage – greater tendency for resorption, replacement with fibrous tissue, ossification and more infection compared with autologous tissue.
- Homologous bone – acts generally as scaffold for formation of new bone; slower to become incorporated and revascularized.
- **AlloDerm** (Lifecell Corp.) – a homologous/cadaveric dermis that has been processed to remove cellular elements, it becomes incorporated into the host.

Cadaveric skin allograft

Allograft can be used by itself as a dressing (see above) or laid over 3:1 (or wider) meshed autograft (Alexander technique). Burns patients are immuno-suppressed so rejection of allograft is usually delayed, in some cases up to 85% viability at 1 year.

- The skin must be retrieved within 24 hours of death from a refrigerated cadaver under aseptic conditions (screening serology for hepatitis B virus (HBV), hepatitis C virus (HCV), human immunodeficiency virus (HIV) and skin samples for culture of bacteria, yeast and fungi). It is stored in nutrient media at 4 °C for up to 1 week or cryopreserved (controlled freezing at 0.5–5 °C/min to –196 °C with liquid nitrogen and a cryoprotectant solution). When needed, it is rapidly rewarmed to 10–37 °C (~3–4 min).
- Donor exclusion criteria: high-risk categories for HIV i.e. homosexuals, drug abusers, those with tattoos, prostitutes and haemophiliacs, those with infection/sepsis, neoplasia and autoimmune disease. Only two cases of viral transmission in

3 million tissue transplants (including skin) have been described.

Skin banking in the UK: the need for proper organization
Freedlander E. *Burns* 1998;**24**:19–24.

The Sheffield skin bank was set up in 1991. They use similar inclusion/exclusion criteria as above (based on the guidelines of the American Association of Tissue Banks) using a one-page questionnaire requesting information on past medical and social history.

- Preservation media of 15% glycerol in phosphate buffer saline (PBS) with penicillin, streptomycin and amphotericin B added. Intracellular viruses are destroyed. Skin is banked in 15% glycerol at –80 °C (viable) or in 98% glycerol at room temperature.

Prepared in this way, the cadaveric skin has a 2-year shelf-life but is non-viable, effectively acting as a biological dressing. The paper goes on to describe the logistical difficulties in the running of the skin bank, and increasing demand coming from outside of the original catchment area, leading to the transfer of the service to the National Blood Service in 1996.

Xenografts

- Surgisis® – derived from pig small intestine mucosa. It is often used for fascia replacement; the acelullar matrix allows tissue ingrowth. There are no good clinical data for its effectiveness.
- Integra® – outer silicone layer covers bovine collagen cross-linked with shark chondroitin-6-sulphate that is revascularized and acts as a template for dermal regeneration (vide supra).

Alloplasts

Alloplasts have wide availability/supply without donor site morbidity, but tend to be expensive and elicit a host reaction of some sort as they are foreign materials.

- Metals e.g. stainless steel, vitallium alloy, titanium alloys (10 times stronger than bone and well tolerated but has low fatigue tolerance).
- Medpor (high density porous polyethylene) – allows vascular ingrowth and reduced tissue reaction, but it is expensive and can be difficult to remove.
- Hydroxyapatite – a calcium phosphate salt available in dense (high pressure compaction) or porous hydroxyapatite. A natural source of hydroxyapatite comes from coral. It allows a degree of vascular ingrowth but is brittle and can be difficult to shape. Also available for use as a tissue filler, Radiesse®.
- Silicone is a silicon polymer and its physical state depends on the amount of cross-linking. It is generally inert which means it tends to be encapsulated rather than incorporated.
- Expanded polytetrafluorethylene (ePTFE), Gore-Tex is available in many different forms. It shows reduced tissue ingrowth.

The following are resorbable (unlike the previous examples):

- Polylactide compounds e.g. Lactosorb plating system used in craniofacial surgery, poly-L-lactic acid (PLLA) tissue fillers (Sculptra®). These are completely resorbed and thus have fewer long-term risks.
- Polyglactin – is available as a suture (Vicryl), film or mesh.

II. Necrotizing fasciitis

Necrotizing fasciitis was first described by Wilson in 1952. It is a life-threatening infection (mortality rate up to 53%) that progresses along fascia and subcutaneous tissues. Some describe type I (polymicrobial) and type II (monomicrobial). In most, there is bacterial synergism as lytic toxins increase the spread of anaerobic organisms.

- **Mixed** anaerobe (*Escherichia coli*, *Bacteroides*) and aerobes (*Staphylococcus aureus*, *Streptococcus pyogenes*, *Enterococcus faecalis*). In most cases, *Streptococcus* and/or *Staphylococcus* are the initiating agent.
  - *Vibrio vulnificus* is often seen in those with chronic liver disease and may follow raw seafood ingestion as well as injuries in fishmarkets. This type of disease classically has subcutaneous bleeding.
- Group A beta haemolytic streptococcal (e.g. *Streptococcus pyogenes*) infection – group A *Streptococcus* is carried in the nose/throat of 15% of the population. It can contribute to type I infections or be responsible for type II (most cases are streptococcal but more recently methicillin-resistant *Staphylococcus aureus* (MRSA) has been

found in some cases). There are a number of virulence factors:

- Exotoxin e.g. streptococcal pyrogenic exotoxin A (SpeA); this superantigen causes systemic upset.
- Streptokinase that activates plasminogen and fibrinolysis.
- Hyaluronidase.
- Haemolysins.
- M proteins that inhibit opsonization by alternative complement pathway.

- Clostridial 'gas gangrene'. Sometimes called type III. 80% *Clostridium perfringens* (Gram-positive rods) although it can be caused by other species. Local tissue hypoxia leads to activation of spores with alpha (exo)toxin i.e. lecithinase production that breaks down cell plasma membranes. Classically there is subcutaneous emphysema, crepitus (also found in around half of non-clostridial gangrene) and 'dish-water' exudate.
  - Similar onset and sick patient, but there is characteristic surgical emphysema (crepitus). The bloody blisters contain *Clostridium welchii* if aspirated.
  - High mortality: aggressive surgical approach needed with some evidence to support role of hyperbaric oxygen.

Meleney's synergistic gangrene is rare but rapidly progressive due to synergism between aerobic haemolytic *Staphylococci* (*aureus*) and microaerophilic non-haemolytic *Streptococci*. (Described and detailed in 1924 by Frank L. Meleney, a US surgeon working mostly at Columbia University in New York; he was also one of the first to use bacitracin.)

Risk factors

- Surgery and even intravenous infusions or intramuscular injections have been associated with necrotizing fasciitis.
- Insulin-dependent diabetes mellitus (IDDM).
- NSAIDs e.g. ibuprofen – recent studies show an association with necrotizing fasciitis, during varicella zoster virus infections.

Clinical features

- **Local** swelling and redness, intense pain. There is very rapid spread subcutaneously, the dissemination of infection through tissue planes causes thrombosis of blood vessels and violaceous skin changes with dusky/grey hue and haemorrhagic bullae, with crepitus and anaesthetic zones due to nerve necrosis. The underlying fascial necrosis is more extensive than overlying skin changes.
- **Systemic toxicity**: apathy, confusion and septic shock, that is classically out of proportion to the skin disease. The elderly may be unable to mount a pyrexial response.

Management

Early recognition of the condition and early treatment is vital.

- **Tissue biopsy** (rapid Gram stain of tissue from the periphery/deeper tissues – surface biopsies may detect other bacteria that do not actually contribute to the disease) during early debridement is the mainstay and should not be delayed by radiology or other studies. The so-called 'finger test' is said to demonstrate the loosened tissue planes, cloudy exudate and lack of bleeding via a 2 cm incision but is very much dependent on the experience of the physician.
- **Radiology** - subcutaneous gas on plain X-rays that are usually of little value; computed tomography (CT) may demonstrate gas and fascial thickening. Magnetic resonance imaging (MRI) has been used more recently – fascial necrosis is demonstrated by the lack of gadolinium enhancement on T1 – in general, the sensitivity of MRI exceeds its specificity. Doppler ultrasound or bedside ultrasound may be superior to clinical assessment alone.

Treatment

- Resuscitation including ITU supportive therapy: ventilation/oxygenation, inotropic support and dialysis where necessary.
- Intravenous antibiotics e.g. clindamycin (stops the production of toxins and M proteins), gentamicin (covers Gram negatives), third generation cephalosporins (covers Gram negatives) and imipenem. Immunoglobulins may be given to those with streptococcal toxic shock syndrome.
  - Many propose gentamicin with clindamycin as standard coverage, adding ampicillin if Gram stain shows enterococci.
  - Anaerobes suggested by 'foul-smelling' lesions are covered by clindamycin or metronidazole.

- Radical surgical debridement to healthy tissues, with a 'second look' at 24 hours.
- Hyperbaric oxygen (HBO) has been proposed for clostridial types of infection.

Necrotizing fasciitis of the face and neck

Sepulveda A. *Plast Reconstr Surg* 1998;**102**:814–817.

The head and neck are not common sites for necrotizing fasciitis, being much less common than trunk and perineum (Fournier's). In this series, the cultures usually contained a mixture of *Streptococcus*, *Staphylococcus*, Gram-negative bacilli and anaerobes; some followed pharyngeal or tonsillar abscesses.

Treatment follows the same protocols as necrotizing fasciitis elsewhere, i.e. extensive debridement, systemic antibiotics and HBO, though the authors comment that vital structures in the head and neck makes radical debridement difficult.

Necrotizing fasciitis of the upper extremity

Gonzalez MH. *J Hand Surg* 1996;**21**:689–692.

Cases in this series were all associated with intravenous substance abuse or diabetes, with HIV positivity in 60% of patients tested. The isolated organisms were β-haemolytic *Streptobacillus* or mixed aerobic/anaerobic infection or both.

These cases had an insidious onset with rapid spread along tissue planes; myonecrosis in five patients. Effective debridement was followed by a rapid clinical response; an average of three total debridements were needed, including shoulder disarticulation.

Necrotizing fasciitis of the breast

Shah J. *Br J Plast Surg* 2001;**54**:67–68.

The diagnosis was made based upon clinical features with a high index of suspicion including crepitus due to gas-forming organisms diagnosed by aspiration Gram-stain microscopy. There were Gram-positive cocci – peptostreptococci, Gram-positive rods – clostridia and Gram-positive rods – coliforms. Breast reconstruction was delayed for several months after the acute episode.

III. Clotting and haemostasis

There are four components to clotting and haemostasis.

- **Vasoconstriction** – contraction of vascular smooth muscle both as a local reflex and in response to thromboxane release from platelets.
- **Activation of platelets** – with disruption of the endothelium, platelets adhere to the underlying tissue and the intrinsic pathway is activated. Aggregated platelets promote local thrombin and fibrin generation.
- **Coagulation** – intrinsic pathway (involves normal blood components) and extrinsic pathways (requires tissue thromboplastin from damaged cells) both activate factor X. Most coagulation factors are made in the liver except for VIII and thromboplastin (also calcium and platelets).
- **Fibrinolysis** – i.e. fibrin removal. This comes from the action of plasmin (plasminogen activators from endothelial cells promote conversion of plasminogen to plasmin).

Disorders of coagulation

- Congenital.
  - Haemophilia A – VIII deficiency that is X-linked.
  - von Willebrand's disease – autosomal dominant deficiency of von Willebrand factor (vWF) that will also reduce VIII somewhat (as it normally protects VIII from breakdown). It is the commonest inherited abnormality of coagulation and is actually a collection of conditions with a reduction of vWF rather than a single disease entity.
- Acquired
  - Vitamin K – deficiency of the vitamin inhibits synthesis of II, VII, IX and X; warfarin also inhibits their production (as well as protein C and S).
  - Liver disease – reduced synthesis of clotting factors and reduced/abnormal fibrinogen.
  - Disseminated intravascular coagulation (DIC) – simultaneous coagulation and fibrinolysis, causes reduction of platelets and fibrinogen, but increase in *fibrin* degradation products.

Disorders of haemostasis

- Thrombocytopaenia – due to either reduced production, increased destruction or abnormal function e.g. aspirin (blocks platelet cyclo-oxygenase) and clopidogrel (reduces platelet aggregation by inhibiting ADP binding).
- Blood vessel abnormalities e.g. due to Cushings syndrome/steroids, Henoch–Schönlein purpura (HSP).

Hypercoagulability states

Between 5% and 15% of venous thromboses are caused by inherited deficiencies. Some causes include:

- Activated protein C resistance (APC) (factor V Leiden mutation) – APC normally inactivates factors V and VIII. This is one of the most common inherited causes.
- Antiphospholipid antibody.
- Homocysteinaemia.
- Elevated factors VIII and XI.

B. Pressure sores

I. Aetiology and risk assessment

Pure pressure sores begin with tissue necrosis near a bony prominence leading to a cone-shaped area of tissue breakdown with its apex at the skin surface. Affecting this situation is the additional soft tissue damage caused by moisture, infection and shear forces, etc. (see below).

- ~10% of patients in acute care facilities develop pressure sores (mainly sacral); up to 24% in chronic hospitalized patients.
- 66% of elderly patients with neck of the femur (NOF) fractures and 60% of quadriplegic patients develop pressure sores.
  - Supine patients develop sacral and heel sores whilst the wheelchair/chair bound develop ischial sores.
  - Lying on one side causes trochanteric sores.
  - Occipital sores can also result.

Risk assessment

Many different systems have been described.

- Braden Scale

  The threshold value is usually 18 out of a maximum of 23 (but depends on setting; original threshold was 16); those with a minimum score of 6 have a high risk of developing pressure sores. The scale takes account of sensory perception, skin moisture, activity, mobility, friction, shear and nutritional status.

- Norton Scale for elderly patients
- **Waterlow score** – pressure sore risk assessment chart.
- Body mass index (BMI).
- Continence.
- Mobility.

- Nutrition.
- Skin changes/type.
- Sex/age.
- Adverse wound healing factors/tissue malnutrition.
- Neurological deficit.
- Major surgical intervention(s)/trauma.
- Drugs (steroids, cytotoxics, anti-inflammatory).

Necessary actions

- Regularly reassess pressure damage risk.
- Regularly inspect pressure areas.
- Plan of care: regular repositioning, minimize shear/friction etc.

Pathogenesis

Prolonged unrelieved pressure leads to **ischaemic necrosis** if the tissue pressure is greater than perfusion pressure; the damage is proportional to the pressure and its duration. Muscle is more susceptible than skin to pressure necrosis.

Altered sensory perception contributes as well as:

- Incontinence and exposure to moisture (maceration and breakdown).
- Friction and shear force (traction on perforator vessels to the skin) can lead to subcutaneous degloving.
- Infection causing exacerbation of the sore (apart from causing tissue damage by itself, infection increases susceptibility to pressure, whilst pressure increases susceptibility to infection).

Intrinsic factors may also contribute:

- Ischaemia, sepsis and vascular disease (peripheral vascular disease (PVD), diabetes mellitus, smokers), reducing perfusion.
- Loss of protective sensation.
- Malnutrition and reduced wound healing.

Grading of pressure sores

Grading was originally described by Shea in 1975 and has been modified/updated into various sets of guidelines.

European Pressure Ulcer Advisory Panel grading system (2005).

- Grade 1: **non-blanchable erythema** of intact skin. Discolouration of the skin, warmth, oedema, induration or hardness may also be used as indicators, particularly on individuals with darker skin in whom it may appear blue or purple.

- Grade 2: **partial thickness** skin loss involving epidermis, dermis or both. The ulcer is superficial and presents clinically as an abrasion or blister. Surrounding skin may be red or purple.
- Grade 3: **full thickness skin** loss involving damage to or necrosis of subcutaneous tissue that may extend down to, but **not through underlying fascia**.
- Grade 4: extensive destruction, tissue necrosis, or **damage to muscle, bone**, or supporting structures with or without full thickness skin loss. Extremely difficult to heal and predisposes to fatal infection.

However, it is important to appreciate that the surface appearance does not reflect the underlying extent of the sore.

National Pressure Ulcer Advisory Panel (2007). (American version)

- **Suspected deep tissue injury:** purple/maroon localized area of discoloured intact skin or blood-filled blister. The area may be preceded by tissue that is painful, firm, mushy, boggy, warmer or cooler as compared with adjacent tissue.
  - Deep tissue injury may be difficult to detect in individuals with dark skin tones. Evolution may include a thin blister over a dark wound bed or this may further evolve and become covered by thin eschar. Evolution may be rapid exposing additional layers of tissue even with optimal treatment.
- **Stage I:** Intact skin with non-blanchable redness of a localized area, usually over a bony prominence. Darkly pigmented skin may not have visible blanching; its colour may differ from the surrounding area.
  - The area may be painful, firm, soft, warmer or cooler as compared with adjacent tissue.
- **Stage II:** Partial thickness loss of dermis presenting as a shallow open ulcer with a red pink wound bed, without slough. May also present as an intact or open/ruptured serum-filled blister.
  - This stage should not be used to describe skin tears, tape burns, perineal dermatitis, maceration or excoriation. Bruising indicates suspected deep tissue injury.
- **Stage III:** Full thickness tissue loss. Subcutaneous fat may be visible but bone, tendon or muscle are not exposed. Slough may be present but does not obscure the depth of tissue loss. There may be undermining and tunnelling.
  - The depth of a stage III pressure ulcer varies by anatomical location. The occiput and malleolus do not have subcutaneous tissue and stage III ulcers can be shallow. In contrast, areas of significant adiposity can develop extremely deep stage III pressure ulcers. Bone/tendon is not visible or directly palpable.
- **Stage IV:** Full thickness tissue loss with exposed bone, tendon or muscle. Slough or eschar may be present on some parts of the wound bed. Often include undermining and tunnelling.
  - Again the depth of a stage IV pressure ulcer varies by anatomical location. They can extend into muscle and/or supporting structures (e.g. fascia, tendon or joint capsule) making osteomyelitis possible. Exposed bone/tendon is visible or directly palpable.
- **Unstageable:** Full thickness tissue loss in which the base of the ulcer is covered by slough (yellow, tan, grey, green or brown) and/or eschar (tan, brown or black) in the wound bed.
  - Until slough and/or eschar is removed (at least partly) to expose the base of the wound, the true depth, and therefore stage, cannot be determined. Stable (dry, adherent, intact without erythema or fluctuance) eschar on the heels serves as 'the body's natural (biological) cover' and should not be removed.

II. Management

General

- Optimize nutrition including correction of anaemia, optimize blood glucose, stop smoking.
- Prevention and treatment of infection.
- Catheterize to avoid exposure to moisture if incontinent.
- Relief of spasm – baclofen, diazepam or dantrolene or treatment of contracture – Botulinum toxin, tenotomy, **amputation**, **neurosurgery** e.g. cordotomy/rhizotomy.
- Relieve pressure by regular turning and using a suitable bed; also take care during transfer and pad pressure points.
  - Effective pressure relief for 5 minutes every 2 hours (seated patients should lift themselves

every 10 minutes). Reducing head elevation, i.e. less than 45 degrees, will reduce sacral shear forces/pressure.

- **Beds**
  - ○ Clinitron – ceramic beads fluidized by warm air, i.e. **air fluidized bed** - aims for pressures less than 20 mmHg.
  - ○ Mediscus **low air loss beds**, made of cells which inflate and deflate independently; the Gore-Tex material allows rapid evaporative fluid loss to keep patient dry. It aims to exert less than 25 mmHg at any point.
- **Electronic mattresses**
  - ○ Pegasus – alternating pressure system.
  - ○ Nimbus – dynamic flotation system.

Many dressings for pressure sores have been described; negative pressure (NPWT) dressings can be used in larger defects after debridement until the patient is ready for definitive surgery – the wound can be improved or reduced, but only a minority of cases will avoid the need for surgery.

Investigations

- Blood – albumin, FBC, ESR, U and Es, glucose.
- Wound swabs.
- X-ray to identify bony sequestra; MRI is better if osteomyelitis is suspected (97% sensitive, 89% specific).

Planning and treatment within the context of a multi-disciplinary team environment

- Nursing staff: Waterlow grade and turning, dressings, care of other pressure areas.
- Physiotherapist: treatment of contractures, mobilization, passive joint movement.
- Community nurse (provision of a mattress at home), occupational therapist (provision of gel cushions) and dietician (dietary assessment and nutrition optimization).

III. Surgery

Principles

Surgery is best suited to the well-motivated patient (able to adhere to post-operative measures) with a stable condition (or liable to improve). Proper patient selection is particularly important.

- 'Oncological' debridement of the sore (including osteomyelitis) i.e. 'pseudotumour technique' – some use methylene blue or a betadine pack inserted into the cavity to guide the completeness of excision. **All devitalized tissue should be removed**, along with the pseudobursa.
- Excision of bony prominences (caution with ischial tuberosities).
- Wound closure with healthy tissues, **without significant dead space**. Choice of flap/closure depends on the site of the sore and may be modified by the patient's ambulatory status.
  - ○ Direct closure if **no tension** but in general avoid leaving the suture line in the area of pressure.
  - ○ A range of local flaps have been described; it is important to maintain future flap options as the pressure sore is likely to recur. Flaps should be designed to be as **large as possible**.
  - ○ Free flaps e.g. latissimus dorsi, are usually a last resort for large defects or where local options have been exhausted. The superior gluteal artery (5 mm diameter) is a common recipient artery exposed by a curvilinear buttock incision.
  - ○ Tissue expansion brings in healthy **sensate** tissue and is fairly well tolerated but involves prolonged treatment.

Post-operative care

There is a high rate of recurrence (40–60%) that may be reduced to 25% by optimizing rehabilitative care.

- Skin care optimized pre-operatively (with general management measures mentioned above).
- No pressure on the reconstructed area for at least 2 weeks post-operatively.
- Use of drains and antibiotics.
- Patients should be discharged only after home assessment and mattress in place.
- 2–3-weeks immobilization on a Clinitron bed, during which time patients receive physiotherapy, then a graduated 7–10-day sitting programme to aim for three 4-hour periods of sitting per day with pressure-relieving manoeuvres every 15 minutes.
- Patient education.

Common complications include: haematoma, infection, dehiscence and recurrence.

Specific pressure sores

Ischial pressure sores (28%)

These are the commonest sores in paraplegics who sit in wheelchairs and are the most difficult type of sore to treat. They have a slightly higher recurrence rate than sacral sores.

- **Posterior thigh FC flap** (medially or laterally based) based upon the descending branch of inferior gluteal artery that can be rotated or used as a transposition flap with SSG. This is also known as the gluteal thigh flap and can be 12 × 30 cm.
- **Hamstring V–Y advancement** based upon the long head of biceps (type II – profunda femoris branch). This is classically a musculocutaneous flap but avoid using the muscle in the ambulatory; a fasciocutaneous flap can be harvested instead.
- **Gluteal fasciocutaneous/musculocutaneous flap**.
- The tensor fascia lata (TFL) is a type 1 flap based on the transverse or descending branch of the lateral circumflex artery. The landmarks are anterosuperior iliac spine (ASIS) to lateral patella, the pedicle enters about 10 cm from ASIS. The flap can be sensate (lateral femoral cutaneous nerve) but the distal third is unreliable (stop within 5–8 cm of the knee joint) and may not reach. Some have suggested delaying distal end (Zufferey J. *Eur J Plast Surg* 1988;**11**:109–116) 3 weeks before.
- Gracilis – a relatively flimsy flap.
- Pedicled vertical rectus abdominis muscle (VRAM) flaps can be used for recalcitrant/recurrent sores of the ischium and trochanter.

Ischial pressure sores: a rationale for flap selection
Foster RD. *Br J Plast Surg* 1997;**50**:374–379.

The **inferior gluteus maximus island flap** was the most commonly used flap for reconstruction in this series, with the highest success rate, which was attributed to less tension with hip flexion. The use of this flap was first reported in 1979 (Mathes SJ, Nahai F. *Clinical Atlas of Muscle and Musculocutaneous Flaps*) and modified subsequently by Scheflan M (*Plast Reconstr Surg* 1981;**68**:533–538) and Stevenson TR (*Plast Reconstr Surg* 1987;**79**:761–768).

- Other flaps used in this study included gluteal thigh flap, hamstring V–Y, TFL and gracilis.

Mean time to healing was 38 days with complications in 37%: wound infection, edge dehiscence, partial flap necrosis most common (nearly half) in TFLs (distal part of flap too unreliable for coverage of the ischial area; delay to the tip increases viability or expand prior to transfer) and less in V–Y hamstring.

- Predictors of poor outcome included large sore size with previous surgery and adverse wound healing factors.

Trochanteric sores (19%)

- TFL
- Vastus lateralis (type 1) based on descending or transverse branch of the lateral circumflex femoral artery (10 cm from ASIS) which is detached distally and can cover greater trochanter, pubis and lower abdomen.
- Lateral thigh fasciocutaneous flap which can be posteriorly or anteriorly based, based on the first lateral perforator of the profundis femoris artery.
- Rectus femoris.

Sacral sores (17%)

Buttock rotation flap(s) (fasciocutaneous or musculocutaneous) are straightforward and reliable to use; they can be raised again and advanced further if the sore recurs. Bilateral flaps can be used.

- Gluteus maximus muscle flap: the upper half of the muscle is supplied by the superior gluteal artery whilst the lower half is supplied by the inferior gluteal artery. The muscle is exposed using a buttock rotation flap incision and the insertion on the femur is detached to allow the muscle to be reflected as a **turn-over flap** into the sacral defect (and can also close lower lumbar defects). An SSG is needed.
- **Gluteus maximus rotation flap** is similar to the buttock rotation flaps but is raised in the plane between gluteus maximus and medius, the muscle origin is divided off the gluteal surface of the ilium and the edge of the sacrum to allow rotation into the defect. The arc of rotation may be limited by the superior gluteal vessels but these can be divided and the flap will survive on the inferior gluteal vessels alone.
  - Muscle can be raised segmentally or completely, and can be re-rotated.
- Superior GAP flap i.e. a flap pedicled on a perforator of the superior gluteal artery.
- V–Y gluteus maximus myocutaneous flap, however it 'burns bridges' as it cannot be easily raised again.

Modification of the gluteus maximus V–Y advancement flap for sacral ulcers: the gluteal fasciocutaneous method
Ohjimi H. *Plast Reconstr Surg* 1996;**98**:1247–1252.

The conventional gluteus maximus V–Y flap requires mobilization of the insertion ± origin of the muscle which sacrifices function in the ambulant patient. The authors describe a modification which raises a V–Y skin paddle but the medial portion is elevated in a fasciocutaneous plane. This provides the mobility required to reach the midline with the muscle advanced as a result.

Perforator-based flap for coverage of lumbosacral defects
Masakazu A. *Plast Reconstr Surg* 1998;**101**:987–991.

The authors described their experience using:

- S-GAP flap pedicled upon its dominant perforating vessel.
- Lumbar perforator flaps.

Long-term outcome of pressure sores treated with flap coverage
Yamamoto Y. *Plast Reconstr Surg* 1997;**100**:1212–1217.

The generally accepted view is that ischial sores typically have large dead spaces and are more likely to need muscle flaps whilst sacral sores have smaller dead spaces and can be closed with fasciocutaneous (FC) flaps. However FC flaps seem to exhibit less recurrence than myocutaneous/muscle flaps:

- Muscle flaps provide good early cover but the muscle becomes atrophic.
- Muscle is more susceptible to ischaemia (thus all pressure points in the body are naturally covered by skin-fascia not muscle).

Their conclusion was that muscle flaps are inadequate for the surgical management of pressure sores in the long term.

Management of pressure sores by constant tension approximation
Schessel ES. *Br J Plast Surg* 2001;**54**:439–446.

The authors describe their management of chronic pressure sores by:

- Wound excision with partial suturing and continued dressings to residual wounds.
- The remainder of the wound is closed by using a constant low-grade tension Proxiderm® device that acts on subcutaneous tissues,

based on the principle of 'internal tissue expansion'.

Time to healing in a mixture of wounds was 5–42 days with a success rate of about 70–80%. The advantages put forward include the avoidance of major surgery in debilitated patients. Contraindications include an inflamed wound, wounds with excessive discharge or contamination (faeces) or a deep cavity.

Surgical reconstruction of paediatric pressure sores
Singh DJ. *Plast Reconstr Surg* 2002;**109**:265–269.

Pressure-sore risk factors in this series included spina bifida and cord injury/tumours. Myocutaneous flap reconstruction was preferred and the authors used gluteal flap, posterior thigh flap and total leg flap. The recurrence at mean follow-up of 5.3 years was 5% at the same site and 20% at another site.

IV. Negative pressure wound therapy

The use of negative pressure for wound closure was first described by Argenta LC (*Ann Plast Surg* 1997;**38**:563–576) and Banwell PE (*J Wound Care* 1999;**8**:79–84).

The principle is that negative pressure is used to convert a wound into one that may be healed by a lesser surgical procedure than before. 125 mmHg subatmospheric pressure is commonly used (higher pressures supposedly cause collapse of vessels and decreased blood flow). Dressings are changed every 48–72 hours depending on the clinical situation. It can be used in the community with portable/home machines.

Negative pressure wound therapy (NPWT) is used on a variety of wounds including pressure sores (stages III and IV) and chronic, subacute and acute wounds. Some suggest the use of intermittent therapy (5 min on/2 min off) for chronic wounds after the first 48 hours – the **cyclical loading phenomenon**.

Suggested mechanisms of action include:

- Removes chronic oedema from tissues that facilitates oxygen delivery and removes wound fluid that inhibits fibroblast and keratinocyte activity and contains matrix metalloproteins responsible for collagen breakdown.
- Encourages formation of granulation tissue.
- Increases local blood flow.
- Decreases bacterial colonization.
- Encourages wound contraction – analogous to tissue expansion relying upon creep; exert

mechanical deformational forces upon the extracellular matrix and upon cells.

The worldwide licence to the VAC® (vacuum assisted closure) system belongs to KCI (Kinetic Concepts, Inc.). The basic setup consists of:

- Evacuation tube placed within polyurethane foam dressing tailored to fit the wound.
- Airtight seal created by overlying occlusive dressing.
- Vacuum pump connected via a canister for collection of wound 'effluent'.

Alternative negative pressure wound therapy systems are now available from other manufacturers e.g. Smith and Nephew (Renasys) and ConvaTec (Engenex).

All **non-viable material should be debrided** from the wound before vacuum therapy; acute wounds respond more rapidly than chronic wounds.

- Residual **tumour** in the wound is the main contraindication to therapy as increased blood flow may cause increased growth.
- Fistulae used to be a contraindication but studies have shown that NPWT can be used in selected cases to treat **explored fistulae**.

The list of indications/wounds for the use of NPWT is increasing and includes:

- To secure skin grafts particularly in awkward areas e.g. perineal or in complex wounds; lower pressures are used i.e. continuous subatmospheric pressures of 50–75 mm Hg for 4–5 days.
- 'Burst abdomen' from acute loss or dehiscence – the dressing should not be placed directly on abdominal viscera – an intervening layer should be used e.g. mesh, tulle dressing or omentum; a cheap alternative is a split IV fluid bag (Bogota bag).
- Wounds with small areas of exposed orthopaedic metalwork, bare bone, mesh or other prosthetics; NPWT allows granulation tissue to cover the defects whilst keeping the wound clean and moist.
- Venous ulcers generally need lower pressures ~50 mm Hg in continuous mode with or without cultured keratinocytes or SSG applied to granulating tissue.

Complications:

- Pressure necrosis of adjacent skin if the patient lies on the vacuum tube.
- Maceration of surrounding intact skin if the sponge inadvertently overlaps it.

- Pain is mainly related to venous ulcers – turn down the suction and gradually increase.
- Over-granulation with ingrowth into sponge – traumatic dressing changes with bleeding. Some suggest using a non-adherent layer such as paraffin gauze or silicone dressings e.g. mepitel.
- Large volumes of exudate may be removed from larger acute wounds – so monitor fluids and electrolyte balance if this happens.

Topical negative pressure for treating chronic wounds: systematic review

Evans D. *Br J Plast Surg* 2001;**54**:238–242.

This is a systematic review of studies entered on the Cochrane Wounds Group Specialist Trials register evaluating topical negative pressure (TNP) in the management of patients with chronic wounds. There were only two randomized controlled trials published and examined in detail:

- Joseph E. *Wounds* 2000;**12**:60–67. Significant reduction in wound volume at 6 weeks in favour of TNP.
- McCallon SK. *Ostomy/Wound Manage* 2000;**46** (8):28–34. Decreased time to healing in favour of TNP.

Both studies provide weak evidence in support of TNP compared with saline gauze dressings as both are open to criticism over potential selection and observer bias. The conclusion was that there is little current evidence base to support TNP and more randomized controlled trials are required.

An update to the review was published in 2008 (Ubbink DT. Cochrane Database of Systematic Reviews 2008, Issue 3. Art. No.: CD001898. DOI: 10.1002/14651858.CD001898.pub2) which included a further five trials. The data did not show that TNP increases the healing rate of chronic wounds compared with modalities such as hydrocolloid gel, hydrogels and alginates. They concluded that the studies have methodological flaws and that better-quality research is needed.

Vacuum-assisted closure for abdominal dehiscence with prosthesis exposure in hernia surgery

de Vooght A. *Plast Reconstr Surg* 2003;**112**:1188–1189.

Four patients were treated by VAC for abdominal wall dehiscence following hernia surgery leaving exposed prosthetic mesh. With this method three patients avoided removal of the mesh; the patient who failed to heal was receiving chemotherapy. The mean time to healing with VAC was 24 days; two patients needed split skin grafts.

Treatment of open sternal wounds with the vacuum-assisted closure system
Harlan JW. *Plast Reconstr Surg* 2001;**109**:710–712.

The use of VAC in the management of sternal dehiscence is well established. In addition to the usual effects, it also:

- Stabilizes the wound, improving the mechanics of ventilation.
- Reduces the size of the defect in preparation for flap reconstruction e.g. superiorly pedicled VRAM, pectoralis major flaps.

The authors describe use of a silicone sheet sutured to the underside of the sponge to prevent adherence to deep tissues.

The use of vacuum-assisted closure for the treatment of lower extremity wounds with exposed bone
DeFranzo AJ. *Plast Reconstr Surg* 2001;**108**:1184–1191.

Continuous negative pressure (125 mmHg) was used in the management of patients with open wounds on the lower limb exposing bone or orthopaedic metalwork; preceded by wound debridement until necrotic tissue was eliminated. The dressings were changed and the wounds inspected every 48 hours.

There was rapid decrease in limb oedema within 3–5 days and successful wound closure in 95% of patients and wounds remained stable at up to 6 years follow-up.

C. Scar management

I. Scar formation

Regeneration
Formation of lost tissue without scarring
- Labile cells – divide and proliferate throughout life, e.g. epithelia, blood.
- Stable cells – normally quiescent but can be stimulated to replicate, e.g. liver cells, bone cells.
- Permanent cells – once lost are never regained, e.g. neurones, cardiac muscle.

All tissues heal with some degree of scarring in adult life except perhaps liver and the blood.

Normal scar formation
Dermal injury triggers a cascade that results in the deposition of a vascular collagen matrix that, as it accumulates, becomes a red, raised **scar** – fibrous connective tissue formed when healing by repair. As the matrix matures and remodels, the scar will become flatter and paler after 9 months (takes longer in children).

Classification of scars
(Mustoe TA. *Plast Reconstr Surg* 2002;**110**:560–571.)

- **Immature**: red and lumpy, itchy or painful, matures to become pale and flat (occasionally hyper- or hypopigmented).
- **Linear hypertrophic**: arise within weeks of surgery and grow over 3–6 months and have rope-like appearance with maturation within 2 years. They are possibly due to excessive tension or delayed wound healing; external taping is proposed by some surgeons to reduce risk but the efficacy is unknown/doubtful.
- **Widespread hypertrophic**: widespread raised, red itchy scar; typically a burns scar that remains within the borders of the burn.
- **Minor keloid**: focally raised, red, itchy scar that extends beyond the borders of the original injury. It may take up to a year to develop and fails to resolve; excision is typically complicated by recurrence. There may be genetic and anatomical influences.
- **Major keloid**: as for minor keloid but may continue to extend over years.

Factors influencing a fine scar
Surgical factors
- Atraumatic technique.
- Eversion of wound edges.
- Placement of the scar: adjacent to or within contour lines (e.g. nasolabial fold), within or adjacent to hair-bearing areas (e.g. facelift, Gillies lift) and parallel to relaxed skin tension lines (facial wrinkles).
- Shape of the scar: 'U'-shaped scars tend to become pin-cushioned/trapdoor, e.g. bilobed flap.
- Ellipse length should be 4× its width to avoid dog-ears.

Choice of suture
- Cutting versus non-cutting needle.
- Monofilament vs. braided. Braided sutures are more 'traumatic' and may increase infection risk. There are antibiotic-coated sutures on the market e.g. Vicryl plus with Triclosan.

- Absorbable vs. non-absorbable: absorption by proteolytic enzymes; non-absorbable sutures tend to cause less tissue inflammation.
  - Vicryl is polyglactic acid: tensile strength gone by 30 days, absorbed by 90 days. It is braided.
  - PDS i.e. polydioxanone: loses tensile strength at 60 days, absorbed by 180 days i.e. both double that for vicryl. It is a monofilament.

Patient factors

- Age – infants and the elderly – good scars.
- Region of the body.
- Skin type – glabrous skin results in more scar hypertrophy.
- Individual's scar-forming properties – hypertrophic/keloid scar former.

Factors that contribute to suture marks

It is important to note that the suture itself (silk vs. ethilon vs. staples, etc.) is not so important. Suture marks are partly due to epithelialization of the suture track; in some cases it may be related to local pressure necrosis, or infection including 'stitch abscesses'.

- Length of time the suture is left in place: sutures removed within 5–7 days do not leave stitch marks whilst sutures removed at 14 days will.
- Tension on the wound edges, defect too large and/ or skin sutures tied too tightly. Skin wound tension can be relieved by deeper stitches which bring the skin edges together in apposition.
- Region of the body: hands rarely affected by stitch marks whilst trunk, upper extremities more commonly affected.
- Infection: remove infected sutures or will leave a mark; braided sutures harbour more bacteria (*Staphylococcus*). Minimize the number and weight of sutures. Rate of absorption also related to size of the suture; mucous membranes absorb faster than muscle.

II. Hypertrophic and keloid scars

Both keloids and hypertrophic scars are raised erythematous scars; characterized by an excessive accumulation of collagen, particularly type III.

When interpreting the literature, it is important to note than many studies did not distinguish between hypertrophic scars and keloids. Other possible methodology problems include short follow-up times (see

imiquimod studies; keloid studies should have a follow-up of at least a year) and different populations. These can lead to much confusion which has been perpetuated by literature reviews that often do not refer to the original articles. For example, many articles state that surgery alone for the treatment of keloids has a recurrence rate of 45–100%. The relevant references are:

- Berman B. Adjunctive therapies to surgical treatment of keloids. *Dermatol Surg* 1996;**22**:126–130. This is a review and cites Lawrence 1991 and Edsmyr 1974.
- Berman B. Keloids *J Am Acad Dermatol* 1995;**33**:117–123. This is another review and cites Lawrence 1991 and Cosman 1961.
- Darzi MA. Evaluation of various methods of treating keloids and hypertrophic scars. *Br J Plast Surg* 1992;**45**:374–379. This Indian study included 58 'keloids' treated with radiation alone, surgery with pre- and post-operative radiation, surgery with post-operative radiation or intralesional triamcinolone. No patients were treated with surgery alone.
- Lawrence WT. In search of the optimal treatment of keloids: report and a review of the literature. *Ann Plast Surg* 1991;**27**:164–178. This study compared 27 keloids treated with surgery and triamcinolone vs. 28 treated with surgery and colchicine. No patients were treated with surgery alone. The author reviewed seven studies which reported cure rates of 7% to 55%, and many of these studies had limited long-term follow-up. The 45% recurrence rate refers to Conway 1960.
- Mathangi Ramakrishnan K. Study of 1000 patients with keloids in South India. *Plast Reconstr Surg* 1974;**53**:276–280. This Indian study included 108 cases treated with surgery with 80% recurrence, with no mention of adjunctive treatments, histological evidence or follow-up period.
- Edsmyr F. Radiation therapy in the treatment of keloids in East Africa. *Acta Radiol Ther Phys Biol* 1974;**12**:102–106. The author found that 80% of keloids treated with excision and post-operative radiation did not recur.
- Cosman B. Correlation of keloid recurrence with completeness of local excision. *Plast Reconstr Surg* 1972;**50**:163–166. This study had four of 18 keloid surgeries without post-operative radiotherapy, and there was one recurrence in the average follow-up period of 1 3/4 years i.e. 25%.

- Cosman B. The surgical treatment of keloids. *Plast Reconstr Surg* 1961;**27**:225. This retrospective review had 340 cases of keloid over 1932–1958 with an overall recurrence rate of 38.5% whilst 25 cases excised with no radiation had a 54% recurrence rate.
- Conway H. Differential diagnosis of keloids and hypertrophic scars by tissue culture technique with notes on therapy of keloids by surgical excision and decadron. *Plast Reconstr Surg* 1960;**25**:117–132. This study investigated the adjunctive effect of decadron. The recurrence rate with surgery alone was 45%.

Thus articles quoting a recurrence rate with **surgery alone** with these references must be referring to a study of Indian patients in 1974 (n = 58, 80%) or American patients in 1972 (n = 4, 25%), in 1961 (n = 25, 54%) and in 1960 (45%).

Hypertrophic scars

- Hypertrophic scars are raised scars limited to the initial boundary of the injury.
- There seem to be sites of predilection including anterior chest, shoulders and deltoid.
- They tend to occur soon after injury and show spontaneous regression over months/years.
- They may be related to wound factors such as tension and delayed healing.

A study relating wound tension to scar morphology in the pre-sternal scar using Langer's technique
Meyer M. *Br J Plast Surg* 1991;**44**:291–294.
The authors demonstrated that areas of high tension with

- Pull in multiple directions causes a hypertrophic scar.
- Pull in one direction causes a stretched scar.

Keloid scars

Greek 'cheloide' from 'chele' for crab claw.

- These can extend beyond the original boundary.
- They tend to occur later after injury (months/years).
- They do not show any significant regression without treatment.
- They seem to be better correlated with dark skin colour (15× more common in dark-skinned people).

Patients with keloid scars tend to be of a younger age and there are instances of a familial tendency.

- There may be accelerated growth during pregnancy; it may resolve after the menopause.
- Some believe keloid scars to be caused by an immune response to sebum and thus may be secondary to damage of pilosebaceous structures.
- Histologically there are large collagen bundles with less cross-linking and more disorganization than hypertrophic scars.

Affected wounds do not have to be under tension – e.g. earlobes may also be affected in addition to the sites. It has also become apparent that not all keloids behave in the same way, for example, ear keloids are more amenable to surgery than sternal keloids, further complicating any discussion that lumps all sorts of scars together.

Management

The conventional therapies are intralesional steroid, pressure, topical silicone and surgery in selected cases. The exact mechanisms of action are not known:

- Pressure – 24–30 mmHg 18–24 hours a day for 6–12 months; thus compliance may be an issue. It possibly acts by decreased collagen synthesis and increased collagen lysis (collagenase).
- Silicone – hydration of the wound.
- Steroids – decreased collagen synthesis/stimulates collagenase production, reduced inflammation.

Keloid scars tend to respond poorly to surgery except perhaps ear lesions and overall there is less success with topical silicone. Surgery may be contemplated in conjunction with post-operative radiotherapy (25% recurrence surgery plus radiotherapy, surgery alone > 50–80% recurrence).

Other treatments

Imiquimod 5% cream has been used to prevent recurrence after surgery (see below). It is an immune response-modifying agent; chemically, it is an imidazoquinolone compound that stimulates the production of interferon α, TNF and IL-2 by binding to surface receptors (e.g. Toll 7) on macrophages and other inflammatory cells including T-cells.
Pilot study of the effect of post-operative imiquimod 5% cream on the recurrence rate of excised keloids
Berman B. *J Am Acad Dermatol* 2002;**47**:S209–S211.

Imiquimod 5% cream (Aldara) applied once daily for 8 weeks following excision of keloid scars in 12 patients with stable keloids. No recurrence observed at 24 weeks. Seven scars showed mild hyperpigmentation; two patients had mild irritation and erosions.

This study was supported by an educational grant from 3M Pharmaceuticals, manufacturers of Aldara.

Imiquimod 5% cream for prevention of recurrence after excision of presternal keloids
Malhotra AK. *Dermatology* 2007;**215**:63–65.

This case study included three patients with sternal keloids excised by radiofrequency and then left to heal by secondary intention with imiquimod applied daily. They remarked that there was no recurrence after a follow-up of 12 weeks, and that on stopping the cream, all keloids recurred.

Failure of imiquimod 5% cream to prevent recurrence of surgically excised trunk keloids
Cacao FM. *Dermatol Surg* 2009;**35**:629–633.

This study included nine patients with trunk keloids, with imiquimod treatment started on the night of surgery for 8 weeks, and then followed up at regular intervals. In total, eight keloids recurred – seven of them by the 12th week after surgery.

Treatment of keloid scars post-shave excision with imiquimod 5% cream
Berman B. *J Drugs Dermatol* 2009;**8**:455–458.

This is a prospective double-blind, placebo-controlled study with 20 keloids randomized to imiquimod or vehicle cream for 8 weeks; only 12 completed the 6-month study. There was greater pain and tenderness in the imiquimod group. There were 3/8 recurrences in the imiquimod group compared to 3/4 in the control.

International clinical recommendations on scar management
Mustoe TA. *Plastic Reconstr Surg* 2002;**110**:560–571.

Keloid scars:

- **Intralesional steroid** is the first-line treatment option e.g. triamcinolone 40 mg/ml. Side-effects include dermal atrophy, telangiectasia and depigmentation. Topical steroid is generally less efficacious.
- Topical silicone gel sheeting.
- Pressure therapy.
- Surgery.
  - ○ Surgery alone – recurrence in 45–100%.
  - ○ Surgery + intralesional steroid – recurrence < 50%.
  - ○ Surgery + radiotherapy – recurrence 10%.
  - ○ Radiotherapy carries a small risk of cancer induction. It is generally reserved for resistant keloid in adults.
- **Laser:** recent reports of success using Nd:YAG for flattening keloid scars and pulsed dye laser reduces redness.

Hypertrophic scars

- **Silicone gel sheet is** often the first-line treatment option. Some suggest *prevention* by starting within days of wound healing. It does need to be used for a minimum 12 hours per day (ideally 24 hours) with twice daily washing.
- Intralesional steroid.
- Pressure therapy: 24–30 mmHg for 6–12 months.

The current use of intralesional steroid (concentration, dosages and timing) is mostly based on the findings of Ketchum (1974) who gave largely empirical advice.

More recently, there has been a plethora of intralesional treatments suggested for keloids (and hypertrophic scars) that are largely case reports/small case series:

- Interferons.
- 5-fluorouracil.
- Imiquimod.
- Bleomycin.
- Doxorubicin.
- Verapamil.
- Retinoic acid.
- Tacrolimus.
- Tamoxifen.
- Botulinum toxin A.
- TGF beta.
- Interleukins.
- Onion extract (*Allium cepa*).
- Vitamin E.

A review of the effectiveness of antimitotic drug injections for hypertrophic scars and keloids
Wang XQ. *Ann Plast Surg* 2009;**63**:688–692.

This reviews the studies looking at steroids, 5-fluorouracil, bleomycin, mitomycin C, retinoic acid and colchicine.

The emerging role of antineoplastic agents in the treatment of keloids and hypertrophic scars
Shridarani SM. *Ann Plast Surg* 2010;**64**:355–361.

This paper reviews the studies investigating the role of interferon, bleomycin, mitomycin C, 5-fluorouracil in particular.

Both of these reviews have similar conclusions, that there are substances of 'promise/potential'. However the studies, in general, suffer from problems with methodology (small numbers, short follow-up) with most patients having had other therapies in addition to the one of interest.

Burns

A. Acute burns

I. Relevant anatomy

- Skin surface area ~0.2–0.3 m^2 in the newborn and 1.5–2.0 m^2 in the adult.
- Thickness of epidermis from 0.05 mm (eyelids) to 1 mm (sole of the foot).
- Dermis is approximately 10× thicker than epidermis site for site.

The skin has many different functions:

- Mechanical barrier to bacterial invasion.
- Control of fluid loss.
- Thermoregulation.
- Immunology and metabolism e.g. vitamin D.
- Neurosensory and social interaction.

Epidemiology

- 0.5–1% of the UK population sustains burns each year. 10% of these will require admission and of these, 10% are life threatening.
- 45% of admissions in the USA are scalds in children < 5 years of age. The kitchen and bathroom are the commonest locations for injury in the home in the USA/UK whilst in Hong Kong epidemiological studies have shown that the living room is the commonest location for paediatric scalds.
- Burns sustained during road traffic accidents have a high incidence of concomitant injury.

Outcome

- A plot of burn size vs. mortality shows a sigmoid distribution – 0% with low total burn surface area (TBSA) and plateauing at 100% mortality rate with 100% burn.
- There are many different formulae that calculate the risk of mortality following burns. Most of these are based on statistical analysis of an institution's retrospective data – thus will be most applicable to that institution's demographic and local practice. These should be applied with caution to clinical care of patients; clinical decision-making particularly the withdrawal of treatment in massive burns should be based on the clinical response to treatment rather than calculated figures.
  - The most consistent risk factors are size of burn, age and inhalational injury.
- LD$_{50}$ (% TBSA resulting in death of half the cohort) in 1950 for 21-year-olds was 45%; in 1990 this had increased to 85%. The simple rule of thumb that

adds the patient's age to the percentage area burnt continues to be quoted frequently but is woefully out of date and should not be used any more.

The improvements in the mortality rate have been due to multiple factors including:

- Early and effective resuscitation.
- Control of sepsis, antibiotics/antimicrobials.
- Improved management of inhalation injury.
- Early wound excision and grafting.
- Development of alternative wound closure materials.

Blisters

Damage around the dermo-epidermal junction will lead to the leakage of plasma from heat-damaged vessels causing the epidermis to separate from the dermis i.e. form a blister. Osmotically active particles within the blister fluid contribute to its progressive enlargement with time.

Blister fluid may contain potentially harmful inflammatory mediators and probably should be considered as an open wound since the overlying skin has lost the normal functions of skin. Thus in general, larger blisters can be de-roofed (also reduces pain) though smaller blisters can probably be left alone.

- Increased adenosine concentrations (has potent anti-inflammatory action). Shaked G. *Burns* 2007;**33**:352–354.
- Increased prostaglandin levels in the first few hours. Sugiyama S. *Biomedicine* 1978;**29**:51–53.
- Burn blister fluid decreased keratinocyte replication and differentiation. Garner WL. *J Burn Care Rehabil* 1993;**14**:127–131.

Eschar

Again, an eschar-covered wound can be regarded as an open wound because it retains none of the normal functions of skin. In addition, it is:

- A medium for bacterial growth.
- A source of heat-derived **inflammatory mediators** and toxins which may compromise distant organ function and exacerbate immunosuppression.
- A compromising factor in wound healing.
- A consumer of clotting factors, fibrinogen and platelets.
- A continued source of protein loss including complement.

If the eschar is circumferential, it may impede distal circulation and thoracic and thoraco-abdominal eschars may compromise ventilation.

- **Pseudoeschar** may form in deeper burns after the use of topical antimicrobials which somehow react with the wound exudate; this includes silver sulphadazine (SSD; some suggest that it is due to the polypropylene glycol carrier) and flammacerium (SSD plus cerium nitrate, a more leathery dry pseudoeschar). It can lead to confusion over the depth of the burns in inexperienced hands.

II. Assessment, resuscitation and initial management of burns

First aid at the scene:

- **Stop the injury, which depends on the type of injury** i.e. extinguish any flames ('stop, drop and roll'), switch off/interrupt electrical power source, remove involved clothing, dilute acids and alkali by irrigation rather than neutralization, etc.
- **Cool the burn wound** (but warm the patient) to reduce the tissue damage. Though this is most useful in the first half hour, it is still worth considering even up to 2 hours post-burn and will also reduce pain. Timely cooling reduces direct thermal trauma and stabilizes mast cells, reducing release of histamine and other inflammatory mediators. Use running tap water ~15 °C (avoid ice or iced water, which will cause vasospasm and further compromise of tissue perfusion); wet gauzes or hydrogel dressings can be placed on the wounds afterwards for continued pain relief.

In the A&E department, the approach is basically the same in principle as for any multiply traumatized patient i.e. ABC/primary survey. It is important to remember that seriously burnt patients may suffer additional injuries aside from the burns due to the original incident such as an explosion/car crash or events afterwards such as jumping out of windows to escape from a house fire. The following sequence applies to a 'major' burn:

Airway with C-spine control. A simple check for airway patency is to talk to the patient (and get a response).

- Open airway with chin lift/jaw thrust manoeuvre. Use a Yankhauer sucker to remove debris from mouth and **secure the airway** with:
  - Guedel airway (size approximately with nose to angle of mandible distance).
  - Nasopharyngeal airway (exclude cribriform plate or base of skull fracture).
  - Endotracheal tube: adults size 7 (female) or 8 (male) on average, children – a formula may be used: (age/4) + 4 uncuffed (3 cuffed) or size of nostril/little finger nail.

Breathing (Look, feel, listen) – provide 100% oxygen.

- Exclude life-threatening chest injuries such as tension pneumothorax (place large-bore cannula mid-clavicular line second intercostal space).
- Emergency chest decompression (escharotomy) if circumferential full thickness burns limit respiratory movements (elevated ventilation pressures will drop rapidly with appropriate decompression).

Circulation with haemorrhage control.

- Apply pressure to actively bleeding wounds.
- Insert and secure two large-bore cannulae preferably through unburned skin – consider intraosseus infusions in children < 2 years of age. Commence crystalloid infusion according to fluid deficit as gauged by clinical condition (peripheral and central pulses and BP) and adjust to resuscitation formula after the primary survey.
- Take blood for FBC, U&Es, glucose, group and save/cross-match, arterial blood gas and carboxyhaemoglobin.

Disability: AVPU is a simple method of assessing the approximate level of response:

- Alert.
- Responding to Voice.
- Responding to Pain.
- Unresponsive.

Exposure

- Remove all clothing but maintain a warm ambient temperature; remember to log roll the patient to **check the back**. Hair may need to be trimmed to aid assessment as well as to make dressings easier; this is particularly important in chemical burns. Remove all jewellery particularly those that may potentially cause constriction.
- Assess the burn:
  - **Estimate % TBSA** according to Wallace rule of nines, 'patient's palm' or a burn chart. Remember not to include erythema – it is a reversible hyperaemia that will fade over several hours and has little/no pathophysiological consequences.
  - Estimate depth by clinical characteristics (vide infra).

Secondary survey

- **AMPLE** history (allergies, medications, past medical history, last meal and events and environment of injury).
- Head-to-toe examination for non-life-threatening injuries, assess need for decompression (see below).

Depth assessment

Erythema is a sign of an epidermal injury e.g. sunburn. It is red, very painful, blanches/refills quickly but without blisters. It should not be included in estimates of the burnt surface area as it is not associated with a significant inflammatory response or systemic upset; it usually resolves after a few hours.

Burns can be divided into injuries that are full-thickness or not.

- Superficial partial thickness.
  - Painful with blisters.
  - Skin blanches and refills.
  - Hair follicles are still intact.
- Deep partial thickness.
  - May be less painful/sensitive.
  - Small or no blisters.
  - Fixed staining in tissues.
- Full thickness.
  - Waxy white or charred eschar.
  - Insensate, less pain (there is some pain due to reaction around full thickness burns).
  - No blisters.

Initial management of the burn wound i.e. in the emergency department

- Toilet the wound with saline (aqueous chlorhexidine is not necessary except in grossly contaminated wounds).

- The wound can be dressed with clingfilm or saline-soaked gauzes prior to transfer to definitive unit – as SSD can compromise accurate wound assessment, it should only be considered if the burn wound is contaminated, there will be an anticipated delay in transfer and agreed by the receiving burns unit. SSD is contraindicated in pregnant or nursing mothers and children < 2 months due to risk of kernicterus from the sulphonamide moiety. Although its role in reducing burns infection is undoubted, there is evidence that it actually impedes re-epithelialization (i.e. decreased speed of healing by an adverse effect on keratinocyte DNA) and may increase scarring due to pro-inflammatory effects.
- Tetanus prophylaxis should be considered as per protocols but antibiotics are not usually required.
- Adequate analgesia is an important part of modern burns management: slow IV infusion or incremental doses of morphine e.g. 0.1 mg/kg repeated after 5 minutes as needed.

Criteria for transfer to a burns unit

- Burns > 10% in children or 15% in adults.
- Burns at extremes of age unless minor.
- Full thickness (FT) or deep partial thickness (PT).
- Inhalation injury.
- Burns of special areas: face, perineum and hands/feet.
- Electrical or chemical burns.
- Burns requiring decompression.

Local criteria may differ but in general, an experienced burns unit/centre should treat patients with a large burn, full thickness burn, burn in a special area or a complicated burn (requiring decompression, ICU care, concomitant injuries etc.).

III. Resuscitation regimens

Resuscitation

Initial intravenous resuscitation for burns over 15% in adults (10% in children) – remember that the threshold is somewhat arbitrary.

- Calculate fluid requirement according to the Parkland formula:
  - **2–4 ml/kg body weight/% TBSA**
  - Give half (Hartmann's/Ringer's lactate) in the first 8 hours, calculating from the time of the injury (replacing deficits as quickly as practical) and the remaining half over the next 16 hours.
  - Give colloid in the second 24 hours usually 5% albumin, 0.5 ml/kg in addition to crystalloid.
  - It is common to give more fluid (50% more) if there is an inhalational injury or with electrical injuries. More fluid may also be needed in those with pre-existing dehydration e.g. due to a delay in transfer or concomitant injury causing loss of circulating volume.
- Children will need to be given maintenance fluid in addition; dextrose saline is usually used but hypoglycaemia (due to low hepatic glycogen stores) and hyponatraemia (use half normal saline if transfer is delayed) may occur.
  - 100 ml/kg up to 10 kg.
  - 50 ml/kg up to 20 kg.
  - 20 ml/kg up to 30 kg.

Remember that in the end, whatever fluid formulae you use, these are **only guides** and provide a starting point for fluid administration – it is important to monitor the effectiveness of resuscitation constantly and to respond accordingly and speedily. The trend is to begin at the **lower end** e.g. 2 ml/kg/% TBSA to reduce the risk of **fluid creep** (clinicians are much better at increasing fluids for low urine output than reducing them for high urine output) with '**colloid rescue**' typically 12–24 hours after the burn.

The phenomenon of 'fluid creep' in acute burn resuscitation

Saffle J. *J Burn Care Res* 2007;**28**:382–395.

Fluid creep is a significant problem in modern burns care. It occurs when burns patients receive more resuscitation than predicted by the Parkland's formula, and more than is actually required. The increased fluid has been related to progressive oedema and serious complications such as abdominal compartment syndrome. The reasons put forward for fluid creep include:

- Parkland formula is not accurate in large burns.
- Clinicians are slow/reluctant to reduce fluid infusions when urine output is high.
- Opioid creep – opiates have significant cardiovascular effects including partial antagonization of the adrenergic stress response.
- Influence of goal-directed resuscitation.

Overall, the aim is to give the least amount of fluid required to maintain tissue perfusion i.e. **prevent** burns shock, whilst avoiding the dangers and complications of over-resuscitation. There are many formulae in use and they seem to work reasonably well; however whichever one is used, they are only guides.

Choice of resuscitation fluids

- **Crystalloid** e.g. Hartmann's solution in Parkland formula, is recommended by the BBA and is the most commonly used resuscitation fluid.
  - Hartmann's: Na^+ 130 mmol, K^+ 4, Ca^{2+} 1.5, Cl^- 109, lactate 28. Variable composition between manufacturers. Original solution by Sydney Ringer (British physician and physiologist, 1836–1910) and then lactate added as a buffer i.e. Lactated Ringer's or Ringer's lactate.
  - Normal saline: 154 sodium and 154 chloride.
  - 5% dextrose: 50 g glucose in 1 litre of water.
- **Colloid** e.g. Muir and Barclay formula: % TBSA × weight kg/2 = one ration.
  - Give one ration 4 hourly in the first 12 hours, then give one ration 6 hourly in the next 12 hours and give final ration over 12 hours.
  - There are concerns that the protein may leak out of the circulation and potentiate third space losses (although non-burned tissues re-establish normal permeability shortly after injury).
- **Hypertonic saline** regimes have been described with the aim of reducing the volume of fluid required; however it can cause a shift of intracellular water to the extracellular space causing intracellular dehydration. In addition, it may also be complicated by excessive Na^+ retention and hypernatraemia.
- **Dextran** is a high-molecular-weight polysaccharide (polymerized glucose) available in different sizes e.g. 40, 70 and 150 kdalton molecules. 40% is excreted in the urine whilst the remainder is slowly metabolized. It is not commonly used in burns resuscitation and there are problems associated with its use.
  - Dextran 40 improves flow by reducing red cell sludging (and is thus sometimes used in microsurgery) whilst dextran 70 causes more allergic reactions and compromises blood grouping.
- **Fresh frozen plasma** can be used in children (hypoproteinaemia develops rapidly in paediatric patients) being particularly useful in treating toxic

shock. It delivers passive immunity though with the risk of viral transmission.

Enteral feeding can be used for fluid maintenance in selected cases with the advice that the potassium requirement be doubled. Fluid resuscitation regimens should replace sufficient salt (lost into burn tissue from the extracellular fluid) though this is usually a secondary issue in practice.

Albumin debate

There is a frequently quoted report in the *British Medical Journal* (July 1998) from the Cochrane Injuries Group reporting on a meta-analysis of 30 studies comparing albumin with crystalloid resuscitation fluid in the three groups of hypovolaemia, burns and hypoproteinaemia. They found that the risk of death was higher in albumin-treated groups – for every 17 patients treated with albumin there is one additional death (six for every 100).

- Relative risk for hypovolaemia was 1.46.
- Relative risk for burns was 2.40.

This has often been used as justification for regarding colloids as being dangerous in burns resuscitation. However, there are several important criticisms of the report:

- The studies used in the meta-analysis were very dissimilar and the indications and regimens for giving albumin in these studies were not standard policy in UK burns units.
- Only three burns studies were included (1979, 1983, 1995) with less than < 150 patients included in total.
- There has been a generally good experience with the use of albumin in the USA, where reports demonstrate that 80% of paediatric burns > 95% TBSA given albumin survive.

SAFE (saline versus albumin fluid evaluation) study

SAFE investigators. *Br Med J* 2006;**333**:1044–1046.

This study recruited 6045 patients in 16 ICUs in Australia and New Zealand and found no difference in mortality with resuscitation with either 4% albumin or normal saline irrespective of baseline albumin. Note however that the study excludes burns patients.

Fluid replacement after 24 hours

By this point, the increase in capillary permeability/tissue oedema is said to have peaked and there is a need to restore serum albumin. If crystalloid was given in the first 24 hours, then protein (5% albumin) may be given according to the Brooke formula: 0.5 ml/kg/% TBSA. Some suggest changing Ringer's lactate to D5W; maintenance fluid can often be given via enteral feeding (double K^+ requirements to 120 mmol/24 h).

- If hypertonic saline was used, then the next stage requires free water to reduce serum hyperosmolality.

Other potential issues include:

- Glucose intolerance (due to anti-insulin stress hormones) causes hyperglycaemia, then glycosuria leading to osmotic diuresis.
- Disturbances of ADH secretion (inappropriate ADH, diabetes insipidus).
- High respiratory water loss.

During this second period, **the urine output is a less reliable guide to volaemic status** due to glucose intolerance (osmotic diuresis), SIADH and increased respiratory losses. It may be better to monitor hydration by plasma sodium and urea concentration.

Monitoring in major burns

- Pulse, BP, respirations and core temperature.
- Pulse oximeter (beware CO poisoning).
- ECG if necessary.
- Urine output is the single most sensitive non-invasive parameter – insert urinary catheter for hourly monitoring in major burns. Note that the urine output is not a reliable indicator of the volaemic state in the second 24 hours.
  - 0.5–1.0 ml/kg/h in adults.
  - 1.0–2.0 ml/kg/h in children; weighing nappies is an alternative in infants.
- If output falls then consider administering a **fluid challenge** of 5–10 ml/kg and to increase the rate of fluids in the next hour by 150%; avoid overhydration ('fluid creep').
- Manage haemoglobinuria by encouraging a high urine output e.g. forced alkaline diuresis, keeping urine specific gravity 1.010–1.020.
  - 12.5 g/l mannitol.
  - 25 mmol/l $NaHCO_3$.

Burn wound dressings and topical agents

The ideal burn wound dressing does not exist. Desirable properties of a burn dressing would include:

- Protect against trauma and infection.
- Reduce evaporative heat and water loss.
- Absorb wound exudate.
- Pain relief.

To reduce colonization/infection, the burn wound eschar should be cleansed with aqueous chlorhexidine at each dressing change. Common organisms affecting burn wounds include *Staphylococcus aureus*, Gram-negative bacteria including *Proteus* and *Klebsiella* and mixed anaerobes including *Escherichia coli*.

Mafenide acetate may be used as a topical antiseptic but it can cause pain on application and, through inhibition of carbonic anhydrase, may contribute to a metabolic acidosis.

0.5% silver nitrate is active against *Staphylococcus*, *Pseudomonas* and other Gram-negatives. It is usually used as a solution to wet gauze dressings – over-concentrating beyond 0.5% is toxic to normal cells; there is a risk of toxicity by systemic absorption but this is limited by its insolubility. It is a very effective burn wound dressing, however:

- Leaching of electrolytes, especially sodium, may occur from the burn wound and oral supplements are essential especially in children to avoid rapid hyponatraemia.
- It may rarely cause methaemoglobinaemia.
- It stains fabric brown/black.

Silver sulphadiazine (SSD) has a broader spectrum of antimicrobial activity compared with silver nitrate – it is active against all of the above and also active against *Pseudomonas* and *Candida*. The cream is applied daily and leads to the formation of a pseudoeschar which may complicate wound depth assessment. It is therefore usually only used once a decision is made on the burn depth and need for surgery or otherwise.

However, it penetrates burn eschar poorly and like silver nitrate, it is **not suitable for treating invasive infection in an eschar, only for prophylaxis**. There is a risk of side-effects:

- **Transient neutropenia** (5–15%) may occur 2–3 days after initiation of treatment; the neutrophil count does recover even if SSD is not withdrawn and there is no reported increase in infection rates. The monitoring of white cell counts is important.
- Maculopapular rash (5%).
- Haemolytic anaemia in patients with G-6-PD deficiency.

- Generally it is not used on the face due to the risk of silver deposits (low); it can cause kernicterus in children < 2 months old and is also avoided in pregnant and breastfeeding women.
- **Methaemoglobinuria** is a rare side-effect, where there is oxidation of Fe^{2+} (ferrous) to Fe^{3+} (ferric) form of haemoglobin which is inactive. Normally, 3% of all haemoglobin is composed of methaemoglobin and is converted back by methaemoglobin reductase (an inherited deficiency of this enzyme has been described). It can be treated with 1 ml/kg 1% methylene blue.
- It may inactivate enzyme-debriding agents (varidase) if used concurrently.

Principles of perineal burns treatment

This is an awkward area to treat and usually the emphasis is for conservative therapy (exposure and topical SSD) and to treat late complications e.g. vaginal stents, late release of scar contractures rather than early aggressive surgery.

- Urinary diversion (remember that a urinary catheter is a potential portal for infection).
- Prevention of infection – daily bath/shower rather than prophylactic systemic antibiotics.

Prophylactic antibiotics for burns patients: systematic review and meta-analysis

Avni T. *Br Med J* 2010;**340**:241–251.

This literature review included 17 trials (two independent reviewers extracted the data) and demonstrated that prophylactic systemic antibiotics reduced overall mortality. There was a decrease in pneumonia and wound infections. However the reviewers comment that the overall methodological quality of the included trials was poor and **do not recommend** antibiotic prophylaxis in severe burns except perioperatively.

IV. Mechanisms of burn injury

Burn wound

Jackson's burn wound model (Jackson D. *Br J Surg* 1953;**40**:588–596) has been used to describe the different types or zones of injury occurring in a burn wound.

- Zone of coagulation – the central part is characterized by coagulative necrosis.
- Zone of stasis

  - The aim of effective acute burns treatment is to allow this zone to recover by restoring capillary microcirculation and thus re-establish tissue perfusion, limiting the production of free radicals.
- Zone of hyperaemia – burns that are > 25% BSA incorporate/involve the whole of the body in the zone of hyperaemia.

Systemic effects of a major burn

A major burn can have many effects including:

- Reduced cardiac output, due to
  - Decreased myocardial contractility – a myocardial depressant factor has been proposed. This reduced function can persist despite adequate resuscitation.
  - Decreased venous return and inadequate preload.
  - Increased afterload – increased systemic vascular resistance.
- Increased systemic vascular resistance.
  - Catecholamines and sympathetic activity.
  - ADH and angiotensin II, neuropeptide Y.
- Pulmonary oedema.
  - Increased pulmonary vascular resistance.
  - Increased capillary pressure and capillary permeability.
  - Left heart failure.
  - Hypoproteinaemia.
  - Direct vascular injury following inhalational injury.
- Renal – decreased renal perfusion, increased antidiuretic hormone (ADH) and aldosterone, and increased sodium and water retention.
- Liver/pancreas
  - Glucose intolerance.
  - Protein catabolism especially muscle.
  - Increased metabolic rate.
  - Growth inhibition.
- Gastrointestinal (vide infra)
  - Stress ulceration – Curling's.
  - Gut stasis, ischaemic enterocolitis (rare) and bacterial translocation (treat/prevent with selective gut decontamination).
  - Gall bladder and acalculous cholecystitis.

Mediators of burn wound injury

Inflammatory mediators are local and systemic factors that are responsible for the pathophysiological reaction to (thermal) injury. They are also responsible for changes in the capillary microcirculation promoting **burns oedema:**

- Increased capillary hydrostatic pressure (leading to vasodilatation).
- Increased capillary permeability, leading to:
- Decreased capillary oncotic pressure (due to loss of albumin from the circulation).
- Increased tissue oncotic pressure (albumin leaks out of circulation and large proteins break up into more osmotically active units).
- Decreased tissue hydrostatic pressure (unfolding of damaged macromolecules causes a loosening effect).
- Generalized impairment in cell membrane function leading to swelling of cells.

Burn oedema is biphasic – immediate (first hours of a burn) and late oedema (12 to 24 hours). Mediators can be local (e.g. histamine and prostaglandins, kinins) or systemic (e.g. catecholamines, angiotensin).

Histamine

Histamine is released from mast cells in heat-injured skin and is responsible for:

- Early phase of increased capillary permeability (early peak/first hour of oedema).
- Arteriolar dilatation and venular constriction.
- Pain (and itch).
- Histamine and its derivatives stimulate xanthine oxidase pathways in endothelial cell membrane (hypoxanthine to xanthine) and generation of oxygen free radicals with reperfusion (vide infra).

Prostaglandins, leukotrienes and thromboxanes

These are products of the arachidonic acid pathway and act primarily at a local level.

- Prostaglandins and leukotrienes are released from neutrophils (arriving 4–5 days post-burn) and macrophages (follow arrival of neutrophils). Neutrophil-blocking antibodies given post-burn have been shown to reduce oedema.
  - **PGE2 is the most important prostaglandin in the pathogenesis of burn wound oedema** and increases vascular permeability.
  - PGI2 is a vasodilator and also increases capillary permeability.
- TXA2 is produced locally by platelets; it is less important in oedema formation but through vasoconstriction it may extend the zone of coagulative necrosis. Increased serum TXA2: PGI2 ratios have been found in burn patients. Systemic ibuprofen in sheep reduces post-burn tissue ischaemia by blocking TXA2 production but has little effect on burn wound oedema.

Free radicals

Oxygen radicals are moieties with unpaired electrons and consequently are strong oxidizing agents. These include the superoxide anion (O^{2-}), H_2O_2 and hydroxyl ion (OH^-).

- Hydroxyl ion is the most damaging ($Fe^{2+} + H_2O_2 \rightarrow Fe^{3+} + 2OH^-$).
- Catalase neutralizes H_2O_2 while superoxide dismutase neutralizes O^{2-} and iron chelators (desferrioxamine) may be protective against OH^- formation.

Reperfusion injury results as flow is re-established to a zone of stasis, providing oxygen to drive renewed free radical production through a variety of mechanisms:

- Phospholipase A_2 acts on free phospholipids (from cell injury i.e. burn), converting them along arachidonic acid pathways to products that are chemotactic to neutrophils, which are a source of oxygen free radicals that injure further membrane lipids and stimulate further phospholipase A_2 etc.
- Xanthine oxidase catalyses the conversion of hypoxanthine to xanthine in endothelial cells and free radicals are released as byproducts of this process. Histamine stimulates xanthine oxidase hence cromoglycate, H_2 receptor antagonists and allopurinol (inhibits xanthine oxidase) may all be beneficial.

Angiotensin II and vasopressin

- A fall in renal perfusion pressure stimulates the release of renin from juxtaglomerular cells (afferent arteriolar cells) that monitor renal perfusion. **Renin** converts a circulating α-globulin, angiotensinogen, to angiotensin I, which is in turn converted in the circulation (mainly by pulmonary endothelial cells) by angiotensin-converting enzyme to angiotensin II (AII).
- AII acts upon the hypothalamus to release vasopressin (**ADH**) (which is also released by the hypothalamus due to stimulation of osmoreceptors monitoring plasma osmolality),

which promotes water re-absorption from the collecting ducts.

- ○ AII acts at the adrenal cortex (zona glomerulosa) to release **aldosterone** (also released due to sympathetic efferent discharge) which then increases sodium (and water) retention at the distal convoluted tubule.
- ○ AII causes vasoconstriction including the efferent renal arterioles.
- ○ AII induces thirst.

Others
- Bradykinins increase capillary permeability.
- Serotonin causes vasoconstriction but increases permeability.
- Catecholamines are part of the **stress response** (along with glucagon, ACTH and cortisol). The systemic vasoconstriction that they cause affects vessels in non-burned skin, muscle and viscera. The use of inotropes e.g. in ICU can adversely affect burn healing.

Macrophages and post-burn immune dysfunction
Schwacha MG. *Burns* 2003;**29**:1–14.

Macrophages are major producers of inflammatory cytokines after a burn including:

- PGE2, interleukin 6, TNF alpha, nitric oxide.
- Cytotoxic and cytostatic effects including lymphocyte suppression.

Increased macrophage activity seems to be central to the development of immune dysfunction after a burn.

Nitric oxide, inflammation and acute burn injury
Rawlingson A. *Burns* 2003;**29**:631–640.

Nitric oxide (NO) is produced by many types of cells including vascular endothelium through the oxidation of L-arginine by nitric oxide synthetase. It has been demonstrated to be an important regulator of vasomotor tone as well as:

- Increasing capillary permeability.
- Inhibiting platelet aggregation.
- Systemic effects as a neurotransmitter.

It reacts with superoxide free radicals to produce the highly reactive **peroxynitrite molecule**. It is required for leukocyte-mediated killing and may contribute to resistance to infection and wound healing at later stages of inflammation.

It has been implicated in both the local burn wound inflammation and the systemic inflammatory response to a major burn including pulmonary and cardiovascular dysfunction; dysregulation of NO production is associated with multiple organ failure.

V. Causes of burn injury

The commonest cause of a burn is heat. Other causes include:

- Electrical.
- Cold injury.
- Chemical and extravasation.

Electrical burns

Approximately 1000 deaths occur per year due to electrical injury in the USA, including 80 due to lightning.

The **Joule effect** (or Joule's first law) is the conversion of electrical energy into heat: $J = I^2RT$, where J is heat produced, I is current, R is resistance and T is duration of current.

Hence, the greatest generation of heat occurs when electrical energy passes along a tissue of high resistance, e.g. bone (nerve and blood vessels have least resistance). Other important parameters include frequency of the current and pathway through the body taken.

- Cardiovascular effects – cardiac dysrhythmias are diagnosed in up to 30% of high-voltage injuries (RBBB, SVTs and ectopics). If cardiorespiratory arrest occurs, prolonged resuscitation may be worthwhile.
- Neurological effects – repeated or severe injuries that are not fatal often cause neuropathic sequelae. With current travelling through the head, there is a rapid loss of consciousness – (electrical stunning); a fact that is made use of in slaughterhouses.

Classification of electrical burns
Low voltage (< 1000 V)

This causes local tissue necrosis similar to thermal injury. Injury with an AC power supply can cause cardiac arrest/ventricular fibrillation at a much lower current than a DC current. DC currents tend to cause continuous muscle contractions that lead to deeper injury, as the victim cannot let go.

High voltage (> 1000 V)

This often causes **deep muscle injury** and **compartment syndromes**, leading to haemochromogenuria. There are entry and exit wounds on the skin surface.

- Cardiorespiratory arrest.
- Fractures/dislocations
- Perforation of bowel or paralytic ileus.
- Physiological spinal cord transection in up to 25%.

Lightning injury (very high voltage, very high current, short duration).

- Direct strike (from highest point to ground).
- Ground splash (lightning hits a relatively poor conductor first e.g. a tree or the ground, and then the discharge jumps to make secondary contact with the victim).
- Stride potential (when lightning strikes the ground and spreads laterally, the victim in contact with the ground, induces a potential difference between the legs, cause current to flow through legs and lower trunk).

Lichtenberg figures ('lightning flowers') are fern-like patterns on the skin and are pathognomonic of a lightning strike. Victims of a strike may have fractures/ dislocations and corneal injury and tympanic perforation.

Burn wounds in electrical burns can occur:

- At **entry and exit points** (contact and grounding point; this is actually a misnomer of sorts as in AC currents, the flow is back and forth – with very high voltages, there may be multiple exit sites). Most of the damage will be deeper, particularly at the 'exit' point since the injury is from in to out.
- Due to arcing (up to 80% of injuries related to electricity are due to the arc flash).
- Due to thermal burns following ignition of clothing.

General management

- ABC.
- ECG. Continuous cardiac monitoring for 24 hours is usually suggested for those with high-voltage injuries particularly with current that passes through the chest/heart e.g. hand-to-hand current flow is more risky than hand-to-foot. The assumption being that the transcardiac current may have permanent/chronic effects on the conducting system of the heart, predisposing to late/delayed arrhythmias.
- Monitor for **haemochromogenuria** (haem in urine that is either due to haemoglobulin or myoglobin) and **compartment syndrome** (decompression as needed).

- Debridement and definitive wound closure after 24–72 hours.
  - Salvage of devitalized tissues with emergency free flaps that bring in additional blood supply. Consider vein grafts to ensure that anastomoses are performed outside the zone of injury.
  - Amputation where necessary.

Cardiac monitoring of high-risk patients after an electrical injury
Bailey B. *Emerg Med J* 2007;**24**:348–352.

This was a multicentre (21) prospective study with 134 patients over 4 years. 11% had abnormal ECGs on admission but no patients developed potentially lethal late arrhythmias during cardiac monitoring for 24 hours. The authors conclude that asymptomatic patients with normal initial ECG do not require cardiac monitoring if there has been no loss of consciousness and if less than 1000 V, even if transthoracic.

Most literature supports the view that a normal initial ECG in a low-voltage injury is associated with a low risk of late arrhythmias but the evidence for high-voltage injury is unclear.

Experience of 14 years of emergency reconstruction of electrical injuries
Zhu ZX. *Burns* 2003;**29**:65–72.

The authors review 14 years' experience with 155 patients. Good results were possible with their suggested protocol of CURA (comprehensive urgent reconstruction alternative):

- Early (70% within 1 hour of admission) conservative wound debridement but preserving vital structures (nerves, tendons, bone) even where viability is in doubt.
- Flap cover (including vascularized transplantation of nerves etc.) within 48 hours.
- Then continuous irrigation of the wound bed beneath the flap with a solution of lidocaine and chloromycetin in saline for up to 72 hours post-reconstruction.

Delayed complications
- Cardiac dysrhythmias.
- Neurological problems.
  - Central (from 6 months) epilepsy and encephalopathy.
  - Brainstem dysfunction.

- ○ Cord problems including progressive muscular atrophy, amyotrophic lateral sclerosis and transverse myelitis.
  - ○ Peripheral (from months to up to 3 years) – progressive neural demyelination.
- Cataracts (from 6 months) – occur in up to 30% of patients with high-voltage electrical burns involving the head and neck.

Cold injury

Cold injury can either be local (frostbite) or systemic (hypothermia). The latter is usually due to exposure of the body to cold temperature with **lowering of the core temperature** whilst the former is usually due to focal exposure of body parts to cold (slow cooling) or agents such as dry ice or liquefied gases (fast cooling).

Common acute symptoms are coldness and numbness with pain on rewarming.

Predisposing factors for hypothermia:

- Extremes of age.
- Alcohol (peripheral vascular dilatation).
- Mental instability.
- Low ambient temperature with strong air currents (wind chill).

Predisposing factors for frostbite:

- Temperature, wind chill factor and duration of contact.
- Pre-existing hypoperfusion (atherosclerosis, etc.) and smoking (vascular spasm).
- Moisture content versus oil content of the skin.

Four phases of cold injury:

- **Prefreeze** (3–10 °C) before ice crystals have formed; there is increased vascular permeability.
- **Freeze–thaw** (−6 to −15 °C) Extra- and intra-cellular ice crystals form at −4 °C, i.e. when the skin is supercooled, which is necessary owing to the generation of background metabolic heat. At −20 °C, 90% of all available water is frozen.
- **Vascular stasis** with dilatation and coagulation thus shunting blood flow away from the affected part.
- **Late ischaemic** phase with cell death and gangrene.

Effects of thawing

- Initial reversible **vasoconstriction** then hyperaemia with restoration of the dermal circulation.

- **Endothelial cell damage** and formation of **microemboli** leading to distal occlusion and thrombosis (no reflow).
- Liberation of **inflammatory mediators and oxygen free radicals** which contribute to the frostbite injury causing oedema and formation of blisters and later an eschar.

Management

- Avoiding rubbing frozen parts. It is preferable to rapidly rewarm by immersion in circulating water at 40–42 °C for ~30 minutes with analgesia (NSAIDs).
- Leave blisters alone, elevate and splint extremities.
- Tetanus and antibiotic prophylaxis is advisable.
- Delay amputation for as long as possible; the line of demarcation may be indeterminate for many weeks.

Victims often achieve good recovery in the long term but possible long-term sequelae include:

- Residual burning sensations for up to 6 weeks, usually precipitated by warming.
- Cold intolerance/Raynaud's phenomenon.
- There may be permanent sensory loss.
- Hyperhidrosis is one manifestation of altered sympathetic activity.
- Localized areas of bone resorption and joint pain and stiffness.

Chemical burns

Approximately 3% of burns centre admissions are due to chemical burns with most being work-related (depending on the local population), affecting men and the upper extremities.

- Civilian chemical burns – mainly acids and alkalis.
- Military chemical injuries – mainly white phosphorus.
- Industrial:
  - ○ Acid burns are commonest in plating or fertilizing industries. Nitric acid burns have a characteristic yellow staining.
  - ○ Alkali burns commonly seen following use of oven cleaners or soap manufacture.
  - ○ Dyes, fertilizers, plastics and explosives manufacture associated with phenol burns.
  - ○ Hydrofluoric (HF) burns – etching processes, petroleum refinement and air conditioner cleaning.

A feature of chemical burns is that there is usually continued tissue damage long after the initial exposure. The severity is related to:

- Concentration and duration of exposure.
- Type of chemical action.
- Site affected.
- Industrial accidents may have an inhalational component; be on the guard for **eye** injuries.

Emergency management

- Removal of contaminated clothing and copious lavage with running water (care with 'run off' injuries) whilst avoiding hypothermia. In the industrial setting, 'decontamination' procedures and facilities are usually of a high standard, thus injuries often tend to be less severe than household injuries where the problem may be 'ignored' (due to lack of awareness and lack of protective measures) until it is too late.
- Check blood pH/gases and correct acidosis with IV $NaHCO_3$.
- Encourage diuresis with mannitol to prevent renal complications.
- Emergency debridement to reduce the chemical load (and thus to reduce the final damage) is emerging as an alternative to the traditional method of waiting for demarcation. It is particularly relevant in extravasation injuries, (cyto)toxics and HF.

Alkalis e.g. NaOH, KOH, lime

Mechanism of injury:

- Saponification of fat – liquefactive necrosis which means that alkalis are capable of deep penetration.
- Tissue desiccation – burns often look 'shrunken' or 'indented'.
- Protein denaturation.

The pain is usually severe. Severe eye injury may result including scarring, ulceration and opacification of the cornea.

Cement i.e. calcium oxide

There is an exothermic reaction with water e.g. sweat to form CaOH (alkali). The typical injury involves cement getting inside the victim's boots, causing desiccation injury with the prolonged exposure. Symptoms and presentation are thus typically delayed.

Drain cleaners

The common drain cleaners found in supermarkets are usually composed of alkalis (sodium or potassium hydroxide, with or without bleach); some are enzyme based (usually marketed as eco-friendly). Acid drain cleaners are available but primarily intended for use by plumbers due to the hazards including a violent reaction with water.

Acids

Tissue damage occurs mainly by coagulative necrosis.

Formic (methanoic) acid

This chemical is found in industrial descalers and hay preservatives. The wound has a greenish colour with blistering and oedema. Absorption from the skin may lead to metabolic acidosis, haemolysis and haemochromogenuria; serious sequelae such as blindness (due to optic nerve damage caused by systemic absorption), acute respiratory distress syndrome (ARDS) and necrotizing pancreatitis may result.

Hydrofluoric acid (HF)

This chemical is used in the glass industry for dissolving silica. It is capable of causing severe injury.

- F^- binds to Na/K ATPase resulting in K^+ efflux from cells and hyperkalaemia.
- F^- **complexes with cations** including Ca^{2+} and Mg^{2+}, and by binding intracellular Ca^{2+} leads to cell death. Thus it can cause desiccation, corrosion, protein denaturation, liquefactive necrosis and bone decalcification; unrecognized injuries inevitably progress to extensive tissue destruction. Hypocalcaemia leads to cardiac dysrhythmia and refractory (fatal) ventricular fibrillation (VF) may be induced by the action of fluoride on the myocardium. Even 2% TBSA involvement may be **fatal**.

The concentration affects speed with which signs appear:

- < 20% – injury becomes apparent after 24 hours.
- 20–50% – injury becomes apparent after several hours.
- 50% – injury immediately painful.

Management

Emergency management.

- Dilution by copious irrigation.

- Chelation of fluoride ions with calcium preparations.
  - **Topical** calcium gluconate gel ± **injection** of calcium gluconate solution into deeper tissues beneath the burn with a 27-gauge needle, from the periphery of the burn inwards. Injection of calcium reduces wound pain, thus the subsequent return of pain may indicate need for repeat injections.
  - In some cases, injuries may require digital fasciotomy or intra-arterial **infusion** of calcium gluconate via the radial artery.
  - Inhaled HF should be treated by respiratory support and nebulized calcium gluconate.
- Correct systemic hypocalcaemia and hypomagnesaemia – IV calcium chloride. Cardiac monitoring is needed – beware prolonged QT interval due to hypocalcaemia.
- Elimination of fluoride may be improved by:
  - $NaHCO_3$ – alkalinizes urine to promote excretion.
  - Haemodialysis.
  - Wound debridement/excision may be necessary.

Alkyl mercuric compounds

These are most commonly ethyl and methyl mercuric phosphates, and the blister fluid contains liberated free mercury, which can be absorbed and lead to systemic poisoning. Consequently blisters should be de-roofed and the wounds washed copiously.

Hydrocarbons

These cause cell membrane injury by dissolving lipids which leads to erythema and blistering. The skin injuries are usually superficial but systemic absorption of the compounds can lead to respiratory depression e.g. petrol exposure has three potential mechanisms of injury:

- Lipid solvent action causing endothelial cell membrane injury.
- Leaded petrol leads to lead absorption (binds CNS lipids).
- Ignited petrol causes thermal injury.

Phenol

Otherwise known as carbolic acid, phenol is used commonly as a disinfectant but is a component of some deep facial peels. Phenol is also a component in tar which may be removed with toluene.

- Contact can cause dermatitis and depigmentation whilst prolonged exposure may lead to necrosis and gangrene.
- It binds irreversibly to albumin and ingestion of 1 g may prove fatal.
- Treat with copious water irrigation followed by polyethylene glycol (antifreeze).

Hot bitumen burns: 92 hospitalized patients
Baruchin AM. *Burns* 1997;**23**:438–441.

This was a 10-year retrospective review – most were occupational injuries. Bitumen or tarmac is a mixture of petroleum-derived hydrocarbons, mineral tars and asphalt. It needs to be heated to 100–200 °C before use, thus it can cause thermal and chemical injury.

- Cool the burn wound at the scene and the bitumen then becomes cold and hard. There is some debate regarding whether adherent bitumen should be removed as this may cause additional trauma, however in most cases (gentle) removal is advised as it does allow early evaluation of the injury.
- There are numerous methods described such as liquid paraffin which slowly dissolves the bitumen.
  - Sunflower oil. Turegun M. *Burns* 1997;**23**:442–445.
  - Baby oil. Juma A. *Burns* 1994;**20**:363–364.
  - Butter. Tiernan E. *Burns* 1993;**19**:437–438.
  - Neomycin with Tween 80 (polyoxyethylene sorbitan). Demling RH. *J Trauma* 1980;**20**:242.

Highly reactive elements

White phosphorus is a military agent but is also found in fertilizers. It ignites on contact with air and will cause cutaneous burns until covered in water. The burns are typically painful, necrotic yellow wounds.

- Systemic toxicity (hepatorenal).
- Hypocalcaemia and hypophosphataemia.

Suggested management is irrigation of the wound and to remove particles – UV light may help whilst irrigation with 0.5% copper sulphate causes a black film to form (cupric oxide). ECG monitoring is advised with electrolyte imbalance.

Extravasation injury

Severe extravasation injury: an avoidable iatrogenic disaster?
Burd A. *Br Med J* 1985;**290**:1579–1580.

This study quotes two older studies, suggesting that up to 11% of children and 22% of adult patients receiving IV fluids experience some form of extravasation injury. Patients at extremes of age are most at risk. The dorsum of the hand and the foot are at particular risk, as they are more likely to be dislodged with movement. The extent of the resultant damage depends on the chemical composition of the infusate, in particular radiological contrast media, hypertonic solutions and cytotoxic drugs may cause extensive soft tissue necrosis.

The escape of drugs from the veins into subcutaneous tissues is a well-known adverse event associated with intravenous therapy; it occurs in approximately 0.1 to 6% of patients receiving intravenous chemotherapy. Cancer patients are inherently at high risk:

- Often require multiple venipuncture sites and optimal intravenous sites may be reduced due to previous chemotherapy, radiotherapy changes, and lymphedema secondary to surgery.
- Veins are thin and fragile.
- Systemically unwell including malnutrition.

Cytotoxic agents generally cause two types of local cutaneous reactions:

- Irritants – these cause a short self-limited phlebitis and there is a tender, warm, erythematous reaction at the site.
- Vesicants – e.g. doxorubicin and mitomycin. The reaction caused by vesicants is often called chemical cellulitis – initially it is similar to irritation but may worsen, depending on the amount of extravasation and necrosis may follow large-volume extravasations. The wound usually heals poorly and may progress, necessitating surgery. Some vesicants may bind to DNA which may allow them to be recycled and retained in the tissue, prolonging damage.

Signs may range from discomfort and mild erythema to severely painful skin necrosis, ulcerations and invasion and damage of deep tissue structures. The extent of tissue damage largely depends on the concentration, volume and nature of the extravasated agent.

Management

- Stop the infusion promptly.
- Attempt aspiration of residual drug through the cannula and then remove the catheter.

- Local cooling and elevation of the affected extremity may help in preventing ulceration. Heat is recommended for the vinca alkaloids.
- Antidotes – this is controversial as some e.g. sodium bicarbonate may be harmful, and any benefit may be related to dilution – e.g. injection of saline has some success.
- Local injection of steroid – variable success (which may be expected as reactions with antineoplastics are not usually associated with significant inflammation).
- Local injection of GM-CSF – has been used for mitomycin injury. Shamseddine AI. *Eur J Gynaecol Oncol* 1998;**19**:479–481.
- Topical DMSO (free radical scavenger). Bertelli G. *J Clin Oncol* 1995;**13**:2851–2855.

Conservative treatment is preferable for most extravasations as it can be difficult to predict how they will heal, however early excision may be favoured with more harmful chemicals with grafts or flaps (though there is a risk that any residual chemicals may damage the graft/flap).

Extravasation injuries
Gault DT. *Br J Plast Surg* 1993;**46**:91–96.

The paper describes two techniques, liposuction and saline flushout – skin incisions around the area are made with a no. 11 blade – hyaluronidase 1500 units in 10 ml normal saline followed by further irrigation. Analysis of the flushout confirmed the presence of the agent i.e. being removed. In this way 86% healed without soft tissue loss.

Liposuction and extravasation injuries in ICU
Steinmann G. *Br J Anaesth* 2005;**95**:355–357.

The article presents two cases of extravasation injury (thiopentone and contrast media) treated with liposuction within 6 and 2 hours of the injury respectively. Both healed uneventfully.

VI. Paediatric burns

There are many differences to consider. Children tend to suffer different types of burn injuries – two-thirds of paediatric burns are scalds. In addition, children will have different premorbid conditions, e.g. more asthma, less/no angina. There should be a high index of suspicion for non-accidental injuries.

- The skin is thinner hence burns for a given energy insult will be deeper. 65 °C for 2 seconds will cause FT burns in adults (Moritz AR. *Am J Pathol*

1947;**23**:695) but in children lower temperatures will cause FT burns.

- The surface area will need to be considered differently due to the body proportions (larger head and smaller lower limbs): either a modified Wallace's rule of nines or a Lund and Browder chart. A child with an uncomplicated 95% burn has ~50% chance of survival.
  - ○ Modified rule of nines – for a 1-year-old, each year over take 1% from head and neck and add it to the lower limb.
    - – Head and neck 18%.
    - – Lower limb 14%.
    - – Upper limb 9%.
    - – Anterior trunk 18%.
    - – Posterior trunk 18%.

Airway

The airway in children is narrower (in addition, there may be occlusion by tonsils and adenoids) and thus the paediatric airway develops more resistance for a given degree of swelling compared with adults. Children have a shorter, larger floppy epiglottis; they are more prone to laryngomalacia and more prone to bronchial irritability and thus spasm.

Breathing

Children rely more upon diaphragmatic respiration hence thoraco-abdominal burns, even if not circumferential, may require decompression.

Circulation

The relative paediatric circulating volume is larger at ~80 ml/kg compared with the adult 60 ml/kg.

- The heart rate is less reliable as an indicator of volaemic status. Children normally have a lower resting BP than adults (~100 mmHg systolic) which is maintained well until late when up to 25% of circulating volume has been lost. Delayed refill, pallor, sweating, obtunded consciousness are ominous late signs. Cardiac output is more closely related to heart rate than filling pressure.
- Inadequate intravenous access may require an intra-osseus infusion which may allow delivery of up to 100 ml/h of fluid – there is a low marrow fat content hence the risk of fat embolus is rare.

Resuscitation should start at **4 ml/kg/% TBSA** along with maintenance fluid – 5% dextrose or half dextrose/ half saline i.e. 0.45% saline and 4% glucose (77 mmol sodium, 77 mmol chloride and 50 g glucose).

- First 10 kg – 100 ml/kg.
- Second 10 kg – 50 ml/kg.
- Thereafter – 20 ml/kg.

Some use formulae based on the body surface area e.g. Galveston Shriner's:

Total volume (24 hours) = 5000 ml/m^2/BSA burn + 2000 ml/m^2/total BSA.

It is important to avoid volume overload which may easily precipitate right heart failure or pulmonary oedema. The kidneys are immature with less concentrating ability and **urine output continues despite hypovolaemia**. Children need a higher minimum urine output 1–2 ml/kg/h.

Be aware of the risk of hypoglycaemia (due to less stored glycogen) and hyponatraemia (cerebral oedema). Resuscitation is accompanied by a diuresis which washes out potassium – it is common to replace with potassium phosphate since hypophosphataemia may also occur.

Deficit and exposure

Children are less able to cooperate with examination which should be done quickly and efficiently – give adequate analgesia:

Maintenance.

- Paracetamol 10–15 mg/kg four times daily, max 5 doses a day.
- Ibuprofen 5–10 mg/kg 3 times a day, maximum 40 mg/kg/day.
- Morphine IV 0.2 mg/kg 4 to 6 times a day.

Before dressings e.g. morphine.

- 0.1 mg/kg IV – 10 minutes before, can titrate with boluses.
- 0.2 mg/kg IM – if only a single dose anticipated.
- 0.2 mg/kg orally – 60 minutes before. However cannot titrate and there is usually prolonged sedation afterwards.

Entonox has been used in many units for dressing changes for many years, however it has limited analgesic properties. Sadly, analgesia is probably under-used in paediatric burns (Singer A. *J Burn Care Rehab* 2002;**23**:361–365).

It is important to maintain ambient temperature of ~30 °C as the larger surface area to volume ratio means that children lose heat more quickly and have less thermoregulation response (no shivering reflex in neonates, less insulating fat, poorly developed piloerection). This all results in a tendency towards hypothermia (note that burn patients normally have a temperature ~38 °C) which may lead to:

- Ventricular arrhythmias, CNS and respiratory depression.
- Oxyhaemoglobin dissociation curve shifted to the left.

Minimizing the time of exposure will also reduce evaporative water loss and heat loss.

Longer-term considerations in children after burns include:

- There is an inhibition of growth during the 3 years post-burn without subsequent compensatory catch-up. There is a reduction in respiratory reserve where there has been inhalation injury up to 2.5 years post-burn.
- Breast development may be unimpaired, even where there is burn to the nipple–areolar complex and circumferential truncal burns do not cause problems during later pregnancy in adult life.
- Joint contractures appear to be more of a problem in children than adults, more so where excision has been to fascia rather than fat.
- Psychosocial problems.

Non-accidental injuries

Non-accidental (or intentional) burns mostly occur in children as a form of child abuse but may also occur in the elderly, including those in institutional care. There may be clues that suggest an injury to be non-accidental but there is no single feature that can be relied upon.

- Injuries may be due to 'neglect' rather than 'abuse' per se.

A systematic review of the features that indicate intentional scalds in children
Maguire S. *Burns* 2008;**34**:1072–1074.

This is a literature review that included 26 studies reviewed independently by two burn specialists. Some distinguishing features were identified:

- Intentional scalds are often immersion affecting extremities or the buttocks/perineum.
- Immersion injuries have clear upper margins.
- There may be associated or old injuries such as fractures or other unrelated injuries.

- In contrast, accidental scalds tend to affect the upper body with irregular margins and depth.

Other clues include:

- Explanation offered is not compatible with the injury sustained, often blaming a sibling.
- Unexplained delay in presentation.
- Apparent lack of parental concern.
- Apparent lack of parent–child bonding.
- Passive, introverted child.

B. Surgical management of burns

I. Burn surgery

In simple terms, the aim in deeper burns is for timely surgical removal of non-viable tissues and closure of the wound with autografts. There are many variables to consider.

Timing of burn surgery

- Immediate – escharotomy, tracheostomy if required as an emergency.
- Early (< 72 hours usually, though this is rather arbitrary as some use the definition of 1–2 days post-burn) – tangential excision and grafting (intermediate if > 72 hours).
- Late e.g. post-burn reconstruction.

The trend has been to favour early excision, and this is associated with:

- Improved survival rate.
- Decreased hospital stay (< 1 day per % BSA) and reduced expenditure.
- Reduced blood loss.
- Fewer metabolic complications.

The benefit of early surgery has been confirmed by a number of studies:

- Burke JF. Primary burn excision and immediate grafting. *J Trauma* 1974;**14**:389–395.
- Herndon JN. Comparison of serial debridement and autografting and early massive excision with cadaver skin overlay in the treatment of large burns in children. *J Trauma* 1986;**26**:149–152.
- Pietsch JB. Early excision of major burns in children. *J Paediatr Surg* 1986;**20**:754–757.
- Tompkins RG. Prompt eschar excision. *Ann Surg* 1986;**204**:272–281.

- Herndon DN. A comparison of conservative versus early excision therapies in severely burned patients. *Ann Surg* 1989;**209**:547–553.
- Müller MJ. The challenge of burns. *Lancet* 1994;**343**:216–220.

Hot water scalds in children are an exception to the rule of early excision due to the depth often being mixed and indeterminate in the early stage. Thus, to reduce the excision of viable tissue, excision could be delayed until after 2 weeks. At this stage, it will be easier to determine which areas are truly non-viable and by allowing some healing to occur a smaller area is grafted. This will reduce blood loss, which is also reduced by avoiding the inflammatory phase (blood loss averages $0.4\,\text{ml/cm}^2$ if surgery is performed within 24 hours but increases to $0.75\,\text{ml/cm}^2$ between 2 and 16 days post-burn).

However, the disadvantage is that ungrafted or delay-grafted deep PT burns are more likely to form hypertrophic scars.

Level of excision

- **Tangential excision** was first described by Janzekovic in 1975 and basically involves the shaving of thin layers of eschar until viable/bleeding tissue is reached. The major issue with this technique is excessive blood loss.
  - To reduce blood loss, adrenaline can be injected subcutaneously (with or without hyalase) before excision, adrenaline soaks (1:10 000) can be placed on the punctate bleeding points and/or tourniquets can be used where possible for the limbs.
- **Fascial excision** is indicated where the burns are deep, i.e. at least full thickness and the fat layer is deeply involved. There is less bleeding with this technique and graft take is very good. However, the cosmetic appearance is poor and lymphoedema can be a long-term problem.

General intra-operative patient care

- Monitor core temperature: keep ambient temperature high, which can make it somewhat hot and uncomfortable for the surgeons.
- Avoid hypo- or hypervolaemia: monitor urine output, consider CVP monitoring and arterial lines.
- Blood loss should be reduced as much as possible with meticulous haemostasis: cautery, topical thrombin spray, and/or pressure dressings. Blood loss should be accurately assessed.
- Donor sites are traditionally dressed with Kaltostat (calcium alginate).

Wound closure has the benefits of:

- Reducing water, electrolyte and protein losses.
- Reducing pain and wound infection.

Grafting

- Sheet graft (with handmade fenestrations) is preferred for the hands, face, flexural creases whilst meshed skin can be used for other areas. Another choice for the face is to harvest FTSG from the abdomen or thigh, and to apply SSG to the donor areas.
- The grafts can be fixed with staples, sutures or glue. They can be dressed (paraffin gauze) or under some circumstances left open.
- Scalp, scrotum and axillae may be the only available donor areas in those with massive burns.

II. Recent advances

A guide to biological skin substitutes

Jones I. *Br J Plast Surg* 2002;**55**:185–193.

There are many commercial products available for **wound cover** (which is useful for clean superficial partial thickness burns or split skin graft donor sites; alternatively they can provide temporary cover of excised deeper burns):

Biobrane

- Silicone sheet over a nylon mesh that is coated with porcine collagen; the sheet is peeled away as the wound heals over 10–14 days.

Transcyte

- Similar to Biobrane but the collagen-coated nylon mesh is seeded with neonatal fibroblasts that synthesize fibronectin, type I collagen, proteoglycans and growth factors during the manufacturing process whilst subsequent cryopreservation renders the fibroblasts non-viable.
- It is suited to the treatment of partial thickness burns but it is expensive and there is no proven benefit compared with Biobrane.

Apligraft

- Cultured allogeneic neonatal keratinocytes (they fail to express MHC type II antigen after 7 days of culture) on a gel matrix of bovine type I collagen seeded with viable neonatal fibroblasts.

- The main indication for Apligraft is for healing of chronic wounds (e.g. venous ulcers) but it is very expensive. In clinical use, it seems to function more as a wound modulator rather than a composite skin.

Dermagraft

- Cultured human fetal fibroblasts in polyglycolic acid (Dexon) or polyglactin-910 (Vicryl) mesh; the fibroblasts remain viable despite cryopreservation. Supposedly the material stimulates the in-growth of fibrovascular tissue from the wound margin/bed and migration of host keratinocytes.
- It is mainly used in the treatment of diabetic and chronic ulcers. It may be useful as a dermal replacement beneath a split skin autograft for excised burn wounds, with the aim of reducing contracture.

AlloDerm

- Human cadaveric skin with epidermis removed and the cellular components extracted to remove immunocompetency.
- It functions similarly to that of Dermagraft i.e. as dermal replacement only with a split-skin autograft required. It has also been used as interpositional material or a tissue-filler (micronized).

Xenograft – most commonly porcine skin that can be bought in or prepared by well-equipped burns units/ skin banks.

There are also products available for **wound closure**, i.e. to provide permanent coverage of a wound:

Integra

- This is a dermal matrix composed of bovine collagen and shark proteoglycan (chondroitin 6-sulphate) and covered with a silicone elastomer membrane. The silicone is removed after about 3 weeks after in-growth of fibroblasts and vascular endothelial cells, and is then covered with thin epithelial autograft. It can be meshed to improve drainage or contouring. It is an expensive material but definitely has its uses.
  ○ A favourable bed is needed though there are reports that the slow 'revascularization' of the product means that it can 'bridge' over small avascular areas or be used in irradiated tissues.

- The supposed advantages are less hypertrophic scarring and contracture; the skin remains pliable. Overall take is ~80% on average with good cosmetic and functional outcomes. The main risk is of infection (particularly when used in large burns) and it is common to cover it with antimicrobial/antiseptic soaks such as povidone iodine or silver dressings such as Aquacel silver.

Cultured epithelial autografts (vide infra)

Effect of growth hormone therapy in burns patients on conservative treatment
Singh KP. *Burns* 1998;**24**:733–738.

This paper reports the benefits of recombinant human growth hormone (rhGH) (0.2 mg/kg) given subcutaneously once daily for 2 weeks.

- Improved donor and burn wound healing.
- Reduction in weight loss with preservation of serum albumin, induces positive protein balance.
- Shorter hospital stay.

Potential problems:

- Transient hypercalcaemia.
- Albuminuria.
- Hyperglycaemia – one-third require insulin.

Growth hormones, burns and tissue healing
Lal SO. *Growth Horm IGF Res* 2000;**10 Suppl. B**:S39–S43.

The authors state that growth hormone may reduce some of the deleterious effects of the prolonged hypercatabolic state after major burns. A dose of 0.6 IU/kg/day (same as above) reduces wound healing times – possibly through the stimulation of IGF-I growth factors as seen in animal studies.

Other studies demonstrated:

- 3–10× increase in basal laminin and type III and VII collagen.
- 2× increase in protein synthesis.
- Increase blood flow in extremities.

Although there are data to demonstrate improvement on wound healing, the side-effects/complications have limited its wider use, in particular the anti-insulin effects meaning that glucose is less efficiently used and hyperglycaemia is deleterious. A multicentre European study of critically ill (mainly post-operative cardiac surgery) patients demonstrated a doubling of mortality with hGH.

The role of anabolic hormones for wound healing in catabolic states

Demling RH. *J Burns Wounds* 2005;**4**:46–62.

Most studies have concentrated on oxandrolone which has the greatest anabolic and least androgenic effects; it is the only anabolic steroid approved for restoration of lost body weight and lean mass, and has been used with some success in burns patients (it also improves wound healing). The most common side-effect is liver dysfunction (variable severity but commonly a transient increase in aminotransferases).

C. Complications of burns

I. Pathophysiology of smoke inhalation and effect on respiration

Eighty per cent of fire-related deaths are due to inhalation injury.

- Maximum upper airway oedema and narrowing occurs ~24 hours post-injury.
- Inhalation injury in an adult worsens mortality rate by 40%.
- Inhalation injury plus pneumonia worsens mortality rate by 70%.

Inhalational injury can be subdivided into:

- Supraglottic – primarily thermal injury to the upper airways above the larynx.
- Subglottic – primarily chemical injury to alveoli due to dissolved acidic products of combustion.
- Systemic – primarily toxic effects of inhaled poisons.

Symptoms

- Shortness of breath/dyspnoea.
- Brassy cough and wheezing.
- Hoarseness.

Signs

- Circumoral soot and burns.
- Increased respiratory rate and effort of ventilation.
- Stridor.
- Altered consciousness.

Pathophysiology

Injury leads to release of inflammatory mediators causing

- Increased pulmonary artery blood flow.
- Bronchoconstriction (TXA2) and increased airway resistance.

In turn, this leads to

- V–Q mismatch.
- Decreased pulmonary compliance (increases risk of barotrauma if ventilated).
- Interstitial oedema, fibrin casts within the airways act as a culture medium to promote infection and cause distal atelectasis.

Later on

- Formation of a pseudomembrane during the healing phase ~18 days post-injury.
- Permanent airway stenosis/fibrosis.

Carbon monoxide toxicity

Carbon monoxide is a colourless, odourless, poisonous gas produced by the incomplete combustion of hydrocarbons. It has a 200–250 × greater affinity for haemoglobin (Hb) than oxygen and shifts the Hb-O_2 dissociation curve to the left.

The half-life of COHb is ~250 minutes in a patient breathing room air but is reduced to 40–60 minutes with the administration of 100% oxygen; HBO further accelerates the breakdown of COHb (30 min at 3 atm).

- COHb levels > 5% (threshold higher by 10% in smokers) are indicative of an inhalation injury but do not provide an accurate measure of the severity. Toxic symptoms generally appear at levels > 20% (headache) with progressive deterioration until death at levels > 60%.
- CO also directly binds cytochromes, i.e. sick cell syndrome (reduced Na+/K+ pump function). Cytochrome-bound CO is washed out after ~24 hours causing a secondary rise in serum COHb and possibly post-intoxication encephalopathy. Late neurological deterioration can occur several months afterwards.

Hydrogen cyanide toxicity

Cyanide compounds are released when certain plastic materials burn. They bind to and inhibit cytochrome oxidase thus uncoupling oxidative phosphorylation. It is rapidly fatal at inspired concentrations > 20 ppm and serum levels > 1 mg/l whilst smokers have background levels of ~0.1 mg/l.

- ST elevation.
- Increased ventilation via stimulation of peripheral chemoreceptors makes toxicity worse.

Treatment

- 100% O_2.
- The *safest* option is probably **hydroxycobalamin** which acts as a chelating agent that complexes free cyanide to aid its renal excretion.
- **Sodium thiosulphate** provides the sodium substrate for conversion of cyanide (bound to Hb) to thiocyanate (SCN) by hepatic rhodanase. It acts slowly and the SCN produced is excreted in the urine resulting in an osmotic diuresis.
- **Amyl nitrite** traps cyanide onto Hb rather than the cytochromes:
  - Hb (Fe^{2+}) + amyl nitrite to Hb (Fe^{3+}).
  - Hb (Fe^{3+}) + cyanide to cyanohaemoglobin.

Other toxic gases that may be produced in fires include:

- HCl – alveolar injury and pulmonary oedema.
- NO – pulmonary oedema, cardiovascular depression.
- Aldehydes.

Investigations in suspected inhalational injury

- Arterial blood gases with carboxyhaemoglobin.
- Fibreoptic bronchoscopy – features range from soot deposition, swollen mucosa to frankly burnt tissues.
- Chest X-ray – typically few signs early on.

General management of inhalational injury

- Give supplementary humidified O_2 and intubate early if significant inhalational injury is **suspected.** Chest physiotherapy, sputum culture and bronchoalveolar toilet.
  - Elevate head of bed to reduce pulmonary oedema and pressure on the diaphragm by abdominal viscera.
  - Increase the fluid resuscitation requirement for concomitant cutaneous burns.
- Mechanical ventilatory support may be needed, but it is important to try to avoid barotrauma (pneumothorax, pneumomediastinum and surgical emphysema), even if it means that the $PaCO_2$ is slightly high. High-frequency (jet) ventilation reduces tidal volume and airway pressures.
  - Aerosolized or systemic bronchodilators as needed.
  - Aerosolized acetyl cysteine – it is a powerful mucolytic but its exact role is not defined.
  - Avoid tracheomalacia and long-term tracheal stenosis by ensuring cuff pressures of < 20 cm H_2O and conversion from ET to tracheostomy if period of supported ventilation is prolonged.
- Treat only recognized infective complications rather than prophylactically. The commonest source of infection is either from ET tube or opportunistically from patient's GI and skin commensals. Over-use of antibiotics will predispose to over-population with opportunistic organisms.
- Stress ulcer prophylaxis with either sucralfate or H_2 receptor antagonists does not affect pneumonia rates. (Cioffi W J. *Trauma* 1994;**36**:541–547.)

Extracorporeal membrane oxygenation in the treatment of inhalation injury
O'Toole G. *Burns* 1998;**24**:562–565.

Conventional ventilation does not always ensure adequate oxygenation and ECMO has been used to treat severe but reversible cardiorespiratory failure. The experience with two paediatric burn cases was reported – right internal jugular vein to ECMO and back to right carotid artery, for 72 and 144 hours respectively. Patients must be able to tolerate limited heparinization; ECMO may be indicated if they are not responding to maximal conventional therapy, usually defined as 7 days or more of high-pressure ventilation for studies.

Patton reported a case with successful use of ECMO in an adult burn patient with ARDS, (Patton ML. *Burns* 1998;**24**:566–568) in the same issue of the journal.

II. Dietetics as relating to burn-injury metabolism

The basal metabolic rate (BMR) increases dramatically during the acute injury phase, up to 180% for burn injuries more than 40% TBSA. Oxygen consumption and CO_2 production steadily increase over the first 5 days post-injury:

- Associated increase in protein, fat and glycogen catabolism.

- Post-receptor insulin resistance.
- Enhanced glucose delivery to cells including fibroblasts, inflammatory cells and endothelial cells at the burn wound. Carbohydrate metabolism is greatly altered with increased glucose uptake and gluconeogenesis.

Burned patients continue to catabolize protein during the first week post-burn despite aggressive feeding. This causes:

- Weight loss.
- Impaired wound healing and immunity.

The BMR remains higher than normal for up to 12 months post-injury. The negative nitrogen balance persists up to 9 months post-injury and there may be growth delay in children for up to 2 years.

Daily calorie requirements

Most believe that a half to two-thirds of the non-protein calorie intake should be provided by carbohydrate, the rest as fat and protein (20% protein, 28% fat, 52% carbohydrate). A high carbohydrate regimen stimulates protein synthesis and improves lean body mass. Children have less body fat and a smaller muscle mass, hence need proportionately greater intake of carbohydrates.

- There are many formulae used to estimate requirements including the Sutherland formulae (Sutherland AB. *Burns* 1976; **2**:238–244):
  - Adults – 20 kcal/kg + 70 kcal/% TBSA
  - Children – 60 kcal/kg + 35 kcal/% TBSA
- **Harris–Benedict** – BMR calculated with formulae derived from measurements in healthy volunteers and an injury factor of 2.1 is recommended for burns. More recent studies have shown that resting energy expenditure (REE) rarely exceeds the Harris–Benedict predicted BMR by more than 50% in burns of more than 45% BSA when treated with modern techniques.
- See below for Curreri and Hildreth formulae.

However, **indirect calorimetry** provides the most accurate figure. The respiratory quotient is the ratio of CO_2 production to O_2 consumption, and the normal fasting ratio is 0.70–0.85. The recommendation is for twice weekly measurements to be made to assess nutrition started at 120–130% of measured REE.

- Increased respiratory quotient (RQ) results from an increased CO_2 production, i.e. increased carbohydrate metabolism. There is a danger that increased CO_2 production may complicate respiratory function.
- Decreased RQ usually indicates an inadequate calorie intake.

Protein needs:

- Greatest nitrogen losses between days 5 and 10; 20% of calories to replace that lost in a burn wound should be provided by protein.
- Davies formulae:
  - Children – 3 g/kg + 1 g/% TBSA
  - Adults – 1 g/kg + 3 g/% TBSA

The aims of **early feeding** are to minimize net protein loss and to protect the gut from bacterial translocation, prevent gastric ileus and avoid Gram-negative septicaemia.

Nutrition and anabolic agents in burned patients
Andel H. *Burns* 2003;**29**:592–595.

Enteral feeding is superior to parenteral feeding in the burns patient.

- TPN is associated with impaired mucosal immunity and enhanced endotoxin translocation. It is also associated with up-regulated expression of TNF-α which adversely affects survival.
- Enteral nutrition preserves mucosal integrity, protects against bacterial translocation in the gut and is associated with improved regulation of the inflammatory cytokine response.

Duodenal feeding is preferred over gastric feeding, as there is less regurgitation of feed and this may reduce aspiration pneumonia. Overfeeding with high calorie enteral nutrition should be avoided – it may lead to impairment of sphlanchnic oxygen balance in septic burns patients and hyperglycaemia.

Early intragastric feeding of seriously burned and long-term ventilated patients: a review of 55 patients
Raff T. *Burns* 1997;**23**:19–25.

Where gastric ileus is established tubes may be sited in the duodenum or jejunum but hormonal stimulation of the liver and pancreas is greatly reduced when the feed is not placed in the stomach.

It is sensible to begin feeding at low infusion rates (check absorption by aspirating the tube). Shock decreases gut blood flow, thus feeding in the presence of shock may make the gut even more sensitive to the effects of relative ischaemia. Tube feeding may be complicated by inadvertent dislodgement, diarrhoea and pulmonary aspiration.

Their review of 55 patients showed decreased mortality in those successfully fed – 20–40 ml bolus feed per hour with 20 ml water flush, success was defined as residual volume less than feeding rate. Metoclopramide and cisapride were used to assist gastric emptying in selected cases. An interval of more than 18 hours before is unfavourable and decreases the success rate.

Support of the metabolic response to burn injury
Herndon DN. *Lancet* 2004;**363**:1895–1902.

The article describes strategies to reducing the hypercatabolic response:

- Preventing infection.
- Early wound closure, preferably autograft but also includes biosynthetic skin substitutes and cadaveric allograft.
- Raising the ambient temperature to 33 °C so heat for evaporation derives from the environment and less is used by the patient in trying to maintain the raised body temperature (the body tries to increase body temperature to 2 °C above normal).

In addition:

- **Nutritional support.** The BMR can remain elevated for a year after the burn. The catabolic response requires nutritional support and in the main, continuous enteral feeding is preferred, using parenteral feeding only if there is a prolonged ileus or intolerance of enteral feeding.
  - **Adults:** 25 kcal/kg (usual body weight) + 40 kcal/% BSA per day (Curreri PW. *J Trauma* 1971;**11**:390–396). The maximum BSA that this can be applied to is 50%. Although it is commonly used, some feel that it tends to overestimate. Some have also modified this into a 'Curreri Junior' formula for children.
  - **Children:** 1800 kcal/m^2 body surface area + 2200 kcal/m^2 burn area (surface area can be extrapolated using nomograms) per day (Hildreth MJ. *Burns Care Res* 1982;**3**:78–80).
- **Hormonal administration.** The hormonal response can be modulated e.g. by provision of **anabolic hormones** such as growth hormone.
  - rhGH (0.2 mg/kg/day) reduces wound healing time.
  - rhGH (0.05 mg/kg/day) in children improves growth for up to 3 years post-burn.

- Side-effects include hyperglycaemia (but not in children).
- Other potentially useful hormones:
  - Insulin, insulin-like growth factor-1.
  - Oxandrolone (weak testosterone analogue).
  - β-blockade – propranolol (to block the raised catecholamine response) lowers heart rate and thus the oxygen requirement.
- **Physical exercise** as part of post-burn rehabilitation has also shown to improve muscle mass.

III. Burns shock and sepsis

Burns shock and oedema
Normal Starling's forces indicate a slight filtration pressure overall, with this being matched by lymphatic drainage. In an acute burn, soft-tissue oedema develops due to:

- Increased capillary permeability (inflammatory mediators).
- Increased capillary hydrostatic pressure – nearly doubled (hyperaemia, inflammatory mediators, post-capillary sludging of erythrocytes, venular constriction).
- Decreased tissue hydrostatic pressure (unfolding of complex macromolecules including collagen).
- Decreased plasma oncotic pressure (loss of albumin into the tissues).
- Increased tissue oncotic pressure (accumulation of albumin in the tissues and breakdown of protein macromolecules into smaller and more osmotically active subunits).

Large protein molecules, such as fibrinogen and globulins, tend to be retained in the circulation while smaller proteins including albumin leak out, even though capillary pore sizes are larger than the largest proteins. This may be due to the capillary basement membrane remaining intact despite injury to the endothelium. With larger burns severe and sustained oedema also develops in non-burned tissues. The development of oedema is biphasic:

- Immediate formation of oedema within the first hour of injury.
- Second phase of fluid sequestration at 12–24 h post-burn.
- Resolution phase begins ~48–72 h.

Burns sepsis

Methicillin-resistant *Staphylococcus aureus* versus the burns patient
Cook N. *Burns* 1998;**24**:91–98.

Methicillin-resistant *Staphylococcus aureus* (MRSA) was first identified in 1961 and currently accounts for up to 50% of all nosocomial infections in the USA. Strain typing can be useful to monitor spread of infection and response to treatment. MRSA carry a *mec-A* gene encoding low-affinity bacterial cell wall penicillin-binding proteins with reduced affinity for β-lactam. Some strains produce an enterotoxin leading to toxic shock syndrome.

MRSA is a common cause of nosocomial infection in burns patients, probably due in part to a combination of the open wounds and relative immunosuppression, and also indiscriminant use of quinolone antibiotics and ciprofloxacin. There is a high incidence of environmental contamination in burns units; close proximity to infected patients and inadequate hand washing by healthcare personnel are other risk factors for spread.

Around one-quarter of *Staphylococcus aureus* wound swabs in burns patients grow MRSA (Lesseva MI. *Burns* 1996;**22**:279–282). Burn wound colonization may lead to loss of skin grafts and systemic sepsis. Burns patients should be screened and barrier-nursed. Other measures to prevent/reduce infection include:

- Hand washing and alcohol hand rubs (act by protein denaturation and are rapidly bactericidal in vivo with slow regrowth).
- Environmental decontamination (disinfection).
- Isolation of infected patients and decolonization with 5-day course of: nasal bactroban, chlorhexidine throat gargle, bactroban wound ointment and triclosan skin cleanser daily.

Treatment

It is important to eradicate *Staphylococcus aureus* infection regardless of methicillin sensitivity or resistance.

- Early wound closure – the presence of MRSA is not a contraindication to wound closure by split skin graft or other means.
- Topical mupirocin (resistance now being reported).
- Topical silver sulphadiazine.
- Systemic vancomycin alone or in combination with fucidin/rifampicin. Resistance is reported in Japan where there is a very high incidence of MRSA (60–90% of all *Staphylococcus aureus* infection)

alone or in combination. High spontaneous mutation rate and development of resistance to vancomycin has followed increased use of the antibiotic.

MRSA in burns patients – why all the fuss?
Reardon CM. *Burns* 1998;**24**:393–397.

Whilst many studies show increased morbidity and prolonged hospital stay with MRSA infection, there is some contradictory evidence. This retrospective review showed that there was no difference in length of stay, number of operations or mortality rate between MRSA-positive and age and burn-matched control MRSA-negative patients. In addition, excessive isolation of MRSA patients compromises nurse contact, rehabilitation and patient morale.

What's new in burn microbiology?
Edwards-Jones V. *Burns* 2003;**29**:12–54.

Infection accounts for over 50% of deaths from major burns. Infective complications may be mistaken for the hypermetabolic response to the burn injury.

There is significant immunosuppression especially with burns > 30% TBSA, which when coupled with warm ambient temperature and a moist environment leads to increased infection risk. To counteract this, most burns units advocate early wound debridement and grafting and SSD wound dressings, with other commonly used topical antimicrobial agents including povidone iodine and cerium nitrate (+ SSD = Flammacerium™).

- *Staphylococcus aureus* accounts for up to 75% of infections.
  - Damage from collagenases and proteinases, enterotoxins A, B and C and exotoxin, e.g. toxin shock syndrome toxin-1 (TSST-1).
  - MRSA showing increasing resistance to vancomycin.
- *Pseudomonas aeruginosa* often accompanies *S. aureus* mainly at large wound sites and is found in up to 25% of burn wounds. It produces a toxin pigment pyocyanin as well as exotoxin A.
- Other pathogens
  - *Streptococcus pyogenes*.
  - Coliform bacilli.
  - Fungi including *Candida* and *Aspergillus*.

Toxic shock syndrome
Toxic shock syndrome (TSS) was originally described in 1978, and may be associated with a genetic predisposition. The condition is related to the production of

TSST-1 toxin that causes an overstimulation of the immune system. The toxin is produced by many strains of *Staphylococcus aureus* including MRSA. Most people develop the antitoxin by age 30 due to exposure throughout life.

Symptoms of TSS:

- Pyrexia.
- Rash.
- Diarrhoea and vomiting.
- Hypotension.

Mortality rates of up to 50% have been reported. It is not related to size of burns and has been reported in small burns (<10%) in children. Thus treatment has to be rapid and focused:

- Early targeted antibiotic therapy.
- Anti-TSST-1 immunoglobulin/pooled gammaglobulin/fresh frozen plasma contains the antibodies against the toxin. Patients treated rapidly will improve quickly.

The paper also describes some novel therapeutic measures in treating burns infection that are mostly of research interest currently:

- **Bacterial interference** – harmless strains are used to prevent colonization by more virulent ones.
- **Novel agents:** sugar and honey (high sugar content and hydrogen peroxide), papaya fruit (also desloughs).
- Methods for **detecting infections** earlier: PCR, Aromascan technology, intact cell mass spectrometry.

IV. Other complications

Acalculous cholecystitis

This is a very rare complication (<0.5% of burned patients, with an average burn size ~50%) with a high mortality and presents typically as fever, right upper quadrant pain and tenderness and a raised white blood cell count 2–4 weeks post-burn. The diagnosis can be made by ultrasound and is treated by cholecystectomy.

Curling's ulcer

This condition occurs more frequently in the presence of sepsis.

- Only one-third report pain and patients usually present with haematemesis; 12% perforate. Gastric

ulcers tend to be multiple whilst duodenal ulcers are solitary.
- The risk can be reduced from 86% to 2% with effective fluid resuscitation and prophylaxis with antacid therapy/mucosal protectants e.g. sucralfate and enteral feeding.

Ischaemic enterocolitis

This condition is characterized by mucosal ischaemia and bacterial translocation with high mortality. Some suggest selective digestive tract decontamination (SDD) e.g. with cefotaxime, tobramycin, polymixin or amphotericin B but this may increase Gram-positive colonization including MRSA.

Suppurative thrombophlebitis

This occurs mainly at peripheral cannulation sites and is related to duration of placement. It is usually occult and only one-third show clinical signs presenting as sepsis/positive cultures with 'unknown' source. Commonly involved organisms include:

- Non-burns patients – *Staphylococcus, Klebsiella, Candida*.
- Burns patients – same as those cultured from the burn wound.

Heterotopic ossification after severe burns: a report of three cases and review of the literature
Richards AM. *Burns* 1997;**23**:64–68.

By definition, heterotopic ossification (HO) is the formation of lamellar bone in soft tissues where it does not normally form. Myositis ossificans (MO) is HO in muscles and other soft tissues, and strictly it is a misnomer and should be termed fibrodysplasia ossificans progressiva (sometimes MOP). It can occur with or without previous injury.

It is a rare autosomal dominant disease that begins at age 5 on average. Non-hereditary MO is uncommon in children and occurs from direct muscle trauma with ossification confined to the muscle. Ectopic calcification is mineralization but histologically is not bone forming.

The overall incidence of heterotopic ossification in burns is approximately 1–3% and the exact aetiology is unclear, though it is more common in patients with >20% TBSA. It occurs most commonly in the area between the olecranon and the medial supracondylar ridge of the humerus. The calcification increases as long as wounds remain open/granulating. It seems to be related to movement and joints underlying areas of FT burn may be at increased risk; it may be associated with **aggressive passive mobilization** of shoulder and elbow.

- The typical time of onset is between 3 weeks and 3 months.
- Serum calcium and phosphate remain unchanged, alkaline phosphatase may rise but these are unreliable indicators.
- Early radiographic signs (calcification) may be reversed by effective burn wound closure.

Once matured (decreased activity on bone scan indicative of maturation of bone scan, usually >12 months after), excision typically does not lead to recurrence.

- NSAIDs may help – possibly by preventing osteoblastic differentiation of mesenchymal cells, and may be indicated in high-risk cases.
- Diphosphonates bind calcium and phosphates to prevent hydroxyapatite crystallization, thus bone matrix is not mineralized; however, it does become mineralized after treatment is stopped. It is controversial and routine use is probably not indicated.

Marjolin's ulcer

See skin cancer.

Hypopigmentation

Management of hypopigmentation following burn injury

Grover R. *Burns* 1996;**22**:627–630.

Hypopigmentation after a burn is usually permanent; supposedly the post-burn scar is a barrier to melanocyte migration and melanosome transport from melanocyte to keratinocyte. Hypopigmentation is most common in the hands and head and neck and is most obvious in pigmented races.

Vitiligo is distinct (autoimmune phenomenon) although there is some overlap with Koebner's phenomenon – induction of vitiligo by trauma.

Treatment options:

- Dermabrasion and thin SSG.
- Particulate grafting – morcelization of skin graft and spread over dermabraded wound bed (Harashina and Iso technique).
- Melanocyte transplantation – culture melanocytes (and keratinocytes) from a trypsinized skin biopsy, and applied to dermabraded wound bed.
- Tattooing/camouflage make-up/natural dyes e.g. henna, especially for Asian skin.

D. Burns reconstruction and rehabilitation

I. Burn scar management

A scar will result whenever a wound heals by the process of repair but scars can be normal or abnormal. Over a period of months, normal scars go through a sequence where the scar may appear red, raised and firm as the vascular matrix accumulates before a plateau period that is followed by remodelling/maturation to become softer, flatter and paler.

Principles of burn scar management

There is a distinction between scar minimization and scar treatment.

- **Scar minimization**
  - Early burn excision and wound closure.
  - Maintain a full passive range of movement and optimize active joint **mobilization**.
  - **Splint** in a position of function throughout early treatment and later rehabilitation.
- **Scar treatment**
  - Early ambulation and **exercise**. This maintains joint movement, muscle mass and bone density.
  - Massage and compression/**pressure garments**.
  - Topical treatments such as steroid injections, silicone, laser therapy and ultrasound.
  - Avoid the development of permanent joint changes by early scar release.

Hypertrophic scars

- Post-burn hypertrophic scarring generally becomes apparent 6–8 weeks after grafting. They tend to develop at sites of delayed wound healing e.g. deeper burns, infected wounds or those allowed to heal by secondary intention. There are also certain high-risk skin types and anatomical locations.
- These scars have an abundance of disorganized type 1 collagen and a high TGF-β3:TGF-β1 and TGF-β 2 ratio.

Management of hypertrophic scars

The hypertrophic scar is a common consequence of burn injury; it follows a qualitatively similar time line to the normal scar although both the accumulation of the matrix and the duration of abnormality are usually much greater.

- Pressure therapy (15–40 mmHg) accelerates maturation of the scar by a process linked to a reduction in tissue perfusion and oxygenation. Pressure garments should be commenced within 2 weeks of grafting and maintained as long as the scar is immature or hypertrophic (> 1 year) – head and neck compression devices in children have been shown to impair mandibular growth in some studies.
- Silicone gel sheet softens scars.
- Intralesional triamcinolone enhances collagenase activity and dampens fibroblastic activity.
- Massage.
- Excision for selected scars – e.g. if clearly related to a predisposing cause such as delayed healing, or if causing significant problems with function.
- Axsain cream (capsaicin) is effective against scar itching – substance P inhibitor.

Pulsed dye laser in burn scars: current concepts and future directions
Parrett BM. *Burns* 2010;**36**:443–449.

This is a review of the use of pulsed dye laser (PDL; either 585 or 595 nm) for hypertrophic scars. The erythema associated with these scars may be due to multiple dilated microvessels occluded by endothelial cells; vascular proliferation plays a key role. Pulsed dye laser causes photothermolysis when laser energy is absorbed by haemoglobin causing coagulation, and tissue hypoxia leading to collagen realignment and remodelling. Clinical studies have demonstrated that PDL flattens/decreases scar volume, increases pliability, reduces erythema and improves texture, usually after 2–3 treatments and recurrence is usually not seen. The most common side-effect is purpura for a week or so; pigmentation problems may occur in darker-skinned patients. Both acute and established hypertrophic scars are suitable for treatment but PDL is **less effective in thick scars** though it can be combined with other modalities. The authors suggest that PDL should be considered before surgical excision.

II. Burn reconstruction

Rehabilitation is the process by which a person attains their maximal potential following injury; it involves both surgical and non-surgical treatments (vide supra). Reconstruction should generally be postponed until all wounds have matured unless there is a progressively deforming force, e.g. eyelid ectropion.

Priorities:

- Prevention of deformity.
- Restoration of active function.
- Restoration of cosmesis.

Timing of reconstruction
- **Emergency.** Urgent surgery is needed when vital structures are exposed e.g. the cornea.
- **Essential.** Problems that are not urgent but will significantly improve the patient's final function or appearance if performed early e.g. contractures that prevent the activities of daily living, limiting range of movement (ROM) and not responding to non-surgical measures. Similarly scarring in children adversely affecting growth should be treated early. Microstomia or other perioral scarring that limits dietary intake is another example.
- **Elective.** Most cases of burn scarring will fall into this category; many will be focused primarily on aesthetics.

Reconstructive surgery using an artificial dermis (Integra): results with 39 grafts
Dantzer E. *Br J Plastic Surg* 2001;**54**:659–664.

This is a review of patients who underwent Integra grafting for functional reconstruction of a scarred area. The authors state that good functional reconstruction was possible – treated areas are supple and non-adherent to underlying structures with uniform skin colour and texture, with little/ or no hypertrophic scarring.

The authors suggest that for best results, a well-vascularized wound bed with good haemostasis is needed. Meshing was avoided and hand fenestration was preferred when drainage was needed. The Integra was secured with stitches or staples with a tie-over dressing for mobile sites. Ultra-thin split skin grafts replaced the silicone layer after a mean of 22 days. The most common complication was infection (5/31), however the transparent silicone allows easy identification of infected areas, which are excised and antibiotics started.

Reconstruction of special areas
Head and neck

Facial burns are generally treated conservatively initially due in part to their superior healing potential.

- Reconstruction should follow aesthetic units either with FTSG where required or thick unperforated sheet SSG e.g. from the scalp. **Quilting and exposed grafting** are useful techniques – inspect grafts twice daily and aspirate haematomas as required. Pressure therapy should be started early.

- Useful FTSG donor sites are pre-/postauricular area, supraclavicular fossa, upper eyelid and nasolabial folds. Other sites tend to produce colour/texture mismatch.

Total face reconstruction with one free flap
Angrigiani C. *Plast Reconstr Surg* 1997;**99**:1566–1575.

The authors present their experience with this technique in five patients with severe facial burns. Bilateral extended scapular–parascapular free flaps were used to reconstruct five full-thickness full-face burns (nose required separate technique). Bilateral microvascular anastomoses of superficial circumflex scapular arteries to facial vessels were performed. The donor area on the back requires grafting.

Pre-expanded ultra-thin supraclavicular flaps for (full) face reconstruction with reduced donor-site morbidity and without the need for microsurgery
Pallua N. *Plast Reconstr Surg* 2005;**115**:1837–1844.

The authors present their experience of facial reconstruction in 12 patients. Large tissue expanders were placed under the area of the flaps, from the transverse cervical artery to the shoulder. They were able to harvest thin flaps up to 30×14 cm.

Burn syndactyly

This most commonly affects the first web. There is usually **web reversal** with the dorsal web being more distal and there may be limitation of abduction. Treatment options include Z-plasty type flaps: jumping man flap, VM-plasty or 4-flap-plasty etc. Recurrence is not uncommon despite splintage.

Scalp alopecia

Burns to the scalp often lead to areas of hair loss.

McCauley classification

- Type I – single alopecia segment.
  - a – <25% – single expander.
  - b – 25–50% – single expander with over-inflation.
  - c – 50–75% – multiple expanders.
  - d – >75% – multiple expanders.
- Type II – multiple areas of alopecia amenable to tissue expansion correction.

- Type III – multiple areas of alopecia not amenable to tissue expansion.
- Type IV – total alopecia.

Serial excision can deal with alopecia up to 15% of total scalp. For larger areas of hair loss, tissue expansion is a useful technique; the scalp can be expanded to twice its area before noticeable reduction of hair density occurs.

Trunk and genitalia

Burns to the nipple–areolar complex in adolescence may disturb breast growth however the breast bud lies quite deep and so is relatively preserved. Nevertheless scar contractures may impair development and typically, the burned breast tends to be flatter and lacks natural ptosis necessitating mastopexy of the uninjured side and multiple scar releases.

- Implants if required should be placed subpectorally.
- Nipple reconstruction can be considered with local flaps such as skate flap though the risk of necrosis is increased due to the scarred skin.

Perineal burns should be managed conservatively in general; excision of penile skin especially should be avoided. Avoid long-term urethral catheterization; suprapubic catheters are preferred.

Reconstruction of the burned breast with Integra
Palao R. *Br J Plastic Surg* 2003;**56**:252–259.

Childhood-burn breast scars were reconstructed using Integra. The authors recommend careful preservation of the inframammary fold, and overlapping of Integra to avoid scar hypertrophy. The Integra is dressed with gauze impregnated with povidone iodine and nitrofurazone and these were changed twice weekly. Antibiotic prophylaxis was standard. Unmeshed autografts were used for the second stage on around day 28 on average. The authors reported 100% Integra take with no infections with this technique and concluded that it provided good aesthetic reconstruction and improved scar quality.

Adnexal structures do not regenerate in Integra so some patients complain of dryness but can be managed by moisturizing creams.

Burned breast reconstruction by expanded artificial dermal substitute
Tsoutos D. *J Burn Care Res* 2007;**28**:530–532.

This case report describes the multistage treatment of a female patient who had chest wall burns at age of

27 months, which were treated conservatively resulting in contracture and breast hypoplasia.

- In the first stage, the contractures were released and the defect covered with Integra whilst a submuscular expander was inserted.
- 4 weeks later, the silicone layer was removed and the expander injected; further injection continued until the desired volume was reached.
- 6 months later, the expander was exchanged for a silicone implant.

The study demonstrates that Integra can be expanded like normal skin, though the mechanism for this is unclear.

Hands

Although reconstruction of the hands is a high priority compared with other body sites, with a life-threatening major burn, the priority is to close as wide an area as possible i.e. trunk and lower limbs.

Late dorsal scar contracture can treated by full scar excision, extensor tenolysis and soft tissue coverage with thin flaps such as lateral arm or radial forearm free flap – with the latter, the PL tendon can be included for grafting.

Post-operatively, vigorous physiotherapy and appropriate splinting, avoiding wrist hyperextension (develop compression neuropathies) is important.

Burns of the hand and upper limb – a review
Smith MA. *Burns* 1998;**24**:493–505.

Deep partial thickness and full-thickness burns should be debrided (with preservation of fat and dorsal veins) as soon as possible, ideally within 72 hours. Early surgery has been shown to result in better function and less need for re-operation. Either sheet SSG or unexpanded mesh is suitable.

- Palmar burns are treated conservatively and rarely need debridement; thick SSG is used if absolutely necessary.
- Non-viable digits may be allowed to separate rather than debrided – mummified tips are rarely a source of infection. The PIPJ is the most commonly exposed joint; cover exposed tendons and joints with free, pedicled or local flaps. Primary arthrodesis may be needed in certain conditions.

Proper positioning and mobilization post-injury and post-operatively is important.

- Limb elevation and splints.

- Physiotherapy – active and passive movements – whilst avoiding precipitating heterotopic bone formation by over-aggressive mobilization of shoulder and elbow. Regional anaesthesia to encourage movement (brachial plexus block) may be needed.

The above paper does state escharotomies should be painless and can be performed at the bedside. However, there are many advantages to performing the procedure under controlled sterile conditions in an operating theatre unless there is an anticipated long delay to surgery.

Psychiatric considerations

Established psychiatric disturbances may have led to the initial burn injury, e.g. suicide attempt, or altered perception due to substance abuse or withdrawal may have contributed to the injury. In addition, delirium may be a psychological reaction to injury or a manifestation of metabolic derangement, e.g. hypoglycaemia, hypoxia, sepsis or pain. The following problems have been described:

- Psychosis, delusions, hallucinations or paranoia (rare in children).
- Post-traumatic stress syndrome.
  - Poor sleep, hypervigilance, flash-backs, nightmares.
  - Depression, panic attacks, guilt (e.g. sole survivor).
- Longer-term problems.
  - Self-consciousness and poor self-esteem.
  - Phobias and anxiety.

Children and adolescents appear to become well adjusted eventually.

Is there still a place for comfort care in severe burns?
Platt AJ. *Burns* 1998;**24**:754–756.

With the improvements with burn care, even those with massive burns may survive. This was a questionnaire-based survey of 'comfort care' policy in the UK and found that priorities for determining suitability for resuscitation were:

- Age and % TBSA.
- % TBSA full-thickness burn (including special areas).
- Smoke inhalation.
- Preburn morbidity.

Suicidal intent was not an important factor in decision-making. Although patients' wishes were taken into account, often treatment had already been initiated including sedation and intubation by that time. The choice for 'comfort care' was usually a joint decision between consultant and relatives.

The authors specifically state that it is important to emphasize that 'comfort care' does not equate to 'no care'. In most 'borderline' cases, a trial of full resuscitation to assess the patient response allows time for the family to become involved in a decision 'in the light of day'.

III. Burns itch

Pruritis is a common complaint after burn wounds have healed and it is often used as a marker of scar maturation.

Burns itch is poorly understood and can be difficult to treat. It tends to begin at the time of healing and peaks at 2–6 months but can persist for a long time – in one study, at 4 years 29% had persistent itch and at 12 years 5%.

Itch is transmitted by C-fibres though it may involve a separate subset distinct from pain fibres; some say that itch is conveyed by epidermal fibres whilst pain goes by the dermal fibres. There are many substances that are said to be involved including histamine, as well as serotonin, proteases, kinins and neuropeptides including substance P.

Some have reported good results with PDL for burn scars in terms of redness, size, texture and itchiness whilst others have shown marginal effects in these except itchiness (effective after a few days and lasts for weeks). Overall, the evidence base is rather scanty. Clinical psychologists may have a role, teaching better coping strategies to patients.

Strategies

First line – **antihistamines** (chlorpheniramine, diphenhydramine, cyproheptadine – using non-sedatives during day, piriton at night) in combination with:

- Emollients e.g. simple moisturizers and aloe vera.
- Pressure garments (thought to decrease histamine release).
- Opioids and sedatives as needed.

Second line – it is perhaps sensible to choose simple methods with few side-effects though they may not work that well, e.g. massage, silicone (may take 3 months or more before effects evident), TENS, Unna boots, hypnosis, capsaicin cream and topical silver.

Third line – use possibly more efficacious treatments but with side-effects that may persist e.g.

- Topical antihistamines (e.g. Anthisan, a cream for bites).
- H1 and H2 antagonists – some studies suggest that H1 and H2 blockade may be synergistic.
- Topical steroids (skin thins due to inhibition of collagen production).
- Doxepin (a TCA) in Zonalon and Zepin is effective, probably due to the affinity of doxepin for H1 and H2 receptors and action on muscarinic receptors. It may have a slight burning sensation.
- Gabapentin works in some but may cause behavioural problems in children.
- Dothiepin cream. This is a sedating TCA.
- Tacrolimus.

Head and neck

A. Principles of diagnosis and management of maxillofacial trauma

I. General

The most common aetiological factors in head and neck trauma are assault (nasal > mandible > zygoma) and road traffic accidents (though the introduction of seatbelts has reduced facial injuries from 21% to 6%).

Important points to take note of in the history include:

- Degree and direction of force.
- Loss of consciousness, if any.
- Previous maxillofacial injuries, eyesight and occlusion.

General evaluation

ABC (primary survey) to detect life-threatening injuries.

- Airway obstruction.
  - May be caused by segmental mandibular symphyseal fractures being pulled backwards into the oropharynx along with the tongue by the unopposed action of geniohyoid and digastric muscles.
  - Haemorrhage may occur from fracture sites such as pterygoid plexus of veins, maxillary or ethmoidal arteries, or rarely from the internal carotid artery into the tonsillar fossa. If required, this may be treated with posterior nasal packing and or immediate fracture reduction; angiography and selective embolization may be needed for continued

bleeding (in stable patients, unstable patients may need ligation of the external carotid).
  - Oedema.

Specific assessment of fractures as part of the secondary survey

- Look, feel and move – examine in sequence, either up-to-down or down-to-up.
- All fractures cause bruising, swelling and tenderness ± loss of function.
  - Look also for asymmetry.
  - Palpate for step deformities and crepitus.
  - Remember to check intra-orally – inspect and palpate maxillary buttresses.
- Take note of associated injuries.
  - 25% of orbital fractures have globe injuries.
  - 15–20% of facial fractures have cervical injuries.
  - Neurological injuries.
    - Primary due to initial injury.
    - Secondary due to response to injury e.g. hypotension, hypoxia.

Upper face

- Forehead.
  - Forehead sensation.
  - Crepitus indicating frontal sinus fracture.
  - CSF rhinorrhoea (anterior cranial fossa fracture).

Mid-face

- Orbits.
  - Ocular dystopia, **restricted eye movement**.
  - Exorbitism or enophthalmos.
  - Pupil size and reactivity.
  - **Diplopia**/field defects.
  - Raccoon eyes (anterior cranial fossa fracture).
- Zygoma.
  - **Malar flattening** when viewed from above with palpable step along inferior orbital rim.
  - Trismus.
- Nasal bones – palpable deformity, check specifically for septal deviation/haematoma.
- Maxilla.
  - Infra-orbital nerve numbness and malar flattening.
  - **Increased mobility** (grasp anterior maxilla whilst fixing the face at the nose), however impacted fractures may not move.

  - Maxillary alveolus moves but nasofrontal area does not – Le Fort I.
  - Maxillary alveolus *and* nasofrontal area move – Le Fort II.
  - Entire mid-face moves – Le Fort III.

Lower face

- Mandible.
  - **Malocclusion, abnormal bite** and trismus.
  - Lower lip numbness due to inferior alveolar nerve injury.

Others

- Laryngotracheal injuries – cricoid/thyroid cartilage fracture.
- Ears
  - Haemotympanum and signs of middle cranial fossa fracture i.e. CSF otorrhoea, Battle's sign and conductive or sensorineural hearing deficit.
- Soft tissue injuries.
  - Examine for facial nerve injury.
  - Parotid duct division.

Investigations

Computed tomography (CT) scan is the investigation of choice for all maxillofacial trauma except perhaps for isolated mandibular injuries i.e. CT for mid and upper facial injuries.

- Orthopantomogram (OPG).
- AP mandible open and closed.
- Reversed Towne's view for the condyles.
- OM views for mid-facial injury.

Principles of surgical management

- Early one-stage repair with access to all fracture fragments.
- Rigid fixation with immediate bone graft if needed.
- Definitive soft tissue cover.

II. Frontal sinus fractures

The frontal sinus drains via the nasofrontal duct to the middle meatus. It is absent unilaterally in 10%, bilaterally in 4%.

Severe force to the glabellar area is needed for the frontal region to be fractured. There may be a palpable deformity and paraesthesia of the forehead. X-ray may demonstrate a fluid level but CT (axial and coronal) may be needed to delineate the fracture clearly.

Late complications include sinusitis, mucocoeles and meningitis, thus prophylactic antibiotics are often given.

Anterior wall – thicker than posterior.

- Non-depressed fractures do not need specific treatment.
- Depressed, but not comminuted, elevate via subbrow incision and low profile plate/wire; some have used cyanoacrylate glues.
- Depressed and comminuted, elevate via bicoronal or butterfly (subbrow and nose), may need cranial bone graft. If there is extensive disruption of mucosa, it is better to obliterate the sinus (parietal bone, abdominal fat, temporalis fascia).

Posterior wall

Cerebrospinal fluid (CSF) rhinorrhoea (confirm with ß2-transferrin test or bedside ring test) and pneumocephalus may follow. Urgent neurosurgical consultation is needed.

- If the mucosa and duct (test drainage with methylene blue) are undamaged then the fracture can be fixed.
- Injury to nasofrontal ducts may cause mucocoeles, sinusitis and meningitis and it is necessary to remove all the mucosa (burr down), block off the duct (fat, bone or pericranial flap) and to **cranialize** the sinus; if only one nasofrontal duct is injured, removing the midline septum may help.

III. Orbital fractures

The orbit is composed of seven bones, with the thinnest part being the lamina papyracea of the ethmoid bone that makes up the lower part of the medial wall.
General symptoms and signs.

- **Diplopia** and **ophthalmoplegia** (decreased movement), e.g. inferior rectus tethering.
  - ○ **Ocular dystopia** refers to the position of the globe and in trauma results more commonly from a change in the volume of the orbit compared with the globe, e.g. enophthalmos.
  - ○ **Orbital dystopia** – bony orbits either do not lie on the same horizontal plane (vertical dystopia) or too close/far i.e. hypotelorism/hypertelorism, and this is usually the result of craniofacial developmental anomalies.

- – Telecanthus – inner canthi are widely separated, which may or may not be associated with hypertelorism.
- **Enophthalmos** is due to a discrepancy between ocular tissue and orbital volume causing the globe to sink in, e.g. blow-out fracture. Compare this to exophthalmos which is the result of increased ocular tissue but normal orbital volume.
- **Exorbitism** (proptosis) is the result of normal ocular tissue but decreased orbital volume – which may be due to retrobulbar haemorrhage, tumours or a blow-in fracture.
- Bruising, oedema, subconjunctival haemorrhage (may be due to bleeding from fracture site if the posterior extent cannot be seen).
- The **afferent pupillary defect** is an important clinical finding – if optic nerve is damaged then its consensual response (which remains intact) will overcome its direct response and will cause paradoxical dilatation when light is shined in affected eye (and not in normal eye which causes a consensual dilatation). Also known as Marcus Gunn pupil.
- Rupture, vitreous and anterior chamber haemorrhage and lens dislocation.

The latter in particular require assessment by an ophthalmologist and consultation for an assessment within 24 hours is essential – 25% of orbital fractures are associated with globe injury.

Blow-out fracture

Wall displacement away from the globe increases orbital volume and causes enophthalmos (although superimposed haemorrhage and oedema may cause exorbitism).

- Fracture of the medial thin lamina papyracea of the ethmoid – often treated conservatively.
- Superior wall fractures – may also have anterior fossa, frontal sinus and frontal bone fractures.
- Lateral wall fractures – usually have an associated zygoma fracture.

Indications for surgery include:

- Floor defect greater than 2 cm.
- Positive forced duction testing.
- Low vertical position of globe.
- Need to treat other fractures.

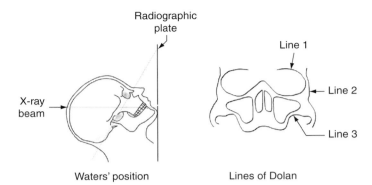

Radiographic plate

Line 1

Line 2

Line 3

X-ray beam

Waters' position

Lines of Dolan

Figure 3.1 Waters' view: Waters' position (Charles Alexander Waters 1888–1961, American radiologist). The arrow shows the direction of the X-ray beam; inclination brings the petrous bones below the floor of the maxillary sinus. The Waters' view provides the single most comprehensive projection with good views of the maxilla, maxillary sinuses, zygoma (and arches), orbital rims and nasal bones. Lines of Dolan (see main text).

Blow-in fracture is where wall displacement decreases orbital volume and may cause exorbitism. These fractures may impinge on the recti which can be tested with forced duction test.

Orbital floor fractures

- There may be suspensory ligament and inferior rectus injury.
- Surgery (ORIF) may be required to correct increased orbital volume/enophthalmos, muscle entrapment or ocular dystopia. Access to the orbital floor is gained via lower lid, subciliary or transconjunctival incisions with lateral canthotomy.
- Identify infraorbital rim, incise periosteum and elevate to identify fracture.
- Lift herniated tissue carefully and reconstruct the orbital floor.

The floor is reconstructed if necessary with alloplastics (Medpor or titanium mesh) or bone graft; a Teflon or silastic sheet may be sufficient for small defects. In other situations, a BIPP pack can be inserted into the maxillary antrum to support the orbital floor and can be left *in situ* for many months pending definitive floor reconstruction.

Imaging of orbital fractures

Computed tomography is the mainstay, particularly fine cut coronal slices. Common X-rays are OM, Waters' and Caldwell views.

- Medial orbital wall fractures are virtually undetectable on plain X-ray.
- Anterior orbital floor fractures may have a **teardrop sign** but many of these can be treated conservatively – only the posterior floor fractures need treatment for enophthalmos.
- Endoscopic evaluation is of current interest.

The main indications for surgery are enophthalmos or restriction of eye movement causing diploplia (which may be partly caused by oedema, thus it may be worthwhile waiting for swelling to settle).

Lines of Dolan

- Line 1 (orbital line, from lateral to medial) – fractures of lateral orbit or diastasis of frontozygomatic suture, fracture of orbital floor.
- Line 2 (zygomatic line) – fractures of lateral orbit and zygomatic arch.
- Line 3 (maxillary line) – fractures of lateral wall of maxillary sinus and zygomatic arch.

Strategies for the management of enophthalmos
Grant MP. *Clin Plast Surg* 1997;**24**:539–550.

When a patient presents with enophthalmos, the orbit needs to be imaged to define the bony abnormalities – as little as 5 mm displacement of the orbital rim can cause significant enophthalmos.

- Surgery requires **good access**: mobilize soft tissues over the fracture and slightly beyond, multiple incisions may be required.
  - Bicoronal: superior rim, roof, upper medial and lateral walls.
  - Conjunctival: floor, inferior parts of walls.
  - Gingivobuccal: inferior rim.
- **Reposition the bony fragments** – first the rim then the internal walls. The superior and inferior rims are the most amenable to fixation, whilst the walls may be onlay grafted with split calvarial (less resorption) or split rib grafts, alloplastic materials can also used.
- **Restore soft tissue attachments**, closing periosteal layers to avoid periosteal 'slippage' and resultant soft tissue deformity.

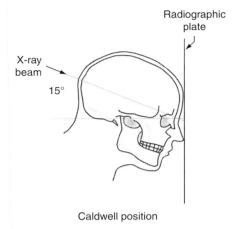

Figure 3.2 Caldwell position. The arrow shows the direction of the beam; the inclination removes the petrous ridges from a view of the orbital structures and is thus useful for imaging fractures of the orbital margins, frontal bone and zygomaticofrontal sutures.

Eye injuries

Superior orbital fissure syndrome

- Structures passing through this fissure are III (also has parasympathetics), IV and VI to extraocular muscles, V1, ophthalmic veins. Fracture, oedema or haemorrhage causes pressure within the muscular cone formed by the recti.
- Symptoms include exorbitism, **ophthalmoplegia**, **dilated pupil** (loss of III parasympathetic constrictor tone leading to unopposed SNS dilator activity), **ptosis** (loss of SNS supply to Müller's muscle that travels with lacrimal branch), anaesthesia in V1 territory. Fracture reduction may be needed with gradual recovery in weeks–months.

Orbital apex syndrome

- Fracture through the optic canal with division of the optic nerve at the apex of the orbit may cause neuritis, papilloedema or **blindness**. Early steroid therapy may be indicated.

Traumatic optic neuropathy

- This is the loss of vision without external or internal ophthalmoscopic evidence of eye injury – the optic atrophy appears weeks later and is usually said to be secondary to a direct globe injury, then retinal vascular occlusion, orbital compartment syndrome and injury to proximal neural structures. Treatment is usually conservative; the 1999 International Optic Nerve trauma study (*Ophthalmology* 1999; **106** (7):1268–1277) demonstrated no clear benefit of high-dose steroids or surgical decompression of optic canal (increase in acuity in 32%, 52% and 57% of surgery, steroid and **observation** groups respectively) but it was non-randomized.

Sympathetic ophthalmia

- The problem (an inflammatory response) affects both eyes and may cause complete blindness. The aetiology is unknown but may occur secondary to a penetrating eye injury or after intraocular surgery. Some speculate on a cell-mediated response (to melanin-containing structures from retina) and suggest prevention by enucleation of severely injured and sightless eyes within 2 weeks; evisceration is cosmetically more pleasing but may be less effective.

Traumatic carotid cavernous sinus fistula

A fracture may cause tears in vessels and formation of a fistula which leads to proptosis, injection and chemosis. There may be an ocular bruit and a dilated ophthalmic vein on CT angiography. There may be embolic or ischaemic events (due to steal phenomenon). Some fistulae may close spontaneously but others may need either carotid ligation or coil placement to obliterate the fistula.

IV. Maxillary fractures

Anatomy

The body of the maxilla contains the maxillary sinus that is fully formed by 15 years. The maxilla has four main processes:

- Alveolar (becomes resorbed in the edentulous patient).
- Frontal – supports the nasal bones.
- Zygomatic – articulates with the zygoma.
- Palatine – articulates with vertical/horizontal plates of palatine bone.

Consider the **four vertical pillars** of the face which transmit forces from the maxilla to the skull base, and are the best areas for bony fixation:

- **Nasomaxillary (canine) buttress** – alveolar process of maxilla opposite canine to the frontal process of the maxilla and nasal bones i.e. medial to the orbit.

- **Zygomatic buttress** – alveolar process of the maxilla (opposite first molar tooth) to the zygomatic process of the frontal bone i.e. lateral to the orbit.
- **Pterygomaxillary buttress** – posterior body of the maxilla to the skull base via the sphenoid (including the pterygoid plates).
- Mandibular buttress – ascending ramus to the skull base via the temporomandibular joint (TMJ).

And the **five horizontal buttresses:**

- Supra-orbital bar.
- Infra-orbital rim.
- Zygomatic arch.
- Palate.
- Body of the mandible.

Maxillary fractures usually present with **malocclusion** (consider pretraumatic class II or III malocclusion) as well as **malar flattening** with loss of height. Mid-face fractures are often comminuted.

- **Cracked tea-cup sign**: percussion of an upper tooth with an instrument may produce a distinctive note (compared with a solid metallic resonance) if a tooth is broken or if the maxilla is fractured. This should be used with caution as it may exacerbate matters.
- Look for palatal fractures.

About one-third of Le Fort II and III fractures are complicated by **CSF rhinorrhoea** due to fractures of **the naso-ethmoid area** (cribriform plate); 95% resolve within 3 weeks but antibiotic prophylaxis of meningitis is advisable. Persistent leaks may need repair of the dural tear via craniofacial approach.

Le Fort classification

- **Le Fort I**: a horizontal fracture that separates the alveolar and palatine processes from the body of the maxilla. Note that the pterygoid plates are usually affected in Le Fort I fractures but are left intact in Le Fort I osteotomies (pterygomaxillary disjunction).
- **Le Fort II**: a **pyramidal** fracture similar to I but the fracture line passes through the zygomaticomaxillary suture/maxillary antrum, the orbital floor, medial orbital wall and across the nasofrontal area. It incorporates the nasal skeleton

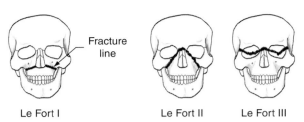

Figure 3.3 Types of Le Fort fractures.

(nasal bones and septum) and the infra-orbital foramen (nerve may be injured).
  - Disruption of the medial canthal ligament, attached to the frontal process of the maxilla may lead to telecanthus.
  - The maxillary segment displaces back and up causing an **anterior open bite**.
- **Le Fort III**: a transverse fracture that passes through the frontomaxillary junction, orbit and frontozygomatic junction to separate off the whole of the maxilla and mid-face from the skull base (**craniofacial disjunction**) with a 'free-floating' maxilla with mobility at ZF suture and nasofrontal region.
  - There is an anterior open bite as for II and anaesthesia of maxillary teeth that usually resolves.

Maxillary fractures may also be **dentoalveolar** involving the teeth and supporting bone only.

Surgical treatment

Nasotracheal intubation may be needed to allow access to the lower mid-face and teeth, and possible need for IMF, otherwise a tracheostomy may be needed (a basal skull fracture needs to be excluded). The first step is to re-establish bite and correct facial deformity. The mandible is fixed first if fractured to provide a stable base.

- **Rowe or Tessier disimpaction forceps** to move the maxillary fragment, being watchful for haemorrhage from descending palatine arteries.
- Fracture immobilization/fixation.
  - Intermaxillary fixation (IMF) (use the patient's dentures if edentulous) to reduce fractures and restore/maintain occlusion whilst a superior gingival sulcus incision is used to expose the fracture in a Le Fort I – take care to identify and preserve the infraorbital nerve.

- o Intra-osseous wires or miniplates (1.5–2.0 mm) and screws – aim for four (bilateral medial and lateral buttresses) points of fixation.
  - o External fixation used for mid-face fractures particularly those requiring anterior traction, those with severe comminution and cases with concomitant fracture/dislocation of both condyles.
- Uninjured or healthy teeth in the fracture line do not need to be removed – the fracture line usually passes through or around the tooth socket.
- Soft tissue closure.

Other issues.

- Additional miniplate fixation to reconstruct the injured buttresses reduces duration of interdental wiring which is usually maintained for 4–6 weeks.
- Le Fort I fractures in the edentulous patient may need no treatment.
- Le Fort II require intra-oral incision as above for lateral buttress and subciliary incision for the infraorbital rim.
- Le Fort III – beware of cribriform (meaning like a sieve – Latin *cribrum*, not cribiform) plate fracture (care with/avoid nasogastric tubes). A bicoronal incision may be needed as an alternative to a combination of lateral brow, subciliary and/or nasofrontal incisions to fix ZF and nasofrontal regions.
- Panfacial fractures are difficult to manage surgically as then there is no stable frame for fracture reduction to be based on. Conventionally the mandible is reduced first, then moving upwards. The AP position of the zygoma needs careful checking to maintain facial projection.

Complications include malocclusion, mal/non-union or maxillary sinusitis. Le Fort III fractures may also be complicated by eye problems – blindness, epiphora, hypertelorism or CSF leak.

V. Temporal bone fractures

Temporal bone fractures may be associated with facial fractures, presenting with haemotympanum, Battle's sign (mastoid area bruising), otorrhoea (25%, but most resolve within 24 hours) or facial nerve palsy. Classification includes:

- **Longitudinal** (usually anterior and extralabyrinthine) – 80–90%: facial nerve injury in

1/5 (usually horizontal segment distal to the geniculate ganglion) and hearing loss in 2/3 (usually conductive). It is bilateral in up to 1/3. Common causes include temporal/parietal impacts.
- **Transverse**: facial nerve injury in 2/5 and hearing loss in almost 100% which is usually sensorineural. Commonly caused by frontal or parietal forces.

Immediate complete **facial nerve palsy** should be explored immediately, whilst delayed complete paralysis has a better prognosis and is usually only explored if there is electrical evidence of degeneration. Incomplete palsy is usually treated conservatively.

- **Sensorineural hearing loss** may result from disruption of the membranous labyrinth and tends not to improve, with few treatment options except hearing aids/cochlear implants.
- **Conductive loss** usually improves as long as the ossicular chain is intact (wait 2 months for other causes such as TM perforation or haemotympanum to resolve).
- **Vestibular disruption** may accompany transverse fractures – nystagmus (fast component away from injured side) and vertigo, that tends to improve after a few weeks, steadily decreasing for the next few months until compensation by about 6 months.

VI. Zygomatic fractures

The zygoma contributes to the lateral orbital rim at its articulations with the sphenoid and frontal bones, and also contributes to the orbital floor where it articulates with the maxilla. Thus the zygoma is fractured in blow-out or blow-in fractures of the orbit.

Classification – Knight and North
- Undisplaced.
- Arch fracture.
- Depressed body fracture.
- Depressed body fracture with medial rotation.
- Depressed body fracture with lateral rotation.
- Comminuted fracture.

Examination
- Look.
  - o Swelling, bruising and conjunctival haemorrhage lateral to the limbus.
  - o **Malar flattening** when viewed from above – the zygoma tends to be inferiorly displaced which may lead to the lateral canthus (attached

to Whitnall's tubercle) descending, causing a downsloping palpebral fissure.
  ○ There may be enophthalmos with an associated blow-out fracture.
- Feel – tenderness, fracture mobility and step-off. Infra-orbital nerve paraesthesia.
- Move – trismus may be present.

X-rays

- Submentovertex (for zygomatic arches).
- Occipitomental views at 0°, 15°, 30° and 45°.

These are tetrapoid rather than 'tripod' fractures:

- Infra-orbital rim, to the floor, often through the infra-orbital foramen.
- Lateral orbital wall – zygomaticofrontal suture.
- Zygomaticomaxillary buttress.
- Zygomatic arch – usually at the thin part posterior to the zygomaticotemporal suture.

The articulations of the zygomatic bone with its neighbouring bones need to be assessed; high-energy injuries may cause comminution. The **zygomaticofrontal** suture is the strongest and the last of the articulations to fracture completely – if it is disrupted, then ORIF is usually indicated. Undisplaced fractures may be treated conservatively (with regular re-evaluation), however the fracture is usually **unstable** due to the pull of the masseter and the vast majority need fixation to avoid late recurrence of deformity (malar flattening).
  Access to the zygoma for ORIF:

- **Upper lid incision** allows access to the temporal process and supra-orbital rim, i.e. ZF suture can be stabilized with a miniplate.
- **Subciliary incision** allows access to sphenoid process (infra-orbital rim) and arch.
- **Buccal sulcus incision** to the maxillary process to visualize the zygomaticomaxillary buttress.

Important points of fixation are the ZF suture (most important landmark to ensure accurate reduction), infra-orbital rim and zygomaticomaxillary buttress in particular. Severe high-energy injuries may need a coronal incision to allow greater exposure. Incisions and dissection may cause numbness in the distribution of zygomaticotemporal and zygomaticofacial nerves. Periosteal resuspension of soft tissues may prevent malar ptosis.

Gillies lift

This is the standard approach to zygomatic arch fractures – which are mainly aesthetic problems with palpable/visible contour deformities, with or without trismus.

- An incision through the scalp of the hairy temple, 2–3 cm behind the hairline.
- The superficial temporal fascia (temporoparietal fascia) is continuous inferiorly with SMAS and superiorly with galea. The deep temporal fascia splits to encircle the zygoma, thus access needs to be gained to the plane under this fascial layer. The muscle should be visible through the wound.
- A Rowe's elevator (or Bristow or Kilner elevator) is inserted and tunnelled deep to the zygomatic arch and a lifting action used to reduce fracture while the head is stabilized.

This approach, with the elevator placed behind the anterior attachment of the arch behind the body of zygoma, may also be used to disimpact the bone.

ORIF complications

- Early.
  ○ Diplopia (usually resolves within 24 hours).
  ○ Bleeding including retro-orbital haematoma.
  ○ Nerve injury.
- Late.
  ○ Plate infection, extrusion, migration.
  ○ Scars and cicatricial ectropion.
  ○ Bone healing/union problems – delayed, malunion, non-union.
  ○ Sinus problems.

The most common cause of post-reduction enophthalmos is inadequate reduction of the fracture (with increased volume of the bony orbit).

VII. Mandibular fractures

The mandible is fractured in more than half of all facial fractures and only nasal bone fractures are more common. Most fractures of the mandible are **open** (into the mouth) and thus should be covered against *Staphylococcus aureus* and anaerobes with antibiotics as well as antiseptic mouthwashes; fractures near the root of a tooth are also considered open.

Classification according to anatomical location of the fracture

In order of frequency but exact figures depend on the predominant cause of trauma e.g. road traffic accident (RTA), sports or assaults, which can vary between different study populations:

- Condyle (35–40%) – thin condylar neck (about 2/3 of fractures in those under 10 years of age, second only to nasal fractures in this age group).
- Angle (20%) – where the root of the wisdom tooth represents a weak area.
- Parasymphysis (10–15%) – where the long canine root is lined up with the mental foramen.
- The body fractures more often in the elderly as it thins due to resorption.
- Ramus and coronoid process 3% and 2% respectively.

Other classifications include: open vs. closed, displaced vs. non-displaced, favourable vs. unfavourable and single vs. multiple. An effort should also be made to look for *contre-coup* fractures.

Look for:

- Pain, swelling, trismus (normal 3.5–5 cm, first 2 cm is rotatory, 2–3 cm is combination of rotation and translation and final 2 cm is translation) and mental nerve numbness.
- **Intra-oral haematoma** – the mental nerve exits the mental foramen below the second premolar, about halfway down in the dentulous mandible.
- **Malocclusion, missing/loose teeth**.
- Chin deviation in those with a fractured condyle.

Palpate:

- Bimanual examination of mandible stability/ mobility and focal tenderness.

- The condyles may be palpated between fingers in the preauricular region and external auditory meatus (EAM).

X-rays:

- OPG and PA mandible provide the most useful information.
- Reversed Towne's view demonstrates the condyles well.
- 3D CT provides useful information on the mandible and teeth including those in the line of the fracture, particularly easy visualization of fracture displacement.

Muscle action on the mandible

Depending on the configuration of the fracture, muscle forces may act to distract or compress a fracture site. **Unfavourable fractures** are those which are likely to become displaced due to muscle action on the fracture fragments.

Parasymphyseal fragment is:

- Pulled down by geniohyoids.
- Pulled down and laterally by the digastrics.
- Pulled backwards by genioglossus.

Body of the mandible is:

- Pulled up by masseter.
- Pulled up and backwards by temporalis.
- Pulled backwards by the pterygoids.

Most fractures require some form of reduction and immobilization but some can be treated **conservatively** (soft diet etc.):

- Undisplaced fractures including the condyle.
- Greenstick fractures.
- Normal occlusion with minimal trismus.

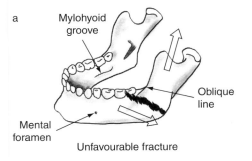

a Mylohyoid groove
Oblique line
Mental foramen
Unfavourable fracture

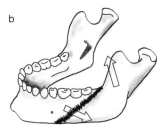

b
Favourable fracture

Figure 3.4 Mandibular fracture. (a) Unfavourable fracture. Displacement is likely. Upward arrow represents pull of the temporalis, masseter and medial pterygoid muscles whilst the downward arrow represents the digastric and mylohyoid muscles. (b) Favourable fracture. Displacement is unlikely as muscle forces tend to compress fragments together.

In most cases, the aim is to restore occlusion and reduce the fracture by dental wiring (intermaxillary fixation) first, followed by definitive fixation e.g. miniplate:

- Unicortical fixation via intra-oral approach (avoid incising in the depths of the sulcus).
- Two plates anterior to the mental foramen to stabilize against complex muscle pull – larger inferior and smaller superior plates.
- One plate at the angle that must be on the upper border since this is the tension side of the fracture that tends to pull open (Champy).

The occlusion is then reassessed after removal of the IMF wires, they can be replaced (or elastics) if required.

Caution is needed in children

- IMF is often not stable enough (mixed dentition with missing teeth, small teeth).
- Miniplates need to be used cautiously – screws may disrupt permanent tooth buds; absorbable plates may be considered, although these may not be available, are more expensive and have a higher profile. Imperfect restoration of occlusion tends to self-correct over ~2 years.

There are two main fixation systems in use:

- **Champy** – monocortical miniplates. The underlying concept is that only tensile stress (stress leading to expansion) is harmful to fracture healing therefore need abutment of bone to bone in the fracture segment; excessive mobility will lead to bone resorption and ingrowth of fibrous tissue.
- **AO** – this uses a tension band and stabilization plate (rather bulky) – small plate on the alveolar border to neutralize tensile force whilst the larger inferior border plate neutralizes compression and torsion stresses. Reconstruction plates can be used for segmental bone loss or severe comminution.

Angle fractures may need to be approached via a submandibular incision:

- 2 cm inferior to the lower border of the mandible to preserve the marginal mandibular nerve and dissect over the submandibular gland at the level of the investing fascia (i.e. much the same as a neck dissection). Some cases may need percutaneous placement of screws.

  - 1 plate on upper border for fractures posterior to mental foramen, 2 plates if anterior (i.e. mandibular border).
- **Angle fractures have the highest complication rate**; ORIF vs. IMF rates are comparable.

Isolated coronoid process fractures are rare and are treated conservatively unless displaced:

- Dental wires for 2 weeks with liquid/blended diet then mobilize.
- Malocclusion is the main complication – patients tend to function well despite the chin deviation/ malocclusion.

Treatment of mandibular fractures using bioabsorbable plates

Kim YK. *Plast Reconstr Surg* 2002;**110**;32–33.

Although rigid internal fixation of mandibular fractures reduces the need for intermaxillary fixation, titanium plates may be complicated by infection, localized long-term tissue damage and may be palpable. Poly-L/DL-lactide plates slowly transfer stress forces to healing bone as they absorb (helps to prevent bone atrophy). Complications (mostly infection) occurred in six patients following the use of bioabsorbable plates (without compression) in 69 mandibular fractures.

Potential complications include inflammatory reactions and partial resorption. Absorbable plates are bulky, expensive, and may not be suited to comminuted fractures or patients with poor oral hygiene.

Indications for ORIF of condylar fractures

- Failure of IMF to correct occlusion after 2 weeks.
- Bilateral fractures – fix one side.
- Foreign bodies.
- Head-injured patients/mental retardation and unable to tolerate IMF.
- Significant displacement especially laterally or into middle cranial fossa – intracapsular fractures are usually stable.

Surgery can be difficult – access is difficult, there is a risk of facial nerve injury and the small fracture fragments make standard ORIF techniques a problem. In general:

- No malocclusion – soft diet and observe for developing malocclusion which then requires IMF with elastics.
- Malocclusion – closed reduction (IMF with elastics) except for lateral anterior open bite which

probably requires ORIF, especially if displaced, if bilateral or if there are panfacial fractures.

High fractures of the condyle or ramus are approached via a Risdon incision combined with a pre-auricular incision. Early active ROM exercises are needed to rehabilitate the TMJ.

Multiple fractures

The mandible has a tendency to splay/widen; it may need external fixation for complex multiple fractures.

- **Guardsman's fracture** is the commonest type of multiple fracture and is caused by a fall or blow to the middle of the chin resulting in bilateral condylar fractures and para/symphyseal fracture. It is seen in the elderly, epileptics and occasionally in soldiers who faint on parade. There may be retraction of the mandible with an anterior open bite. Generally the symphysis is fixed along with only one condylar fracture after IMF used to gain initial occlusion. IMF is left in place for 2 weeks to treat the other condylar fracture.

Intermaxillary fixation

IMF can be used alone to treat comminuted mandibular fractures or where there is contamination; if used alone then it should be maintained for 6 weeks, however IMF fitted to incisors over a long period may lead to loosening of teeth, thus molars should be chosen if possible.

- Need to prestretch wires.
- Stop turning when a secondary twist develops or it will break.
- Gunning splints for the edentulous patients – held in with wires passed around the mandible and through the maxillary sinus.
- Can be used to stabilize dentoalveolar fractures.

Teeth

Position:

- 'Mesial' describes the position towards the central incisors i.e. towards the midline.
- 'Distal' describes the position away from the midline.

Surfaces of a tooth:

- Buccal vs. lingual.
- Occlusal vs. apical.

Reasons for removal of a tooth in fracture fixation

- Grossly mobile, complete displacement from socket.
- Periodontally compromised.
- Root fracture or exposed at apices.
- Evidence of periapical lucency.
- Functionless tooth i.e. not opposing tooth.

Edentulous fractures

The lack of teeth compromises the accuracy of reduction. May need:

- Transfacial approach.
- Reconstruction plate.
- Bone grafting acutely.

VIII. Nasal and nasoethmoid fractures

Nasal fractures

These are the commonest facial fractures; the nose is a prominent feature and a frequent recipient of trauma either due to interpersonal violence or personal injuries such as falls, sports or RTA. The nasal bones usually fracture in their lower half where the bone is thinner. Experiments by Clark in 1970 showed that the nasal bones are more likely to break (i.e. less force required) from a lateral blow than a frontal blow. Numbness at the tip of the nose indicates anterior ethmoidal nerve injury. Diagnosis may be difficult if the patient presents during the oedematous phase. It is important to rule out a nasoorbitoethmoid (NOE) fracture.

Stranc & Robertson classification of lateral injuries (relating to increasing forces) (*Ann Plast Surg* 1979;**2**:468):

- Plane I – just the ipsilateral bone, with a depression usually at the junction of the upper two-thirds and lower one-third (fracture site in 80%; Kazanjian & Converse's *Surgical Treatment of Facial Injuries*, 1959).
- Plane II – ipsilateral depression, contralateral nasal outfractured and/or impacted into frontal process of maxilla.
- Plane III – forces sufficient to fracture frontal process of maxilla and lacrimal bone with possible lacrimal duct injury. There may be multiple fragments.

There is a similar Stranc & Robertson classification for frontal injuries.

Manipulation under anaesthetic (MUA) is performed within 2 weeks:

- Asch forceps for correction of septal deviation.
- Walsham forceps for in-/out- fracture of nasal bones, release/disimpact.

Post-operatively:

- Nasal packs may be used to splint fracture fragments and septum.
- Nasal POP/splint used to maintain position after reduction of fracture.
- Any late correction will need formal rhinoplasty; secondary reconstruction should be delayed for at least 6 months.

Nasoorbitoethmoid fractures

These fractures involve the area between the medial canthi.

- **Telecanthus** as medial canthal ligaments displace laterally/rupture – bowstring test, and **saddle nose deformity**.
  - Normal intercanthal distances:
  - Male 28 ± 4 mm.
  - Female 25 ± 3 mm.
- Lower orbital rim step-off may be present – medial segment is lower due to the fragments sinking under gravity (compare this with zygomatic fractures where lateral segment is pulled down by the masseter).
- Enophthalmos, +/- diplopia.
- Subconjunctival haemorrhage.
- Loss of dorsal nasal projection, with periorbital oedema and ecchymosis.

Markowitz classification based on central fragment bearing medial canthal tendon:

- Type I – single central fragment without medial canthal ligament disruption.
- Type II – comminuted central fragment without medial canthal tendon disruption.
- Type III – severely comminuted with disruption of medial canthal tendon.

Management

It is a difficult fracture to repair. It is important to reconstruct the intercanthal relationship as well as the nasal dorsal projection and internal orbital structures.

Medial canthal tendon

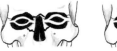

Type I Type II Type III

Nasoethmoidal fractures

Figure 3.5 Types of nasoethmoidal fractures.

- Access via **coronal flap** or medial orbital (Lynch) incision.
- Fracture stabilization with miniplates if possible.
- Medial canthal tendon reconstruction with transnasal wiring (transnasal canthopexy).
- Calvarial cantilever bone graft for nasal dorsum.
- Redrape soft tissues paying particular attention to the nasoorbital valley.

IX. Soft tissue facial injuries

Simple lacerations involving skin only

Direct pressure is the preferred method to control bleeding in the emergency situation; 'blind' clamping is discouraged, as it may damage important structures.

- **Irrigation of the wound** with copious amounts of saline is a vital step and should be performed as soon as possible; its importance is often underestimated and omitted by emergency staff.
  - High-pressure irrigation has been shown to be more effective in reducing bacterial numbers than low-pressure irrigation, but it may increase tissue damage; using a 20–50 ml syringe with a 16–19 G cannula is sufficient in most cases. Antiseptics such as chlorhexidine are not necessary except perhaps in grossly contaminated wounds and may actually damage tissues.
- It is preferable to close wounds within 6 hours, but the good vascularity of facial soft tissue means that a slight delay is still acceptable (up to 24 h). Most 'civilian' wounds can be closed after debridement with the exception of delayed presentation, bites, crush/avulsions and those with impaired wound healing.

Regional blockade is preferred to local infiltration of local anaesthetic where possible to reduce distortion of anatomical landmarks that are useful for accurate reconstruction; avoid injecting directly into the wound. Debride skin sparingly, even if 'questionable'-looking, but trim grossly irregular or 'shelved' edges. Conservative debridement is suggested especially around the lip, commissures, eyelid and distal nose where 'devitalized tissues' often recover and may be difficult to reconstruct.

- **Meticulous closure in layers:** deeper absorbable sutures should allow skin closure with precise apposition without tension and use anatomic landmarks to aid proper alignment.
- With tissue loss, complex flaps are not indicated at the initial stage due to unreliable survival of flaps and wound edges especially in crush/avulsion injuries. Areas that cannot be closed primarily are most appropriately treated with skin grafts or dressings. Abrasions are superficial wounds and will heal quickly, but need to be scrubbed thoroughly to avoid permanent **traumatic tattooing** that would be difficult to treat subsequently.

The wound is waterproof after 48 hours. Clean wounds several times a day with solutions or ointments; the value of antimicrobial ointments in clean incised wounds is not proven.

- **Antibiotics** are not needed unless the wound is contaminated or grossly infected; a lower threshold is sensible in those with immunosuppression, e.g. those taking steroids or in diabetics (the thickened basement membrane limits vasodilatation whilst there is reduced neutrophil/monocyte function and reduced fibroblast proliferation). Prophylaxis has been shown to be effective (Cochrane review) at reducing infections in dog, cat and human bites with Augmentin being adequate in most cases.
- Sutures should be removed early (after 5 days for the face, after 3–4 days for the eyelids).

Alternatives to sutures include:

- **Tissue adhesives** (cyanoacrylates such as Histacryl or Dermabond), which are particularly useful in children but it is important not to get the glue into the wound, as it is cytotoxic. Histacryl is N-2-butylcyanoacrylate and sets after 30 seconds. The blue dye is toluidine based and is used as an indicator. Several studies have demonstrated efficacy e.g. a controlled study with paediatric facial lacerations with low tension (Quinn JV. *Ann Emerg Med* 1993;**22**:1130–1135). Steristrips are not as strong and come off easily when wet and are thus not suited for lacerations around the mouth.
- **Steristrips.** Avoid using traction when applying the strips (applies to adhesive dressings in general) otherwise erythema (may be mistaken for 'allergy') or blistering particularly in the elderly may occur. Some emphasize that strips should be touching/ slightly overlapping so that even distribution of force occurs across the incision as fibroblast activity is sensitive to direction of stresses (Eastwood M. *Proc Inst Mech Eng H J Eng Med* 1998;**212**(2):85–92).

Maximal wound strength (80%) is reached at 8 weeks but at time of suture removal it is only 5–10% of normal skin strength. Some recommend steristrip support after suture removal but the actual efficacy is unknown.

Deeper lacerations

Knowledge of the underlying anatomy is invaluable for the plastic surgeon dealing with trauma:

- **Cut muscle bellies** can be apposed with a modified Kessler or similar stitch without excessive tension that would otherwise strangulate the tissues or 'cut through'. Muscle healing with useful but not normal function has been demonstrated in animal models: dense scar forms, segments that are denervated undergo variable atrophy and fibrosis, with 50% tension and 80% shortening at 12 weeks after total transection, but this is much better than no repair.
- **The parotid duct** lies along the middle third of a line joining the tragus to the midpoint of the philtrum; it travels with the buccal branch of the facial nerve (often damaged as well) and the transverse facial artery. It pierces the buccinator at the upper third molar and enters the oral cavity at upper second. In cases of suspected duct trauma, the duct can be cannulated for injection of air or methylene blue (may stain tissues); alternatively use a thick prolene suture. The duct should be repaired with fine sutures (8'0 or 9'0) over a stent that is either looped out of the mouth, taped to the face or cut short and secured intra-orally (as difficult as it sounds). The stent is left in place for 5–7 days. If the duct cannot be repaired:

○ **Stump ligation** is recommended for proximal injuries. This will lead to temporary painful swelling with a small risk of infection; the gland subsequently atrophies after a couple of weeks. In general, the use of vein grafts to reconstruct the duct has been unsuccessful.

○ In distal transection, the duct stump can be diverted to the oral cavity, but it is a difficult and sometimes unrewarding procedure.

○ Isolated parenchymal lacerations can be repaired; use pressure dressings and administration of glycopyrrolate if needed. Some say that parenchymal lacerations do not need to be sutured as salivary fistulae are rare and tend to close conservatively within a few days/weeks.

B. Head and neck malignancy

I. Staging

Head and neck cancers form 7% of all cancers; one-third of these patients will die from their tumours whilst one-fifth will have synchronous tumours. It occurs in males more frequently; smoking and alcohol increases the risk of squamous cell carcinomas (SCCs) by up to 15 times.

The AJCC divides head and neck cancers into the following categories:

● Lip (page 114) and oral cavity (page 70)
● Pharynx (page 79)
● Larynx
● Paranasal sinus (page 82)
● Salivary gland (page 83)
● Thyroid
● Oesophagus

Staging

The TMN (tumour, metastases, nodes) classification system is more useful than the overall stage in most instances as the latter is much broader e.g. T3N0 and T1N1 are both stage III but are very different clinically.

TMN classification system

Basic staging system

Tumour

● TX – primary tumour cannot be assessed.
● T0 – no evidence of primary tumour.
● Tis – carcinoma *in situ*.

● T1, T2, T3 and T4 – increasing size and extent of primary tumour.

Nodes

● NX – regional nodes cannot be assessed.
● N0 – no evidence of regional lymph node involvement.
● N1 – regional lymph node involvement.

Metastasis

● MX – distant metastasis cannot be assessed.
● M0 – no evidence of distant metastases.
● M1 – distant metastases.

Staging of intra-oral cancers

This is a 'typical' system.

Tumour

● T1 – < 2 cm.
● T2 – 2–4 cm.
● T3 – >4 cm.
● T4 – extension to bone, muscle (including extrinsic muscle of tongue), skin, neck, etc.

Nodes

● N0 – no evidence of regional lymph node involvement.
● N1 – mobile ipsilateral node < 3 cm.
● N2.
 ○ N2a – ipsilateral node 3–6 cm.
 ○ N2b – multiple ipsilateral nodes.
 ○ N2c – contralateral or bilateral nodes.
● N3.
 ○ Any node > 6 cm.
 ○ Fixed nodes.

Metastasis

● M0 – no evidence of distant metastases.
● M1 – distant metastases.

Additional nomenclature includes:

● p = **pathological staging** which is preferred if available, to clinical (c) stage. This also makes the distinction between the cTNM before treatment based on examination and investigations and the pTNM – the pathological or post-surgical TNM which adds information from surgery and pathological examination. This is the dual classification with cTNM guiding treatment whilst pTNM helps with prognosis; when TNM is used without a prefix it implies the clinical classification.

- m = multiple tumours – the tumour with the highest T is classified with the multiplicity or total number of primary tumours indicated in parentheses e.g. T2(m) or T2(5).
- y = following multimodal/neoadjuvant therapy.
- r = recurrent tumour when reclassified after a disease-free interval.
- a = autopsy findings.

Overall staging (also 'Roman numeral staging').

- Carcinoma *in situ* is stage 0.
- In the absence of metastasis, overall stage follows tumour stage; T1 is stage I whilst T4 is stage IV.
- Any nodal involvement is at least stage III: N1 is stage III when the tumour is not T4 and there are no distant metastases, whilst N2 or above is stage IV.
- Any distant metastasis is stage IV.

Tumours should not be restaged, if a patient without distant metastasis at presentation and before treatment then shows evidence of distant spread then it does not change from M0 to M1.

Work-up of patients with head and neck cancer

- Complete examination of head and neck – 20% have synchronous tumours especially larynx and nasopharynx.
- Panendoscopy – DL, rigid bronchoscopy and rigid oesophagoscopy.
- Metastatic work-up – CXR/CT, basic blood tests including liver function and calcium. Others depending on symptoms.

II. Premalignant conditions

Definition – these are skin lesions that are not malignant but may become malignant.

Leukoplakia

Schwimmer first used this term in 1877, though Paget was the first to recognize the malignant potential of the lesion. Oral lesions are strongly associated with smoking and betel nut chewing, less so with intra-oral sepsis (caries), drinking spirits and chronic irritation (less important now – the classic chronic cheek bite lesion does not transform) i.e.

multifactorial. Truly idiopathic leukoplakia may be more at risk of malignant change. It affects males twice as frequently.

The lesions of leukoplakia are typically white–grey verrucoid plaques (though can vary), mostly found in the oral cavity including the tongue and are usually painless. There are three stages:

- Earliest – non-palpable, with white slightly translucent discolouration.
- Later slightly elevated - opaque white with granular texture.
- May progress to thick white lesions with induration and fissuring.

The clinical diagnosis is one by exclusion (i.e. exclude candidiasis, lichen planus, biting/friction, lupus etc.); it is not a specific disease entity – rather it is a keratotic white plaque that cannot be scraped off and cannot be given another specific diagnostic name. The term carries no histological definition but has classical histological features of hyperkeratosis, parakeratosis (thickened keratin layer containing nuclear remnants) and acanthosis. Dysplasia is not a feature of simple leukoplakia but is more likely to be found in erythroplakia.

About 15–20% undergo malignant transformation into aggressive SCCs; though some studies say that it is as low as 0.6%. Chronic lesions may have greater risk of transformation. The highest risk seems to be associated with lesions that are long-standing, verrucous, have erosion/ulceration, the appearance of a nodule particularly with hard periphery or located in the anterior floor of mouth and under surface of the tongue.

Erythroplakia up to 50% risk of transformation. There are two main types of leukoplakia:

- Uniform white plaques (homogeneous) with low malignant potential.
- Speckled/verrucous leukoplakia with more malignant potential.

Some are mixed white and red (speckled or erythro-leukoplakia). **'Hairy' leukoplakia** is an unusual form seen mostly in HIV-positive patients. It is associated with opportunistic Epstein–Barr virus (EBV) infection and seems to have a very low risk of malignant transformation with tendency to spontaneous resolution. There are some trials with antiviral therapy, podophyllin, tretinoin and cryotherapy.

Treatment

Biopsy; repeat as necessary being wary of sampling error.

- Excision if precancer or cancer detected.
- Alternatively, treat by avoiding precipitating factors. Many may regress if the source is removed especially smoking (over half disappear within one year).
- CO_2 laser or surgery.

Cochrane review 2001 (reassessed 2006)

This review assessed RCTs on the subject. Treatment with beta-carotene, lycopene, vitamin A or retinoids was successful but high rate of relapse was common. The conclusion was that to date there are no effective treatments in preventing malignant transformation of leukoplakia.

III. Reconstruction

Recipient vessels

Choice of recipient artery in the head and neck.

- The commonly used arteries are the facial and superior thyroid arteries.
- Others: lingual, superficial temporal and occipital depending on the site.

Choice of recipient vein in the head and neck.

- **Internal jugular vein** end-to-side or end-to-end to a branch close to the main trunk.
- **External jugular vein** which is formed by the posterior auricular vein joining the posterior division of the retromandibular vein (superficial temporal vein and the maxillary vein) and drains into the subclavian vein. It crosses the sternocleidomastoid muscle.
- **Facial vein**. The common facial vein is formed by the junction of the anterior facial vein with the anterior division of the retromandibular vein. It divides into two – one drains into the internal jugular vein while the other receives the anterior jugular vein before draining into the external jugular vein.

Vessel-depleted neck

Suitable recipient vessels can be in short supply e.g. in the irradiated head and neck or repeat surgery.

- Arteries.
  - Often can use the transverse cervical (found in the bottom lateral corner of posterior triangle)

or (pectoral branch of) thoracoacromial vessels (can be used even if pectoralis major has been raised before).
  - The external carotid itself can be used with a side clamp with good proximal and distal control.
- Veins
  - The cephalic vein can be turned over.
  - There is some evidence that 'reverse flow' in certain arteries with significant collaterals e.g. facial and superior thyroid can be used – according to Batchelor, any artery with pulsatile flow can support a flap whether anterograde or retrograde, may be useful where geometry unfavourable e.g. kinking more likely with using proximal portion.

Vein grafts may be needed when there is insufficient vessel length. The length of the vein graft does not seem to affect patency per se, but increasing the length increases the risk of thrombosis and kinking.

IV. Oral cancer

This group forms 30% of all head and cancer tumours and overall 2–3% of all tumours (in places like India, it constitutes 40% of all cancers). More than 90% of intra-oral tumours are SCCs.

- Other tumours include salivary gland tumours (sublingual and minor) that are likely to be high-grade malignancies including muco-epidermoid and adenoid cystic tumours. Intra-oral adenoid cystic tumours tend to excite little inflammatory response and invade the mandible without radiological change; they also show aggressive perineural spread with tendency for skip lesions.
- Less common are lentiginous melanoma (usually superficial) and sarcomas.

History

- Age and general health.
- Smoking history which has implications for pulmonary function but not microsurgical success.
- Alcohol history and likelihood of withdrawal symptoms.

Risk factors include the 'S's: smoking, spirits, spices, sharps, syphilis and sunlight. 75% are most closely related to smoking and alcohol; in some cultures betel nut chewing is an important factor e.g. India and Taiwan. Overall the 5-year survival is 50%.

Relevant anatomy

The oral cavity is the area from the lip vermillion to the junction of the hard and soft palates superiorly and circumvallate papillae inferiorly.

- The oropharynx lies from the circumvallate papillae of the tongue to the tip of the epiglottis (or hyoid bone level) and includes the soft palate, tonsils, ariepiglottic folds and valleculae.
- The hypopharynx from the aryepiglottic folds to the origin of the oesophagus (cricoid cartilage level). Important subsites are postcricoid region, piriform fossa and posterior pharyngeal wall.

Examination:
Assess the size (T status) and site including fixity to tongue, mandible and floor of mouth, as well as the presence of any trismus and patient's dental status.

- **Synchronous** tumours – detected within 6 months – up to 15%.
- **Metachronous** tumours – detected at > 6 months – 40% in those who continue to smoke compared with 6% in those who quit.

Common sites affected in both categories include oropharynx, lung and oesophagus.
Investigations:

- Chest X-ray, blood tests.
- MRI/CT scan of tumour and neck for staging and planning.
- Panendoscopy.
- Local anaesthetic (LA) biopsy of lesion for histology.
- Fine needle aspiration (FNA) of any neck masses.

Leukoplakia vs. erythroplakia vs. *Candida*

- Leukoplakia is dysplastic/keratotic mucosa; it must be biopsied for a histological diagnosis. Malignant change occurs in about 5%.
  - It can be excised in the case of small lesions; dysplasia also responds to CO_2 laser.
  - Close observation is an option, particularly if only keratotic. Tobacco is the most common risk factor and must be stopped.
  - Ulceration is an indication of invasive SCC.
- Erythroplakia has a higher malignancy potential than leukoplakia (up to 50%) and can be

considered as an *in situ* SCC. It tends to affects the 'sump' areas of the oral cavity. It can be treated with surgery (treatment of choice) or laser ablation; the use of retinoids has been described for both leukoplakia and erythroplakia – they may help but have significant side-effects. Lesions with a mixture of leukoplakia and erythroplakia are often called 'speckled leukoplakia'.
- *Candida* (lichen sclerosis) usually scrapes off, is less keratotic and can be differentiated on biopsy. The pre/malignant potential of this is controversial.

Treatment

Oral lesions rarely metastasize below the level of the clavicle.

- T1N0M0 lesions may be effectively treated using either surgery or radiotherapy alone.
- **Surgery first debulks 99%+ of tumour mass and allows accurate staging; free tissue transfer facilitates post-operative radiotherapy.**
- **Radiotherapy by comparison only debulks the tumour by ~25%.** It also delays surgery and eliminates the possibility for further radiotherapy if surgical margins are narrow or involved. Late effects include fibrosis and telangiectasia (i.e. >2 years).
- Chemotherapy can be offered as part of a controlled trial, as palliation or as neoadjuvant to reduce the tumour bulk prior to surgery.

General treatment by stage

- T1N0
  - Excision or radiotherapy only; the neck can be observed – there is a 20% risk of occult disease (Hicks 1997 vide infra).
  - T1 and low-volume/mobile T2 tumours can be reasonably treated by radiotherapy alone as long as their distance from the mandible is sufficient to avoid radionecrosis. Results show similar control rates and superior function compared with surgery.
    - T1N0M0 SCC tongue, 80% 5-year survival with either radiotherapy or surgery alone.
    - T3N0M0 SCC tongue, 30% 5-year survival with either alone.
- T2–3N0
  - Excision and reconstruction.
  - Modified radial neck dissection (MRND). There is some debate with T2 tumours – neck

dissection (ND) is suggested for higher-risk areas such as tongue or floor of mouth (FOM) and where the neck would be opened for access.

○ Radiotherapy. This is indicated for incomplete excision, extracapsular spread, perineural invasion and N2/N3 disease i.e. multiple positive nodes (Hicks 1997 vide infra) and also close excision margins (< 5 mm),

- T4N1
  ○ Excision and reconstruction.
  ○ Mandible.
    – Rim resection if tumour abuts.
    – Segmental resection if invading or previous radiotherapy.
  ○ Ipsilateral MRND (types 1–3) or radical therapeutic ND, bilateral ND if the tumour crosses the midline.
  ○ Radiotherapy. As above.

Excision margins

It is important that excision is not compromised to preserve function:

- Well-defined tumours should be excised with margins of at least 1 cm, preferably using Colorado needle-tip cautery.
- Ill-defined tumours, recurrent tumours or those arising in previously irradiated tissues should be excised with margins >2 cm.
- Consider perineural spread along lingual or inferior alveolar nerves into the pterygopalatine fossa and divide nerves as close to the skull base as possible.

Reconstructive options

- Direct closure.
- Split skin grafts are suited to resurfacing hard palate defects.
- Local flaps.
  ○ Mucosal flaps.
  ○ Tongue flaps.
  ○ **Nasolabial flaps** are useful for reconstruction of defects 6 × 3 cm of the FOM, ventral surface of tongue and oral commissure but is more difficult in the dentate. However it is usually a **two-stage** technique with division of the pedicle after 3–4 weeks; de-epithelializing a portion of the flap to make it a one-stage

procedure may compromise flap viability. They can be inferiorly based (supplied by the facial artery) or superiorly based (infraorbital artery), and may be used bilaterally. They are reliable though it has been said that inferiorly based flaps are more reliable except where the facial artery was ligated during simultaneous neck lymphadenectomy (Varghese BT. *Br J Plast Surg* 2001;**54**:499–503).

  ○ Submental flaps.
- Pedicled flaps.
  ○ **Pectoralis major** myocutaneous flap. It is useful for large volume defects but the donor may promote chest infection/basal atelectasis due to donor site pain.
  ○ **Latissimus dorsi** myocutaneous flap. This is also a large volume flap that is reliable and safe however whilst the harvest is simple, it involves turning the patient.
- Free flaps allow flexibility and variability of design. The radial forearm flap is most useful including fascial flaps (+ SSG) for very low volume defects, e.g. hard palate fistulae. The anterolateral thigh flap (especially if thinned) is also commonly used. Free flaps are not acceptable to Jehovah's Witnesses.

Other considerations.

- Airway management: tracheostomy; avoid use of encircling neck tapes and suture instead.
- Flap regime:
  ○ Warm, well and wet – keep well hydrated, and optimize pain management.
  ○ Hourly flap observations – mostly clinical. For objective measures, consider δ-T (temperature difference).
  ○ Early return to theatre is wise if there are concerns; the salvage for a failed free flap is usually another free flap – the indication for this type of reconstruction will not have changed.
- Caution with wound breakdowns and fistulae – the irradiated carotid that is exposed to saliva is at significant risk of blow-out.
- Post-operative nasogastric feeding.
- Infection prophylaxis.

Role of radical surgery and post-operative radiotherapy in the management of intra-oral carcinoma
Robertson AG. *Br J Plast Surg* 1985;**38**:314–320.

Two treatment modalities for floor of mouth and tongue tumours (T_2 and greater, N0–3, M0) were compared:

- Group 1: **radical surgery (including radical LND)** + radical radiotherapy (4–8 weeks after).
- Group 2: non-radical surgery (± LND) + radical radiotherapy.

The 5-year survival rates (%) were:

Tongue		Floor of mouth	
Group 1	Group 2	Group 1	Group 2
44	5	41	10

Squamous cell carcinoma of the floor of mouth 20-year review
Hicks WL. *Head Neck* 1997;**19**:400–405.

T1 tumours have a ~20% risk of occult nodal disease. Elective ND is often performed for reasons of access but is also warranted for occult disease. With surgery alone:

- Involved margins ~40% local recurrence.
- Clear margins ~10% local recurrence.

Other regions
Buccal mucosa/oral cavity tumours
Most tumours occur inferior to the plane of occlusion.

Gingiva/alveolar mucosa particularly the molar area. These tumours tend to invade bone early and have a high incidence of nodal metastasis – 25% in T1 tumours. They are best treated with surgery.

Floor of mouth
Seventy per cent are found anterior to the lingual frenulum and lymph drainage can be bilateral. 15–30% will have invaded the mandible at presentation i.e. T4 with nodes in one-third. T1 tumours can be treated with radiotherapy or surgery, but larger tumours should be resected.

Smaller defects of the ventral tongue/FOM can be closed with buccal mucosal flaps or nasolabial flaps (two-staged, inferiorly based) whilst larger defects will need either a PM flap or free flap.

Retromolar trigone
Retromolar trigone (RMT) is the area between the upper and lower third molar teeth, medial to the ascending mandibular ramus and the medial pterygoid muscle. This is an important site of development of SCC with lymphatic drainage to the jugulodigastric and submandibular nodes. One- to two-thirds of patients present with nodal disease.

Patients almost invariably present with bony involvement (ascending ramus) with infiltration of mandibular canal and inferior alveolar nerve. Involvement of the nearby muscles (medial pterygoid, masseter and tendon of temporalis) will cause trismus.

Tumours tend to spread to the FOM/tongue and to the faucial area more than to the palate or buccal mucosa.

Faucial tumours
Faucial tumours may be SCC or malignant lymphoid tumours (tonsil). SCC can be keratinizing or non-keratinizing; other types of non-keratinizing tumours are lymphoepithelioma and TCC.

They tend to spread laterally through the pterygomandibular raphe/constrictors to invade the medial pterygoid but rarely the mandible; also medially to the FOM/tongue and anteriorly to the retromolar trigone.

T2 tumours or less have a 40% cure rate with radiotherapy alone thus surgery is preferred. The type of resection (of the tumour and involved bone) via mandibular split and swing, depends on degree of invasion:

- Rim resection.
- Rim, anterior ascending ramus, coronoid process; this includes mandibular canal and inferior alveolar N.
- Entire ascending ramus including condyle.

Reconstruction
- Soft tissue with either radial forearm free flap or pectoralis major myocutaneous flap.
- Bone if needed as a strip of radius in the radial forearm flap, but may be unnecessary even where the ramus has been completely removed as posterior defects tend to cause less morbidity.

Tongue
The commonest presentations of a tongue cancer are:

- Tongue ulcer (52%) or tongue mass (19%).
- Neck mass (4%). (69% had a clinically negative neck on presentation; Haddadin KJ. *Br J Plast Surg* 2000;**53**:279–285).

Tumours of the anterior 2/3 are twice as common as the posterior 1/3.

Examination

- Tumour size (T stage): stage at presentation – T1 (23%), T2 (50%) and T3/4 (27%) (Haddadin 2000 vide infra).
- Site.
  - Does it cross the midline?
  - Is the tongue fixed to FOM?
  - Hypoglossal nerve palsy?
- Neck status.

These are investigated similarly to other oral tumours. Examination under anaesthetic (EUA) is often necessary to establish the degree of spread within the mouth whilst MRI imaging, including the neck, is also helpful.

Treatment

The tongue may be approached via:

- Submandibular 'visor' incision and a pull-through technique sparing the mandible.
- Lip split and 'Y' incision (for synchronous neck dissection) combined with a (paramedian) mandibular osteotomy. An en bloc or in continuity neck dissection aims to remove any lymphatic pathways between the primary and superior neck nodes (I and II), but may increase complications such as fistula formation.

If tumour fixes the tongue to the hyoid then the latter also needs to be removed; (re)-suspension will facilitate swallowing. **Frozen section** control of margins should be considered. The mobility of the residual tongue and a well-formed sulcus are important parts of a properly reconstructed tongue. The value of innervated flaps e.g. radial forearm free flap (RFFF) or anterolateral thigh (ALT) is not confirmed particularly in the long term. Ninety per cent of non-innervated flaps regain at least some sensation (probably due to axonal sprouting into the flap); innervated flaps do gain general sensation sooner but it may not be that important for tongue function. Patients generally do not complain of a lack of taste due to taste buds being almost ubiquitous in the oral cavity.

- TisN0 – CO_2 laser.
- T1 tumours can be treated with excision with a 1 cm margin (or radiotherapy only), possibly with direct closure or SSG and no neck dissection.

- T2 tumours usually.
  - Reconstruction with a thin free flap, e.g. radial forearm flap neck. The overall function is related to the residual tongue and its mobility; it is important to avoid tethering but also to maintain volume which prevents shift of the residual tongue and allows the tongue to contact the palate for swallowing and speech. Predictors of poor post-operative function include large defect size, midline defects and post-operative radiotherapy.
  - Ipsilateral MRND.
    - The high incidence of involved neck nodes in tongue cancer means that neck dissection is often needed, even stage I or II tumours have **42% occult metastases in neck nodes**.
    - 60% occult nodes > 5 mm invasion (Fukano 1997 vide infra) and elective neck treatment is strongly indicated; upstaging of clinically negative neck in 36% of patients (Haddadin 2000 vide infra).
    - **Contralateral ND for T2 tip of the tongue tumours** that are clinically N0 (35% incidence of occult nodal disease) or N2c disease.
  - Radiotherapy.
- T3 tumours of the tip of the tongue usually:
  - Tumour excision and reconstruct with bulky free flaps or pectoralis major.
    - If more than 50% is involved then a total glossectomy should be considered (vide infra).
    - Significant involvement of the base of the tongue may require a laryngectomy (vide infra).
  - MRND (types 1–3) is performed wherever possible, otherwise a radical ND.
  - Radiotherapy.
- T4 tumours involve extrinsic muscles of the tongue.

Natural history and patterns of recurrence of tongue tumours

Haddadin KJ. *Br J Plast Surg* 2000;**53**:279–285.

A retrospective study of 226 patients with tongue SCC (Canniesburn) with the following management principles:

- **Surgery:** complete surgical excision wherever possible, with therapeutic ND for palpable disease

and elective ND for 'high-risk' tumours or where the neck is opened for access/reconstruction.
- ○ 36% of clinically negative necks upstaged whilst 7.7% of clinically positive necks were downstaged.
- **Post-operative radiotherapy** for: large and/or infiltrating tumours, narrow excision margins and positive cervical nodes.

The resulting 5-year survival was pT2 79%, pT2 52% and pT3/4 35%.

- The primary site and ipsilateral neck are the most common sites for recurrence (27 and 34 patients), which is more common than contralateral neck recurrence (which is also relatively high – 19 cases).
- Second oral primary occurs in 10%.
- **Disease-related deaths occur in about half** of patients and are mostly due to advanced local disease (80%) rather than systemic spread.

Depth of invasion as a predictive factor for cervical lymph node metastasis in tongue carcinoma
Fukano H. *Head Neck* 1997;**19**:205–210.

- Depth of invasion <5 mm – ~6% incidence of nodal disease.
- Depth of invasion > 5 mm – ~60% incidence of nodal disease.

Overall, clinically negative necks (N0 or stage I and II) had 30% incidence of occult disease. The authors recommend tumour excision with frozen section for measurement of the depth, with an elective ND if there is invasion > 5 mm.

Total glossectomy

Total glossectomy is mainly reserved for:

- T3/T4 tumours.
- Post-radiotherapy recurrence.
- Where > 50% of the tongue is involved (high risk of perineural and perivascular spread) – in such cases, the contralateral lingual vessels and the lingual and hypoglossal nerve are often involved precluding hemiglossectomy.

Reconstruction after total glossectomy

- Bulky flap reconstruction e.g. pectoralis major myocutaneous flap or myocutaneous free flap e.g. rectus abdominis, ALT.

- Laryngeal suspension – hyoid to mandible.

Post-operative speech therapy is needed; speech is generally regained by all patients even after total glossectomy.

Oropharynx

The oropharynx lies from the circumvallate papillae of the tongue to the tip of the epiglottis (or hyoid bone level) and includes the soft palate, tongue base, tonsils, ariepiglottic folds and valleculae. Tumours here can spread into the nasopharynx and hypopharynx, particularly **submucosally**, thus tumours are generally larger than they appear clinically.

- Tongue base – often painless. Palpation will help reveal degree of infiltration.
- Soft palate – usually present early.
- Tonsil tumours may be associated with EBV; 1% of tonsil tumours are secondaries. Note that the internal carotid artery is about 2.5 cm away from the tonsillar fossa (posterolateral).
- Posterior pharyngeal wall tumours usually present late and have spread past the midline. They are excised at the level of the prevertebral fascia and bilateral node dissection is often needed.

Principles of excision

- Laryngectomy should be considered for tumours involving a significant part of the tongue base due to the high risk of aspiration; those who keep their larynx should have good pulmonary function.
- Access.
  - ○ Peroral.
  - ○ Slaughter's pull through for delivery into the neck.
  - ○ Access to the posterior pharyngeal wall and the base of the tongue may be gained by a midline/paramedian mandibulotomy with or without a midline glossotomy.
- More than half will have nodal disease at presentation thus neck dissection is indicated even in N0 disease.
- Tracheostomy is usually needed to maintain the airway.

A major part of the surgical morbidity is related to the impact on the structures involved in swallowing such as:

- Bolus preparation.
- Transport – tongue contacts hard palate.
- Oropharyngeal component.

- ○ Tongue base moves posteriorly.
- ○ Velopharynx closes off.
- ○ Hyoid moves anteriorly elevating the larynx.
- ○ Cricopharyngeus relaxes.

Reconstruction

- Allow small defects of the posterior pharyngeal wall to granulate or close primarily if possible.
- Flap closure.
  - ○ Free flap, e.g. radial forearm flap or ALT.
  - ○ Pectoralis major myocutaneous flap.
  - ○ Temporalis muscle flap or temporoparietal fascial flap.

Inadequate reconstruction of the soft palate may lead to velopharyngeal incompetence (VPI) and hypernasality, thus it is usually preferable to have a bulky flap (with or without a pharyngoplasty) if static, or to have a dynamic flap, which is attached to working muscle.

V. Mandible reconstruction

Mandible in oral cancer

The main blood supply to the mandible comes from the periosteum from the buccal and submandibular branches of the facial arteries (especially with advanced age) – the inferior alveolar artery supplies the teeth and alveolar part of the mandible only.

- Alveolar resorption results in loss of alveolar height and approximation of gingival mucosa to the floor of the mouth at the mylohyoid line.
- After dental extraction the cancellous bone is in contact with the mucosa overlying it.

Most intra-oral tumours **do not** involve bone but access to excision of intra-oral tumours may require:

- Splitting the mandible – lip split and mandibular osteotomy.
- Slaughter's pull-through technique (stripping floor of mouth structures off the mandible by subperiosteal dissection and delivering them through a submandibular incision).

Mandibular osteotomy

The lip split in the midline with an incision curving around the chin – this is the most aesthetic and preserves sensation and motor control best. There are choices for the osteotomy site:

- Symphyseal.
- Paramedian – anterior to mental foramen and allows genioglossus and geniohyoid muscles to remain attached to the mandible helping to maintain tongue stability. It provides good exposure.
- Lateral – posterior to the mental foramen and so divides inferior alveolar neurovascular bundle.

Technique of osteotomy:

- Vertical osteotomy e.g. between the second incisor and the canine – one looks for a suitable gap between teeth, an X-ray/orthopantomogram (OPG) may be useful in planning.
- **Step osteotomy** risks exposing the dental roots but allows good osteosynthesis with two plates.
- Sagittal split leads to inevitable exposure of the dental roots.

Miniplate and screws are most commonly used for fixation; some use intra-osseus wires. Preplating of the osteotomy sites allows better fixation and compression.

Patterns of spread of squamous cell carcinoma within the mandible
McGregor AD. *Head Neck* 1989;**11**:457–461.

Routes of entry of squamous cell carcinoma to the mandible
McGregor AD. *Head Neck* 1988;**10**:294–301.
  Direct infiltration.

- Dentate mandible – via the periodontal membrane at the occlusal surface; invasion is heralded by loosening of teeth.
- Edentulous mandible – via the alveolar surface at tooth gaps; following dental extraction, the cortical bone does not regenerate so that cancellous bone is in contact with the overlying mucosa. The periosteum is resistant to tumour invasion but fails to protect the edentulous occlusal surface.
- Post-irradiation mandible may be invaded at several sites.

Tumour can spread within the mandible either through the medulla or permeative spread along the mandibular canal. Trismus (pterygoid involvement) and pain radiating to the ear or temple (auriculotemporal nerve) or lower lip (mental nerve) are poor prognostic signs.

Imaging

Orthopantomogram, CT or MRI – suggestive changes include new bone formation (except on the occlusal surface) and loss of haemopoietic marrow seen in involved areas of bone. However, changes secondary to radiotherapy can be difficult to distinguish from tumour.

Principles of mandibular excision

It can be difficult to determine degree of invasion of the mandible by tumour but generally, excision should be limited to what is required for adequate margins – approximately 1 cm controlled by frozen section. The degree of involvement and the vertical height of the mandible determine the choice between either rim resection or segmental resection – a shorter vertical height increases need for segmental resection whilst T3 or T4 tumours generally require segmental resection.

- **Rim resection** is generally only feasible in the non-irradiated mandible for early tumour spread (T1–2) or because stripping of overlying densely adherent mucosa is difficult/impossible. In the former scenario, the resection level should be below the mandibular canal such that the entire canal from mandibular foramen to mental foramen is resected, preventing tumour permeation along the inferior alveolar nerve.
- **Segmental resection** for short vertical height, larger tumours and prior mandible irradiation (makes it more difficult to clinically determine the degree of involvement and also leads to poor bone healing at osteotomy sites). The size of the segment may be small or a total mandibulectomy; the TMJ should be preserved if possible during hemimandibulectomy. A (sub)total mandibulectomy may cause an 'Andy Gump' deformity.

Immediate reconstruction with post-operative radiotherapy is the general management after resection. Virtually all mandibular resection is accompanied by synchronous neck dissection irrespective of the presence of palpable disease.

Reconstruction of the mandible

Aims:

- Enable normal chewing and swallowing, maintain oral competence.
- Denture rehabilitation and aesthetics.

Jewer classification of mandibular defects (modified by Soutar):

- **Central segment** – from mental foramen to mental foramen, subdivided by the midline into left and right; requires a curvature/osteotomy in the reconstruction.
- **Lateral segment** – from mental foramen to the lingula preserving the posterior ascending ramus and the condyle; may be reconstructed with a straight piece of bone.
- **Ascending ramus.**

Segmental loss is best treated with vascularized bone graft as it allows rapid union and additional tissue can be imported; the use of non-vascularized bone grafts will need rigid fixation and good soft tissue cover. Longer sections of segmental loss are associated with a higher complication rate – 7% if < 5 cm vs. 80% if > 5 cm. The choice of reconstruction in a particular individual depends on many factors but in general:

- **Young patient** with non-malignant process: rigid fixation and non-vascularized bone grafts are an option, whilst distraction is particularly useful for developmental abnormalities (and also trauma or to revise previous vascularized bone grafts). Vascularized bone grafts may be needed particularly for more complex defects.
- **Elderly patients** with poor premorbid health, poor prognosis: **soft tissue only** reconstruction with or without a reconstruction plate. Allografts such as freeze-dried bone or non-vascularized autografts may be combined with vascular flaps in selected patients.

Non-vascularized bone grafts

- **Bone segment** from iliac crest or rib grafts – aims to re-activate the osteogenic potential of periosteal progenitor cells. There is vessel ingrowth and removal of dead bone cells and repopulation of the existing Haversian canal network.
- **Particulate bone and cancellous marrow (PBCM)** can be harvested from the ilium and provides marrow mesenchymal cells and endosteal osteoblasts. It still undergoes the same resorption–replacement cycle but with a lesser degree of resorption.

Grafts must have adequate vascular soft tissue cover. Graft survival may possibly be enhanced using pre- and post-operative hyperbaric oxygen. In irradiated tissues this promotes vascularization from 30 to 80% of normal tissue levels and should be considered whenever operating on bone within an irradiated field.

If post-operative radiotherapy is contemplated, then mandibular reconstruction by non-vascularized bone may need to be delayed unless there is a symphyseal defect (where the pull of the pterygoids can cause sleep apnoea). Delaying radiotherapy to allow bone healing may compromise 'cure'.

Complications:

- Resorption: Calvarial bone is retained longer than other bone grafts and may be related to the differences between intramembranous vs. endochondral ossification.
- Poor take due to hostile recipient bed (including previous radiotherapy – hypovascular, hypocellular and hypoxic tissues).

Vascularized bone

Osteomyocutaneous flaps

- **Lateral trapezius with spine of scapula** – the flap is based on transverse cervical vessels which should be preserved during ipsilateral neck dissection (but not always); it incorporates bone from the spine of the scapula and a skin paddle over the acromioclavicular joint which can be orientated horizontally or vertically. It is important to preserve the suprascapular nerve during dissection – it supplies supraspinatus, which initiates shoulder abduction.
- **Pectoralis major with fifth rib or edge of sternum** (Ariyan S. *Surg Oncol Clin N Am* 1997;**6**:1–43) – this is based on pectoral branch of thoraco-acromial artery (50% of pectoralis major blood supply); the muscle is also supplied by lateral thoracic and superior thoracic arteries, 40% and 10% respectively). It is traditional to plan incisions to allow for a deltopectoral flap as salvage i.e. 'defensive incision'. The skin island is of limited size if primary closure of the donor area is required. Rarely, pleura is taken for intra-oral lining (requires post-operative chest drain). Its use is supposedly contraindicated in cases of pectus excavatum.
- **Sternocleidomastoid with medial segment of clavicle** (up to 8 cm) – it is based on occipital vessels (with supply also by the superior thyroid artery and the thyrocervical trunk) with the skin paddle overlying clavicle available with a viability

of ~35% but is increased if the middle vessel is preserved. The arc of rotation is determined by point of entry of the XIth nerve. It is contraindicated by cervical nodal disease which requires radical neck dissection, although the flap may be used where there is a single level I node treated by suprahyoid dissection. It is thus usually indicated for benign defects in the mandible, dysplasia or primary mandibular tumours. A bilateral flap incorporating the intervening manubrium has been described.

Osseus flaps – the 'gold standard' particularly for osteoradionecrosis (ORN)

- **Fibula** – this flap provides the longest length of bone available (~25 cm) that also readily accepts osseo-integrated implants; the bone is straight and thus requires multiple osteotomies for subtotal mandibular reconstruction. The overlying skin paddle is useful for FOM reconstruction but may be unavailable in up to 10% due to the vascular configuration. This flap is probably the most common choice for mandibular reconstruction. Whilst the pedicle vessels are of a good size they are rather short (discarding the proximal bone may 'lengthen' the pedicle). The rare peronea magna or dominant peroneal artery is something to be aware of; elderly patients may rely upon the peroneal artery for supply to the foot. The major pulses need to be checked pre-operatively and angiography may be indicated in selected patients.
- **Radial forearm flap** – Its use in mandibular reconstruction was originally described by Soutar 1983. It is a reasonably good option for lateral and central segmental defects but the low bone volume makes it less suited when osseo-integrated implants are planned. The bone segment ~12 cm lies between the insertion of pronator teres proximally and brachioradialis distally, and one should remove less than a third of the cross-sectional area to avoid subsequent fracture. The periosteal supply comes from perforators in the lateral intermuscular septum and vessels which pass through FPL. The thin pliable skin island (up to 6 cm can be closed primarily) is suited for mucosal and skin reconstruction but the thin weak bone functions more or less as a spacer and may need to be combined with a reconstruction plate.
  - Doppler the skin perforators pre-operatively. 6–10 cm of bone should be left proximally and

distally to reduce joint disruption. Open wedge osteotomy is both easier and more precise.

- **Deep circumflex iliac artery (DCIA)** - the bone segment (15×6 cm both cortical and cancellous) can accommodate osseo-integrated implants, is naturally curved and thus requires no osteotomy, making it **an almost ideal bone flap particularly for hemimandible reconstruction** but has a precarious skin paddle (10% risk of failure) and is often too bulky. The donor site can be quite painful with a risk of hernia later on (close the external oblique meticulously). A portion of the internal oblique muscle based on the ascending branch of the DCIA can also be harvested for intra-oral lining.
  - The DCIA comes off the iliac artery at the same level as the deep inferior epigastric artery and runs below the line of the inguinal ligament towards the ASIS. Harvest with a sandbag under the hip.
  - Refinements – avoiding harvest of muscle will reduce the donor site morbidity and the bone can be combined with the groin flap skin paddle as a chimeric flap with a thinner skin island than the classical DCIA. Depending on the position of the recipient vessels – the contralateral hip is most suited for an ipsilateral anastomosis due to the vascular configuration.
- **Scapula flap** – a thin, straight 12×3 cm bone segment is available from the lateral border of the scapula along with a reliable skin paddle based on the subscapular artery. It is suitable for central (symphyseal) defects but the thin bone cannot accommodate osseo-integrated implants. The patient has to be turned during the operation.

Alloplastic materials

- Metal plates including reconstruction plates (3 screws either side) may be used, usually as temporary support as the metal will fatigue eventually. They have been used in selected cases where functional demands are low.
- Allogeneic bone may be useful as a crib for PBCM autograft – mandible allografts must be hollowed out and packed with autograft; holes are burred through the cortex to enable fixation of host soft tissues and the ingrowth of vessels.
- Bone substitutes such as hydroxyapatite are rigid, do not remodel and cannot support a prosthesis.

Reconstruction of posterior mandibular defects with soft tissue using a rectus abdominis free flap
Kroll SS. *Br J Plast Surg* 1998;**51**:503–507.

A 'simpler' soft tissue-only flap may be used in patients with poor tumour prognosis or poor general health, particularly if the TMJ has been excised as it would be very difficult to reconstruct. Posterior defects cause less morbidity than anterior defects; good aesthetics and functional outcome have been reported.

Overall:

- **No reconstruction** – may be considered for lateral defects or defects of the ascending ramus. The chin will be deviated to the deficient side but speech and swallowing is usually satisfactory, and it reduces the surgical time.
- **Reconstruction plates** may be appropriate for those with poor prognosis/low demand (extrusion and fracture are almost inevitable) but should be limited to lateral defects as anterior defects reconstructed in this way have a high extrusion rate. This obviates the need for a bone donor site.
- **Non-vascularized bone** can be used for smaller defects (< 6 cm) except in cancer patients who are likely to need radiotherapy (which will lead to an extrusion/infection/resorption rate of 50–80%).
- **Vascularized bone** is the gold standard treatment for larger (> 9 cm) or complex (soft tissue) defects, and in irradiated tissues.

Secondary lengthening of the reconstructed mandible by distraction osteogenesis
Yonehara Y. *Br J Plast Surg* 1998;**51**:356–358.

Mandibular distraction osteogenesis was originally described by McCarthy (1992). This paper reports two cases where the mandible was reconstructed with free fibula flaps that were initially inadequate in length. Lengthening was achieved by a midline osteotomy with gradual widening by distraction.

Dental restoration is usually delayed. Osteointegrated implants can be placed in fibula or DCIA flaps where there is more than 6 mm bone height; other favourable features are provision of well-vascularized bone and soft tissue cover particularly a thin intra-oral lining.

VI. Hypopharynx

The hypopharynx is the region from the aryepiglottic folds to the origin of the oesophagus (cricoid cartilage level). Important subsites for tumours are postcricoid region (10%), piriform fossa (70%) and posterior pharyngeal wall (20%).

T staging:

- T1 – One subsite and less than 2 cm wide.
- T2 – More than one subsite or 2–4 cm without hypopharynx fixation.
- T3 More than 4 cm or with hypopharynx fixation.
- T4a – Invades mid-line thyroid/cricoid, hyoid, oesophagus, strap muscles.
- T4b – Invades prevertebral fascia, mediastinum or encases carotid.

Hypopharyngeal tumours have a tendency to spread submucosally and have **skip lesions**. The majority of patients (80%) present with advanced disease (stage III/IV) and 17% have distant metastases. T1 tumours can be treated with radiotherapy alone, but few patients present at this early stage; later stages require excisional surgery – laryngectomy is usually needed, reconstruction and post-operative radiotherapy.

- If there is adequate mucosa then primary closure is an option as long as a 34F catheter can be passed.
- If there is inadequate mucosa then reconstruction requires either a free jejunum or a tubed fasciocutaneous flap e.g. RFFF or ALT, or a tubed pectoralis major. Tubed flaps are said to have a higher incidence of fistulae compared with the jejunal flap (the bulk of the pectoralis major can make tubing it difficult). Preservation of a strip of pharyngeal mucosa e.g. back wall is generally associated with better functional results compared with complete circumferential reconstructions.

Pharyngeal reconstruction using free jejunal flaps was first reported by Seidenberg in 1959. Using the jejunum has the advantages of a flexible and self-lubricating tubed reconstruction that preserved near-normal swallowing fairly well. The flap has average donor vessel diameters of artery 1.2 mm, vein 3.0 mm – a single pedicle allows perfusion of a segment of jejunum up to 40 cm in length (Huang JL. *Ann Plast Surg* 1999;**42**:658–661). However, a laparotomy is required with its attendant possible complications and may be contraindicated e.g. with previous abdominal surgery.

- The bowel can be opened out along anti-mesenteric border as a 'patch' for reconstruction of intra-oral mucosal defects.
- A segment with its mucosa removed can be skin grafted to reconstruct overlying soft tissue defects

if needed (Carlson GW. *Plast Reconstr Surg* 1996; **97**:460–462)

Technique

- Open or laparoscopic approach (Gherardini G. *Plast Reconstr Surg* 1998;**102**:473–477).
- Isolate the second or third jejunal loop (or 40 cm) beyond the ligament of Treitz on a 'V'-shaped mesentery containing an artery and a vein. Re-anastomose the cut small bowel but leave the raised jejunal flap *in situ* until ready to transfer (to shorten ischaemic time).
- When ready (i.e. recipient vessels prepared) divide the jejunal flap and inset, proximal anastomosis first, in an isoperistaltic direction. Tack the posterior surface to the prevertebral fascia. The upper end may be too narrow to anastomose to the wide distal pharyngeal stump: a reverse L end–side anastomosis or jejunal expansion with a patch flap may be considered (Yoshida T. *Br J Plast Surg* 1998;**51**:103–108).
- Then perform the microvascular anastomosis – superior thyroid artery and external jugular vein are ideal recipients. The reperfused bowel will produce secretions. The distal mucosal anastomosis is made with a V inset anteriorly to reduce the formation of strictures. Excessive redundancy may lead to problems swallowing and should be avoided by careful tailoring of the length of the flap, and insetting inferiorly with the neck in a near-neutral position.

Flap monitoring (buried flaps)

- Exteriorizing a minor segment of the flap (~2 cm) to observe colour, secretion and peristalsis (Katsaros J. *Br J Plast Surg* 1985;**38**:220–222), a 4–5 cm segment produces initially ~100 ml/24 h (decreasing to ~10 ml/24 h at 2 weeks) that can be collected in a stoma bag (Giovanoli P. *Microsurgery* 1996;**17**:535–54). This segment is excised ~5 days under local anaesthesia.
  - A similar method can be used for tubed fasciocutaneous flaps e.g. ALT with multiple perforators.
- A window can be created in the neck skin flap to expose the serosa of the underlying jejunal flap which is tacked to the skin and covered with a thin SSG (Bafitis H. *Plast Reconstr Surg* 1989;**83**:896–898).

- Endoscopic/fibreoptic examination of the major segment.
- Implantable Doppler probes; some have described the use of hand-held surface Doppler probes to monitor the pedicle/anastomosis after marking its position on the skin – a 'venous hum' is said to be more specific.

Gastrograffin swallow is usually performed on day 7 to define any leaks and then oral intake is accordingly reinstated (note that contrast swallow tests do not provide information on the viability of the flap). In the uncomplicated case, post-operative radiotherapy can be commenced ~5 weeks post-reconstruction.

Success rates (flap viability) are generally ~95% with most thromboses occurring within the first 24 h. If one flap fails another can be harvested, whilst avoiding leaving a segment of jejunum between two donor sites as denervation of this segment leads to motility disorders.

Speech restoration

- Artificial larynx – electronic box.
- Oesophageal speech.
- Tracheo-oesophageal fistula and valve e.g. Provox, Blom-singer.
- Autologous valve free flap e.g. ileocaecal.

The speech following a jejunal flap is often described as being 'wet'.

Reconstruction of the head and neck
Ariyan S. *Surg Oncol Clin N Am* 1997;**6**:1–43.

The 5-year survival for hypopharyngeal SCC is < 25% regardless of mode of treatment:

- Gastric pull-up is palliative but allows rapid return to oral feeding.
- Jejunal free flaps are technically more difficult with more complications.

VII. Tumours of the nasal cavity and paranasal sinuses

Nasal polyps

These are relatively common, occurring in about 1% of the normal population (up to half of cystic fibrosis sufferers – suspect this disease if nasal polyps occur in children). The risk of malignant change is thought to be very low and nasal polyposis is not regarded as being a premalignant condition. There is no reliable way to distinguish benign from malignant clinically although unilateral solitary polyps are more likely to be malignant.

Biopsies prior to definitive treatment are not a routine procedure for simple polyps, but should a biopsy prove to demonstrate a malignant lesion then a wide local excision via lateral rhinotomy and post-operative radiotherapy is needed. Ethmoidectomy is usually achieved by piecemeal excision. Post-operative epiphora due to blocked nasolacrimal duct is not uncommon.

Nasal cavity tumours

These tumours usually present with epistaxis, obstruction or rhinorrhoea. Radiotherapy is a common treatment in order to avoid potentially mutilating surgery. Fifteen per cent will develop a second primary, approximately half in the head and neck.

Nasopharyngeal carcinoma (NPC)

The nasopharynx is the region behind the posterior choanae, up to the palatal plane (soft palate to posterior pharyngeal wall). NPC is common in Chinese and also North and sub-Saharan Africans. In other populations, it comprises 0.25% of all carcinomas. Risk factors apart from ethnicity (HLA linkage) include EBV and dietary nitrosamines, whilst smoking and alcohol are not major aetiological factors.

- The vast majority are SCCs – keratinizing (I), non-keratinizing (II) or undifferentiated (III).

Early-stage symptoms may be trivial; common methods of presentation are cervical lymphadenopathy (upper jugular or level V, 70% have nodes at presentation), otitis media, obstruction or epistaxis. Thus many are relatively advanced at presentation. Some patients may have skull base symptoms i.e. cranial nerve palsies or distant metastases but are relatively rare. There are attempts to find disease at earlier stage i.e. screening with EBV IgA.

T staging

- T1 – Nasopharynx.
- T2a – Extension to oropharynx, nasal cavity without parapharyngeal extension.
- T2b – Tumour with parapharyngeal extension.
- T3 – Bony structures or paranasal sinuses.
- T4 – Intracranial extension, cranial nerve involvement, infratemporal fossa, hypopharynx, orbit, masticator space.

Investigations

- Endoscopic exam and biopsy – may be predominantly submucosal.
- Neck node FNA.
- Imaging: CT/MRI with contrast agent (especially for parapharyngeal involvement).

Accurate staging is important for determining the neck status and RT planning. The tumour is typically very radiosensitive and even extensive disease may regress completely; IMRT may allow better shielding of normal tissues and allow higher doses to be used. Therefore, most cases are treated with RT with or without concomitant chemotherapy depending on their state of health. Salvage surgery is then offered for recurrences; most recurrences occur in first two years.

- Stage I – radiotherapy to primary and neck.
- Stages II–IV – radiotherapy or chemoirradiation.

Hypothyroidism is a common complication of irradiation. Twenty to 60% will develop distant disease.

Paranasal sinus tumours

These are rare tumours (~1/100 000) in the USA, comprising 3% of all head and neck malignancies and most are SCC (80%) with adenocarcinoma making up most of the remainder. Sinus tumours are more common in Japan and Uganda, most frequently affecting males in the over 60-year age group.

- 55–60% occur in the maxillary antrum.
- 25–35% nasal cavity.
- 9–14% ethmoid sinuses, 1% sphenoid and frontal sinuses.

These patients usually present late (T3/4). Possible risk factors include: smoking and alcohol (synergy seems to exist), occupational causes such as wood dust, chromium and nickel, cyanide chemicals as well as radiation and possibly human papilloma virus (HPV).
Investigations:

- EUA and biopsy – biopsy can be performed directly through medial wall of the maxillary sinus for example or via Caldwell–Luc approach.
- Facial X-rays, orthopantomograph (OPG).
- Staging with MRI or CT for definition of soft tissue and bony involvement respectively.

Most of these tumours are treated by surgery followed with post-operative (brachy) radiotherapy. Notable exceptions to this being:

- Sarcomas – chemotherapy then surgery.
- Lymphomas – chemotherapy and radiotherapy.

Maxillary sinus tumours

The maxillary sinus may be affected by primary tumours or may be invaded from neighbouring regions e.g. palatal tumours. Primary tumours often present with tooth pain (first and second premolars) or cheek numbness (due to involvement of the infra-orbital nerve), i.e. usually advanced disease at the time of presentation.

The periosteum of the orbital floor is an effective barrier to tumour spread but the anterior and posterior bony walls are thin and readily eroded; posterior extension into the pterygopalatine fossa can lead to surgically inoperable disease due to involvement of the maxillary nerve and artery.

Presentation:

- Facial symptoms: swelling, pain and infraorbital/ cheek paraesthesia.
- Dental symptoms: gingival or palatal mass, pain or unhealed extraction socket, fistula.
- Nasal symptoms: epistaxis, discharge, obstruction, pain.
- Ocular symptoms: proptosis, epiphora, eyelid swelling, impaired vision, pain.

Staging:
Tumour staging

- T1 – mucosal involvement only.
- T2 – bony involvement including inferomedial spread (hard palate, nasal cavity) but not posterior wall extension including pterygoid plates.
- T3 – bony involvement superolaterally (orbit, anterior ethmoidal sinuses) or posterior wall of maxillary sinus, subcutaneous tissue involvement.
- T4a – anterior orbit, skin of cheek, pterygoid plates, infratemporal fossa, cribiform plate, sphenoid or frontal sinuses.
- T4b – orbital apex, dura, brain, cranial nerves other than maxillary division, nasopharynx or clivus.

Nodes and metastases as for oral cavity.

Ohngren's line is a plane that lies diagonally connecting the inner canthus with the angle of the mandible. Maxillary sinus tumours invading above this line carry a worse prognosis. Overall,

- Local recurrence 45% especially in the first year.
- Nasal disease and distant disease in approximately 1/5.
- 40% 5-year survival.

Or based on symptoms related to the degree of spread:

- Stage 1: symptoms due to swelling itself: swelling, numbness and pain.
- Stage 2: symptoms related to inferomedial spread: tooth pain/numbness/loosening, nasal bleeding/discharge/obstruction.
- Stage 3: symptoms related to superolateral spread above Ohngren's line: ocular pain, ophthalmoplegia or impaired vision.

Treatment

In general, most maxillary sinus tumours are best treated by surgery then radiotherapy (thus pre-operative dental evaluation is usually routine). Other factors include nutritional support as well as encouraging the patient to stop smoking.

- Resect as much maxilla as is required for tumour clearance. **Maxillectomy** is usually carried out via an excision via Weber–Fergusson lateral rhinotomy approach ± subciliary Dieffenbach extension or craniofacial bicoronal approach. Tumours affecting the inferior half of the maxilla may be assessed via a lip-split whereas facial degloving is usually needed for superomedial tumours. Selected cases may need orbital or transcranial approaches.
  - Extensive maxillectomy requires ipsilateral insertion of grommets to prevent secretory otitis media.
  - Prevent post-operative trismus by excision of the coronoid process.
- Prefabrication of an **obturator** to close oronasal fistula (preferably with pre-operative assessment) or reconstruct (immediate or delayed) palate using a free bone flap e.g. fibula or DCIA or simply close off space with a flap, e.g. muscle – free rectus or fasciocutaneous – ALT.
  - The **orbital floor** may require reconstruction with bone graft e.g. rib or iliac crest, or with titanium plate. Frank orbital involvement is more problematic particularly at the apex – dural seal, cavernous sinus and the ophthalmic artery need to be considered.
  - Skin of the cheek may need to be replaced – flaps such as the RFFF are usually a poor colour

match, so some suggest a second step consisting of de-epithelialization and a scalp SSG.
- Lymph node metastases are rare (except for tumours of the maxillary sinus that also involve buccal mucosa) as poorly supplied by lymphatics.

Suarez had the following comments about the orbit (Suarez C. *Head Neck* 2007;**30**:242–250):

- The periorbitum is a good barrier to invasion although the lamina papyracea may be destroyed quite quickly, and the orbital contents may be preserved with close observation.
- Exenteration is required once the periorbitum has been breached. Tumour types with aggressive behaviour such as adenocarcinoma or SCC compared to esthesioneuroblastomas should have a lower threshold for exenteration.
- Orbital wall reconstruction is need if two or more orbital walls are involved to prevent displacement.

Other sinus tumours

- Ethmoid sinus tumours: surgical access via a lateral rhinotomy or craniofacial approach.
- Sphenoid sinus tumours: the sinus lies below the optic chiasm and the pituitary fossa within the body of the sphenoid bone, thus these tumours are treated mainly by radiotherapy alone.
- Frontal sinus tumours: 4% of individuals do not have a frontal sinus. Surgery via a craniofacial approach followed by radiotherapy.

Malignant tumours of maxillary complex: 18-year review

Stavrianos SD. *Br J Plast Surg* 1998;**51**:584–588.

Treatment with the combination of surgery with post-operative radiotherapy results in 68% and 64% 5-year control and survival. This is better in comparison than:

- Radiotherapy alone, 39% and 40% respectively.
- Surgery alone – survival 30%.

Differential diagnosis of facial/cheek swellings:

- Benign, e.g. dermoid cyst, ossifying fibroma.
- Malignant, e.g. squamous cell carcinoma, adenocarcinoma, lymphoma.

VIII. Salivary glands

The salivary glands can be described as being serous or mucous in nature:

- Parotid gland is mainly serous (P-S).
- Submandibular gland is a mixture.
- Sublingual gland is mainly mucous.
- Minor salivary glands entirely mucous.

Eighty per cent of all salivary gland tumours are found in the parotid (80% are benign):

- 75% are pleomorphic adenomas (PA, roughly 80% for the 80–80–80 rule).
- 10% are adenolymphomas (proportions vary depending on ethnicity – more common in Chinese).
- 3% mucoepidermoid carcinoma (most common malignant tumour of parotid and of salivary glands overall).
- 3% adenoid cystic (most common non-parotid malignant tumour).
- 9% other carcinoma including carcinoma ex-PA.

Salivary malignancies comprise 3% of all head and neck tumours and all pre-auricular masses in adults should be regarded as a parotid mass until proven otherwise. **Haemangiomas** are the most common parotid tumour in children.

Other salivary glands:

- 10–15% of all salivary gland tumours are found in the submandibular gland: a smaller proportion (65%) are pleomorphic adenomas with other types being relatively more common. Half of the tumours in submandibular glands are malignant (80% of parotid tumours are benign whilst 80% of minor salivary gland tumour are malignant).
- 10% are found in the sublingual glands (70% malignant) or the minor salivary glands – especially of the hard palate.
- The smaller the salivary gland the more likely that a tumour is malignant and the more likely that a malignant tumour will behave aggressively.

Parotid gland

The gland is ectodermal in origin and is enveloped by the parotid fascia that is derived from the investing fascia of the neck. The deep and superficial lobes (75% of the gland) are divided by the facial nerve; there may be an accessory gland that is anterior and superficial to the masseter. From superficial to deep pass the following structures:

- Facial nerve, its upper and lower divisions and the *pes anserinus*.

- Retromandibular vein (posterior and anterior branches to post-auricular/external jugular and anterior/common facial veins respectively).
- External carotid artery and its two terminal branches.

Other structures in the gland include:

- Pre-auricular lymph nodes.
- Fibres of the auriculotemporal nerve.

The parotid duct (of Stenson, 5 cm long) turns around the anterior border of masseter to pierce buccinator opposite the third upper molar and travel obliquely forward to open into the oral cavity opposite the second upper molar.

Nerve supply to the parotid:

- Sensation – auriculotemporal nerve, which is a branch of the mandibular nerve (V3) and emerges anterior to the tragus. It also supplies the upper part of the pinna (lower half is supplied by the great auricular nerve; the posterior auricular nerve is a preparotid branch of the VIIth nerve and is motor to occipitalis).
- Sensation to the parotid fascia – great auricular nerve (C2, 3).
- Secretomotor – preganglionic fibres from the inferior salivary nucleus (glossopharyngeal nerve/tympanic branch of IX/lesser petrosal nerve/otic ganglion/post-ganglionic fibres in the auriculotemporal nerve). The otic ganglion is closely applied to the mandibular nerve beneath the foramen ovale in the infratemporal fossa.

The posterior belly of digastric is on the deep inferior surface of the gland and is a guide to the location of the facial nerve as it emerges from the stylomastoid foramen.

Submandibular gland

The gland is composed of superficial and deep parts which are separated by the free border of mylohyoid. No structures pass **through** the gland. The submandibular lymph glands lie in contact with or within the gland.

- Superficial part is grooved posteriorly by the facial artery.
- Deep part lies between the lingual nerve above and the hypoglossal nerve below.

The duct (Wharton's) emerges from its superficial (inferior) surface, is 5 cm long and passes deep to mylohyoid and geniohyoid to open in the mouth next to the frenulum.

Nerve supply: the preganglionic fibres in the superior salivary nucleus/nervus intermedius/facial nerve/chorda tympani/via petrotympanic fissure go to the lingual nerve/submandibular ganglion and postganglionic fibres then pass directly to the gland.

Salivary gland tumours

Tumours usually present as localized painless nodules ± fixity. Differential diagnoses (for a parotid lump) include: sebaceous cyst (punctum and discharge), sialolithiasis (the whole gland is swollen and is related to meals), autoimmune conditions e.g. Sjögren's or lymphoma (examine nodes).

- **Pain** is suggestive of malignancy but may be due to other reasons such as infection/inflammation.
- **Short history** is suggestive of malignancy also (steady growth then rapid growth suggests carcinoma ex-PA).
- Parotid tumours may involve the **facial nerve** and weakness is a strong indicator of malignancy, as is bleeding from the parotid duct orifice. Note that sarcoidosis of the parotid may also present with nerve palsy.
- Lymphadenopathy and skin changes are other features suggestive of malignancy.
- Tumours in children and the elderly are more likely to be malignant.

Biopsy is largely contraindicated in the major salivary glands unless the features of the lump and history are strongly suggestive of pathology other than pleomorphic adenoma. In contrast, biopsy of the minor salivary glands is indicated because it is less likely that the lump will be a pleomorphic adenoma – more likely to be a carcinoma for which treatment will be based on the results of the biopsy.

Examination should include:

- Lump including intra-oral and bimanual.
- Full head and neck examination including:
  - Facial nerve function.
  - Lymph nodes and other possible draining areas e.g. external auditory meatus, and scalp.

Classification of salivary gland tumours

There are many different types. Metastatic tumours (up to one-third of parotid malignancies) have most commonly spread from scalp or ear tumours particularly SCCs, but prostate and kidney metastases have been described.

Adenoma

- **Monomorphic** (adenolymphoma, **Warthin's** tumour) is a benign tumour accounting for 10% or more of parotid tumours and is most commonly found in older male patients, particularly smokers. Tumours are composed of uniform epithelial tissue, with lymphoid stroma. They may be multifocal or bilateral (10–15%) and a 10% recurrence rate after surgery (**10% rule**).
- **Pleomorphic adenoma** (PA) is composed of different types of epithelial tissue and different types of stroma – chondroid, myxoid, mucoid, hence the name. It is typically found in middle-aged women. It typically exhibits slow growth and incomplete excision (e.g. due to bosselations) or seeding leads to recurrence. The 2–10% risk of malignant change is the main reason for surgery.
- **Myoepithelioma** is a tumour of minor salivary glands that is similar to pleomorphic adenoma, usually presenting as a large intra-oral swelling with a characteristic slow growth over many years. It is usually said that biopsy should be avoided; MRI defines tissue planes and resectability. Treatment may not be required though secondary middle ear obstruction and effusion may require grommet insertion.
- **Mucoepidermoid tumour** displays squamous and mucous metaplasia within ductal epithelium and behaves variably, low to high grade (or well, intermediate or poorly differentiated) – tumours in major glands tend to be low grade like PAs, whilst in the minor glands, they behave more like adenoid cystic carcinomas. There is rarely a discrete capsule and recurrence after excision is fairly common.

Carcinomas (epithelial tumours)

- Adenocarcinoma.
- Squamous carcinoma.
- Anaplastic carcinoma.
- **Carcinoma in pleomorphic adenoma (carcinoma ex-PA)**. The diagnosis is suggested by a sudden increase in the rate of growth with the development of fixity in a previously mobile swelling that has been present for many years (typically over 10 years). There may be facial nerve weakness or paralysis. The tumour behaves like anaplastic

carcinoma with a poor prognosis but can be unpredictable at times.

- Adenoid cystic carcinoma (ACC).

Malignancies are generally divided into low (mucoepidermoid, acinic cell) or high grade (mucoepidermoid again, ACC, SCC, AC and anaplastic/undifferentiated).

Adenoid cystic carcinomas

The smaller the gland, the more likely that a tumour arising within it might be an ACC. These tumours have a Swiss cheese pattern histologically with **no capsule**, the tendency for marked **perineural spread, perivascular invasion** and infiltration of tissue planes without a lymphocytic response and the occurrence of **skip lesions** means that excision is followed by 'inevitable' recurrence.

There are several **histological subtypes**: solid (10%, worst prognosis), cribriform ('classic' presentation seen in more than half) and tubular (best prognosis).

Adenoid cystic carcinomas present most commonly in the fifth decade, with a slow rate of growth and typically have a protracted disease course, being prone to local recurrence (especially where there is perineural invasion) and late metastatic potential e.g. 25 years later as lung metastasis.

- Embolic spread to lymph nodes is very rare but nodes may be involved due to direct invasion.
- Haematogenous spread to the lungs and bones is more common (36%).

Adenoid cystic carcinoma of the head and neck
Chummun S. *Br J Plast Surg* 2001;**54**:476–480.

In this series of 45 patients, the commonest sites were nose/paranasal sinuses and parotid and submandibular salivary glands. Most patients were treated by combined surgery and radiotherapy but there was incomplete resection in almost two-thirds of patients. There was local recurrence in 20% of patients after surgery. The commonest site for distant recurrence was the lung and overall survival at 5 years was 65%.

Facial nerve sacrifice and radiotherapy in parotid adenoid cystic carcinoma
Iseli TA. *Laryngoscope* 2008;**118**:1781–1786.

This is retrospective review of 52 cases showed that selective nerve sacrifice (for pre-operative nerve dysfunction or encased nerve at surgery) improved local control and survival (not statistically significant) but worse quality of life. Cummings (1970) was one of

the first to advocate nerve preservation with postoperative radiotherapy (as long as the pre-operative nerve function is intact), thus an alternative is to accept a higher recurrence rate but with improved quality of life. These issues need to be carefully discussed with patients. Patients who had radiotherapy after surgery had better local control. N0 patients rarely went on to develop lymphadenopathy. In contrast to SCCs, ACCs cannot be considered cured after 5 years of disease-free survival.

Lymphoid tumours (malignant lymphomas) have a typical history of a diffuse rapidly enlarging swelling with **no facial nerve involvement** in a previously normal gland. It may occur in a gland affected by Sjogren's syndrome. The diagnosis is made by biopsy, and the treatment is chemotherapy rather than surgery.

Investigations

- If the lump is thought to be separate from the parotid gland (e.g. sebaceous cyst) use ultrasonography (USG) to confirm.
- Sialography if thought to be sialolithiasis.
- If the lump is truly a parotid swelling then FNA to obtain a tissue diagnosis – FNA can diagnose pleomorphic adenomas in 95% or more of cases; it can diagnose malignancy accurately, just not the type. Core biopsies have a greater risk of facial nerve damage. Open biopsy is generally contraindicated due to the possible risk of tumour seeding.
- MRI to determine the extent of the tumour: superficial or deep lobes or both, to assess the neck nodes and relationship of the tumour to the facial nerve. CT shows less soft tissue detail but is still a reasonable option.

Some surgeons argue that there is little/no need for FNA, that a superficial parotidectomy with frozen sections is the 'biopsy' that is therapeutic in most cases. However there are also valid arguments for pre-operative investigations that allow better planning particularly for malignant tumours that may require radical surgery with neck dissection, facial nerve grafting or flap reconstruction.

T staging

- T1 < 2 cm.
- T2 2–4 cm.
- T3 > 4 cm.
- T4 > 6 cm or invasion.
  - a – skin, mandible, ear canal or facial nerve.

○ b – skull base, pterygoid plate or encasing carotid.

Radiological imaging in primary parotid malignancy
Raine C. *Br J Plast Surg* 2003;**56**:637–643.

Magnetic resonance imaging is capable of diagnosing malignant parotid disease (i.e. poorly defined tumour boundary with radiological evidence of local tumour invasion) with up to 93% sensitivity.

- It is a useful tool in conjunction with the clinical history, examination findings and fine needle aspiration cytology for the **diagnosis** of malignant parotid lumps and facilitates staging of the neck.
- It defines the relationship of the tumour to the facial nerve.

Management

- Parotid.
  ○ Benign or low-grade tumours:
    - Superficial lobe – superficial parotidectomy (lobectomy) e.g. mucoepidermoid.
    - Deep lobe – total parotidectomy preserving the facial nerve.
  ○ High-grade malignancy:
    - Radical parotidectomy sacrificing the facial nerve and surrounding involved structures including masseter, medial pterygoid, styloid process and associated muscles and the posterior belly of digastric. Overlying skin may also need to be sacrificed.
  ○ Submandibular.
    - Benign or low-grade tumours – submandibular gland excision.
    - High-grade tumours – excision of gland plus excision of surrounding structures including platysma, mylohyoid and hyoglossus muscles, hypoglossal and/or lingual nerves.
- Minor gland tumours – radical local excision.

Note that even where there is an extensive adenoid cystic or mucoepidermoid tumour for which surgery (with or without reconstruction) would only be palliative, surgery may still be worthwhile because recurrent disease may take many months or years to become apparent and is often painless. Nerve grafts may be required where branches of the facial nerve have been sacrificed (greater auricular nerve, sural nerve).

Neck dissection is suggested for salivary gland tumours when:

- Clinically positive neck including MRI-diagnosed disease (MRND).
- Recurrent tumours.
- High-grade malignancy.
- Extensive involvement of the deep lobe of the parotid with a malignant tumour.

Radiotherapy

Salivary gland tumours tend to respond poorly to radiotherapy therefore one should assume that surgical resection is the only chance of cure. Adjuvant radiotherapy may be indicated in cases of residual or recurrent disease or high-grade or advanced (T3/4) malignancies.

Radiotherapy has no place in the management of PAs which should be adequately excised; radiotherapy actually may increase risk of malignant change.

- Neutron therapy may be of some benefit with adenoid cystic carcinoma.

Parotidectomy

Typically a Blair incision is used (some have described limited incisions or face-lift incisions for selected lesions). The great auricular nerve is preserved if at all possible (6 cm below tragus lying on the SCM) as the subplatysmal/SMAS skin flaps are raised.

Identification of the facial nerve, if a nerve stimulator is to be used then no muscle relaxant is used:

- At the stylomastoid foramen.
- Posterior belly of digastric which can be followed back to the digastric groove.
- Tympanomastoid suture – the nerve is 6–8 mm deep to the inferior end of this.
- Triangular projection of the tragal cartilage points to the nerve which is 1 cm deep and anterior inferior.
- The buccal branches run alongside the parotid duct.
- The inferior trunk/marginal mandibular branch accompanies the retromandibular vein as it emerges from the inferior surface of the gland.
- Marginal branch runs below the inferior border of the mandible and over the facial artery.

Sometimes the tumour size/position makes **retro-grade nerve dissection** necessary.

Management of the facial nerve

- If the tumour is close, carefully dissect out and consider post-operative radiotherapy.
- If the nerve is involved:
  - If the patient is under 60 then reconstruct the nerve (interpositional/cross facial with great auricular/sural/medial cutaneous nerve of the forearm).
  - If the patient is over 60, then consider instead a temporalis transfer with fascia lata extensions, gold weights or endobrow lift/mid-face lift.

Excision of the tumour

- Superficial parotidectomy for PA or mucoepidermoid of superficial lobe.
- Facial nerve-sparing total parotidectomy.
  - Resection of superficial lobe first then deep lobe; chasing deep lobe tumour into the parapharyngeal space may require dislocation of the TMJ or mandibular osteotomy. The external carotid artery and retromandibular vein are ligated and excised with specimen.
- Radical parotidectomy sacrifices the facial nerve and this may be needed in high-grade tumours. Immediate nerve grafting and temporary lateral tarsorrhaphy is recommended under such circumstances.

Neck dissection

- If N0 (clinically/MRI) then observe.
- Positive neck (unusual) or highly aggressive tumour – synchronous lymphadenectomy.
- If the parotid tumour is a metastasis from a face/scalp primary – lymphadenectomy.
  - The parotid is a relatively common site for regional metastases – lymph nodes are incorporated into the gland due to the delay (embryologically) in the formation of the capsule. These nodes receive lymphatic drainage from wide areas of skin as well as the orbit, external ear and posterior oro/pharynx.

Complications

- Intra-operative – facial nerve palsy, retromandibular vein damage.
- Early.
  - Skin flap necrosis, infection, haematoma.

  - Sialocoele or salivary fistula.
- Late.
  - **Frey's syndrome** i.e. gustatory sweating occurs because post-ganglionic parasympathetic secretomotor fibres destined for the parotid hitch-hiking in the **auriculotemporal nerve** (sensory nerve to the ear and temple) are divided by surgery. Nerves degenerate to the level of the cell bodies in the otic ganglion and then regenerate along the auriculotemporal nerve and link up with sweat glands, so that subsequent eating induces sweating in the distribution of the auriculotemporal nerve. Variably reported incidence (10–40%, many cases may be subclinical); can be treated with antiperspirants, dermofat graft/Alloderm interposition, tympanic neurectomy or botulinum toxin.

Malignant tumours of the parotid gland: a 12-year review
Malata CM. *Br J Plast Surg* 1997;**50**:600–608.

Parotid malignancies are relatively uncommon, affecting 1–4 in 100 000 in the UK. This study included 51 patients with just over one-half having T3 or T4 disease on presentation. Carcinoma ex pleomorphic adenoma was common (transformation in up to 10% reported).

- FNA had a 88% sensitivity in diagnosing malignancy.
- MRI more useful than CT (especially for imaging neck nodes).

Generally, fixed tumours without facial nerve palsy are treated by either:

- Total parotidectomy (sparing all or part of the nerve) and post-operative radiotherapy or
- Radical parotidectomy and facial nerve reconstruction (five patients).

Neck dissection was reserved for palpable disease or positive MRI findings or where the neck is entered for access purposes. Immediate temporary tarsorrhaphy was performed for palsied patients to prevent exposure keratitis.

Overall, three-quarters received post-operative radiotherapy (including all patients with adenoid cystic carcinoma), some of these had had immediate nerve grafting after radical parotidectomy.

Poor prognostic factors included:

- Males.
- Incomplete excision.
- Pre-operative facial palsy.

Metastatic parotid tumours were usually located in nodes in the superficial lobe of the parotid and suited to superficial parotidectomy. Free flap coverage of a fungating tumour is acceptable for palliation.

Malignant tumours of the submandibular salivary gland:15-year review
Camilleri IG. *Br J Plast Surg* 1998;**51**:181–185.

Submandibular gland malignancy accounts for 8% of all salivary gland malignancy.

This was a review of 70 patients (mean age 64 years) with the main presenting symptom being a painless enlarged gland (average duration of symptoms 3 months). FNA was 90% sensitive. The commonest tumour in this series was adenoid cystic followed by carcinoma ex pleomorphic adenoma. The prognosis was related to TMN status at presentation.

The standard treatment was primary surgery plus post-operative radiotherapy. However, they found that malignancy was sometimes an incidental finding, diagnosed after removal of an enlarged gland previously assumed to be due to duct obstruction.

Salivary duct carcinoma:clinical characteristics and treatment strategies
Guzzo M. *Head Neck* 1997;**19**:126–133.

This aggressive tumour histologically resembles invasive ductal carcinoma of the breast and mainly affects the parotid duct, presenting as a rapidly enlarging swelling with pain and facial nerve paralysis. Nodal and distant metastases are common at presentation.

Surgery and post-operative radiotherapy is the treatment of choice but the local recurrence rate is high. It is commonly fatal within 2 years though some patients, in whom ductal carcinoma occurs in association with a pleomorphic adenoma, may have a more indolent form.

Management of parotid haemangioma in children
Greene AK. *Plast Reconstr Surg* 2004;**113**:53–60.

This is a retrospective review of 100 children and demonstrated that females were affected much more frequently (4.5×). Most patients (86%) had combined skin and parotid involvement. 10% required treatment for complications including narrowing/obstruction of the auditory canal.

- Small haemangiomas may be managed by intralesional steroid injection whilst systemic steroid is recommended for larger lesions. There is a response to interferon in up to 80% but potential for neurological complications limit its use.
- Surgery for a **proliferating** parotid haemangioma risks excessive blood loss and facial nerve injury. Patients with larger lesions were more likely to require surgery during the involutional phase later in childhood e.g. resection of fibrofatty tissue overlying the parotid with facelift-type mobilization and resection of affected skin.

Hyperbaric oxygen therapy for wound complications after surgery in the irradiated head and neck
Neovius EB. *Head Neck* 1997;**19**:315–322.

Hyperbaric oxygen (HBO) aims to increase oxygen tension in hypoxic tissues e.g. after radiotherapy especially radionecrosis of the mandible and post-surgical, post-irradiation wounds and fistulae. Some suggest **prophylactic** pre-operative therapy (20 pre-operative sessions, 10 post-operative) before surgery in irradiated tissues.

A session of HBO treatment usually consists of exposure to 2–3 bar, 100% oxygen for 75 min and 30–40 daily treatments may be required. Proposed benefits include:

- Increased fibroplasia and angiogenesis to aid wound healing.
- Facilitate oxygen-mediated phagocytic killing of pathogens to reduce infection.
- Bactericidal effect on anaerobes.

Complications include temporary myopia, barotrauma and oxygen toxicity and seizures.

There is apparently no effect on cancer cells.

Prediction of outcomes in 150 patients undergoing microvascular free tissue transfers to the head and neck
Simpson KH. *Br J Plast Surg* 1996;**49**:267–273.

The authors had a 5% flap failure rate. Some risk factors included:

- Glyceryl trinitrate (GTN) therapy for angina was predictive of thrombosis of the venous anastomosis, possibly a reflection of generalized vascular disease.

- Bronchodilator therapy, with higher ventilation pressures post-operation and coughing possibly leading to higher blood pressure.
- Diuretic therapy predictive of thrombo-embolic problems, may be related to dehydration and decreased venous tone.

There was **no correlation** of flap failure with:

- Extremes of age, gender or ASA status.
- Smoking or alcohol consumption.
- Previous radiotherapy or chemotherapy – recipient vessels unaffected by radiotherapy.
- Diabetes.
- Duration of surgery.

They also reported a 20% re-exploration rate which was increased in those using NSAIDs.

The overall mortality rate was 4.7%; mortality and strokes were commoner in patients with pre-existing vascular disease (especially previous myocardial infarction) and steroid treatment.

- The incidence of chest infection is proportional to age and commoner in men whilst patients taking bronchodilators had more hypoxaemia.
- Donor site problems were related to anaemia, previous radiotherapy and peripheral vascular disease. Donor and recipient site infections were both related to hypertension that the authors related to more bleeding and a reflection of vascular disease.

IX. Orbital tumours

Most orbital tumours (89%) are secondary tumours (breast, lung, prostate and melanoma) – due most frequently to local invasion e.g. from paranasal sinuses.

Primary malignant tumours include:

- Lymphosarcoma and rhabdomyosarcoma.
- Meningioma and glioma.
- Orbital malignant melanoma (MM), which can have several origins:
  - Extrascleral extension of posterior uveal MM e.g. from choroid or ciliary body.
  - Extension of adnexal MM e.g. from eyelid or conjunctiva.
  - Primary orbital MM – melanocytosis of the meninges of the optic nerve.
  - Metastatic melanoma i.e. haematogenous spread from a skin primary.

Other conditions include:

- Inflammatory – thyroid, autoimmune, orbital pseudotumour, mucocoeles.
- Vascular – haemangioma.

Childhood conditions affecting the orbit:
The most common lesion is a dermoid cyst whilst the most common malignancy is a rhabdomyosarcoma. Other lesions include:

- Haemangioma.
- Optic nerve glioma.
- Teratoma.

Investigations

- Plain X-ray, CT, MRI.
- Biopsy (division of lateral canthal ligament allows access behind the globe).

Full ophthalmological examination should be part of the assessment.

Proptosis is a common symptom – protrusion of > 21 mm beyond orbital rim or > 2 mm relative to the other side. The direction of displacement is important e.g. lacrimal tumours tend to displace the globe inferior and medially.

- A proptotic eye that is not adequately protected can lead to exposure keratopathy.
- Severe stretching may compromise the optic nerve.
- Proptosis secondary to a mass/tumour can cause compressive optic neuropathy.

Surgical approaches to the orbit

In general, anteriorly placed lesions are best treated via transorbital approaches whilst lesions of the posterior 1/3 are best treated via extraorbital routes, though this is not absolute.

- The medial wall can be approached via a Lynch incision, transcaruncular incision or endoscopic endonasal approach.
- The orbital floor can be approached via subciliary, transconjunctival or transantral approach (a buccal gingival sulcus incision).
- The lateral orbit can be approached via upper eyelid crease, lateral canthal, lateral orbital rim or coronal incisions.

Lateral orbit

- The **upper lid skin crease incision** (Harris added extension past the lateral canthus) allows access to the orbital apex and upper 2/3. When using this route, it is important to avoid damaging the levator aponeurosis by going superiorly when the orbital septum is reached.
- **Lateral canthotomy** (straight incision introduced by Berke) allows lateral wall access and is especially usefully in children.
  - Lateral triangle flap joining an upper lid skin crease and lateral canthotomy raised as a medially based flap allows access to the lateral orbit.
  - Lateral orbitotomy may be needed for apical/large masses.
- **Lower lid swinging flap** – allows access to the lower 2/3 of the apex. The lid may need to be shortened (transversely) when closing to reduce the risk of lid retraction/ectropion. The flap can be subclassified as low or high.

Types of excision

- **Evisceration** – removal of contents within the scleral shell (e.g. with an evisceration spoon). This is not suitable for tumour surgery and may provoke **sympathetic ophthalmia**.
- **Enucleation** – removal of the globe from the orbit preserving muscles and eyelids; prostheses can be inserted with muscle reattachment. It is suitable for treatment of intra-ocular malignancy, e.g. uveal tract melanoma without extrascleral spread.
- **Total exenteration** – removal of the entire contents of the orbit along with the eyelids and bony orbital walls. This is reserved for life-threatening malignancies within the orbit or for extensive involvement of the orbit especially globe or extra-ocular muscles by paranasal tumours. In the latter case, the resection of the primary sinus should occur en bloc with the orbital contents.
- **Subtotal exenteration** – excision that clears peri-orbita and fat but spares the globe and extra-ocular muscles, often resulting in enophthalmos, dystopia and diplopia e.g. for:
  - Slow-growing eyelid malignancies including recurrent basal cell carcinomas (BCCs) of the inner canthus invading the lacrimal sac or
  - Tumours of the paranasal sinuses that have invaded into the orbit but not breaching the peri-orbita (periosteum/membranes of the orbit).
- **Limited exenteration** – removal of sections of the bony wall of the orbit with the overlying peri-orbita and fat that may be suited for cases of localized invasion by paranasal sinus tumours.

Reconstruction

- **Split skin grafts** – may be used to cover exposed fat following subtotal exenteration or to line the bony orbit following total exenteration. One advantage of this method is that it does not mask recurrence. Mucosal grafts are alternatives.
- **Temporalis muscle flap and SSG**. The muscle is tunnelled through a bony window created in the lateral orbital wall to line the orbit after total exenteration without bony resection. The socket is maintained and accommodates a prosthesis, however it may mask recurrent tumour and leaves a temporal hollow. Other local flaps include the forehead flap and the TPF flap.
- **Pectoralis major**. The myocutaneous flap is pedicled on the thoraco-acromial vessels and tunnelled beneath the clavicle and through maxillary defect to provide lining to the exenterated orbit. It can be used for large defects following maxillectomy but there is a significant risk of tip necrosis due to the long excursion.
- **Free flaps**
  - Latissimus dorsi, rectus abdominis can provide skin and muscle bulk to fill the orbital defect.
  - Thinner flaps such as the RFFF or ALT are also being used.

Reconstruction of the orbit
Spinelli HM. *Surg Oncol Clin N Am* 1997;**6**:45–69.

The orbital septum forms a barrier to haemorrhage, infection, inflammation and neoplasia.

The authors suggest that orbital reconstruction should be guided by the **likelihood of tumour recurrence**: coverage by skin grafts or healing by secondary intention allow observation but if definitive surgery i.e. with curative intent has been performed, and there is no specific need to observe closely, then immediate reconstructive surgery can be performed.

- Healing by secondary intention takes weeks to months and is not practical in irradiated tissues. It may lead to a shallow socket.

- Skin grafts can take directly on to orbital bone and heal quickly, in addition grafts inset on top of subgaleal fascial flaps allow for closure of sinus fistulae and dural defects.
- Dermis/fat grafts can be used for enucleated sockets but are prone to resorption. If the extra-ocular muscles gain insertion on the dermis then they can move a prosthesis.
- Pedicled muscle flaps e.g. frontalis, temporalis and pectoralis major (some suggest a two-stage procedure with an exteriorized pedicle, ligated at 2 weeks is an alternative to the tunnelling described above). The temporoparietal fascial flap based on the superficial temporal vessels is made of the layer continuous with SMAS and can be tunnelled subcutaneously into orbit or used as a free flap. However it may lead to hair loss, and risk facial nerve injury.
- Free muscle flaps are good fillers, particularly useful for irradiated beds. They can combat infections and seal off sinus fistulae/dural leaks.

Bony reconstruction

- Free split calvarial bone grafts.
- Bone composite free flaps.
- Alloplastic materials – titanium plates.

Considerations for orbit reconstruction in children:

- The orbit is almost adult size by 2 years and fully adult ized by 7 years. Children do not have fully formed sinuses and the roots of the maxillary teeth abut the infra-orbital rim (thus at risk).
- Alloplastic materials should not be used in children wherever possible. Autologous bone is preferred though the cranium is thin and more cancellous and splitting should not be attempted until > 9 years of age. The iliac crest and rib grafts are alternatives.

Prosthesis

- None – simply use an eye patch.
- Adhesive, with or without glasses.
- Osseointegration.
- Obturator prosthesis when eyelids have been preserved.

Skull base tumours

Investigations:

- Nasendoscopy.
- CT scan with and without contrast.
- MRI scan.
- MRI angiography – assess vascularity of tumour; pre-operative embolization may be considered.
- Metastasis screen.

Surgery may be combined with radiotherapy for some tumours (although there are reports of BCC and SCC invading bone, becoming more aggressive after irradiated).

Access to the anterior skull base:

- **Weber–Fergusson** (lateral rhinotomy) incision extended onto the forehead ('facial split') provides good access to the maxilla and anterior skull base.
- **Bicoronal flap** gives excellent exposure of the anterior skull base – **even when the patient is bald** as the scars heal well and can be combined with a facial split incision. The plane of dissection proceeds in the subgaleal level to a point ~1.5 cm above the supra-orbital rim, then the dissection is subperiosteal.
  - Excision of the anterior cranial base is required for resection of ethmoidal and sphenoidal sinuses – central craniotomy with osteotomy proceeding along the supra-orbital rim, through the medial orbital walls and linked by a nasal osteotomy.
  - Exposure osteotomies (removing segments of the craniofacial skeleton with replacement later) include Le Fort III osteotomy that provides exposure of the posterior nasopharynx for resection of clivus tumours via a buccal approach.

Access to the lateral skull base:

- Lateral temporal approach for access to the middle cranial fossa, the infratemporal fossa and the petrous temporal bone. This uses a facelift incision extended around the temporal region.
  - Orbitotemporal exposure osteotomy: frontal and temporal craniotomies and removal of bone blocks, e.g. supra-orbital rim, orbital roof and lateral orbital wall.

Complications of excisional surgery:

- Death.
- Blindness.
  - Raised intra-orbital pressure can be treated by steroids, mannitol and lateral canthotomy.

- Severe haemorrhage.
- Infection (potentially fatal) – due to communication between the nasopharynx and the intracranial space.
- Cerebrospinal fluid leaks.
  - Dural tears may be closed by direct suture and fibrin glue (this is made from pooled serum and poses a potential infection risk).
  - Dural deficits are reconstructed with free pericranial or fascial grafts, with free fascial flaps for large defects.

X. Principles of skull base reconstruction

Some suggest that reconstruction should be delayed until margins have been confirmed as clear and when there has been no early recurrence. Reconstruction of the bony skull base is rarely required as brain herniation (encephalocoele) is uncommon but **soft tissue reconstruction** is needed to obliterate the dead space and to close off intra- and extracranial communication.

- Local pedicled flaps.
  - **Galea frontalis myofascial flap** – based on supratrochlear and/or supra-orbital arteries at the supra-orbital rim and is raised at a level just beneath the hair follicles down to the full-thickness of galea. It can be turned down to close off the roof of the nasopharynx from the anterior cranial fossa and sutured through drill holes to the bony margins of the defect.
  - **Temporal galeal flap** is a similar flap to the galea frontalis flap but is based on the superficial temporal vessels and can reach to the frontal area to just beyond the midline. There is a risk to the frontal nerve if it is raised too low.
  - **Temporalis muscle flap** – the muscle can be elevated on the superficial and deep temporal vessels down to its insertion on the coronoid process, and can be used to close off the roof of the orbit.
- Free tissue transfer is particularly useful in closing off dead space and providing a good blood supply to an area which has often been irradiated e.g. free latissimus dorsi (LD) or omentum (long pedicle).
- Branemark prosthesis.

Petrosectomy for invasive tumours: surgery and reconstruction
Malata CM. *Br J Plast Surg* 1996;**49**:370–378.

Sixty per cent of tumours of external auditory meatus and petromastoid region have bone involvement at the time of presentation. Fifty per cent present with established nerve palsy (usually VII) and this is a poor prognostic sign.

Radical surgery offers the only hope for cure, and may be achieved in ~20%; **petrosectomy** sacrifices facial and vestibulocochlear nerves and occasionally IX–XII. Salvage petrosectomy following radiotherapy for recurrent disease is largely futile but it may be considered for palliation of pain and fungation.

The procedure involves a combined intra- and extracranial approach and a neurosurgeon is needed. A parotidectomy and neck dissection is commonly performed synchronously.

- Neck dissection also allows dissection of the internal carotid artery and internal jugular vein as they enter the skull base.
- Metastatic parotid tumours are more difficult to treat with radiotherapy than involved neck nodes.

The defects are reconstructed with free flaps with the rectus abdominis being the flap of choice; bone grafts to support the brain are unnecessary. The more common complications include injury to dural sinuses (haemorrhage), CSF leaks and meningitis.

C. Reconstruction of other facial regions

I. Ear reconstruction

Ear anatomy

The Frankfurt (sometimes Frankfort) plane runs from the inferior margin of the orbit (orbitale) to the upper margin of the external ear meatus (porion) and is regarded as the anatomical positional of the human skull, and is close to the horizontal plane of the head in the living subject.

- Distance from lateral brow ~ length of ear.
- Axis of ear to vertical 20 degrees.
- Distance of helical rim to scalp 1.5–2 cm.

Arterial supply comes from the external carotid: postauricular, superficial temporal and occipital arteries.

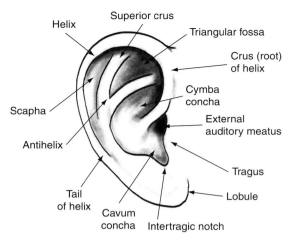

Figure 3.6 External ear anatomy.

Sensation

- Great auricular (C2–3) – lower half of ear.
- Auriculotemporal (trigeminal V2) – lateral part of upper ear, anterosuperior parts of external auditory canal.
- Lesser occipital – medial part of upper ear.
- Auditory nerve of VII to external auditory meatus.
- Arnolds nerve (X) – concha and posterior auditory canal.
- Jacobsens nerve (IX).

Reconstruction of the ear

Seventy per cent of tumours of the external ear are related to actinic damage and are more common in men, supposedly women's ears are protected by their longer hair. Tumours tend to spread locally fairly readily.

- Most tumours are SCC with a higher metastatic potential when compared with other facial SCC and tend to spread to internal jugular and parotid nodes.
- BCCs are uncommon outside the conchal fossa, but may also be found on the posterior surface and lobe.

Other tumours include melanoma and adnexal tumours (adenocarcinoma, adenoid cystic) but these are rare; they generally require amputation of the pinna and possibly neck dissection.

Clinical classification of auricular defects (Tanzer)

- Anotia 1 in 6000 in Whites, 1 in 4000 in Japanese.
- Complete hypoplasia (microtia).
  - With atresia of the external auditory canal.
  - Without atresia of the external auditory canal.
- Hypoplasia of the middle third of the auricle.
- Hypoplasia of the superior third of the auricle.
  - Constricted (cup or lop) ear.
  - Cryptotia (1 in 400 Japanese).
  - Hypoplasia of the entire superior third of the auricle.
- Prominent ears.

Microtia

Microtia occurs 1 in 10 000, being more common in the Japanese and Navajo Indians (0.1%); it is twice as common in males. The proportion of right, left and bilateral microtia is 6:3:1.

- **Causes** include teratogens (thalidomide, retinoic acid) or some intrauterine ischaemic insult (stapedial artery); microtia is a feature of some syndromes e.g. Treacher Collins and hemifacial microsomia/Goldenhars.
- **Associated features** include:
  - Hearing loss – sensorineural less common (10–15%) than conductive (80–90%).
  - Others include facial clefts, micro/an-ophthalmia, limb defects etc.

Nagata classification

- Anotia.
- Lobular type (most common) – lobule remnant and helix.
- Conchal type – lobule remnant, concha, external meatus and tragus.
- Small conchal type – lobule with small concha.
- Atypical microtia – types that do not fit into the above categories.

Reconstruction in microtia

Patients are often referred soon after birth, and screening for other anomalies undergoing or complete. They should be seen annually until ready for surgery.

- Family history.
- Hearing test and imaging including temporal bones, MRI for facial nerve.

The ears are 85% of their final size by 3–4 years of age (close to adult size by 11 years); it is often said that by 6 years of age an adult-sized ear can be reconstructed from rib cartilage. Auricular reconstruction generally precedes any middle ear surgery to ensure that the tissues are virgin. Symmetry cannot be guaranteed in terms of position or size; about half are similar in size, 40% are larger than the normal ear with the remainder smaller.

Auricular reconstruction for microtia: Part II. Surgical techniques
Walton RL. *Plast Reconstr Surg* 2002;**110**:234–249.

Tanzer technique

- Stage one: transverse re-orientation of lobular remnant.
- Stage two: framework carved from contralateral 6–8th costal cartilages and buried beneath mastoid skin.
- Stage three: elevation of framework to create retroauricular sulcus with FTG to sulcus.
- Stage four: reconstruction of tragus by composite graft from normal ear.

Brent technique

Based on the Tanzer technique but modified in sequence; patients aged 4–6 years.

- Stage one: high-profile cartilaginous framework as above and placed into mastoid pocket (use of suction drains to help emphasize underlying cartilage shape).
- Stage two: transposition of the lobule (occasionally combined with stage three).
- Stage three: elevation of the construct as above with placement of a banked piece of cartilage behind the ear to increase projection.
- Stage four: tragus reconstruction (trend to reconstruct tragus with the framework) and excavation of conchal bowl, symmetry adjustment.

Nagata technique

- Stage one: formation and placement of an ipsilateral cartilaginous framework (6–9th ribs, use wire) with transposition of the lobule to include tragal reconstruction.
- Stage two: after 6 months, elevation of the construct with placement of a further crescent of costal cartilage in the postauricular sulcus to increase

projection. Temporoparietal fascial flap and SSG from occipital scalp used to resurface sulcus (or advance retroauricular skin and graft the remainder).

There are only two stages but there is a theoretical greater risk to skin vascularity from the increased dissection and more cartilage is needed leading to significant donor site deformity (supposedly this can be minimized by leaving perichondrium intact). Patients are usually 10 years old or when chest circumference at xiphoid is > 60 cm to allow additional cartilage harvest.

Post-operatively:

- Suction drains and dressings.
- Avoid contact sports (to protect chest and framework).

Complications of ear reconstruction:

- Infection (< 0.5%) and haematoma.
- Skin necrosis and extrusion of the cartilage framework.
- Resorption of the cartilaginous framework.
- Hair resulting from placement in hair-bearing skin where there is a low hairline (standard depilation techniques).
- Thick or inelastic skin compromising aesthetic result.
- Use of a temporoparietal fascial flap causing alopecia/visible scar and numbness.
- Donor site complications e.g. pneumothorax, atelectasis, chest wall scar (some suggest an IMF scar in females) and deformity (more likely with older patients), pain.

Reconstruction following acquired loss

Acquired loss is usually due to tumour (60% SCC, 35% BCC and 5% melanoma) or tumour surgery, occasionally due to trauma or burns (ears are involved in 90% of facial burns).

Conchal/antehelical defects reconstructed by:

- Full thickness skin graft.
- Trap-door flap.
- Islanded retroauricular flap.

Injuries affecting the external auditory meatus (EAM) will have the tendency to heal by stenosis; acrylic moulds used for 6/12 have variable results, as does surgery in the form of FTG or local flaps.

Upper third defects reconstructed by:

- **Helical advancement** (Antia and Buch) generally recommended for defects of 3 cm or less.
- Banner flap – from posterior sulcus based at the root of the helical rim along with contralateral conchal cartilage graft.
- **Pocket technique** (Mladick RA. *Plast Reconstr Surg* 1971;**48**:219–223) – this requires two stages; dermabrade avulsed segment and insert into an adjacent postauricular skin incision with edge of the pocket sutured to the edge of the stump. At the second stage after 4 weeks or so (originally 2 weeks), the ear is released by elevating the skin off the ear and returning it to the retroauricular bed; the denuded ear is left to re-epithelialize or grafted if the process is slow.
- **Chondrocutaneous composite flap** based on skin pedicle from root of helix (Davis J. *Symp Reconstr Auricle* 1974;**247**:9) or on outer border (Orticochea). The donor is covered with a transposition flap with skin grafting to this donor.

Middle third defects reconstructed with:

- Composite grafts of contralateral helical rim.
- Ipsilateral conchal cartilage graft covered both posteriorly and anteriorly by a transposition flap from retro auricular skin.
- Direct closure using either wedge excision or helical advancement (Antia and Buch).
- Large rim defects reconstructed with tubed bipedicled flaps created in postauricular skin, transferred at two later stages i.e. **three-stage tube flap**.
- **Converse tunnel technique** – a tailored piece of cartilage is tunnelled under the mastoid/postauricular skin and joined to the edges of the helical defect. The ear is then separated from the mastoid area in a second stage after 3 weeks with the graft attached, and the defect covered with FTSG.

Lower third defects (lobe reconstruction can be complex):

- Two-stage approach: inset free edge into adjacent skin then release with an adjacent local flap.
- Contralateral composite graft.
- One-stage approach (below).

A combined flap technique for earlobe reconstruction in one stage
Alconchel MD. *Br J Plast Surg* 1996;**49**:242–244.

The anterior skin is used to make the posterior surface whilst posterior skin is used to make anterior surface:

- Reflect rim of skin of antihelix/helix inferiorly to form upper part of posterior surface.
- Medially based islanded skin flap raised from posterior sulcus to make anterior surface and lower part of posterior surface by folding it.

This avoids two-stage approach and the donor defects often close directly (but could be closed with a FTSG if necessary).

Reconstruction of the amputated ear

- Banking of cartilage beneath retroauricular skin but it tends to flatten out (Sexton).
- Banking of cartilage subcutaneously as a prefabricated flap, e.g. forearm for later transfer as a composite free flap (Schiavon M.*Plast Reconstr Surg* 1995;**96**:1698–1701). However flap bulk obscures definition; therefore consider transfer as a fascial/cartilage flap and SSG.
- Dermabrasion of anterior skin and draping with a retroauricular flap (Pribaz JJ. *Plast Reconstr Surg* 1997;**99**:1868–1872).
- Temporo parietal fascial flap coverage of denuded cartilage.
- Fenestration of cartilage and resiting as a composite graft – tendency to fail.
- Excision of posterior skin and cartilage fenestration (Baudet) – reconstruct sulcus 3/12 later with skin graft.
- Microvascular replantation – but technically difficult, to either superficial temporal or the posterior auricular vessels (vide infra).

Total ear replantation
Kind GM. *Plast Reconstr Surg* 1997;**99**:1858–1867.

The distal superficial temporal vessels are dissected and then reflected back into the operative field (however this precludes later use of a temporoparietal flap), allowing direct anastomosis to the superficial temporal vessels. Alternatively the ear vessels can be anastomosed to the postauricular vessels.

Venous drainage is often inadequate because of small calibre and low-flow vessels and vein grafts may be needed. Leeches are often used post-operatively, especially in artery-only ears. Heparinization may be used and this may lead to a need for transfusions.

Management of the burned ear

- Topical antibiotics (sulfamylon – painful and hyperchloraemic acidosis).
- Padding and avoidance of pillow friction.
- Early debridement reduces the risk of infection and chondritis.
- Whilst non-viable areas may separate spontaneously, areas of chondritis should be aggressively debrided and covered (FTSG or fascial flaps).

Correction of the cauliflower ear

Vogelin E. *Br J Plast Surg* 1998;**51**:359–362.

The aim should be to prevent permanent deformity by early drainage of the haematoma. Most regard cauliflower ear (haematoma auris/perichondrial haematoma) as a subperichondrial collection, which by separating the cartilage from its source of nutrition causes necrosis and deformity by fibrosis.

The author says that cartilage splits into two leaves with haematoma in between and untreated haematoma that fails to resorb becomes calcified. They suggest bat ear type of posterior approach, resecting calcified haematoma and posterior leaf of cartilage whilst the anterior leaf is resculpted by anterior scoring to recreate antihelix.

Tissue expansion as an adjunct to reconstruction of congenital and acquired auricular deformities

Chana JS. *Br J Plast Surg* 1997;**50**:456–462.

Tissue expansion can be used to generate additional skin in difficult or salvage situations when large amounts of unscarred skin are not available. If excessive scarring prevents the use of expansion, then a temporoparietal flap may be required but this will reduce the definition of the cartilage framework.

- Retroauricular rectangular expander placed via a remote incision in the temporal hairline.
- Slow expansion commenced after 2 weeks and maintained for 2 weeks before removal.
- Capsulectomy performed and cartilage framework inserted; suction drains used to facilitate skin draping.

There is a complication rate of 30% including extrusion, infection and haematoma; hair growth can be reduced using the ruby laser.

An operation for Stahl's ear

Ono I. *Br J Plast Surg* 1996;**49**:564–567.

Stahl's bar is a 'third crus' projecting from the antihelix with flattening of the helical rim. Options include:

- Anterior stepped wedge excision of skin and cartilage. Closure with helical advancement and a small cartilage graft (from conchal fossa) inset behind approximated cartilage edges.
- Turnover/rotation techniques.
- Splinting from the neonatal period (similar to bat ears).

Posterior Z-plasty and J-Y antihelix-plasty for correction of Stahl's ear deformity

El Kollali R. *J Plast Reconstr Aesthet Surg* 2009;**62**: 1418–1423.

The Z-plasty is used to lengthen the skin on the posterior surface of the affected ear – the short vertical length tends to cause a bow-stringing effect. Posterior scoring and suturing is used to reconstruct the superior crus.

Ear reduction

Gault DT. *Br J Plast Surg* 1995;**48**:30–34.

The aim of ear reduction surgery in this study was to correct asymmetry or to reduce congenitally large ears. The basic technique involved excision of crescent-shaped skin and cartilage from the scaphal hollow and advancement of the helical rim with excess excised at the root of the antihelix.

Cleft/split ear lobe

Many different techniques have been described with or without Z-plasties or similar techniques to prevent notching. Pardue AM (*Plast Reconstr Surg* 1973;**51**:472–473) described a method of reconstructing the hole with a small flap from the cleft, though it may be simpler to simply perform a complete repair and then pierce the ear again subsequently.

Otoplasty

Prominent ears occur in up to 5% of the population. This is inherited as an autosomal dominant trait in some. The main features are:

- Poorly defined/absent antihelical fold.
- Conchal excess e.g. > 1.5 cm.
- Conchoscaphal angle > 90°.

Non-surgical treatment

Neonatal cartilage is malleable, supposedly due to maternal oestrogens/high hyaluronic acid levels and moulding within this early window (within 1–2 weeks) may be successful (Matsuo K. *Clin Plast Surg* 1990;**17**: 383–395) but does entail a significant undertaking for up to 6–8 weeks.

Surgical techniques

History of treatment

- The use of sutures to recreate the antihelical fold described by Mustardé JC. (*Plast Reconstr Surg* 1967;**39**:382–386).
- Open anterior scoring to recreate an antihelical fold described by Chongchet V. (*Br J Plast Surg* 1963;**16**:268–272).
- Transcartilaginous incision originally described by Lucket in 1910.

Options

- Suture techniques – conchoscaphal (recreate antihelical fold; Mustardé), conchomastoid (to reduce conchal projection but may distort meatus; Furnas)
- Excisional – cartilage – conchal reduction, skin.
- Cartilage moulding – **Gibson's Law** 1958 states that cartilage will bend away from scored surface due to release of interlocked stresses. This is utilized in **Strenstrom's** technique (1978) that uses a rasp/otoabrader via a posterior approach and Chongchet (1963) anterior scoring technique with a blade 1/2 to 2/3 of the cartilage thickness. There are open and closed techniques (vide infra).

Otoplasty by percutaneous anterior scoring: another twist to the story

Bulstrode NW. *Br J Plast Surg* 2003;**56**:145–149.

This is a review of patients in whom Mustardé technique was used in combination with percutaneous anterior scoring using a hypodermic needle (alternatives include toothed forceps and endoscopic carpal tunnel instruments). Complications:

- Haematoma nil, infection 3.5%.
- Hypertrophic scarring 1.8%, residual deformity 5.3%.

Otoplasty: open anterior scoring technique and results in 500 cases

Caoutte-Laberge L. *Plast Reconstr Surg* 2000;**105**: 504–515.

This was a review of 500 otoplasty patients.

Pre-operative evaluation:

- Assess degree of (un)folding of the antihelix.
- Depth and size of conchal fossa.
- Prominence of lobe.
- Assess the quality of the cartilage and the angle between auricle and mastoid (males 25°, females 20°).

They excluded those with constricted (lop) ear deformity and note Darwin's tubercle, posterior antihelical crura (Stahl's bar).

The overall satisfaction (very satisfied or satisfied) rating was 94.8%. Ninety-five per cent of cases were bilateral and 59% were performed under local anaesthesia. Complications were not common but included:

- Bleeding 2.6% (haematoma 0.4%).
- Wound dehiscence 0.2%, infection nil.
- Keloid scars 0.4%, inclusion cysts 0.6%.
- Loss of ear sensation 3.9%, tender ears 5.7%.

The incidence of **asymmetry** (18.4%) was quite high, with residual deformity less frequent (5%); both commoner in younger age groups – dual-operator technique is significantly more likely to give rise to asymmetry and since young children usually have a general anaesthetic and two surgeons, this may explain the greater incidence of asymmetry in the young.

In addition, others have described early complications of chondritis and late complications of recurrence/late deformity (24% with Mustardé, 10% with cartilage scoring) as well as scar hypertrophy/sensitivity.

II. Reconstruction of the eyelids and correction of ptosis

Anatomy

- Anterior lamella composed of skin and muscle – orbicularis oculi.
  - Orbital fibres – contraction causes screwing up of the eyes tightly e.g. to resist opening.
  - Palpebral fibres responsible for blinking gently.
    - Pretarsal for involuntary blink and tear film distribution.
    - Preseptal voluntary and involuntary assistance with blinking.
- Posterior lamella composed of lid retractor, conjunctiva (non-keratinizing squamous epithelium) and tarsal plate. The latter are

condensations of the orbital septum and are dense fibrous tissue around Meibomian glands and **not cartilage**. Usually, the upper lid tarsal plate is ~8–12 mm tall and ~2 mm thick. **The orbital septum** is a dense fibrous membrane from periosteum of orbital rim, through the lid to the tarsal plate separating orbital and periorbital tissues. Some describe the orbital septum as the middle lamella; it fuses with the posterior lamella at the tarsal plate.

- ○ Suspensory ligament of Lockwood completes the ligamentous attachments to the globe.
- ○ Numerous glands of Moll.
- ○ Lateral and medial condensations of the tarsal plates form the lateral and medial canthal ligaments.

Orbital fat lies between the lamellae.

Eyelid retractors

- Levator palpebrae superioris
  - ○ This striated muscle (45 mm in length) attaches to the upper tarsal plate via the levator aponeurosis (15 mm in length) to become part of the anterior lamella.
  - ○ It acts to elevate the upper eyelid (10–15 mm); it is supplied by the superior division of the oculomotor nerve. It is crossed by the superior transverse ligament (of Whitnall) in its upper part that acts as a check to levator retraction.
- Müller's **muscle** lies deep to levator.
  - ○ It is composed of smooth muscle and supplied by **sympathetic fibres** travelling in the oculomotor nerve. It maintains the tone of raised eyelids and effects fine adjustment on lid height; paralysis (Horner's syndrome) causes 2–3 mm of ptosis.
  - ○ It is involved in the sympathetically mediated startle response (eye opens wide). It may also help to transmit the action of levator to the tarsal plate.
- **Capsulopalpebral fascia** of the lower lid – this is a condensation of fibrous tissue that is analogous to the levator aponeurosis. It is an extension from the inferior rectus muscle to the tarsus and functions to stabilize the tarsus allowing the eyelid to descend when the eyeball looks down. It splits around the inferior oblique and then reunites to form Lockwood's ligament.

Blood supply

Marginal and peripheral arcades from lid margin.

- Upper lid – branches of ophthalmic artery (internal carotid).
- Lower lid – branches of facial artery (external carotid).

The marginal arcades lies just anterior to the tarsi, 2–4 mm from the lid margin; the superior peripheral arcades lies just superior to the tarsal plate just anterior to Müller's muscle.

Sensation comes from V1 and V2 for the upper and lower lid respectively.

Lacrimal gland

Secretomotor fibres come from superior salivary nucleus that relay in pterygopalatine ganglion and travel in zygomatic branch of VII. There are accessory lacrimal glands:

- Meibomian glands – lubricate lid margins.
- Glands of Zeiss.
- Glands of Moll.

The lacrimal apparatus consists of:

- Lacrimal punctum is located at the medial canthus, upper and lower canaliculi lead from it to the lacrimal sac, travelling beneath the upper and lower limbs of the medial canthal ligament.
- Lacrimal sac drains into the nasolacrimal duct which empties into the inferior meatus of the lateral wall of the nose; the sac is pulled open during contraction of the palpebral fibres of orbicularis oculi and closes by elastic recoil. Valves in the canaliculi prevent reflux.

Causes for dry eyes include smoking, old age (including post-menopausal) as well as antihistamine treatment and sicca syndrome.

Lacrimal gland tumours

Fifty per cent are **pleomorphic adenomas**; they usually present as painless slow-growing lesions with no inflammatory signs.

- There is a high risk of local recurrence due to tumour spillage and generally the advice is not to biopsy, but rather to treat by total gland excision.

Twenty-five per cent are **adenoid cystic carcinomas**.

- These spread diffusely along tissue planes and are locally aggressive, they almost always recur locally.

Surgery requires total gland excision and orbital exenteration.

- Swiss cheese appearance histologically and basaloid changes associated with very poor prognosis (20% survival at 5 years, otherwise 70% at 5 years).

Another 25% are a miscellaneous group including adenocarcinomas, malignant change in a pleomorphic adenoma or muco-epidermoid tumours. In general, these are treated by total gland excision and orbital exenteration.

Eyelid tumours

Consider biopsy to confirm histology before definitive excision under frozen section control and reconstruction.

- The majority of tumours are BCCs (especially lower lids mainly at medial and lateral canthi); only 10% of lid tumours occur on the upper lid. Recurrent BCCs should be excised with frozen section control of margins.
- SCC accounts for ~2% of eyelid tumours (most often upper lid).

General principles

The upper lid is more important for lid function and protection, therefore Mustardé advised against the use of the upper lid for lower lid reconstruction. Suggested methods include:

- Up to 1/3 – direct closure.
- 1/3–1/2 – canthotomy and cantholysis.
- 1/2 to 3/4 – myocutaneous advancement flap.
- >3/4 – tissue from opposite lid or adjacent areas e.g. cheek, temple, forehead.

Partial thickness loss

- Skin – primary closure or FTSG (contralateral lid or postauricular).
- Conjunctiva – advancement of adjacent conjunctiva for small defects, buccal/nasal mucosa for larger areas (nasal mucosa said to contract less, 20% vs. 50%), hard palate, contralateral grafts.
- Tarsus – primary repair, palatal mucosal graft, cartilage graft or allograft (Alloderm).

Eyebrow defects

- Hair-bearing FTSG.
- Pedicled flap based on superficial temporal vessels.
- Hair transplant: pinch or micrografts.

Reconstruction of the lower lid

- Defects between **one-quarter and one-third** of the eyelids can usually be closed directly after wedge excision; repair in layers to avoid notching. A lateral **canthotomy** and cantholysis may be required if closure is overtight providing ~5 mm of extra advancement. For older patients with lax lids, primary closure of up to 40% defects can be achieved.
- If closure is still tight then a **Tenzel flap** – a semicircular rotation flap based high above the lateral canthus, it is combined with a lateral canthotomy and cantholysis and can close defects of up to 60%.
- Greater defects will require the recruitment of tissue from elsewhere. Local tissue provides best colour and texture match. There are many local flaps:
  - Bipedicled **Tripier flap** (includes strip of orbicularis muscle). The pedicle can be incorporated into the defect or divided at 3 weeks. It can be used as an unipedicled flap up to the midpupil point.
  - Upper eyelid transposition flaps (unipedicled Tripier).
  - Fricke flap – a temporal flap of skin above the eyebrow, the skin is thick.
  - Glabellar or forehead flap, the skin is thick.
  - Nasolabial flap.
  - **Cheek advancement flap**, e.g. McGregor (transposition with Z-plasty) or Mustardé (cheek rotation), can provide total lower lid reconstruction. The flap should be raised thin and well-mobilized to reduce retraction.

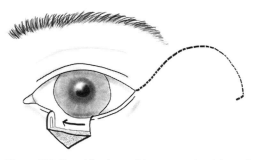

Figure 3.7 Tenzel flap for eyelid reconstruction. It is combined with lateral cantholysis.

Hughes flap

A **tarsoconjunctival flap** from the upper lid is advanced inferiorly to reconstruct the lower lid (sub/total); the flap is taken > 4 mm from the lid margin and includes a small portion of the upper tarsus. The second stage of flap division is performed at 6 weeks, during which the eye would be occluded. The anterior lamellar is usually reconstructed with a skin graft or a local skin muscle flap. Critics say that it is inadvisable to take tissue from the upper lid to reconstruct the lower lid, however the Hughes flap is able to reconstruct defects larger than two-thirds without distorting the canthal angles. The Cutler–Beard flap is similar but from the lower to the upper lid.

An alternative for larger (> 50%) defects is a two-layer composite chondromucosal graft from the nasal septum. The two lamellae need to be considered.

- Cartilage support may not be needed – thick cheek or forehead skin will usually suffice.
- Conjunctiva can be advanced into a lower lid defect to avoid mucosal grafts.

Locoregional flaps

These can be used if there is insufficient good-quality lid tissue, but are not ideal due to the thicker skin that is usually involved and will need separate lining of the inner surface.

One-stage reconstruction of full thickness lower eyelid defects using a subcutaneous pedicle flap lined by a palatal mucosal graft

Nakajima T. *Br J Plast Surg* 1996;**49**:178–181.

A skin island from the lateral cheek is rotated 180° into the lower lid with the pedicle based on the lateral canthus and including a small portion of orbicularis.

The flap is lined with palatal mucosal (leaving periosteum of donor area intact, and dressed with tie-over collagen sponge for 10 days) which is thicker and more durable than oral mucosa.

This method enables reconstruction of the entire skin of the upper or lower lid as an aesthetic unit. A similar flap was described by Heywood AJ. *Br J Plast Surg* 1991;**44**:183–186.

Upper lid reconstruction

Direct closure of defects of up to one-third (more in elderly).

Local flaps are generally required for defects > 25% similar to lower lid reconstruction. There is greater need for chondromucosal septal grafts or grafts of conchal cartilage for upper eyelid.

- **Tenzel flap**, as above up to 60%. A triangular excision of skin and muscle only below the square full thickness defect allows for the advancement/rotation.
- **Hueston lid switch** is an Abbé-type flap from the lower lid which is most suited to defects > 50% of the upper lid. It is a technically complex two-stage technique and the donor defect needs to be reconstructed but may be the **best option** for the large upper lid defect.
- **Cutler–Beard flap** – this is a two-stage procedure capable of reconstructing a whole upper lid. The full thickness of the lower lid is advanced under the lower lid margin and then sutured to the upper lid defect. The bridge is divided after 3 weeks. Support of the upper lid margin is lacking and may require a cartilage graft between conjunctiva and muscle.
- Fricke flap, paramedian forehead flap.

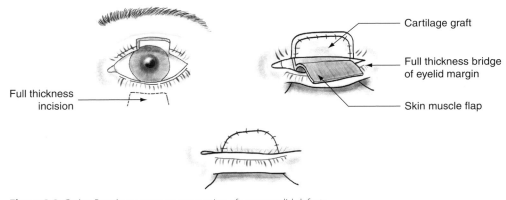

Figure 3.8 Cutler–Beard two-stage reconstruction of upper eyelid defects.

V–Y myotarsocutaneous advancement flap for upper lid reconstruction

Okada E. *Plast Reconstr Surg* 1997;**100**:996–998.

This technique is suited to defects of 25–50% where the lateral canthus remains intact; it advances full-thickness lid tissue except orbicularis which forms the pedicle. Tissue is moved from lateral to medial with the stem of the Y in the lateral canthus. It is a single-stage reconstruction that also avoids the need for chondromucosal grafts.

Surgical reconstruction in cryptophthalmos

Weng CJ. *Br J Plast Surg* 1998;**51**:17–21.

Cryptophthalmos is a feature of Fraser syndrome (1962) (autosomal recessive inheritance, more common in Romany population) and is associated with organ system abnormalities such as genitals, nose, larynx, kidneys, ears and mental disability. It is defined by the presence of at least two of four major characteristics: cryptophthalmos, syndactyly, genital anomalies and one affected sibling. About half of these patients have syndactyly.

The eyelids are fused and a membrane of skin passes from the forehead to the cheek, partially or completely over the affected eye and adheres to the globe. Cryptophthalmos can be complete, incomplete and abortive (eyelid is completely fused and underlying eye does not form). In the first two forms, there is microphthalmia.

Surgery aims to correct improperly fused tissues: eyelid reconstruction in this paper involves a composite chondromucosal graft and flap cover. Most are blind at birth but some have reaction to light/partial vision after eyelid repair.

Intraorbital tissue expansion in the management of congenital anophthalmia

Dunaway DJ. *Br J Plast Surg* 1996;**49**:529–535.

This is a report of ten cases of anophthalmos and microphthalmos.

The developing globe is a stimulus to the growth of the bony orbit and in anophthalmia the stimulus is absent. Growth stimulus may be restored by intra-orbital expansion with a spherical expander positioned within the muscle cone, covered with a tarsorrhapy, and the port tube passed through a hole in the lateral orbital wall and the infratemporal fossa to the scalp.

Releasing osteotomies in children > 2 years reduce the resistance to expansion and help prevent expander extrusion when planning expansion over a shorter time. When planning expansion over a prolonged period, e.g. in neonates and then removed at ~7 years, osteotomies are generally not necessary.

Dermoid cysts

Classification of dermoid cysts:

- Acquired – implantation type – insect bite, minor trauma, etc.
- Congenital teratoma type.
- Congenital inclusion type – at sites of embryonic fusion plates.

Orbitofacial dermoids are of the congenital inclusion type.

The management of midline transcranial nasal dermoids in the paediatric patient

Bartlett SP. *Plast Reconstr Surg* 1993;**91**:1208–1215.

Most facial dermoids are subcutaneous and only a minority have deeper extension. This retrospective review of 84 patients demonstrated that the three commonest anatomical locations were:

- **Frontotemporal** (lateral brow area) commonest with 65% and were generally soft, non-fixed and tended to be slow growing and asymptomatic. They could be resected by splitting the orbicularis oculi and excising down to periosteum. No special work-up was needed.
- **Orbital** (25%). Females were affected twice as frequently. These dermoids could adhere to frontozygomatic or medial sutures but were usually easily dissected free with no transosseous extensions. They rarely need work-up.
- **Nasoglabellar** (10%) – often presented as a mass with or without a punctum (with fine hair growth or sebaceous debris from punctum). The nasal bones may be split.
  - Midline glabellar lesions had no deep extension (*n* = 2) whilst dorsal nasal lesions had occult naso-ethmoid and cranial base abnormalities on CT. Thus **dorsal nasal dermoids** need radiological work-up and may need bicoronal approach.

Ptosis (blepharoptosis)

Normally, the upper eyelid level is such that it covers 1–2 mm of the upper limbus of the cornea. **Ptosis** is an abnormal droopiness of the upper lid that covers more of the cornea.

Beard's classification of ptosis (1981)

- Congenital.
- Acquired.

Frueh classification (1980)

- Neurogenic.
- Myogenic.
- Aponeurotic.
- Mechanical.

Congenital ptosis

Lid lag is common. In most cases, there is an absence of levator palpebrae (the muscle is replaced by fibro-fatty tissue) hence there is a congenital myogenic ptosis; in some the ptosis is due to innervation problems. Most cases are idiopathic but some are genetic with autosomal dominant inheritance being more common.

The problem is usually noticed shortly after birth.

- Reduced palpebral aperture, with **absent or asymmetrical lid crease**.
- Reduced light reflex to upper margin distance.
- Decreased levator excursion (normal 15–18 mm) – remember to immobilize brow/frontalis.
- On downward gaze, ptotic eyelid is held higher due to levator fibrosis preventing lid descent.
- Levator biopsy demonstrates absence of striated muscle, with fibrosis whilst Müller's muscle tends to be normal.

Generally surgery is deferred until ~5 years unless there is:

- Severe ptosis obstructing visual field leading to amblyopia.
- Corneal exposure risking ulceration.

Some conditions are associated with congenital ptosis:

- **Blepharophimosis syndrome** is the combination of ptosis with short palpebral fissures, epicanthus inversus and telecanthus; some may also have mild hypertelorism. The reduced vertical and transverse dimensions of the palpebral aperture may be due to a combination of upper lid ptosis with epicanthic folds and telecanthus. This can occur either in isolation or in association with other anomalies; some show autosomal dominant inheritance.
  - Brow suspension for ptosis.
  - Jumping man flap (Mustardé) for epicanthic folds or Roveda correction.
    - May need craniofacial surgery for hypertelorism.
- **Marcus Gunn jaw-winking syndrome** – there is synkinesis of the upper lid with chewing caused by aberrant trigeminal nerve innervation; it is seen in about 2–6% of patients with congenital ptosis.
- Associated anomalies:
  - Anophthalmos/microophthalmos.
  - Harmatomas/benign tumours e.g. neurofibroma, lymphangioma and haemangioma.
  - Strabismus, amblyopia.

Acquired ptosis

- Neurogenic.
  - Oculomotor nerve lesion.
  - Horner's syndrome (effects reduced with 10% phenylephrine hydrochloride).
  - Demyelination i.e. multiple sclerosis.
  - Traumatic ophthalmoplegia or ophthalmoplegic migraine.
- Myogenic.
  - **Senile/involutional ptosis** – stretching of the levator aponeurosis and muscle with age; actual levator function is usually good. This is the **most common** cause and is often categorized separately.
  - Myaesthenia gravis (worse later in day, Tensilon test is diagnostic – neostigmine or edrophonium), found in young females or older males.
  - Muscular dystrophy.
  - Steroid ptosis.
  - A rare cause of chronic progressive ptosis is **chronic progressive external ophthalmoplegia** (Kearns–Sayre syndrome – as a subset with possible risks of ataxia, deafness, diabetes and sudden cardiac death) which usually presents in young adults as an **adult ptosis with poor levator function** with symmetrical ophthalmoplegia. It has been classed as a mitochondrial myopathy (mitochondrial DNA is transferred maternally) and can be diagnosed by electromyograph (EMG) and thigh muscle biopsy that may show ragged red fibres on Gomori trichrome staining.
- **Traumatic (second most common).**
  - Injury to levator mechanism, e.g. **surgery** including cataracts – may also damage/scar

superior rectus muscle when used for insertion of a stay stitch to immobilize the eye.

- Mechanical.
  - Lid tumour.

Pseudoptosis is the appearance of ptosis rather than true ptosis (i.e. droopy upper lid), for example:

- Globe displacement e.g. with enophthalmos.
- Mechanical lid displacement e.g. inflammation, oedema.
- Dermatochalasis (excess redundant skin).
- Contralateral lid retraction e.g. thyroid eye/Grave's disease.
- Hypertropia, visual axis is higher than the fixating eye; dissociated vertical deviation.
- **Blepharochalasis** – rare condition in young, with recurrent lid oedema and subsequent stretching.
- **Duane syndrome** – absent/hypoplastic abducens and the lateral rectus is innervated by the oculomotor nerve, which leads to limitation of abduction and sometimes adduction. There may also be fibrosis/fibrous attachments of the extraocular muscles. The globe tends to retract into the orbit.
- Blepharospasm.

Assessment

Take a history including patient concerns – functional versus aesthetic, assess general health, medications (aspirin/warfarin), smoking/diabetes, history of dry eyes.
Ascertain cause – is it congenital or acquired:

- **Neurogenic or myogenic**.
- **Mechanical**: any lid swellings?
- **Trauma**: history of injury or cataract surgery or blepharoplasty? A history of atopy (leading to habitual eye rubbing) or hard contact lens use?

In the absence of the above and in an elderly patient, the cause is likely to be **senile** ptosis or **pseudoptosis** due to other conditions. In very simple terms, congenital ptosis is seen soon after birth and associated with poor levator function and absent lid crease whilst involutional ptosis is associated with good levator function and a high crease.

Examination

Look

- **Measure the degree of ptosis** in mm (mild 1–2; moderate 3–4; severe > 4 mm) and compare with other eye. The distance between mid-pupillary point to lid margin is normally ~5 mm.
- Check for brow ptosis (brow level in relation to the supra-orbital rim).
- Dermatochalasis.
- Presence of lid crease – site of aponeurosis insertion is lost in disinsertion syndrome.
- Assess lower lid position e.g. scleral show, lower lid laxity.

Move

- **Levator function** (should be 15–18 mm), measure from down gaze to up gaze with brow/frontalis immobilized: excellent (> 10 mm), good (8–10 mm), fair (5–7 mm) and poor (1–4 mm).
  - **Lagophthalmos** (incomplete closure of the lids) is a sequelae of all surgeries for ptosis; avoid overcorrection in those with pre-operative lagophthalmos during downward gaze (this suggests fibrosis of the levator).
  - **Bell's phenomenon**: eyeballs rotate upwards when the lids are closed. Some patients do not have this and one should be much less aggressive with ptosis correction in these as over-correcting may lead to corneal exposure during sleep.

Test

- Acuity.
- Pupils.
- Extra-ocular movements.
- Dry eyes – these patients are at risk of corneal exposure with post-operative lagophthalmos.
  - History and symptoms.
  - Schirmer's test I and II.
  - Tear film breakup.

Asymmetric ptosis

Correction of one side may unmask ptosis in the other side.

Hering's Law: the levator muscle receives equal innervation bilaterally. Severe ptosis affecting one side creates impulse for bilateral lid retraction but after treatment of the ptosis the impulse for lid retraction will decrease and may reveal ptosis in the contralateral eye.

- Hering's test – aims to reveal contralateral ptosis with brow immobilization in straight gaze; elevate ptotic lid with cotton bud and check for contralateral ptosis.

Surgical options

There are many options, and the choices are largely determined by the degree of ptosis and the levator function. Many authors suggest various formulae to predict the amount of correction, but in general every mm of ptosis correction requires 4 mm of **levator excision/plication/advancement**, whilst tarsal plate resection (for acquired ptosis only and rim must be preserved) is more direct – 1 mm resection for 1 mm elevation.

Good levator function (> 10 mm).

- Mild ptosis < 2 mm –**Fasanella–Servat** procedure: conjunctival approach – invert the tarsal plate, clamp with artery forceps and excise a 2-mm caudal segment (which includes aponeurosis attachment, tarsus, Müller's and conjunctiva) then oversew. The algorithm is 4-mm resection for 1-mm ptosis, 6-mm resection for 1.5 mm ptosis, 11–12-mm resection for 3-mm ptosis. The overall success rate is about 70%.
- Mild-to-moderate ptosis > 2 mm –**aponeurosis surgery**, e.g. resection or plication of the aponeurosis.

Table 3.1 Surgical options for correction of ptosis.

Levator function	Degree of ptosis	Procedure
Good (> 10 mm)	Mild (1–2 mm)	Fasanella–Servat, Müllerectomy
Good (> 10 mm)	Moderate (3–4 mm)	Aponeurosis surgery
Fair (5–10 mm)	Moderate (3–4 mm)	Levator surgery (resection/advancement)
Poor (< 5 mm)	Severe (> 4 mm)	Frontalis suspension surgery

Poor levator function < 10 mm) or **moderate ptosis** > 3 mm.

- Moderate ptosis, poor levator function 4–10 mm – **levator shortening** (resection or plication) **or advancement**.
  - Incise skin at proposed supratarsal fold and expose orbital septum and distal levator mechanism; the latter is incised at the upper border of the tarsal plate and the Müller's muscle dissected free. A lifting suture is placed into the tarsus and levator (4 mm to 1 mm). Fix the crease e.g. anchor blepharoplasty.
  - Levator reinsertion is only indicated in true levator dehiscence which is usually due to trauma.
- Severe ptosis, very poor levator function < 4 mm – **suspension surgery**. The frontalis muscle that normally elevates the brow is used to elevate the upper lid, and does so via a frontalis sling. This is likely to cause lagophthalmos at night thus nocturnal eye protection is very important in this group. In addition, the sling will cause a blemish/indent on downward gaze. In the best hands (Crawford), there is still a 10% recurrence rate over 20 years.
  - Crawford/Fox techniques – **fascia lata** (preserved or autologous, latter is used for recurrent cases or where preserved fascia is not available) sling connecting frontalis to tarsal plate or **palmaris longus** – preferred in children but absent in 15%).
    - Harvest the fascia lata with the knee slightly flexed and rotated internally: a 5.1 cm transverse incision 6.4 cm above the knee reveals the fascia that is incised transversely for 10–12 mm before two vertical incisions either side allow the use of a stripper to harvest 20–25 cm. Late bleeding/haematoma may occur thus rest is advised for several days.

Figure 3.9 Fasanella–Servat procedure.

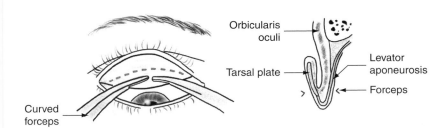

Orbicularis oculi

Tarsal plate

Levator aponeurosis

Forceps

Curved forceps

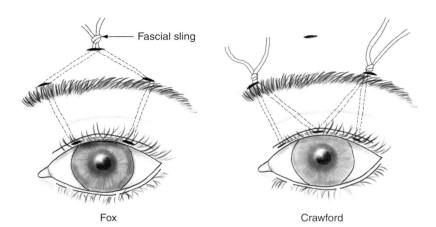

Fascial sling

Fox   Crawford

Figure 3.10 Common techniques of sling repairs for ptosis include the Fox and Crawford techniques; a special 'Wright' needle is used for threading the fascia, palmaris longus or alloplastic material through.

○ Prolene sutures or silicone loops – may be 'adjustable' (many different materials have been used) in congenital cases.
○ Frontalis advancement is an alternative.

Other surgical notes.

● Correcting ptosis will cause an apparent telecanthus post-operatively (as ptosis gives the illusion of a narrowed intercanthal disease).
● Those with a hypoplastic tarsus e.g. in congenital ptosis, are at risk of lid eversion after surgery.
● The levator mechanism tends to dehisce more on the medial side causing a shift temporally, thus ptosis repair should take account of this.
● Local anaesthetic with adrenaline causes partial lid retraction as it blocks somatic innervation of levator muscle and activates sympathetic innervation of Müller's muscle, hence final position of lid needs to include 1–2 mm of over-correction. Common complications include under- and over-correction (with corneal exposure) though some degree of lagophthalmos is to be expected after surgery. Other complications include entropion/ectropion and eyelid crease asymmetry.

Surgical treatment of lagophthalmos in facial palsy
Inigo F. *Br J Plast Surg* 1996;**49**:452–456.

Complications of **lagophthalmos** include dryness leading to corneal keratitis and conjunctivitis. Treatment approaches in facial palsy include:

● Artificial tears drops/ointments, protective lenses.
● Lateral tarsorrhaphy, canthoplasty/canthopexy.

● Gold weight, also platinum weights.
● Cross facial nerve grafts to re-innervate orbicularis (ineffective with long-standing paralysis).
● Temporalis turnover flap (but may cause involuntary closure during chewing).

This paper describes a technique of **levator lengthening** using autologous conchal cartilage graft sutured between tarsal plate and levator aponeurosis successful in 11 out of 12 patients. They demonstrated that the width of graft required to reduce the palpebral fissure by 1 mm is ~4 mm.

New technique of levator lengthening for the retracted upper lid
Piggott TA. *Br J Plast Surg* 1995;**48**:127–131.

Lid retraction may occur with Graves' disease or occasionally following an upper blepharoplasty. There are two main approaches:

● Müller's muscle division via a conjunctival incision.
● Division of levator aponeurosis and Müller's muscle via a skin incision.

The paper describes a technique of lengthening the levator aponeurosis by designing 'castellated' flaps in the aponeurosis and suturing the resultant flaps end on end. The length of each flap should be 1 mm more than the desired correction. The authors note that this technique is not suited to skin-loss problems, e.g. burn scar contracture.

Ectropion
Classification

- **Involutional** – Treat by lid shortening e.g. wedge excision ± lower lid blepharoplasty (Kuhnt–Symanowski).
- **Mechanical** e.g. lid tumour, treat by excising the lesion.
- **Cicatricial** – release scar and reconstruct e.g. Z-plasty, FTSG or flap.
- **Paralytic** e.g. VII nerve palsy, can treat as for involutional i.e. Kuhnt–Symanowski or canthoplasty and sling suspension.

Evolution of the lateral canthoplasty: techniques and indications

Glat PM. *Plast Reconstr Surg* 1997;**100**:1396–1405.

Anatomy

The upper and lower tarsal plates are attached via the lateral canthal tendon ('retinaculum') to Whitnall's tubercle inside the lateral orbital rim. The lateral canthal tendon is continuous with the levator aponeurosis in the upper lid and the suspensory ligament of Lockwood in the lower lid.

The main indications for canthoplasty are:

- Correction of horizontal lid laxity or ectropion from paralysis/atony.
- Prevention of cosmetic blepharoplasty lower lid retraction.

Main techniques:

Tarsal strip procedure (Anderson RL. *Arch Ophthalmol* 1979;**97**:2192–2196)

- This causes **horizontal lid shortening** and is thus used for horizontal lid laxity, paralytic and atonic ectropion. A tarsal/dermis strip is raised and anchored to the superolateral orbital rim with or without a pentagonal wedge excision.
- Scissors are placed at the lateral commissure and a full-thickness cut is made into the lateral canthus; the lower half of the lateral canthal tendon retinaculum is isolated and cut free from its attachment to the bone. An incision is made on the eyelid margin a small distance from the cut tendon, and the tarsal plate is cleared of all adherent skin and conjunctiva which creates a small strip of tarsal plate tissue that will become the new tighter tendon and is fixed by non-absorbable suture (4–0 PDS or Mersilene) to the periosteum just inside the orbital rim and reinforced with dissolving sutures. The anterior skin and muscle flap is dissected inferiorly and the excess is trimmed away.

Inferior retinacular lateral canthoplasty: a new technique

Jelks GW. *Plast Reconstr Surg* 1997;**100**:1262–1270.

The inferior limb of the lateral canthal tendon is suspended to the periosteum of the superolateral orbital rim at the level of the upper edge of the pupil which can be performed via an upper eyelid approach (blepharoplasty) incision.

Cosmetic canthoplasty for mild lid retraction in the lateral segment is often used in blepharoplasty to avoid post-operative lower lid retraction or frank ectropion. Less invasive variations on canthal tendon tightening (canthopexy) involve suturing the soft tissues just below the end of the tarsal plate to the tough periosteum of the orbital bone.

Entropion

- In children, entropion can be left alone as it will usually resolve.
- In adults, Kuhnt–Symanowski blepharoplasty as for involutional ectropion.

Thyroid eye disease

This is primarily an autoimmune reaction in extra-ocular muscles and fat. The management is predominantly medical although emergency orbital wall decompression may be needed in some cases.

- Olivari procedure (Olivari N. *Plast Reconstr Surg* 1991;**87**:627–643): lateral canthoplasty and excision of intra-ocular fat using a blepharoplasty approach to upper and lower eyelids. Average 6 ml from four quadrants. Beware of removing too much intraconal fat as it has a high morbidity.

III. Nasal reconstruction

(See also Rhinoplasty.)

The nose is divided into thirds:

- Proximal – over the nasal bones.
- Middle – over upper lateral cartilages.
- Distal – over nasal tip and alar cartilages (lower lateral cartilages). The columella is formed in part from the medial crura of the alar cartilages.

Skin over the upper two-thirds (dorsum and side-walls, upper two zones) is thin, whilst skin over the lower third (lower zone, tip and alar) is thick, sebaceous and more fixed. The skin may also be divided into convex and flat units; flaps which tend to contract at the edges/trapdoor are good choices to replace convex units whilst flat areas are better replaced by FTSG.

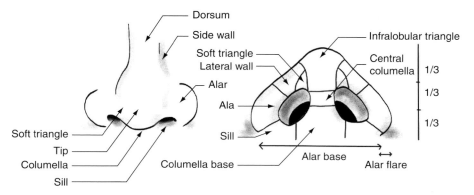

Figure 3.11 Nasal anatomy with subunits (Burget and Menick). The nasal base is often divided into thirds as well as seven subunits.

Sensation

- V1 – radix, rhinion, side-walls (infratrochlear) and skin over dorsum to the tip (nasociliary – external nasal).
- V2 – lateral tissue over lower half of nose, columella and vestibule (infraorbital).

Arterial supply

- Internal carotid – ophthalmic artery to anterior ethmoidal artery, dorsal nasal artery.
- External carotid – facial artery.
  - Superior labial to columellar branch.
  - Angular artery to lateral nasal artery that arises 2–3 mm above the alar groove is the primary blood supply to the nasal tip if transcolumellar incisions are used.

The common reasons for reconstruction are skin cancer, mainly basal cell carcinoma (BCC; 10 times more common than SCC). The aims are good cosmesis combined with good function, primarily a patent airway. Reconstruction of nose needs to consider **skin, support and lining**.

Basal cell carcinoma margins should be ~3 mm minimum for nodular BCCs on the nose, up to ~10 mm for histologically confirmed morphoeic lesions. Bone and cartilage act as barriers to penetration – bone is less commonly invaded than cartilage because there is a loose plane between it and the overlying skin.

- **Cosmetic subunits** (Burget and Menick): dorsum, side-walls, alar lobules, tip, soft triangles and columella. Where there is > 50% skin defect in any one unit, total excision and reconstruction should be considered for optimal results.

Reconstruction needs to consider the defect in terms of its location, the thickness as well as its dimensions.

Reconstruction of the skin

- Healing by secondary intention or primary closure.
  - For example, small defects (< 1 cm square) of the glabella/medial canthus.
- SSG
  - Prone to contracture but makes it 'easier' to monitor recurrence.
  - Consider resurfacing the whole nose as a single cosmetic unit.
- FTSG (pre-/postauricular).
  - Some suggest the use of conchal bowl skin for the tip as the concave skin will mould quite well to the convex tip.
- Composite grafts of skin and cartilage (McLaughlin CR. *Br J Plast Surg* 1954;7:274–278) can be taken from helical rim or root of helix. They are limited to < 1.5 cm in size; the area of dermal contact can be maximized to optimize take.
- Local flaps.
  - **Banner flap** (local transposition flap) for defects < 1 cm^2 of **dorsum/tip**.
  - **Bilobed flap** (Esser JFS. *Dtsch Zschr Chir* 1918; **143**:385; Zitelli JA. *Arch Dermatol* 1989;**125**: 957–959) for defects 1–2 cm^2. Laterally based design flaps can be used for the tip; medial for the lobule. The pivot point should be

positioned away from the alar margin or lower lid to reduce distortion.

- ○ Rieger rotation flap also known as dorsal nasal flap (rotates tissue of whole dorsum inferiorly based on a lateral pedicle – angular artery); similar to a hatchet flap or glabellar flap. This can cover larger defects **up to 2 cm²**.
- ○ Median glabellar advancement flap – needs Burow's triangle excision.
- ○ Nasolabial flap especially **for alar** – superiorly or inferiorly based, one- or two-stage (for best results) or islanded (beware of tendency to trapdoor).
- ○ Cheek advancement flaps **for side-walls** e.g. V–Y cheek flaps.

Pedicled flaps from the forehead

- **'Indian technique'** allows total nasal skin reconstruction, but usually requires 7.5 × 7.5 cm of scalp (35–45% of the forehead).
  - ○ Pre-operative (or intra-operative) subgaleal tissue expansion may be useful but critics point to rebound contraction of flap. Expansion increases vascularity (delay), thins the flap (thus less bulky) and facilitates direct closure of the donor defect.
  - ○ Flap thinning is safe ~1 month post-operation (intradermal steroid injections causing fat atrophy may also be used).
- **Paramedian forehead flap** based on supratrochlear vessels – subperiosteal dissection from a point 2 cm above the supra-orbital rim to the medial canthus helps to preserve them. The flap can be thinned 'distally' (further from the eye) as the vessels become more superficial as they near the hairline. The flap can be canted obliquely for extra length; also it can be based on the contralateral vessel to reduce the arc of rotation.
- **Seagull forehead flap** (Millard) is a modified forehead flap with lateral extensions for covering alae.
- **Scalping rhinoplasty** (Converse, 1942) is based laterally on superficial temporal vessels and makes use of 60–70% of the whole forehead, arching into anterior scalp raised on the subgaleal level. Skeletal elements can be prefabricated with cartilage grafts inset into the flap. The forehead part of the donor is grafted and the scalp donor is dressed. The pedicle is divided after 2–3 weeks and the unused flap returned.

- **Washio temporomastoid flap** – the postauricular skin (and thicker mastoid skin) based on the superficial temporal artery (and its retroauricular branch) is transferred to the nose defect. No delay is required and there are no facial scars.

Technical refinements in the Washio tempororetroauricular flap in reconstruction of the nasal wing Henriksson TG. *Scand J Plast Reconstr Surg Hand Surg* 2005:**39**:295–298.

This is an article reviewing the authors' experience with the flap in seven patients. They included a portion of conchal cartilage in some cases for nostril support.

Distant flaps from the arm

The 'Italian technique' of total nasal skin reconstruction uses a proximally based medial arm skin flap (the original description by Tagliacozzi, 1597 was distally based) with pedicle division after 3 weeks. This technique is of historical interest only.

Free flaps – the commonest choice is a radial forearm flap with or without bone – colour and texture mismatch is a potential issue; microsurgical replantation of an amputated nasal skin has been described. Burget and Menick have described use of the RFFF for the lining whilst using the forehead for the outside coverage.

For total nasal reconstruction free flaps are generally used only when the forehead is not available. The skeletal elements can be prefabricated using cartilage and a lining constructed.

'Distal' dorsalis pedis flap for nasal tip reconstruction
Bayramicli M.*Br J Plast Surg* 1996;**49**:325–327.

The authors used this technique in a patient with tip loss requiring free cartilage grafts and unwilling to undergo staged procedures or have a forehead scar. A skin flap based on dorsalis pedis artery and the long saphenous vein raised from the dorsum of the second toe and the first and second web spaces; the flap was anastomosed to the superior labial artery and facial vein. It may be used with cortex from the second metatarsal to provide support when necessary. It is a thin flap with good aesthetic result (may grow hair) and a very long pedicle, however the donor defect often requires SSG.

Reconstruction of the lining

Small defects will re-epithelialize but the contraction may compromise results (cosmesis and airway);

similarly, SSGs for lining of the inner raw surface of flaps is also not preferred for this reason (some use palatal mucosa).

- In-turning of external nasal skin (similar to a trap-door flap) hinged on the edge.
- Folding of distal part of pedicled e.g. forehead flaps – tends to be rather bulky.
- Nasolabial flaps.
- Intranasal flaps, for example:
  - Septal door/hinge flap (De Quervains) – anteriorly based flap of mucosa and a portion of cartilage (leaving enough septum to provide support) is rotated to close the gap in the external nose/lining at the expense of a septal perforation. The ipsilateral mucosa is removed before it is covered.
  - Septal mucoperichondrial pivot flap – can provide lining and some dorsal skeletal support. The majority of the septum is pulled forward out of the nasal cavity on a narrow pedicle (septal branch of superior labial artery) pivoting near the nasal spine to be folded outward to line the dome area. The raw septal surface in the nasal cavity is left to heal by secondary intention.
  - Mucosal advancement flap for small defects. These can be bipedicled based on septum and piriform aperture.
- Free flaps (see above).

Reconstruction of the skeleton

Ideally, the skeleton should be reconstructed at the same time as skin/lining reconstruction but the vascularity of these tissues (and their ability to support the skeleton) is a consideration e.g. if SSG is used for lining, skeletal elements should probably be deferred to a second stage.

- Midline support.
  - 'L'-shaped costochondral strut (Gillies) from the nasal radix and angulated to contact the anterior nasal spine; the columella tends to be wide with this technique.
  - **Cantilever bone graft** (Converse, Millard) screwed to the nasal radix with a small subjacent bone wedge to provide projection; avoids the problem of a wide columella (Jackson IT. *Ann Plast Surg* 1983;**11**:533–540). Ideally, calvarial graft is used as it is said to be

less prone to resorption and may be harvested via the skin flap incisions
  - Hinged septal flap (Millard) – similar to the 'L'-shaped strut but made from the septum *in situ* hinged superiorly on the caudal end of the nasal bones.
  - Septal pivot flap as above, in combination with a cantilever graft for dorsal support.
- Lateral support – cartilage grafts.
  - Anatomic grafts – supposedly provide improved alar rim correction with less nostril distortion. Autologous cartilage is shaped to resemble the lateral crura and fixed to the residual medial crura or a columellar strut.
  - Non-anatomic.
    - Alar batten grafts for alar collapse and external valve obstruction. Cartilage graft is used to bridge the collapsed area from piriform aperture to lateral third of lateral crura.
    - Lateral crural strut graft – for retraction of the alar rim and malposition of the lateral crura. Long struts are placed between the deep surface of the lateral crus and vestibular skin and sutured, whilst the lateral end extends to the piriform aperture.
    - Alar contour grafts – cartilage buttress is inserted through an infracartilaginous incision into a pocket at the rim.
    - Alar spreader grafts to treat internal nasal valve collapse or pinched tip deformity.
  - Alloplasts – risk implant exposure and infection.
    - Vitallium or titanium mesh.
    - Medpor allows tissue ingrowth, seems to reduce infection rates but is more difficult to remove.

Columellar reconstruction

- Bilateral nasolabial flaps – these can be tunnelled or rolled inwards to line the vestibule and create a central columellar post.
- Forked upper lip flaps – transverse flaps from the upper lip (best for long-lipped patients or the elderly).
- Vestibular flaps (Mavili) – use of internal vestibular skin.
- Forehead flap.
- Chondrocutaneous composite grafts e.g. from auricular for small defects.

- Washio flap (Motamed S. *Br J Plast Surg* 2003;**56**:829–831).

Reconstruction by prosthesis

This is a reasonable choice for debilitated or elderly patients.

- Branemark osseo-integrated prosthesis.
- Prosthesis suspended on spectacles.

Total external and internal construction in arhinia

Meyer R. *Plast Reconstr Surg* 1997;**99**:534–542.

Arhinia is extremely rare and may be associated with CNS abnormalities. Total arhinia includes loss of the entire olfactory system; there is a failure of invagination of nasal placodes hence no nasal cavities (choanal atresia).

Reconstruction is approached in three stages:

- Skin (forehead flap), septum (costochondral graft) and lining (in-turned de-epithelialized flaps and nasolabial flaps).
- Drilling out of the maxilla to provide a communication into the oropharynx and allow nasal breathing while eating; lined by buccal mucosal flaps and reconstruction of alae with composite conchal grafts.
- Widening of nasal airways using a burr, lined with FTSG using fibrin glue and stenting with silicone spacers.

Rhinophyma

This condition is characterized by sebaceous hyperplasia of the nasal skin with erythema and soft tissue enlargement. It is a severe form of acne rosacea and has no association with alcohol intake. It is 12 times more common in males, typically affecting them in middle age and after. There is said to be a risk of malignant change (typically BCC) in up to 15–30%.

Treatment

- Non-surgical – hygiene, tetracyclines, isoretinoin, topical metronidazole.
- Surgical – tangential excision (cold steel, dermabrasion or CO_2 laser) with kaltostat dressing.

IV. Scalp reconstruction and hair restoration

Scalp avulsion occurs in the subgaleal plane. It is usually said that due to the extensive collateral supply, a total scalp avulsion can be replanted on a single set of vascular anastomoses.

Principles

Replace with like tissue

- Use adjacent/remaining scalp if possible; the **parietal scalp is mobile** and the galea can be scored to increase advancement. Flaps should incorporate at least one named vessel.
- Consider tissue expansion – it can be combined with flaps.

Defects should be considered in terms of size, location as well as the causative factor.

- Anterior defects.
  - Smaller – V–Y or rotation advancement (donor site may need grafting).
  - Larger – temporoparietaloccipital flap, Orticochea.
- Parietal defects.
  - Rotation, advancement.
  - Bilobed.
  - Tissue expansion.
- Occipital defects.
  - Rotation/advancement.
- Vertex defects.
  - Pinwheel, rhomboid especially whorl pattern, double opposing rotation/advancement.

Near total defects

- Free flaps are often needed e.g. LD myocutaneous flaps tend to be bulky whilst muscle flaps are thinner and contour well but tend to atrophy and retract (exposing bone) thus need careful tailoring of size. Other options include omentum, RFFF, ALT etc.
- Integra® – can potentially work well over denuded bone, even irradiated bone (as long as it is not actually dead/necrotic), due to its low metabolic requirements.
- Repeated tissue expansion.

Alopecia

McCauley classification

- Type I – single segment of alopecia.
  - A < 25% – use single expander.
  - B 25–50% – use single expander and overinflate.
  - C 50–75% – use multiple expanders.
  - D > 75% use multiple expanders.
- Type II – multiple areas of alopecia amenable to tissue expansion.

- Type III – multiple areas of alopecia not amenable to tissue expansion.
- Type IV – total alopecia.

Calvarial reconstruction

- Autologous.
  - Split clavarial bone especially parietal bone because it is thicker and has fewer underlying sinuses.
  - Split rib – donor sites may regenerate if periosteum is preserved.
- Alloplastic – many choices including methyl methacrylate monomer (MMA) over titanium mesh.

Hair restoration

The average scalp has about 100–150 thousand hairs with more in blondes and less in redheads. Hairs are arranged in **follicular units** – each with 1–4 terminal hairs, 1 vellus hair and approximately 9 sebaceous glands along with perifollicular vessels, nerves and erector pili. The follicles are subcutaneous but the bulb is not absolutely necessary – if the upper two thirds of the follicle survive then 30% will grow.

Hair grows in cycles:

- **Anagen** (87%) this is the phase of active growth that lasts about 3 years or more (longer in females) during which follicular cells proliferate and become keratinized.
- **Catagen** (3%) lasting 3 weeks during which there is degradation of the follicle; the hair base keratinizes and separates from the dermal papillae.
- **Telogen** (10%) this is the resting phase that lasts for about 3 months. Hair is shed (on average 50–100 every day) and the follicle is inactive. With a prolonged telogen and a shortened anagen, hair thinning will result.

Alopecia is hair loss and the commonest cause is androgenic alopecia, i.e. **male pattern baldness** that is relatively common. It is X-linked dominant and related to a defect in the susceptible follicle, either excessive 5 α-reductase activity (testosterone to dihydrotestosterone, DHT) in susceptible (frontal scalp) follicles or excessive sensitivity to DHT. Occipital scalp follicles tend to have reduced activity and are less influenced by hormonal factors making them good donors ('donor dominant') that will grow when transplanted to bald areas.

Other less common causes of alopecia include:

- **Alopecia areata** – unknown cause but involves a perifollicular lymphocytic infiltration. It affects males and females equally. The exclamation point sign is a pathognomonic feature. The natural history is unpredictable, and whilst spontaneous recovery is common so are recurrences.
- **Telogen effluvium** – there is diffuse hair shedding with spontaneous recovery over several months; provoking factors include stress, hormonal upset or medication related.
- Traumatic alopecia – usually related to hairstyle or sometimes trichotillomania (compulsive hair pulling).
- **Cicatricial alopecia** – this subset of alopecia is characterized by the scarring and follicle destruction that occurs. It can be subdivided into secondary causes such as burns, infection etc. or primary cicatricial alopecia (e.g. discoid lupus erythematosus and lichen planopilaris, both uncommon) that is characterized by inflammatory cell infiltrates and can itself be divided into neutrophil-rich, lymphocytic-rich or mixed types. A skin biopsy is usually necessary for diagnosis.

Assessment

Factors that need to be considered include:

- Density of hair – affects donor availability.
- Colour of hair – lighter hair, including grey or 'salt and pepper' allow for more natural-looking results.
- Type of hair – thick or thin, straight or curly (hair with natural wave generally allows better results).

Classification

- Male pattern baldness is most often classified by the **Norwood** modification of the Hamilton classification which has types I (minimal frontotemporal recession) to VII (horseshoe shape).
- Female alopecia is generally classified with the **Ludwig classification** with grades I–III of thinning over the vertex.

Medical therapy for alopecia

These are often used together with surgery.

- **Minoxidil** (Rogaine or Regaine depending on country) – available in 2–5% topical solutions that need to be applied on the scalp twice daily. The main complaint is the 'messiness' but 5% may have skin irritation. Useful results are seen in approximately one-third but it does need to be used indefinitely. It is usually regarded as first-line therapy and there is evidence of a synergistic effect with tretinoin. The exact mechanism of action is unclear though the original medication was intended to treat hypertension; there may be a direct mitogenic effect but it has no antiandrogenic action.

- **Finasteride** (Propecia, Proscar) – this is a 5 α-reductase inhibitor that is effective in reducing further loss but may also increase hair growth in a proportion of patients. There are some side-effects though including 1–2% impotence/reduced libido; it also is rather expensive and needs to be used indefinitely.
- **Spironolactone** being an androgen receptor antagonist also slows down hair loss, and is probably one of the most widely prescribed medications for male pattern baldness.

Surgical treatment

Surgical options include:

- Serial excision (suitable for areas less than 15% of the scalp); scalp reduction may be combined/precede other methods such as hair transplant or local flaps.
- Rotation flaps.
- Tissue expansion – it is said that 50% of defects can be resurfaced this way without noticeable hair thinning.

Scalp reduction i.e. excision of areas of bald scalp can be considered for stable bald areas particularly at the crown/vertex. Serial excision of approximately 4 cm can be performed each time; this can reduce grafting requirements but anterior undermining should be minimized, as this would tend to elevate the brow.

Hair transplantation

Transplantation is contraindicated in:

- Diffuse female pattern baldness.
- Non-donor dominant alopecia.
- Alopecia areata (commonly treated by steroids, minoxidil and phototherapy).
- Active cicatricial alopecia.

The aim of hair transplantation is to achieve natural-looking results whilst minimizing scalp scars – the priority is to achieve a normal anterior hairline. In Norwood types V–VI there is approximately 12.5% of the scalp available as donor areas – the best areas are the occipital and temporal regions. A strip is harvested (some use multi-bladed knifes) and closed directly; the hairs are then divided up into units.

- Micrografts contain 1–2 hairs.
- Minigrafts contain 3–8 hairs.

Smaller grafts are usually placed in the front of the hairline with larger micrografts/minigrafts behind them. Grafts placed in holes e.g. made with needles do not become compressed like grafts placed in slits made by knives, and thus look better – some combine the two together. More than one procedure/grafting session may be needed.

Particular attention must be paid to the direction of the follicles:

- Front/anterior hairline 45–60°.
- Posterior hairline 75–80°.
- Vertex/crown 90° i.e. perpendicular.
- Posterior to crown 45–60° downwards.

Post-operatively, the grafted area is covered with a non-adherent dressing; the hair can be washed by pouring a water-shampoo mix without massage. Normal washing is allowed after 2 weeks.

- No exercise/exertion.
- Avoid direct sunlight.

Four months or more should elapse before judging the results; transplanted hairs grow for about a month before entering telogen for 2–3 months.

Complications

- Lidocaine toxicity.
- Bleeding.
- Infection.
- Scarring.
- Poor growth.
- Poor appearance e.g. unnatural hairline, dolls-head appearance.

V. Lip reconstruction

Anatomy

The upper lip can be subdivided into aesthetic sub-units: lateral and median/philtrum, separated from the cheek by the nasolabial/mesolabial fold.

Muscles

- Orbicularis oris acts to form a whistling expression. The sphincteric activity depends on muscle continuity. The muscle also inserts into dermis and intermingles with nearby muscles.
  - Extrinsic fibres intermingle with buccinator, decussate at the modiolus.
  - Intrinsic fibres – incisive and mental slips.
- Elevators.
  - Levator labii superioris and LLS alaeque nasi (elevates upper lip and flares nostrils).
  - Levator anguli oris.
  - Zygomaticus minor and major (elevates lips).
- Depressors
  - Depressor anguli oris.
  - Depressor labii inferioris.
  - Mentalis (role in lower lip protrusion).
  - Platysma (lowers lower lip).
  - Risorius – from parotid fascia to angle of mouth (draws angle of mouth laterally).

Nerves

- Motor.
  - Upper lip muscles – buccal branch of VII.
  - Lower lip muscles – marginal mandibular branch of VII.
  - Orbicularis oris is supplied by both.
- Sensory
  - Upper lip – infra-orbital nerve (maxillary branch of V).
  - Lower lip – mental nerve (termination of inferior alveolar nerve, mandibular branch of V).

The blood supply comes from superior and inferior labial branches of facial arteries with rich midline anastomoses – a cut labial artery will bleed from both ends. The inferior labial artery branch arises from the facial lateral about 2.5 cm lateral and 1.5 cm inferior to the oral commissure. The artery travels within the orbicularis about 1 mm deep to the white roll.

Lymphatics of the upper lip tend not to cross the midline unless the lesion itself has crossed the midline, going to the preauricular/parotid, submandibular and submental nodes. The lower lip lymph drains to the submandibular and submental nodes. Lymph node metastases are uncommon (10–20% for lower and upper lip respectively) as they tend to occur late and the highly visible nature leads to a relatively early

diagnosis. SCCs and melanomas have a tendency to spread along nerves, which may be suggested by symptoms of numbness or parasthesia.

Pathology

- Most upper lip lesions are BCCs.
- Most lower lip lesions are SCCs (only 5% of SCCs occur on the upper lip) and commissural/mucosal SCCs have a higher propensity for metastasis.

Excision margins should be 5–10 mm for SCCs.

- Tumour size and thickness also correlate with metastatic potential.
- May need to combine surgery with radiotherapy.

T staging of lip SCC

As for intra-oral SCC if involving mucosa.

- T1 tumour < 2 cm.
- T2 tumour > 2–4 cm.
- T3 tumour > 4 cm.
- T4 tumour invades adjacent structures (bone, tongue, skin of neck).

Lip reconstruction

Ideally the reconstructed lip should be competent – it should be sensate and have a complete innervated muscle ring. In addition, for the lower lip in particular, a good sulcus (to prevent drooling). Other considerations include cosmesis (symmetry and preservation of landmarks – particularly the vermilion border – single 'l', derived from the French vermeil, a red dye – classically vermiculum from *Kermes vermilio* the insects that feed primarily on Kermes oak) and speech.

- The defect can be analysed using the size (absolute and relative), depth and involvement of commissure.
- The mucosal incisions can often be shorter than the skin incisions due to its extensibility.
- When using double opposing advancement-rotation flaps for off-centre defects, the contralateral lower lip is made the longer limb to avoid using excessive ipsilateral upper lip tissue.

Local anaesthesia may be sufficient for small to moderate reconstructions:

- Upper lip – bilateral infra-orbital nerve blocks (1 cm below the inferior orbital rim in line with the medial limbus).

- Lower lip – bilateral mental nerve blocks (intra-oral infiltration in line with the lower canines; nerve may be visible by putting the lower lip on the stretch).

Vermilion defects

- A small notch defect can be closed by V–Y advancement of buccal mucosa.
- Partial (up to 50%) defects can be closed by axial sliding musculovermilion advancement, deep to the level of the labial artery. Other options include simple advancement (dissection between mucosa and muscle), V–Y advancement as above or vermilion lip-switch (dividing at 2 weeks).
- Subtotal (50%) defects can be closed with a tongue flap (two-staged muscle mucosa flap) but the aesthetics are suboptimal compared with lip/mucosa.
- Total defects – mucosal advancement provides a good colour match but the mucosa may become dry and scaly.

Lower lip reconstruction

In situ cancer may be treated by lip shave and mucosal advancement (may need incisional release to convert into a bipedicled flap) or CO_2 laser.

Losses of up to one-third of the lower lip may be closed directly (more if elderly) whilst larger defects will require recruitment of additional tissue in the form of various flaps. Wedge excisions can be shield or W (skirting around the mental/labiomental crease) or a so-called 'double barrelled excision' – the lip segment is full-thickness whilst the chin segment is skin/subcutaneous tissue takes only.

Defects one- to two-thirds of the lower lip

- **Abbé flap** – some are loathe to violate the upper lip to reconstruct the lower (vide infra).
- **Abbé–Estlander flap** (defects of the commissure/lower lateral lip) – the flap is designed to be half the width of the defect, pedicled on the contralateral side. Initial descriptions were two-staged, but most commonly it is used for lateral defects and is single-staged but the segment is insensate and the modiolus is distorted affecting animation (may need commissure reconstruction later). The vascularity is more tenuous than the Abbé flap as the pedicle is based on the contralateral artery which is further away.
- **Karapandzic flap is** a neurovascular circumoral advancement flap that transfers skin, muscle and mucosa that achieves correct muscle orientation but requires an intact commissure. The circumoral incision is the height of the defect, and goes through skin and superficial facial muscles (with limited mucosal incision) but preserves neurovascular supply to orbicularis oris whilst dividing radial elevators or depressors. However, preserving nerves means that **advancement is limited** (compared with Gillies/McGregor) and so usually needs to be bilateral for moderate defects. It can be used for lower or upper lip (may need Burow's triangle excision) defects.
  - It introduces no new tissue and hence leads to microstomia though this will stretch to a certain extent.
- **Gillies fan flap** – some regard it as being halfway between a Karapandzic flap and a McGregor flap. It is an insensate myocutaneous flap but the muscle is denervated and is suited for upper or lower lip defects next to the commissure; it can be raised bilaterally for total upper lip reconstruction. There have been many modifications.
  - For the lower lip, the flap is cut back to the nasolabial fold – it **advances** along rather than rotates into the defect and thus the commissure moves medially (and becomes rounded); again no new tissue is recruited – the lower lip is still shortened but less so than with a Karapandzic flap.
  - A Z-plasty modification allows better turning around the commissure (Panje WR. *Otolaryngol Clin North Am* 1982;**15**:169–178) and is similar to a McGregor flap.
- **McGregor flap** is a myocutaneous flap composed of three approximately equally sized squares that **rotates** around the commissure which remains in the same place. As it introduces **new tissue** into the lip, microstomia is avoided.
  - The new lip is devoid of vermilion which can be reconstructed by mucosal advancement or tongue flap.
  - There is a lack of a functionally complete muscle ring but the theoretical risk of drooling is rarely observed.
  - A Nakajima flap is similar but preserves the neurovascular bundle inferolaterally.
- **Johanson's step technique** – a central defect is approximated by creating step cuts in the soft tissue of the chin; it can close defects up to 50%, though with larger defects microstomia will result.

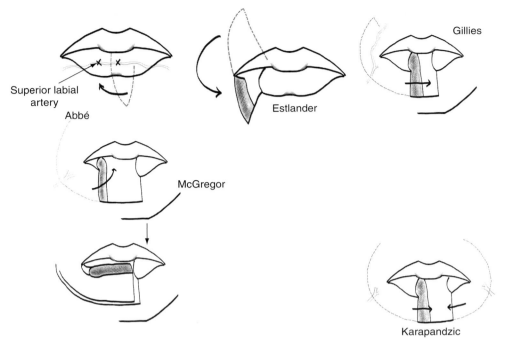

Figure 3.12 Different types of lip reconstruction.

Defects greater than two-thirds of the lower lip

- Bilateral McGregor or other flaps.
- **Webster–Bernard/Bernard–Burow** flaps – **advances cheek and chin tissue**, with excisional triangles (leaving mucosa) on the cheek. The vermilion is reconstructed by advancement of buccal mucosa. There is less microstomia compared with bilateral Karapandzic/Gillies flaps but at the cost of more scarring, and reduced muscle function (thus potentially reducing oral competence) – thus some suggest that it may be more suited for upper lip reconstruction. It is generally advised that simultaneous neck dissection should be avoided in these patients.
- Steeple flap – an islanded composite cheek flap based on the facial artery, but it is denervated, hence there is sensory and motor loss. Simultaneous neck dissection is avoided.
- Free tissue transfer.
  - Thin fasciocutaneous flaps e.g. radial forearm flap with palmaris longus sling (medial cutaneous nerve of the forearm for a sensate flap) or ALT with fascia lata sling. These flaps tend to have a poor colour match (landmarks such as the vermilion border are difficult to reconstruct) and do not have functioning muscle.
  - Myocutaneous flap e.g. gracilis with coaptation of motor nerve.

Upper lip reconstruction

Upper lip cancers are much less common. Defects with an intact vermilion may be closed by nasolabial flaps, though these may disrupt the nasolabial fold (can minimize by subsequent revision) and create a trap-door scar.

- Loss of up to one-quarter of the upper lip may be closed directly.
- For slightly larger defects, simple advancement flaps may be combined with crescentic perialar excisions.
- **Abbé flap** (Robert Abbé 1851–1928, American surgeon and radiologist – he was a good friend of Marie Curie). Whilst midline upper lip defects can often be easily closed directly this will mean the loss of the normal philtral appearance. The Abbé

flap, lip-switch pedicled on the lateral side of the donor lip, is a useful option for central defects, especially in women, and can also be used for lateral defects up to 50% of the upper lip.

- A flap of the same height but **half the width** of the defect along with a skin/subcutaneous only 'Burow's triangle along the mental crease allows easy donor closure. The position of the artery is noted on the free/unpedicled side; a cuff of muscle is left around the pedicle – there is often no recognized accompanying vein and the soft tissue is said to improve venous return. The bridge is divided after 2–3 weeks.
  - With more central defects, the flap that has a rotation point that allows the greatest amount of mouth opening, which usually means that the pedicle is based on the contralateral artery.
  - It theoretically reconstructs muscle continuity, but the segment tends to be rather insensate – some sensation may return after several months in the order of pain, touch and temperature.
- Karapandzic flap (vide supra).
- Estlander (vide supra) is similar to the Abbé flap but used for lateral defects involving the commissure.

For larger defects (greater than two-thirds):

- If there is sufficient cheek tissue for advancement, then Bernard–Burow's – bilateral for central defects or ipsilateral combined with contralateral perialar advancement for lateral defects.
- With insufficient cheek tissue, free flaps need to be considered e.g. RFFF.

Microsurgical replantation of the lip: a multi-institutional experience
Walton RL. *Plast Reconstr Surg* 1998;**102**:358–368.

This is a retrospective review of 13 separate reports of lip replantation all due to bite injuries; upper lip injuries were twice as common. Anastomoses of labial vessels were performed (< 1 mm in diameter) though reconnection of vein was not feasible in one-half of patients. Regardless of venous repair, there was venous congestion in all patients which was treated by leeches (that left visible scars) and systemic heparinization used in 11/13.

All replants survived ultimately and although almost all required subsequent scar revision, the aesthetic and functional results were better than possible with other methods of reconstruction.

Reconstruction of electrical burns of the oral commissure
Donelan MB. *Plast Reconstr Surg* 1995;**95**:1155–1164.

It is very difficult to reconstruct the specialized structure of the commissure:

- Thin mobile lip segment.
- Moves dynamically and symmetrically.

In burns, a conservative approach is usually adopted initially with secondary reconstruction (including scar contracture release) at a later stage. The author describes the use of an anteriorly based **ventral myomucosal tongue flap** to reconstruct the lower lip portion of the commissure with pedicle division at 2 weeks. It provides good volume of tissue but the combination of awkward tongue position and significant swelling post-operatively means that a soft or liquid diet is needed for several days.

The upper lip portion of the commissure is reconstructed with a Gillies–Millard flap which is a superiorly based flap raised from the scarred commissure and rotated upwards to lengthen the upper lip. Scar release is performed through the flap incisions.

VI. Cheek reconstruction

The cheek is divided into three aesthetic subunits or zones:

- Zone 1: **suborbital zone** from the lower eyelid down to the gingival sulcus and from the nasolabial fold to the anterior sideburn.
- Zone 2: **pre-auricular zone** from the tragus to the anterior sideburn and from the junction of the helical rim with the cheek down to the mandible.
- Zone 3: **buccomandibular** – area inferior to the suborbital zone and anterior to the pre-auricular zone.

Suborbital zone

Reconstructive options:

- Direct closure with a vertically orientated scar.
- FTSG.
- Local flaps including
  - Limberg, V–Y, McGregor flap for defects less than 4 cm.
  - Cervicofacial flap for larger defects, with wide undermining and incorporating the platysma into the flap. To reduce the risk of ectropion, the flap should be anchored to the periosteum

at the zygomatic arch and inferior rim of orbit; a lateral canthopexy may be needed.

- ○ Tissue expansion – ideally two or more expanders.
- See also lower eyelid reconstruction.

Pre-auricular zone

Reconstructive options:

- Direct closure (facelift-type undermined flap).
- Local flaps: Limberg flap, hatchet flap, anteriorly based cervicopectoral flaps.
- Distant flaps: pectoralis major (bulky), latissimus dorsi myocutaneous flaps (tunnelled over or through PM), deltopectoral flaps (with delay to increase reliability of the tip, e.g. tie off thoracoacromial perforator a week before).
- Free flaps: particularly if > 10cm – radial forearm, scapular flap, ALT, lateral arm; conventionally fasciocutaneous flaps are preferred as they atrophy less.

Buccomandibular zone (cheek proper)

Reconstructive options:

- Skin only: direct closure, FTSG, local flaps and distant flaps as above.
- Lining: tunnelled nasolabial flap, axial tongue flap (based on a lingual artery), flaps which epithelialize including buccal fat flaps, galeal flaps (with periosteum) and masseter cross-over flaps.
- Skin and lining: double skin paddle pectoralis major, deltopectoral flap, free flaps including radial forearm (± bone, tendon), scapular flap.
- Flaps in combination for reconstructing lining and skin separately.

Cervicofacial flap

This flap can be used for reconstruction of zones 1 or 3.

- Inferiorly based rotation flap moving postauricular skin anteriorly onto the cheek.
- Posteriorly based rotation flap moving neck skin upwards onto the cheek.

The plane of dissection is deep to SMAS and the platysma is included in the flap. The flap should be anchored e.g. to zygomatic or infra-orbital periosteum to prevent ectropion.

Guidelines for head and neck tissue expansion

(Wieslander JB. *Scand J Plast Reconstr Surg Hand Surg* 1991;**25**:47–56.)

- Choose an expander with a length and width at least as large as the defect.
- Choose an incision perpendicular to the direction of planned expansion.
- Fill the expander at the conclusion of the operation to a safe volume to reduce seroma/haematoma.
- Wait 2 weeks for healing before beginning expansion, and then continue weekly.
- Overexpand to 30–50% estimated required volume to overcome flap contraction at the second stage.
- Capsule can be incised to increase stretch but avoid a full capsulectomy.

Contour defects

Cheek contour defects may be part of Romberg's, hemifacial microsomia, facial lipodystrophy (which may be associated with AIDS/HIV treatment) or trauma. Options include:

- Fillers e.g. collagen, semi-permanent (Sculptura – poly-L-lactic acid), dermal/dermofat, fat injections (50% loss).

De-epithelialized flaps e.g. platysma, free flaps as above including omentum.

D. Management of patients requiring radical or selective neck dissection

I. Neck anatomy

Fascial layers

The deep cervical fascia has four components:

- **Investing fascia.** This is the layer of deep fascia that lies beneath the subcutaneous fat and splits into superficial and deep layers as the parotid fascia surrounds the gland. A local thickening forms the stylomandibular ligament.
- **Prevertebral fascia.** This covers the muscles that form the floor of the posterior triangle and forms a layer over which the pharynx and oesophagus can freely slide. It covers the brachial plexus trunks and subclavian artery but **not** the subclavian vein and is pierced by the four nerves of the cervical plexus.
- **Pretracheal fascia.** This separates the trachea from the overlying strap muscles to allow free gliding of

the trachea. It encloses the thyroid gland (pierced by the thyroid vessels) and blends laterally with the carotid sheath.

- **Carotid sheath.** This envelopes the carotid arteries (common and internal), the internal jugular vein (thin) and vagus nerve and is adherent to the deep surface of sternocleidomastoid.

Triangles of the neck

Posterior triangle

The borders are the anterior border of trapezius, middle third of clavicle and posterior border of SCM. The posterior belly of omohyoid subdivides into an upper occipital triangle and a lower supraclavicular triangle. **The investing fascia** forms the roof whilst the floor is composed of the **prevertebral fascia** (overlying the muscles: splenius capitis, levator scapulae, scalenus posterior, medius and anterior; also the three trunks of the brachial plexus).

Contents:

- Lymphatics.
  - Lymph nodes: occipital, supraclavicular and lowermost deep cervical nodes.
  - Thoracic duct enters the junction of internal jugular vein (IJV) and subclavian vein on the left side.
- Nerves.
  - Accessory nerve crosses from upper third SCM to lower third trapezius within the fascial roof.
  - Cutaneous branches of cervical plexus.
    - Lesser occipital C2, greater auricular C2, 3, transverse cervical C2, 3 and supraclavicular C3, 4.
  - Muscular branches of the cervical plexus.
    - C1 travelling with XII forms the superior root of the ansa whilst C2,3 forms the inferior root of the ansa.
    - C2, 3 to SCM.
    - C3, 4 to trapezius.
    - C3, 4, 5 as the phrenic nerve to the diaphragm.
  - The plexus lies on scalenus anterior beneath the prevertebral fascia and may be joined by the accessory phrenic nerve, a branch from the nerve to subclavius (from the brachial plexus).
- Vessels.
  - Transverse cervical and suprascapular vessels from the thyrocervical trunk – these may be

important 'stand-by' vessels in the vessel-depleted neck.
  - Subclavian artery lies low down in the triangle.
  - External jugular vein.
- Muscle – omohyoid.

Anterior triangle

The borders are the anterior border of SCM, lower border of the mandible and the midline; note that it does not meet the posterior triangle being separated by the width of the sternomastoid muscle. The roof consists of the platysma and deep cervical fascia.

It can be subdivided into:

- Submandibular (digastric) and submental triangles by the anterior belly of the digastric muscle.
- Carotid (jugulodigastric) and muscular triangles by the omohyoid muscle.

Contents:

- Lymph nodes: deep cervical nodes (which are closely adherent to internal jugular vein), submandibular and submental nodes.
- Nerves.
  - X lies within the carotid sheath and superior laryngeal branch.
  - Lingual branch of V3 (one of the three sensory branches from the posterior division).
  - XI (at apex of the triangle).
  - XII.
  - Ansa cervicalis.
- Vessels.
  - Common carotid has no branches proximal to its bifurcation at C4 (upper border of thyroid cartilage). The internal carotid artery has no branches in the neck whilst the external carotid has multiple branches.
  - IJV lies lateral to the internal carotid artery; the facial, lingual, superior and middle thyroid veins.
- Muscles.
  - Suprahyoid muscles: digastric, stylohyoid, mylohyoids, geniohyoids and hyoglossus.
  - Infrahyoid strap muscles: sternohyoid and omohyoid superficial, thyrohyoid and sternothyroid deeper.
  - Other soft tissue:
    - Hyoid bone and thyroid cartilage.
    - Thyroid and parathyroid glands.

– Submandibular and sublingual salivary glands.
– Trachea and oesophagus.

Branchial cysts, if present, will lie in the anterior triangle. The classic presentation is as a soft, cystic mass anterior to the sternomastoid that contains straw-coloured fluid with cholesterol crystals. They are usually well encapsulated but can extend to the lateral pharyngeal wall.

Suprahyoid region

This includes the digastric (submandibular) and sub-mental triangles between the mandible, the hyoid bone and the two posterior bellies of digastric.

- Nodes: submental and submandibular lymph nodes.
- Nerves:
  - Lingual nerve spiralling around (crossing twice) the submandibular duct of Wharton.
  - Hypoglossal nerve.
- Vessels: the anterior jugular veins drain into the external jugular veins in the posterior triangle.
- Muscles: supra- and infrahyoids as above.
  - Other soft tissue: submandibular (and duct) and sublingual salivary glands.

The role of MRI scanning in the diagnosis of cervical lymphadenopathy
Wilson GR. *Br J Plast Surg* 1994;**47**:175–179.

MRI is capable of identifying all enlarged nodes > 4–5 mm diameter (i.e. 100% sensitive) but it cannot reliably differentiate between benign and malignant lymphadenopathy (53% specific for malignant lymphadenopathy).

Clinical examination is unreliable in many patients with 30% false-positive and 40% false-negative, and misses nodes up to 2 cm in diameter, especially if deep to SCM.

- Clinically negative neck but high risk: MRI scan to confirm node status.
- Clinically positive neck: FNA with neck dissection if histologically confirmed.

T1-weighted images (relaxation time for protons to align to the magnetic field):

- Tumours generally appear **darker** than normal surrounding tissues.
- Fat has high (bright) signal.
- Fluid has low (dark) signal.

- Contrast (gadolinium) increases T1 relaxation time and so nodes become brighter (more iso-intense with fat) and hence not useful in this context in defining nodes.

T2-weighted images (relaxation time for protons to 'dephase') with opposite tumour, fat and fluid signals (fat dark, fat suppression).

II. Torticollis

Torticollis: *tortus* (twisted) *collum* (neck).

Congenital

Torticollis in children is likely to be congenital (0.5% of births).

- The actual cause is usually unknown; it may be due to a primary fibrosis of sternocleidomastoid. There may be a palpable mass within the substance of the muscle in the first few weeks that then gradually dissipates but may leave an area of fibrosis.
- It is loosely associated with possible birth trauma with difficult deliveries (primparous, breech etc.) in up to 60% of cases and a muscle-specific compartment syndrome either during delivery or perinatal (in utero crowding) is another theory. It may run in some families.
- In some cases it is compensatory e.g. vertical orbital dystopia (craniosynostoses, facial clefts, hemifacial microsomia) – child holds head on one side to compensate and attain stereoscopic vision. These are called **positional torticollis as** opposed to muscular torticollis above (those with a mass or 'tumour' form a separate subcategory).

Rare 'atypical torticollis' e.g. posterior fossa tumours, cervical cord tumours.

In idiopathic cases, the initial treatment is physiotherapy, 5–10% may need surgery (best between 1–4 years of age). Those who have postural torticollis tend not to need surgery for the torticollis itself.

Acquired torticollis

This is torticollis presenting in a previously normal patient. Most cases are idiopathic, though a small number develop it secondarily. In addition, most cases are usually mild with either jerking or prolonged involuntary position.

In adults (25–60 years old), this is most commonly spasmodic and is a form of focal cervical dystonia, a chronic movement disorder. It was previously thought to be a psychiatric illness, but is now viewed as a neurological illness. The aetiology is unknown but may follow trauma. In some families it is inherited (autosomal dominant with reduced penetrance).

- 10–20% of patients may experience remission, but nearly all patients relapse within 5 years and are left with persistent disease.
- Botulinum toxin is the most effective treatment but reports of development of neutralizing antibodies occurs in 5–10% of patients (though this is based on previous older formulations and higher dosage regimes). Anticholinergics and baclofen may also help e.g. 50% relief with anticholinergics but with significant side-effects.
- Sternocleidomastoid (SCM) myoplasty after failed conservative management; selective denervation of the muscles responsible for the abnormal movement or posture.

Musculoskeletal (e.g. cervical spine abnormalities), ophthalmologic (e.g. congenital nystagmus) infectious (e.g. parapharyngeal abscess), neurologic, posterior fossa tumours and trauma (e.g. brachial plexus palsy) and neoplastic conditions may present early with only torticollis thus the first step in evaluation is always a careful and complete physical examination.

Congenital muscular torticollis and associated craniofacial changes

Hollier L. *Plast Reconstr Surg* 2000;**105**:827–835.

In this study, 16 patients with congenital torticollis were assessed for associated craniofacial abnormalities. The left side of the neck was affected in 80%. All patients were initially managed by physiotherapy with surgical release, myoplasty (step lengthening) or resection of SCM in four patients.

Associated abnormalities included:

- Displacement of the ipsilateral ear (backwards and downwards).
- Ipsilateral eye inferiorly displaced.
- Deviation of the nasal tip to the affected side.
- Recession of the ipsilateral zygoma and mandibular displacement (chin points to affected side).

Vertical orbital dystopia

Tan ST. *Plast Reconstr Surg* 1996;**97**:1349–1361.

In this condition, the orbits lie on unequal horizontal planes. Associations include:

- Cranio-facio-cervical scoliosis complex: hemifacial microsomia, torticollis, cervical abnormalities.
- Goldenhar syndrome.
- Unilateral coronal synostosis, asymmetric bilateral coronal synostosis.
- Craniofacial clefts.
- Trauma.
- Fibrous dysplasia.

Treatment requires orbital translocation but not if it is the only seeing eye. The eye on the affected side may be blind or amblyopic.

- Bicoronal approach.
- Osteotomies around the orbit to allow movement in the coronal plane as required; it is easier to elevate the lower orbit, as lowering an orbit requires subjacent wedge resection.
- Medial canthal ligament and lacrimal apparatus are left attached; if impossible, then transnasal canthopexy is indicated.
- If the frontal sinus is inadvertently opened, it is cranialized and the frontonasal duct plugged with diploic bone.

Transient diplopia may occur post-operatively in patients with normal vision pre-operatively.

III. Neck dissection

Management of neck nodes

Surgical education: neck dissection

Chummun S. *Br J Plast Surg* 2004;**57**:610–623.

The occurrence of cervical node metastases in patients with head and neck cancer **reduces survival by 50%**. The presence of any palpable lymph nodes means that the cancer becomes stage III or IV.

Risk factors for metastases:

- Anterior tumours are less likely to metastasize compared with posteriorly located tumours.
- Highest risk of nodal metastases is associated with tongue tumours.
- T-stage and thickness (highest risk >8 mm thick, lowest <2 mm).
- Histology including perineural and perivascular invasion.

Radiotherapy reduces the risk of post-operative neck failure by >50%.

Node levels (Memorial Sloan-Kettering)

- Level Ia   submental triangle.
- Level Ib   submandibular triangle.
- Level II   upper deep cervical/jugulodigastric.
- Level III   mid deep cervical.
- Level IVa   lower deep cervical – deep to sternal head of SCM.
- Level IVb   lower deep cervical – deep to clavicular head of SCM.
- Level Va   posterior triangle – along accessory nerve (omohyoid).
- Level Vb   posterior triangle – along transverse cervical artery.
- Level VI   anterior compartment.
- Level VII   upper mediastinum (this is no longer used).

Patterns of spread

There tend to be typical patterns of lymphatic spread:

- Enlarged supraclavicular node usually indicates a primary site below the clavicle e.g. breast, bronchus, stomach, pancreas.
- Enlarged level nodes III–V usually means a primary site in the mid-neck e.g. thyroid, larynx, pharynx.
- Enlarged jugulodigastric node suggests a primary in the oral cavity, face or scalp.

With multiple enlarged nodes, consider the diagnosis of lymphoma and check other node basins and liver/spleen.

Pattern of lymph node metastases in intra-oral squamous cell carcinoma

Sharpe DT. *Br J Plast Surg* 1981;**34**:97–101.

Radical neck dissection specimens from 98 patients with **intra-oral SCC** were examined. The important conclusions were:

- There were no lymph node metastases in posterior triangle, submental triangle, salivary glands or sternomastoid muscle.
- There were predictable patterns of lymph node involvement:
  - Hard palate and maxilla   level I.
  - Lower lip   levels I and II.
  - Floor of mouth and alveolus   levels I and II.
  - Tongue   levels I and II.
- No lower internal jugular nodes (levels III and IV) were involved in the absence of disease higher up.

- The more anterior the lesion, the more likely that level I nodes would be involved first; the more posterior the lesion, the more likely that level II nodes would be involved first.

The conclusion was that functional neck dissection, preserving the accessory nerve in the posterior triangle and SCM, would be **oncologically safe**.

Classification of neck dissection

A neck dissection removes lymph nodes in a block from the neck. It can be therapeutic and or prognostic (staging). The contralateral neck is usually left alone except for tumours of the tongue tip or those crossing the midline.

Management of nodal disease

- N1 – surgery (if node > 3 cm) or radiotherapy (if node < 3 cm).
- N2 – selective or MRND III.
- N3 – MRND I/RND.

It can be considered in N0 necks (clinical examination is only two-thirds accurate at best):

- Risk of subclinical disease is high.
  - Consider site – lip, sinus, glottis vs. oral cavity/pharynx.
  - Tumour factors such as size, thickness, histology e.g. T3/4 N0 tongue usually selective neck dissection (SND).
- Provides surgical access to tumour or vessels for reconstruction.
- For patients who are difficult to follow up.

Note that level V is rarely involved in clinically N0 necks.

Radical neck dissection (Crile 1906)

All nodes in levels I–V are removed along with the SAN, IJV and SCM.

Indications:

- Recurrent tumours.
- Level II node encasing accessory node ± extracapsular spread.
- Post-irradiation field.

Modified radical neck dissection

The modified radical neck dissection spares some non-lymphatic structures in an effort to reduce the morbidity of the procedure.

- **Sternocleidomastoid** – the concerns are mostly in the cosmetic/contour deformity, though the muscle may offer protection for the carotid artery particularly when flap necrosis or fistula formation occurs. Its loss results in the least morbidity of the three non-lymphatic structures sacrificed during RND thus it is most often sacrificed (subtypes I and II).
- **Internal jugular vein** – bilateral IJV resection is associated with serious complications such as raised ICP, oedema, stroke and death (0–3% mortality for staged RND vs. 10–14% for simultaneous RND – Dulguerov P. *Laryngoscope* 1998;**108**:1692–1696). Some clinicians believe that risks are reduced if the operative time is less than 5–6 hours, but most prefer either staged procedures or IJV reconstruction if bilateral IJV resection is necessary. The IJV is an important recipient vein for microvascular surgical reconstruction. Post-operative patency rates are very high though it may be affected by radiotherapy.
- **Spinal accessory nerve** – nerve injury results in dysfunction of the trapezius muscle causing the shoulder to droop as the scapula is shifted laterally and rotated downward – thus patients have an asymmetric neckline, a drooping shoulder, winging of the scapula, and weakness of forward elevation but complain mostly of shoulder stiffness/discomfort with decreased range of motion, particularly shoulder abduction. Conversely, sparing the nerve reduces shoulder and neck pain and reduces the need for pain medications (Terrell JE. *Laryngoscope* 2000;**110**:620–626).

Suarez presented anatomical work that demonstrated that the lymphatics are generally well compartmentalized away from the non-lymphatic structures by fascial layers. Bocca proposed the term 'functional neck dissection' in 1967; different subtypes and classifications were proposed by Medina, Robbins and Byers in 1989, 1991 and 1994 respectively.

The subtypes are often referred to as 'Medina subtypes':

- Type 1: preserves accessory nerve only.
- Type 2: preserve nerve and the internal jugular vein.
- Type 3: preserve nerve, vein and SCM – this is equivalent to Bocca's 'functional neck dissection'

(although he originally spared the submandibular gland).

The type of MRND performed depends upon clearance of the tumour and is often determined **on-table**. Although formalized indications for MRND have not been created and clinicians vary in their preference, in general terms MRND is indicated wherever possible without oncologic compromise.

The relationship of nodal metastases to the trio of structures is evaluated using inspection and palpation e.g. IJV thrombosis. Inability to develop a clean plane of dissection that preserves the thick reactive fibrous tissue around nodes means that the structures need to be sacrificed.

Selective neck dissection

The selective neck dissection that leaves some lymph node groups based on a predictable pattern of spread was first described in Hanley 1980. It is often performed to gain 'access'.

- Suprahyoid dissection: removes level I submental and submandibular nodes from the suprahyoid region.
- **Supra-omohyoid dissection** is a common option for N0 anterior tongue and FOM tumours. It can be performed *en passant* while gaining access to the tumour and removes nodes in levels I–III along with occipital nodes in the posterior triangle.
  - There is a 3.5% failure rate (Shah JP. *Cancer* 1990;**66**:109–113) but the thoracic duct is not at risk, whilst the SCM, accessory nerve and internal jugular vein is spared (like type 3 MRND).
  - It is not suitable for parotid and tonsillar tumours as these all drain preferentially to level IV and V.
- Posterolateral neck dissection removes occipital nodes along with posterior triangle (V) and jugulodigastric chain (II–IV) – is an option in posterior scalp tumours.
- Anterolateral II–IV for oro/hypopharynx and larynx.

Extended radical neck dissection

This is an RND along with additional resection (additional nodes or non-lymphatic structures).

- Paratracheal dissection (VI and VII).
- Parotidectomy.

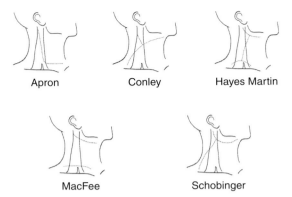

Figure 3.13 The main types of incisions for neck dissections. There are many subtle variations on each type e.g. the Conley-type incisions are often called 'Y-shaped' whilst the Hayes Martin is a 'double-Y'.

Operative technique – modified radical neck dissection

Tracheostomy may be needed for bilateral neck dissection: use either a vertical or horizontal incision through the level of the second tracheal ring, with a cuffed Shiley tube size 8 in most cases.

- Bjork flap – an inferiorly based flap with the edge stitched to the skin, originally introduced for safe reintroduction of displaced tubes, though there are concerns that if sutures cut out then the tube cannot be reinserted. In addition, the stoma is slower to close down and is said to be associated with a higher rate of stenosis.

Position the patient slightly head up with the neck extended (sandbag under the shoulders) and the head turned away from the operative side. Many types of skin incisions have been described but optimizing exposure safely is the priority – most commonly a 'Y' incision (e.g. Conley, or variant) with a curved vertical limb to avoid contracture whilst many prefer an apron type incision to avoid the trifucation. The MacFee incision is advocated if the neck has already been irradiated though some people use it as their 'default'.

- **Raise the skin flaps** deep to platysma to mandible, clavicle and trapezius whilst preserving the marginal mandibular and cervical branches of VII in the upper flap and greater auricular nerve and accessory nerve also. The external jugular vein should be preserved for a venous anastomosis if possible.
- Clear the submental then the submandibular triangles from anterior to posterior, to the

posterior border of the mylohyoid which is then retracted to allow identification of the submandibular gland and the structures around it. Take care to avoid injury to marginal mandibular nerve whilst freeing the submandibular gland; ligating the duct and the facial artery twice in the process. The lingual nerve is deep to the gland whilst the hypoglossal nerve is deep to the posterior belly of digastric as well as Wharton's duct; the superior attachment of the SCM to the mastoid can be divided.

- ○ Digastric muscle – 'Residents friend'.
- ○ Erb's point – where great auricular nerve crosses over posterior border of SCM.
- Elevate the level 1 contents downwards to identify the superior IJV and determine its condition. Identify the SAN and also determine how the nodes relate to it as well as the SCM.
- Then define the posterior border of the posterior triangle (**trapezius**) taking care to leave the great auricular nerve (and accessory) and then elevate the contents in a posterior to anterior direction. Identify the spinal accessory nerve and dissect it free along its course through the posterior triangle from SCM to trapezius. The apical nodal tissue above the nerve is flipped under the nerve. Deep dissection continues on top of splenius and levator scapulae; the phrenic nerve and brachial plexus will be exposed.
- Approach level IV nodes under the SCM muscle if it is to be spared; otherwise divide it at the clavicle to expose the internal jugular vein. During exposure of the carotid sheath, the branches of the cervical plexus going into the specimen need to be divided whilst identifying and preserving the phrenic nerve. The dissection proceeds over the IJV (identifying the vagus nerve in the carotid sheath) and carotid artery. Going upwards, divide the omohyoid from its attachment to the hyoid (absent in 10%) to elevate zones II and III. The hypoglossal nerve is seen again at the top of the IJV.
- The specimen can then be removed and should be marked for histology. The operative field is irrigated with sterile water before close over drains.

There are many variations – major and minor – for example, the dissection can proceed in reverse, starting with clearance of the posterior triangle before the submental/submandibular area.

Complications of neck dissection

There is a 1% mortality rate associated with the operation.

Intra-operative

- Nerve injury: IX–XII, lingual, phrenic and sympathetic chain (Horner's) – manipulation of the carotid bulb may cause bradyarrhythmias/arrhythmias.
- Inadvertent vessel injury – especially internal jugular vein (note risk of air embolus), and if this happens, then:
  ○ Anaesthetist should be informed – ask for head down.
  ○ Control the vein, especially distally to prevent air entering the circulation.
  ○ Then isolate the bleeding point and repair if possible.
  ○ If there is continued oozing, then using the SCM to plug it may help.
  ○ If air embolism has already occurred (reduces cardiac output) then the air may be aspirated with a central line or directly through the skin.

Early post-operative

- Airway problems.
- Infection.
- Seroma/haematoma.
- Carotid blow-out (salivary fistula, previous radiation therapy).
- Skin flap necrosis (especially posterior flap), wound dehiscence (up to 1/4) with the risk of vessel exposure. Previously irradiated vessels are at greater risk of blow-out; protective coverage with a muscle flap should be considered.
- Lymphatic fistula (1–2% of neck dissections):
  ○ Repair if recognized intra-operatively.
  ○ Significant drainage is usually taken arbitrarily as that over 500 ml/day.
  ○ TPN dries up the drainage within 24 hours.
  ○ Low fat diet; control protein levels and electrolytes.

Late

- Scar hypertrophic or contracture.
- Accessory nerve loss – shoulder pain and weakness.
- Glossopharyngeal nerve injury – difficulty swallowing.

- Neuroma.
  ○ Trigger point sensitivity at the site of division of branches of the cervical plexus.
  ○ Shoulder pain syndrome.
- Oedema – facial, cerebral.

Adverse prognostic factors

- Poorly differentiated primary tumour.
- Thick tumour (> 4 mm).
- Lymph node.
  ○ Numbers (and multiple levels, especially lower levels).
  ○ Extracapsular spread.
- Perineural invasion.
- Invasion of carotid artery, other vessels.
- Poor response to radiotherapy or chemotherapy.
- Increased angiogenesis, apoptosis index, non-cohesion.

Radiotherapy after neck dissection

The most common indications for post-operative radiotherapy are:

- Positive neck dissections.
- Single large involved node (> 3 cm).
- Extracapsular spread.

Post-operative therapy to the **primary** may be considered for close/positive margins, perineural or perivascular invasion, > 5 mm tumour thickness, invasion of adjacent soft tissues etc.

If radiotherapy is planned, then a dental check-up is important; any caries should be dealt with prior to radiotherapy as subsequent dental infections/extractions will rapidly involve the mandible and may cause osteoradionecrosis (ORN).

- Brachytherapy is an alternative to external beam radiotherapy; facilitated by the insertion of selectron rods at the time of surgery.
- Radiated tissues lose natural planes making dissection difficult and frozen section histology is unreliable in previously irradiated tissues.
- ~20% of tumours overall will recur despite clear margins whilst 60% of tumours recur if margins are involved.
- Field change in oral mucosa may lead to a high second (or more) primary rate; hypopharyngeal tumours also have a high second primary rate.
- Recurrences after a full course of radiotherapy cannot be given further radiotherapy.

Complications include:

- Eyes (cataracts and dry eyes).
- Hearing (sensorineural loss).
- Salivary glands (xerostomia).
- Hypopituitarism.
- Growth disturbances of the craniofacial skeleton in children e.g. retinoblastomas and orbital hypoplasia; fibrosis of facial soft tissues.
- Injury to dental roots and TMJ ankylosis.

Management of the occult primary

Clinically palpable node – T0N1+

- Full history of age, occupation, smoking, drinking, dental health, drugs, allergies, past medical and surgical history (PMSH), systems review.
- Thorough head and neck examination including intra-oral examination.

Differentiate from a lymphoma (examine other node basins) or primary carcinoma in a branchial cyst.

Investigations

- Blood tests including EBV, IgA.
- FNA (excision if suspicious of lymphoma or if FNA equivocal).
- CXR and OPG.
- Panendoscopy.
  - EUA upper aerodigestive tract e.g. nose, pharynx, oesophagus, bronchus.
  - Biopsy: nasopharynx, tonsil, piriform fossa, base of tongue and FOM.
- MRI scan.
  - Use the information from the above investigations to direct the MRI scan.
  - T2-weighted images detect peri-tumour oedema and so may overestimate size.
  - Sinister features for lymph nodes include:
    - Size > 1.5 cm.
    - Loss of capsule definition.
    - Multiple nodes.
    - Central necrosis.
- CT/PET.

Surgical treatment

- If N1 consider modified radical neck dissection or primary radiotherapy (to neck and likely primary sites).
- If > N1 proceed to modified radical neck dissection with post-operative radiotherapy particularly if there is extracapuslar spread.

Sentinel lymph node biopsy in head and neck cancer

Although sentinel lymph node biopsy (SLNB) is practised in melanoma (Morton DL. *Arch Surg* 1992; **127**:392–399) and breast cancer (Krag DN. *Surg Oncol* 1993; **2**:225–240) in particular, for head and neck cancer it is primarily a research tool and is not commonly performed outside validation trials (Calabrese L. *Acta Otorrhinol Ital* 2006;**26**:345–349; Kuriakose MA. *Curr Op Otol Head Neck Surg* 2009;**17**:100–110).

A multicentre trial (Ross GL. *Ann Surg Oncol* 2004;**11**:690–696) with 134 patients with T1/2 tumours found sentinel nodes in 93%. The sensitivity was 90% (lower in FOM tumours) and it upstaged the disease (positivity) in 48% of anterior tongue and 33% of FOM tumours. The authors concluded that this supported the view that SLNB can be used as a staging tool in T1/T2 tumours of the oral cavity/ oropharynx.

It can be used when the primary is small and thin so that it can be accessed without osteotomy and does not require vessel access in the neck. It is of greater value in N0 necks compared with N1 as the disease may make lymphatic drainage unpredictable.

E. Approaches to management of facial palsy

I. The patient with facial palsy

Congenital or acquired facial palsy

Acquired facial palsy is much more common.

- Spontaneous palsy (Bell's).
- Post-traumatic (facial laceration, head injury).
- Secondary to tumour excision (parotid, acoustic neuroma, glioma).

Important to determine:

- **Level of the palsy** – intracranial, intratemporal, facial.
- Duration of the palsy – wasting of muscles and neuromuscular junction atrophy means that imported muscle will be needed.

Examination

- Temporal ('frontal' branch): Brow ptosis, lack of wrinkling.
- Zygomatic branch (orbicularis oculi): Lagophthalmos, corneal exposure.

- Buccal branch: Lip weakness, lack of a smile.
- Marginal mandibular branch: Drooling, asymmetric.

Basic principles of treatment

Intracranial and intratemporal: no **proximal** stump.

- Less than 1 year: use cross-facial nerve graft (XFNG) to distal nerve stump or directly into muscle (neurotization).
- More than 1 year
  - In younger patients (better nerve regeneration and fit for free flap) use free pectoralis minor or gracilis with cross-facial nerve graft.
  - In older patients (poor nerve regeneration, unfit for major surgery) consider
    - Muscle transfer: temporalis turnover.
    - Nerve transfer: IX, XI, XII.

Other supplementary procedures:

- Static suspension: facelift, fascia lata sling.
- Correction of drooling.
- Gold weight into upper lid.

Extratemporal division: **proximal and distal** stumps available.

- Less than 1 year: direct repair or primary nerve graft.
- More than 1 year: pectoralis minor coapted to ipsilateral nerve stump.

Möbius syndrome

This is a rare congenital anomaly with multiple cranial nerve palsies – most commonly, VII nerve palsy associated with other cranial nerve palsies, most often of VI. The facial vessels are also often abnormal; there are other anomalies of the limbs, face with drooling of saliva, abnormal dentition but almost always of normal intelligence.

There is a high incidence of congenital cardiac disease, spinal anomalies, corneal abrasions and peripheral neuropathies and microglossia.

The aetiology is unknown – genetic or embryopathic (hypoxia, infection or toxic) and the pathogenesis is also unclear – e.g. nervous or muscular aplasia or dysgenesis of the two first branchial arches.

Affected children often present for:

- Correction of strabismus.
- Improvement of limb function.
- Facial reanimation.

  - Harrison uses latissimus dorsi free flap with a pedicle long enough to reach down into the neck.
  - Nerve coaption to one of the nerves to masseter (Zucker).

II. Facial reanimation

Aims

- Symmetry at rest and with voluntary and involuntary motion.
- Control of the ocular, oral and nasal sphincters (may need temporary tarsorrhaphy).

Aetiology – four sites

- **Facial nerve nucleus**
  - Usually infarction (stroke), upper motor neurone signs with contralateral weakness sparing the brow (cross-innervation), i.e. no brow ptosis.
- **Pons and cerebellopontine angle**
  - Tumours: acoustic neuroma, glioma.
  - Vascular abnormalities.
  - Central nervous system degenerative diseases including motor neurone disease.
  - Congenital abnormalities and agenesis including Möbius syndrome.
  - Trauma.
- **Within the petrous temporal bone.**
  - Tumours (including cholesteatoma)
  - Trauma (including iatrogenic).
  - Bacterial and viral infections.
    - **Bell's palsy:** viral infection causing swelling of the facial nerve within the petrous temporal bone. 15% have permanent palsy, rarely bilateral; most recover within 12 months.
    - **Ramsay–Hunt syndrome:** herpes zoster infection of the geniculate ganglion (chorda tympani/taste relay station in the petrous temporal bone).
- **Extracranial.**
  - Tumours (parotid tumours).
  - Trauma (including iatrogenic).

Techniques of facial reanimation

Direct nerve repair: this is usually possible for traumatic or iatrogenic injury to the nerve.

Facial nerve grafting. This is best performed within 3 weeks – 1 year of injury e.g. immediate grafting after ablative surgery (up to 95% response), but some good results as late as 2–3 years post-injury. There is a 6–24-month interval to return of facial movement.

- Donors include branches of the cervical plexus or sural nerve (35 cm); great auricular nerve provides up to 10 cm.
- Expect 20% shrinkage of the graft therefore there should be no tension in the repair and should not be dependent on position.

Epineural repair is comparable if not superior to fascicular repair.

Cross-facial nerve grafting

The best chance for restoring spontaneous facial expression is direct nerve repair or interpositional graft – but this may not be possible, for example following excision of an acoustic neuroma.

The technique aims to provide cross-innervation from the non-paralysed side that is capable of producing appropriate coordination of contraction. The grafts connect distal branches of the donor nerve to the recipient nerve at a site distal to the level of injury. It does depend upon overlap in the innervation of muscles from other nerve trunks on the donor side, allowing donor nerves to be 'spare'. The coaption to the recipients may be done in the same stage or in a second stage after allowing axons to grow across (9–12 months).

- Axonal regeneration occurs at a rate of 1–3 mm/day. Only 20–50% of axons cross the nerve graft; reversal of the sural nerve graft may help reduce axonal escape.
- May use branches of temporal, zygomatic, buccal and mandibular nerves but only 15% success with the 'outer' nerves i.e. temporal and mandibular grafts.

Recovery of facial palsy after cross-facial nerve grafts

Iñigo F. *Br J Plast Surg* 1994;**47**:312–317.

In this study, the cross-facial nerve graft was coapted to facial muscle (neurotization) and the results with this approach were excellent. Alternatively the graft was coapted to the distal stump of the contralateral facial nerve.

Patients referred within 1 year of onset of palsy are suitable for cross-facial nerve graft; worst results are in patients undergoing surgery 4–10 years later.

Nerve crossovers

Glossopharyngeal, accessory, phrenic and hypoglossal nerves can be used as donors to the distal stump. This is an alternative when direct suture or grafting is not feasible, for example facial paralysis resulting from intracranial lesions or disorders of the temporal bone.

However, there is **loss of function** in the donor nerve and the movement produced is uncoordinated (**synkinesis**) – this can be palliated by injections of botulinum toxin around the orbicularis oculi muscle to reduce involuntary closure of the eye when attempting to smile.

Hypoglossal nerve crossover leads to > 50% moderate and 25% severe tongue atrophy; it is most suited to immediate reconstruction of the facial nerve trunk as part of the primary ablative surgery and can also be used to 'baby-sit' the facial musculature awaiting the regeneration of fibres along a cross-facial nerve graft.

Muscle transfers
Local muscle transfers

- Temporalis: a turnover flap originally described by Gillies, alternatively detach the tendinous insertion by an osteotomy of the mandibular coronoid process and pass a strip of fascia lata through the detached bony insertion, anchoring the distal end to nasolabial fold and upper/lower lips. However the impulse for movement originates in the trigeminal nerve therefore not physiological; there is usually significant synkinesis.
- Masseter.
- Sternocleidomastoid – too bulky, pull in wrong direction.
- Platysma – too delicate, not enough power.

Free muscle transfer

The action of zygomaticus major alone nearly produces a normal smile – all surgical efforts are directed at reproducing this action. Normal facial muscles have ~25 muscle fibres innervated by one axon, whereas gracilis and pectoralis minor muscles have ~150–200 muscle fibres to each axon.

For this to be successful requires one of the following:

- Ipsilateral nerve coaption to the stump of the facial nerve on the affected side:
  - ~5% of patients have a proximal nerve stump which allows faster nerve regeneration into the donor nerve.

- ○ Alternatively if this is unavailable and a two-stage operation is to be avoided, a nerve other than the facial nerve can be used, e.g. hypoglossal nerve (but will cause synkinesis).
- Preliminary cross-facial nerve grafting.
  - ○ This is needed for long-standing paralysis and the nerve stump unavailable.
  - ○ 6–12 months before second stage.
- Cross-face vascularized nerve coaption in a single stage (see below).

General principles

- Match size of donor and recipient nerves.
- Leave the donor nerve short to minimize re-innervation time.
- Allow for 50% loss of motor power following transfer.
- Match size and shape of donor muscle to available pocket.

Most commonly used:

Pectoralis minor (described by Manktelow).

Pectoralis minor vascularized muscle graft for the treatment of unilateral facial palsy

Harrison DH. *Plast Reconstr Surg* 1985;**75**:206–216.

The transferred muscle should receive impulses from the uninjured facial nerve if a natural smiling response is to be provided.

Cross-facial nerve grafting has a role in young patients with early palsy. More long-standing palsies (over 1 year) suffer from muscle atrophy, and require importation of fresh muscle. However, considerable loss of muscle power following transplantation is to be expected.

- As a first step, a sural cross-face nerve graft is coapted to the buccal branch of the facial nerve overlying the parotid duct, over the upper lip to a banked position at the contralateral tragus.
- Six months later (when Tinel's sign is positive at the distal end of the graft, 20–50% of axons have reached the other side), the free pectoralis minor muscle flap is raised on medial and lateral pectoral nerves and a direct arterial branch from the axillary artery which is anastomosed to facial vessels on the paralysed side. The nerves are coapted to the sural nerve graft.
- The muscle is inserted into the alar base and the upper and lower lips with a point of origin at the zygoma (with the pedicle orientated superficial to aid microsurgery).
- Pectoralis minor flap has a good donor site scar (anterior axillary fold) with no adverse functional sequelae but only provides the lip elevation part of a smile – lacks depressor function and lateral pull normally achieved by buccinator. Some axons are lost.
- Any lagophthalmos is addressed by insertion of gold weights.

Gracilis (described by Harii)

- Single-stage free tissue transfer is made possible by coaptation of the nerve to gracilis (anterior division of the obturator nerve) across the philtrum to the buccal branch of the intact contralateral facial nerve and **avoids the need for a cross-facial nerve graft** acting as a vascularized nerve graft (Kumar PA. *Br J Plast Surg* 1995;**48**:83–88). However there will be some loss of motor end plates on the donor muscle while awaiting regeneration of axons across the face.
- As the pedicle lies on the deep surface of the muscle, some thinning is possible.
- Long pedicle but muscle is rather bulky.
- Simultaneous harvesting possible.

Irreversible muscle contracture after functioning free muscle with ipsilateral nerve coaptation

Chuang DCC. *Br J Plast Surg* 1995;**48**:1–7.

Four patients underwent free gracilis transfer with nerve coaptation to the ipsilateral facial nerve and irreversible muscle contracture developed with onset between 6 and 12 months.

There is a theory that contracture resulted from over-re-innervation/over-stimulation and it is suggested that this is potentially avoided by using cross-facial nerve graft. However later correspondence suggests that contracture may occur after both techniques and it may be related more to muscle fibrosis before re-innervation.

Free muscle transfer for Romberg's disease (hemi-facial atrophy) rather than facial palsy may result in direct neurotization of the muscle which also leads to contracture.

Latissimus dorsi

- Single-stage reconstruction is also possible as the thoracodorsal nerve reaches over to the other side of the face and the nerve is 'vascularized'.

- Muscle trimming to the required size *in situ* is facilitated by the pedicle being on the deep surface.

Serratus anterior, rectus abdominis and platysma have also been used.

- Bank the cross nerve graft (reversed to reduce axonal escape) at the tragus and perform free muscle transfer 6 months later according to progress determined by Tinel's sign.
- Fascicular nerve stimulation of the donor muscle allows determination of which fascicle supplies which strips of muscle.

Comparative objective and subjective analysis of temporalis tendon and microneurovascular transfer for facial reanimation
Erni D. *Br J Plast Surg* 1999;**52**:167–172.

This study compared McLaughlin's technique for temporalis tendon transfer to a two-stage free tissue transfer using latissimus dorsi, gracilis and pectoralis minor (only offered to patients under 50 years of age). The technique for temporalis transfer was:

- Through a facelift incision, the masseter is split to approach the coronoid process.
- The apex of coronoid process detached with an osteotome and a 6 mm drill hole made through detached segment is threaded with a strip of fascia lata.
- The fascia lata sling is re-routed to the corner of the mouth and anchored to previously inserted conchal cartilage grafts.

Microsurgical reanimations
- Resulted in significantly **better measurements of excursion during smiling** while static symmetry was similar to temporalis transfer.
- Swelling of the cheek soft tissues and skin tethering was more problematic.

Static procedures
- Fascia lata slings.
- Superficial temporal fascia suspension.
- Gold weight to upper lids.
- Botulinum toxin to weaken contralateral (normal) side – effect lasts up to 6 months.
- Facelift/brow lifts.

Treatment of drooling by parotid duct ligation and submandibular duct diversion
Varma SK. *Br J Plast Surg* 1991;**44**:415–417.

The opening of the parotid duct is cannulated and the distal part of the duct is dissected out for ligation; the other parotid duct is left intact.

The openings of both submandibular ducts are cannulated next to the frenulum and ducts are dissected out with a surrounding cuff of mucosa and re-routed backwards in the mouth towards the anterior pillar of the fauces.

This is suitable for cerebral palsy patients with excessive and troublesome drooling. There is usually some transient swelling of the (ligated) parotid and both submandibular glands post-operatively. Submandibular duct obstruction may be complicated by sialolithiasis due to the higher calcium and phosphate content of the (mucous) secretions and gravity affecting drainage.

Marginal mandibular nerve palsy
The lower lip is animated by several muscles:

- Orbicularis oris.
- Depressor labii inferioris, depressor anguli oris.
- Mentalis, platysma.

The marginal mandibular nerve is vulnerable to trauma in the submandibular fossa, lying deep to platysma below the body of the mandible, and injury causes paralysis of depressor anguli oris and depressor labii inferioris:

- Inability to form a natural smile.
- Drooling with elevation of the lower lip at rest, unable to move downwards or evert.

Microsurgical strategies in 74 patients for restoration of the dynamic depressor mechanism
Terzis JK. *Plast Reconstr Surg* 2000;**105**:1932–1934.

Reanimation options:

- If the palsy has lasted less than 12 months (with EMG evidence of depressor activity) then an option is direct neurotization of depressors using a cross-facial nerve graft.
- If the palsy has lasted 12–24 months (EMG still shows some depressor activity) or failure of the above, then a mini XII-to-VII transfer or direct neurotization (incorporates 20–30% of the nerve trunk).
- With long-standing palsy: platysma transfer (if functional) or transfer of the anterior belly of digastric which is supplied by the mandibular

division of V – nerve to mylohyoid (branch of inferior alveolar).

- ○ The tendon is divided and mobilized to corner of mouth whilst the insertion on mandible is then divided and inset to reproduce smile vector.
- ○ In young patients re-education is usually successful in reproducing a physiological smile, but older patients require coaptation to a cross-facial nerve graft.

Paralysis of the marginal mandibular branch of the facial nerve: treatment options
Tulley P. *Br J Plast Surg* 2000;**53**:378–385.
   Treatment options include:

- Anterior belly of digastric transfer (ABDT).
  - ○ Anterior belly is left attached to mandible, posterior belly/central tendon divided and re-routed to the corner of the mouth.
  - ○ Simple and very effective one-stage procedure but generates a scar in the submandibular fossa.
- Two-stage microsurgical transfer of extensor digitorum brevis
  - ○ Complex microsurgical procedure with greater donor and recipient site scarring but is useful

when ABD is absent due to surgical trauma of complex facial hypoplastic syndromes.

- Botulinum toxin injection of contralateral depressors. This produces temporary symmetry and is an alternative to contralateral depressor myectomy.

Depressor labii inferioris resection: an effective treatment for marginal mandibular nerve paralysis
Hussain G. *Br J Plast Surg* 2004;**57**:502–510.
   Careful assessment of the surface marking of depressor labii inferioris on the unparalysed side is undertaken by palpation of the vermilion border while the patient attempts to show the lower teeth.

- A muscle block is undertaken by intramuscular injection of local anaesthetic to simulate the effect of myectomy (alternatively botulinum toxin can be used and lasts 3–4 months). Improvements in appearance, oral continence and lip biting reported.
- The muscle is exposed using an intra-oral incision 0.5 cm above the buccal sulcus, retracting the orbicularis oris fibres, and a segment of muscle is then resected across its entire width.

Cleft lip and palate/craniofacial anomalies

A. Principles of management of cleft lip and palate

I. Embryology and anatomy

Embryological development of the maxillofacial skeleton

During the 4th–5th weeks of development, the **pharyngeal arches** form as ridges in the cranial mesenchyme and are separated by pharyngeal clefts, whilst internally out-pouchings of the foregut are formed called pharyngeal pouches. Skeletal components are formed by inward migration of neural crest cells.

The **stomodeum** is the cranial opening of the foregut (mouth and nasal aperture) and five swellings are formed ventrally:

- Paired mandibular swellings (from first pharyngeal arch).
- Paired maxillary swellings (from first pharyngeal arch).
- Fronto-nasal prominence (downgrowth from primitive forebrain).

First pharyngeal arch

The first pharyngeal arch is of most importance from a cleft perspective.

- The arch artery is the maxillary artery from the external carotid whilst the nerve is the trigeminal: motor from mandibular branch and sensory from all three divisions.
- Muscles: muscles of mastication as well as tensor palati, tensor tympani, anterior belly of digastric and mylohyoid. The mesenchyme of the first arch forms the dermis of the face.
- Cartilaginous components include
  - Maxillary process – the mesenchyme undergoes intramembranous ossification to form the premaxilla, maxilla, zygoma and part of the temporal bone.
  - Mandibular process – Meckel's cartilage forms in the mesenchyme of the mandibular process and most of it eventually regresses to leave only the parts that form the incus and malleus, anterior ligament of malleus and sphenomandibular ligament. The mandible forms by intramembranous ossification using Meckel's cartilage as a

template rather than by direct ossification of the cartilage.

- ○ During further development both of these disappear except for those parts forming the incus and malleus.

First arch syndromes

Treacher Collins

Treacher Collins syndrome is otherwise known as mandibulofacial dysostosis; there is a gene defect in chromosome 5 (5q31–33). There is failure of the first arch neural crest characterized by Tessier 6, 7 and 8 clefts centred around the zygoma. Characteristic features include:

- Defects of lower eyelid – loss of lashes or coloboma (6 cleft).
- Macrostomia (7 cleft).
- Absent or hypoplastic zygoma.
- Maxillary and mandibular hypoplasia; cleft palate.
- Hypertelorism and anti-Mongoloid slant.
- Abnormalities of external, middle and inner ear; hearing defects.
- Broad nasal bridge.

Pierre Robin sequence

This was first described in 1822 and affects one in every 8000 live births. The risk of further children being affected is 1–5%. It can often be part of a larger syndrome, the most common of which is **Stickler syndrome** (vide infra).

- Glossoptosis and airway obstruction.
- Mandibular hypoplasia (retrogenia, also microgenia): mandible will grow to more normal proportions between 3 and 18 months of age, with a normal profile by 6 years of age thus mandibular advancement osteotomy is rarely required.
- Cleft palate (60–90%) – usually closed surgically at 12–18 months.
- Defects of ear and eye.

Airway management – the affected neonate suffers from airway obstruction during sleep and will die of exhaustion if not corrected.

- Try nursing prone first.
- Emergency management: pull tongue forward with stitch/towel clip, nasotracheal intubation.
- More permanent techniques for managing the tongue include suturing to inner surface of lower lip (Routledge) or passing a K-wire through the mandible to skewer the base of the tongue in a forward position.
- The use of distraction osteogenesis has been described but should not be used in those under 2 years of age prior to other methods failing due to risk of permanent dental injury and the bones being too soft.
- Definitive procedure for airway maintenance is tracheostomy but this is rarely required.

A **sequence** is a single developmental defect that results in a chain of secondary defects e.g. Pierre Robin syndrome – mandibular hypoplasia causes posterior displacement of the tongue which leads to airway obstruction and precludes closure of the palatal arches, leading to cleft of the secondary palate. The entire cascade of events is often known in a sequence.

A **syndrome** is a group of anomalies that contain multiple malformations and/or sequences. A given anomaly may be incompletely expressed or absent; the pathogenic relationship of the group of anomalies is frequently not understood.

Stickler's syndrome (hereditary progressive arthro-ophthalmopathy)

This is a connective tissue disorder first described in 1960 by Gunnar Stickler from the Mayo clinic. It is a progressive condition with autosomal dominant inheritance – there are several subtypes: COL2A1 (75% of cases, defect on chromosome 12), type XI COL11A1 and 2 (chromosome 6) and type IX COL9A1 (also chromosome 6, recessive variant). Characteristic features include:

- Severe progressive myopia, retinal detachment, vitreal degeneration, glaucoma.
- Progressive sensorineural hearing loss.
- Valvular prolapse e.g. mitral valve prolapse (MVP).
- Scoliosis.
- Pierre Robin features: **cleft palate** and mandibular hypoplasia – flat face with small nose that tends to improve with age.
- Hyper- and hypomobility of joints, leading to osteoarthritis in later life; variable epiphyseal dysplasia causing joint pain, dislocation or degeneration.

It should be considered in any infant with congenitally enlarged wrists, knees or ankles, particularly when associated with the Pierre Robin sequence (30–40%

of those with Pierre Robin sequence has Stickler's). It should also be suspected in those with features of Marfan syndrome with hearing loss, degenerative arthritis or retinal detachment.

Second arch

- Artery – stapedial artery; nerve – facial.
- Cartilage forms the stapes, lesser horn of hyoid and upper part of the body of the hyoid.
- Bone forms body and ramus of mandible.
- Muscles are muscles of facial expression as well as stapedius, stylohyoid, posterior belly of digastric (Möbius' syndrome – a failure of innervation of facial muscles).

Third arch

- Nerve – Glossopharyngeal.

Cartilage is the greater horn and inferior part of the body of the hyoid.

- Muscles are stylopharyngeus, upper pharyngeal constrictors.
- The thymus and inferior III parathyroids (abnormal in Di-Georges or velo-cardio-facial syndrome) are derived from the third pouch.

Branchial cleft anomalies

Otherwise known as branchial cysts, these are found in the anterior triangle and probably represent remnants of the branch clefts that are entrapped and may manifest as cysts, sinuses or fistulae. Cysts tend to be soft and non-tender but may become abscesses if infected.

- First brachial cleft cysts.
  - Type I duplication of external ear canal – a fistula close to the lower part of the parotid with tracts that may terminate in the ear canal (external or middle ear).
  - Type II – usually in the anterior triangle just inferior to the angle of mandible, with a tract through the parotid (thus closely associated to the facial nerve) to the external ear canal.
- Second branchial cleft cysts – deep to platysma with a tract running between the internal and external carotid arteries up to the tonsillar fossae.

Development of the tongue

The tongue precursors appear at ~4 weeks of development: two lateral plus one median (tuberculum impar) lingual swellings from the first arch mesenchyme form the anterior two-thirds of the tongue. Behind this a median swelling (copula or hypobranchial eminence) of second, third and fourth arch mesenchyme forms the posterior tongue.

- Sensory innervation to anterior two-thirds by the mandibular division of V; to posterior third by IX and X.
- Motor innervation mainly XII – the musculature is derived from occipital somites and all are supplied by XII except palatoglossus which is innervated by the X nerve.

Development of the nose and upper lip

The maxillary swellings lie above the stomodeum whilst the mandibular swellings lie caudal; they are present by the 5th week of development. The frontal process lies in the midline, above the maxillary swellings.

- On each side of the frontal process just above the stomodeum, the ectoderm thickens to form two **nasal placodes**. Swellings develop lateral and medial to each nasal placode which deepens to form the nasal pit.
- By week 7, the maxillary swellings advance into the midline, pushing the **medial** nasal swellings to the midline where they fuse to form the upper lip.

Development of the palate

The undersurface of the fused maxillary and medial nasal swellings forms the intermaxillary segment which contributes to:

- Philtrum of the upper lip.
- Part of the maxillary alveolus bearing the upper four incisors.
- Triangular primary palate.

During week 6, the palatal shelves grow out from the maxillary swellings to lie lateral to the tongue. These shelves then ascend with hydration of glycosaminoglycans and fuse in the midline to form the secondary palate; the vertical movement takes place very rapidly (less than 1 second in rat embryos). The secondary palate fuses anteriorly with the primary palate with the junction marked by the incisive foramen.

- Epstein's pearls are cystic epithelial remnants of the zone of apoptosis between the fusing palatal shelves.

Developmental abnormalities leading to cleft lip and palate

Clefts can be divided into clefts of the primary palate and clefts of the secondary or posterior palate (posterior to the incisive foramen).

- **Primary palate** consists of the lip, alveolus and hard palate anterior to the incisive foramen and clefts represent failure of mesenchymal penetration between medial and lateral palatine processes and **failure of fusion of maxillary and medial nasal processes** (cleft of lip and alveolus between incisors and canines extending to incisive foramen).
- **Secondary palate** consists of the hard palate behind the incisive foramen and soft palate and clefts represent failure of the lateral palatine processes to fuse with each other and the nasal septum/vomer.

Anterior and posterior clefts may appear together or in isolation. Degrees of clefting are observed for primary clefts (e.g. incomplete vs. complete cleft lip) and secondary clefts (wide cleft palate vs. cleft uvula).

- Rare clefts include failure of fusion of medial nasal swellings which gives rise to the very rare median cleft whilst failure of fusion of maxillary and lateral nasal swellings causes an oblique facial cleft.

Anatomy of the palate and pharynx

The hard palate includes the palatal processes of the maxilla and the horizontal plate of the palatine bone with an adherent mucoperiosteum (attached to bone by Sharpey's fibres).

- Blood supply via the greater palatine artery (from the maxillary artery) which enters at the greater palatine foramen and runs towards the incisive foramen. Venous drainage via venae comitantes mostly. Lymphatic drainage to the retropharyngeal and deep cervical nodes.
- Sensory innervation via the pterygopalatine ganglion (branches of the maxillary nerve) – nasopalatine nerves to the premaxillary area and by the greater palatine nerve posteriorly.

Soft palate

- The blood supply to the soft palate comes mostly from the lesser palatine arteries, the ascending palatine branch of the facial artery and the palatine branches of the ascending pharyngeal artery.
- All muscles of the palate are supplied by the pharyngeal plexus (cranial accessory nerve and pharyngeal branch of X) except tensor palati (nerve to medial pterygoid – branch of the mandibular nerve).

There are five paired muscles:

- **Tensor palati** (tensor veli palatini) from the scaphoid fossa of the medial pterygoid plate, the lateral part of the cartilaginous auditory tube and the spine of the sphenoid. It passes around the pterygoid hamulus as a tendon and inserts as a concave triangular aponeurosis to the crest of the palatine bone, blending in the midline with that of the opposite side. It acts to tense the soft palate to form a platform that the other muscles may elevate or depress. It also opens the auditory tube during swallowing.
- **Levator palati** (levator veli palatini) arises from the quadrate area of the petrous bone (anterior to the carotid foramen) and the medial part of the auditory tube and inserts into the nasal surface of the palatine aponeurosis. The paired muscles form a 'V'-shaped sling pulling the soft palate upwards and backwards to close the nasopharynx. It also opens the auditory tube.
- **Palatoglossus** arises from the under surface of the aponeurosis and passes downwards to interdigitate with styloglossus. It forms the anterior fold of the tonsillar fossa and acts as a sphincter to raise the tongue and narrow the transverse diameter of the oropharyngeal isthmus.
- **Palatopharyngeus** has two heads. The anterior head arises from the nasal surface of the hard palate whilst the posterior head arises from the nasal surface of the aponeurosis; the two heads clasp the levator palati muscle insertion. They form the posterior pillar of the tonsillar fossa and the innermost muscle of the pharynx, inserting into the thyroid lamina and blending with the inferior constrictor. The anterior head (arising from bone) acts to raise the pharynx/larynx whilst the posterior head depresses the tensed soft palate. Some fibres, along with fibres from the superior constrictor, contribute to the palatopharyngeal sphincter (forms Passavant's ridge when the soft palate is elevated. This is hypertrophied in cleft

palate patients and in 25–30% of normal individuals).

- Muscle of the uvula.

Pharynx

The pharynx is a 12-cm-long muscular tube that extends from the skull base and becomes the oesophagus at the level of C6. The wall consists of four layers: mucous membrane, submucous (fibrous) layer, muscular layer and the thin outer buccopharyngeal fascia.

- Muscles consist of overlapping superior, middle and inferior constrictors with paired stylo-, palato- and salpingo-pharyngeus muscles. The inferior constrictor has two parts, thyropharyngeus and cricopharyngeus, with a weak area in between called Killen's dehiscence.
- Blood supply comes from the superior and inferior laryngeal arteries, ascending pharyngeal artery, also from the vessels supplying palate.
- All muscles are supplied by pharyngeal plexus (motor fibres in pharyngeal branch of X, IX fibres are purely afferent) except stylopharyngeus (IX) and cricopharyngeus (recurrent laryngeal branch of X).

Tonsils

- The pharyngeal tonsil lies high on the posterior wall of the nasopharynx and enlarges to form the adenoids. The tubal tonsil and the opening of the auditory tube lies on the lateral wall of the nasopharynx.
- The palatine tonsils lie between anterior and posterior pillars in the oropharynx whilst the lingual tonsils along with the tubal, palatine and pharyngeal tonsils form Waldeyer's ring.

II. Genetics

General considerations

Definitions

Cleft lip is a congenital abnormality of the primary palate and may be complete/incomplete/microform, unilateral/bilateral and may coexist with a cleft palate.

Cleft palate is a congenital abnormality of the secondary palate which may be unilateral/bilateral or a submucous cleft.

Incidence and aetiology

~1.5 in 1000 in Europe.

- 1 in 500 in Asia.
- 1 in 1000 in Africa.

Cleft lip ± palate (i.e. cleft lip with or without cleft palate, CL/P) is more common than cleft palate alone (CPO). Cleft lip **and** palate is commonest (approximately 50%) whilst CPO occurs in 30% and CL alone occurs in 20%.

- CL/P is more common in boys whilst there is more CPO in girls.
- The **left** lip is affected twice as often as the right – left : right : bilateral 6 : 3 : 1 (Cleft-left).

Genetic predisposition

Genetic counselling is an important part of the overall management of patients and their families. The inheritance of clefts may be chromosomal, Mendelian or sporadic.

- Chromosomal inheritance includes syndromes such as **trisomy 13 (Patau) and 21**.
- Mendelian inheritance includes syndromes due to single gene defects that will be passed on within families – these may be autosomal dominant (e.g. **van der Woude** syndrome – CL/P, missing teeth and lip pits, and **Treacher Collins** syndrome), recessive or X-linked.
- Sporadic cases may be associated with developmental abnormalities (e.g. **Pierre Robin** sequence) with a low risk of further affected children.

Non-syndromic clefts in general display multifactorial inheritance which may include a genetic **predisposition** plus one or more of the following risk factors. There is a higher incidence in offspring of smoking mothers and there is a possible link with maternal drug ingestion including anti-epileptics, salicylates, tretinoin (retinoids), benzodiazepines and cortisone.

Genetic counselling and genetics of cleft lip and cleft palate
Habib Z. *Obst Gyn Survey* 1978;**33**:441–447.

Non-syndromic cleft lip

- With normal parents, the risk of a child with cleft lip is 1 in 750–1000.
  - Second and third affected child – risk 4% and 10% respectively.

- If one parent has cleft lip the risk of having a child with cleft lip is 4%.
  - Second affected child – risk 17%.
- If a child is born with CPO, the risk of CL/P is still 1 in 750.

For non-syndromic CPO

- Normal parents – risk of affected child is general risk.
  - Second and third affected child – 3.5% and 13% respectively.
- One affected parent, risk of first affected child is 3.5%.
  - Second and third affected child – 10% and 24% respectively.

Epidemiology and etiology of clefts

Fogh-Andersen P. *Birth Defects* 1971;7:51–53.

The overall risk of CL/P is approximately 1 in 700 (= 1.5 in 1000 live births).

- If the father has CP the risk of a child with CL/P is the same.
- If the father has CL/P the risk of a child with CL/P is 4% and second child 10%.

Initial assessment of the baby with a cleft lip

- Breathing: if dyspnoeic then nurse prone to allow tongue to fall from airway. Insert a nasopharyngeal airway and apply tongue stitch if necessary. **Continuous positive airway pressure** (CPAP) may need to be considered.
- Feeding: a trial of breastfeeding is always worthwhile; using a soft teat and a squeezy bottle may be considered. CP babies have worse feeding problems than CL babies; parent education is very important.

Patients should be referred to a multidisciplinary cleft clinic for further assessment, planning and treatment. A typical **treatment** plan for unilateral complete cleft of the lip and palate follows but there are many variations/different operations.

III. Surgery

Timing of repair (parentheses are suggested procedures).

- 6 weeks–3 months.
  - Lip (Millard rotation–advancement for unilateral cleft lip) and primary nose correction (McComb).
  - Vomerine flap to anterior hard palate for alveolar cleft.
  - Synchronous soft palate repair in wide clefts may make subsequent hard palate repair easier.
- 3–6 months.
  - Palate repair (von Langenbeck technique including intravelar veloplasty, vomerine flap to close nasal layer at the level of the hard palate).
  - Grommets if required.
- 5 years.
  - Pharyngoplasty for post-palatoplasty velopharyngeal incompetence (VPI) (superior pharyngeal flap preferred except where there is significant lateral wall immobility – then Orticochoea).
  - Nasal correction – Tajima, if required.
  - Lengthen columella – bilateral forked flaps.
- 3–4 years: Speech therapy commenced if required.
- 6 years: Orthodontics – early dental management.
- 9 years: Orthodontics – alveolar bone graft, when the canine teeth first appear radiologically to prevent their root from collapsing into the cleft.
- 11 years: Orthodontics – management of permanent dentition.
- 16 years.
  - Rhinoplasty.
  - Le Fort I advancement to correct class III malocclusion if required.

Bilateral cleft lip

Additional considerations include:

- Presurgical orthopaedics for the protruding premaxilla.
- Millard bilateral lip repair banking forked flaps.
- Lengthen the columella with forked flaps at the time of pharyngoplasty ~5 years.

Delaire approach

Delaire was a maxillofacial surgeon in Nantes who proposed a so-called 'functional' lip repair at 6 months involving more muscle dissection and part of the rationale for operating at this time was that the muscle was better developed.

- 6 months: lip and soft palate repair.
- 18 months: hard palate repair with medial relaxing incisions possible because palate has been narrowed by previous soft palate closure.

Treatment of cleft lip and palate in the UK

Boorman JG. *Br J Plast Surg* 1998;**51**:167–168.

CSAG = Clinical Standards Advisory Group.

Seventeen of 57 units providing cleft lip and palate care were assessed and of the 457 patients reviewed only two units were judged to be good overall. The conclusion was based on numerous criteria: the unit itself, multidisciplinary team, use of protocols, data collection, experience of team members, morale, assessment of children treated aged 5–6 and 12–13 years at the time of the survey, appearance, dental hygiene, speech, hearing, growth, jaw relationships and patient/parent satisfaction.

- There were no significant differences demonstrated in treatment outcomes between plastic and maxillofacial surgeons.
- There are very few high volume operators – only seven of the 99 surgeons performed ~30 new repairs annually whilst the others performed fewer than 10 new repairs per year. However, the only demonstrable benefit of high volume surgery was in speech outcome.

The recommendations of the group were to reduce the number of units to 8–15 with each surgeon treating 40–50 new patients annually; reducing the number of units would also enable better data analysis and facilitate treatment advances.

Cleft lip repair

Unilateral cleft lip classification

- Incomplete (variable vertical lip shortness, nasal sill intact – Simonart's band).
- Complete (complete separation of the lip, nasal sill and alveolus).
- Microform ('forme fruste' – vertical furrow or scar, notch in the vermilion and white roll, variable vertical lip shortness).

  Aims:

- A cupid's bow and philtral dimple (rearrange tissues and lengthen the medial lip).
- Pouting of the lower portion of the lip (avoiding whistle deformity).
- Reconstruct orbicularis oris (re-approximation of muscle).
- Symmetrical alae (reposition displaced atrophic alar cartilages and alar base).
- A straight columella.

Millard originally described the C flap as a medial superior rotation flap that crossed the nasal sill to inset into the lateral lip element as a lateral rotation advancement flap (type I). He refined the technique to use the C flap to inset into the medial lip element, augmenting the columellar height and creating a more natural flare at the base of the medial footplate (type II). However there is a series of incisions/scars at the base of the columella that may be associated with poor healing if not planned properly. The C flap can be used in either position as requirements dictate.

Management of the protruding premaxilla

- **Premaxillary setback** (but sacrifices incisors and compromises growth – now condemned).
- **Presurgical orthopaedics.** Indicated in particular for wide bilateral clefts. It was pioneered by McNeil (1950), a maxillary obturator was used to reduce alveolar and palatal cleft. This is classed as a passive technique and active techniques were subsequently described by Latham.
  - Presurgical orthopaedics does not enhance maxillary growth and orthodontic benefits are limited. Nasoalveolar moulding – correction of nasal deformity with a nasal moulding plate and stent: columella becomes more vertical, improved nasal tip projection and alar cartilage symmetry. It needs to be instituted within 2 weeks of birth.
- **Lip adhesion.** Skin traction on the maxilla by temporarily closing the cleft lip under tension aims to reduce the size of the alveolar cleft (lip adhesion, excising edges and suturing in three layers), achieves this aim without compromising the definitive lip repair.

Repair techniques – brief principles

Unilateral cleft lip – stencil method

This was described by Tennison CW (*Plast Reconstr Surg* 1952;**9**:115–119) and avoids a straight line scar by fashioning a Z-plasty on each side of the cleft. This was modified by Randall and Skoog, in particular reducing the size of the inferior flap. This method is said to be more suited to wide unilateral clefts and very short lip, but leaves a transverse scar low down on the philtral column.

Complete unilateral clefts of the lip

Rotation–advancement repair was described by Millard DR (*Plast Reconstr Surg* 1960;**25**:595–605).

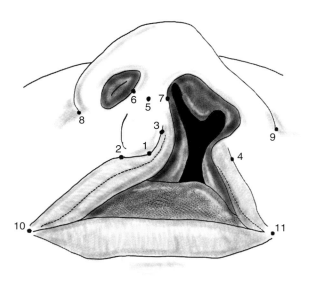

Figure 4.1 The common anatomical landmarks for cleft lip surgery.

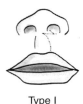

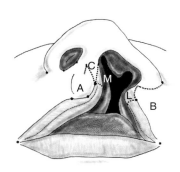

Figure 4.2 Millard advancement-rotation flap is a common choice. A – rotation flap, B – advancement flap, C – columellar base, M – medial mucosal flap, L – lateral mucosal flap. Depending on how the C flap is used, there are subtypes I and II.

The name comes from the fact that it relies upon rotation of a flap (**A** flap) in the philtrum (non-cleft side) downwards and advancement of a flap from the cleft side (**B** flap) to meet the A flap. As the A flap rotates downwards, a small triangular flap above it, the **C** flap, can cross the midline and be inset between the B flap and the nostril sill.

Closure of bilateral cleft clip and elongation of the columella by two operations in infancy
Millard DR. *Plast Reconstr Surg* 1971;**37**:324–331

Presurgical orthopaedics was used for the premaxilla, and lip repair was performed at 1 month of age with banking of forked flaps. Columellar lengthening was performed at a second stage at 3 months.

- The prolabium is deficient of white roll and vermilion and lacks muscle, whilst the columella is short/almost absent. The protruding premaxillary segment is suspended from the nasal septum.
- Poorly formed or absent anterior nasal spine with retruded area under the base of the septal cartilage.
- Broad, flat nose with recession of the foot plates of the medial crura.

The muscle is sutured together from the lateral lip segments in the midline. The prolabial vermilion is turned down and is used for lining behind the muscle repair which adds bulk and helps prevents whistle deformity. The lateral lip segment vermilion and white roll is advanced and joined in the midline.

Bilateral fork flaps are derived from the lateral edges of the prolabium, and each flap is sutured end-on to the alar base to form a standing cone/pyramid. At a second stage an inverted 'V' incision is made in the columella to join the bases of the two fork flaps and the incision is closed as a V–Y to gain columellar length. This technique combines columellar lengthening with advancement of the alar base.

Bilateral incomplete cleft lip

These are typically clefts involving only the lip with a near-normal nose with Simonart's bands across the nasal floors, and a normally positioned premaxilla. They can be repaired using the rotation–advancement technique as for unilateral repair in two stages, one side at a time.

Functional cleft lip repair
Kernahan, Rob and Smith's *Operative Surgery* (*Plastic Surgery*) 4th Edn. 1986.

The flap of skin-mucosa is reflected off each side of the cleft and sutured together whilst the orbicularis oris is mobilized on the cleft side.

Pockets are created on the non-cleft side just beneath the inferior nasal spine and beneath the vermilion border of the lip. The mobilized orbicularis is split into an upper two-thirds and lower third, and these strips are sutured into contralateral pockets. The overlying skin is closed using Z-plasties for lengthening.

Management of whistle deformity

The deformity is largely due to inadequate red margin/vermilion and options include:

- Mucosal advancement from the buccal sulcus including mucosal V–Y advancement (Kapetansky DI. *Plast Reconstr Surg* 1971;**47**:321–323).
- Free graft from lower lip.
- Abbé flap.

Cleft palate repair

The goal of cleft palate surgery is to close the palate with a technique and timing that produce optimal speech and minimize facial growth disturbances.

Veau classification

- Soft palate.
- Soft and hard palate.
- Soft and hard palate and unilateral prepalate.
- Soft and hard palate and bilateral prepalate.

Other classifications

Kernahan's striped Y, further modified by Millard and Jackson, allows the cleft to be located anatomically: 1–3 on the right, 3–6 on the left, from lip anteriorly to the incisive foramen, 7, 8 hard palate and 9 soft palate.

- **LAHSAL classification** that is used by the national database on clefts with the capital indicating complete clefts of: lip, alveolus, hard palate, soft palate, alveolus, lip.

Submucous cleft palate

This occurs in ~1 in 1000 (Kaplan EN. *Cleft Palate J* 1975;**12**:356–368). Signs include

- Bifid uvula ~1–2%.
- Palpable notch in hard palate.
- Blue line/furrow/translucency.

Classic Calnan triad (1954): bifid uvula, shortened soft palate with muscle diastasis and groove in the posterior palate.

Most patients have normal speech and about 15% have VPI which can be the presenting complaint. Others can present with feeding or hearing problems, or else found on routine paediatric examination. If speech and ENT assessment are acceptable, then palatal or pharyngeal surgery can be avoided, otherwise pharyngoplasty is a surgical option.

Interventions for the management of submucous cleft palate

Nasser M. *Cochrane Database Syst Rev* 2008.

Submucous cleft affects 1 in 600. A literature review of randomized controlled trials found **one** methodologically satisfactory trial (Ysunza A. *Plast Reconstr Surg* 2001;**107**:9–14) comparing 72 patients randomized to minimal incision palatopharyngoplasty (MIPP, uncommonly used), pharyngeal flap or sphincter pharyngoplasty. They conclude that there is some weak and unreliable evidence that there is no significant difference between MIPP and other methods.

Aims of cleft palate correction

- Closure of oronasal fistula whilst minimizing maxillary growth retardation.
- Allow normal development of speech whilst facilitating velopharyngeal closure.

Techniques

General anaesthesia with a south-facing endotracheal tube.

- Dingman gag – do not catch the lips and throat packs.
- Mark incisions and infiltrate with local anaesthetic/adrenaline solution.
- Remember to remove the throat packs and Dingman gag at the end of the procedure.

Vomerine flap

This is used to close the anterior hard palate/alveolus at the time of lip repair; it decreases frequency of alveolar nasal fistulae but may worsen maxillary growth retardation.

Types of palatal closure
Flap-less repair

This relies upon movement of mucoperiosteum off the arched palate to lie horizontally to gain enough length for primary closure in the midline without lateral releasing incisions and is only suited for narrow clefts. The closure is under some tension thus a slightly higher fistula rate is expected.

von Langenbeck technique

The palatal tissues are moved towards the midline using lateral releasing incisions that lie lateral to the greater palatine artery (the foramen forms an equilateral triangle with the posterior alveolus and the hamulus). A medial variant described by Delaire uses a releasing incision medial to the greater palatine artery essentially creating random pattern flaps, which are under greater tension leading to more fistulae, but is said to reduce maxillary growth retardation (in comparison to, for example, the Veau technique, due to less disturbance of the anterior palate and its growth centres). Surgicel is packed into the raw areas that heal by secondary intention.

- As part of the technique, the muscle is dissected out from nasal and oral mucosa and swept backwards off the hard palate mobilized to the midline, and then closed. There is no increase in length of the soft palate.
- Delaire used more medially placed incisions/flaps with the aim of reducing maxillary growth inhibition, but is associated with a higher fistula rate.
- The Bardach two-flap palatoplasty was conceived as a modification of the von Langenbeck with the incisions extended anteriorly to allow elevation of two large posteriorly based mucoperiosteal flaps that have good mobility. It is often combined with an intravelar veloplasty.

Soft palate lengthening (Veau–Wardill–Kilner)

These are often described as 'push-back' procedures. The mucoperiosteum of the hard palate is pushed posteriorly while transposing myomucosal flaps based on the greater palatine neurovascular bundles towards the midline, leaving relatively large antero-lateral donor defects. Original descriptions included fracture of the hamulus to release tensor palati but are no longer advocated.

The operation may be performed with or without dividing the nasal mucosa; although dividing the nasal mucosa at the hard–soft palate junction allows greater movement, it does leave a raw area on the nasal surface which may be left to granulate or closed with a variety of local flaps including Z-plasty.

Although palatal musculature is detached from the hard palate, fibres still course **anteriorly** rather than *transversely*. It has been postulated that the 'push-back' techniques may have a greater detrimental effect on future maxillary growth.

Realignment of the palatal muscle

Intravelar veloplasty was popularized by Sommerlad and involved radical muscle dissection, including taking the tensor muscle back to the pterygoid hamulus and repositioning to lie more posteriorly and transversely.

Kriens OB (*Plast Reconstr Surg* 1969;**43**:29–41) provided detailed description of abnormal muscle insertions and directions of pull as well as description of dissection of individual muscles at operation to restore as near normal anatomy as possible.

Two-stage repair (Schweckendiek)

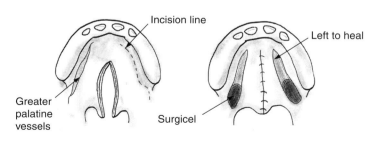

Figure 4.3 Von Langenbeck repair. A bipedicled mucoperiosteal flap is raised by incising behind the alveolus, and mobilized medially whilst preserving the greater palatine vessels.

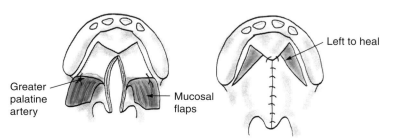

Figure 4.4 Veau–Wardill–Kilner. Mucosal periosteal flaps are raised and sutured together medially leaving areas that are left to heal secondarily. There is retropositioning of the posterior border of the soft back, hence the alternative term 'push-back repair'.

The soft palate is repaired at the same time as the lip at 4–6 months of age with definitive hard palate repair at 12–14 years of age, with an obturator being used in the meantime. The aim of causing less growth inhibition of the maxillary is achieved according to studies with long-term follow-up but at the expense of worse speech with VPI in more than half. A common variation is to repair the palate at 19–24 months.

A technique for cleft palate repair

Sommerlad B. *Plast Reconstr Surg* 2003;**112**:1542–1548.

The author describes a technique of palate repair that combines minimal hard palate dissection with radical retropositioning of the velar musculature and tensor tenotomy. An important feature of this technique is that it is performed using an **operating microscope**. The paper reports 442 primary palate repairs with follow-up of at least 10 years with 80% carried out through incisions at the margins of the cleft and without any mucoperiosteal flap elevation or lateral incisions. Secondary velopharyngeal rates decreased from 10.2 to 4.9 to 4.6% in successive 5-year periods within this 15-year period suggesting that this more radical muscle dissection improves velar function.

The use of the operating microscope for cleft palate repair and pharyngoplasty

Sommerlad B. *Plast Reconstr Surg* 2003;**112**:1540–1541.

The author began using the operating microscope used for all palate and pharyngeal operations in 1991 ($n = 1000$) and reports that it provides a more comfortable position with reliable lighting and variable magnification. As the anatomy is more clearly displayed so the reconstruction is potentially more accurate. In addition, the operating surgeon's view can be displayed through a teaching arm or video screen, for trainees and operating-room staff.

Lengthening the soft palate and reconstruct palatal muscle sling

Cleft palate repair by double opposing Z-plasty
Furlow LT. *Plast Reconstr Surg* 1986;**78**:724–736.

The author described his technique of soft palate repair using double opposing Z-plasty flaps to create a muscle sling across the cleft. In the author's view, this also allows the soft palate to be lengthened without using tissue from the hard palate. It is combined with a Von Langenbeck repair of the hard palate with a midline scar, said to reduce interference with maxillary growth.

The nasal Z-plasty is a mirror image of the oral Z-plasty with the central limb formed by incising the cleft edges. **Anteriorly** based flaps are composed of **mucosa**, the posteriorly based flaps are myomucosal to incorporate palatal **musculature**. The nasal flaps are transposed before the oral flaps and create an overlapping sling of palatal muscle.

- It is reported to produce superior speech and less VPI compared with historical controls.
- The suture lines are at right angles to each other on the nasal and oral layers, reducing the chance of fistulae.

However, subsequent reports suggest that if there is any lengthening with a Furlow's technique, it does in fact do so at the expense of tissue that would be used for closure around the hard–soft palate junction.

Effect of Veau–Wardill–Kilner type of cleft palate repair on long-term midfacial growth

Choudhary S. *Plast Reconstr Surg* 2003;**111**:576–582.

There are concerns that the Veau–Wardill–Kilner type of cleft palate repair causes inhibition of maxillary growth due to the extensive denudation of the palate. The author presents experience with 25 non-syndromic complete unilateral cleft lip and palate patients with an average 12 years of follow-up. Midfacial growth was analysed using 12-year dental models and lateral cephalograms taken before definitive orthodontic treatment. Seventy-two per cent of the patients had a good or satisfactory outcome, 28% obtained a poor score of 4 or 5.

The results suggest that satisfactory long-term midfacial growth can be obtained with Veau–Wardill–Kilner cleft palate repair but did not compare it with other techniques.

Arm restraints in children with cleft lip/palate

Sommerlad BC. *Plast Reconstr Surg* 2003;**112**:331–332.

This randomized trial demonstrated that there was no benefit in using any form of arm restraint.

IV. Complications

Of most concern are the airway and bleeding.

- **Nasal airway obstruction** occurs at two time periods: early due to post-operative swelling and late due to altered nasal morphology (25% decrease in pressure flow through nasal airway).

Fistula (0–34%) that may present as audible nasal escape during speech, hypernasality, nasal regurgitation and deterioration in speech intelligibility.

- Pharyngoplasty rate after palatoplasty up to 20%.
- **Maxillary growth retardation** may be less pronounced in later repair but at the expense of delaying development of normal speech due to late correction of VPI. Growth retardation (Semb G. A study of facial growth in patients with unilateral cleft lip and palate treated by the **Oslo** CLP team. *Cleft Palate Craniofac J* 1991;**28**:1–21) is related to age at surgery; the seniority of surgeon, type of lip repair and pharyngoplasty are not prognostic.
  - Secondary alveolar bone grafting does not inhibit growth but provides a valuable matrix for the eruption of teeth.

Influence of surgical technique on early post-operative hypoxaemia in children undergoing elective palatoplasty

Xue FS. *Br J Anaesth* 1998;**80**:447–451.

Post-operative hypoxaemia is potentiated by oedema of palate, pharynx or tongue along with inability to clear pulmonary and oral secretions and low elastic recoil of thorax and lungs. Children also have comparatively higher oxygen consumption.

Three treatment groups studied 312 patients altogether:

- von Langenbeck palatoplasty.
- Push-back palatoplasty.
- Push-back plus superior pharyngeal flap pharyngoplasty.

Oxygen saturation dips to < 85% were recorded most frequently in patients with combined procedures whilst von Langenbeck repairs were significantly less likely to cause hypoxaemia than the others. Desaturation was most profound within the first 30 min of arrival in the recovery room but depended somewhat on the technique used.

- von Langenbeck palatoplasty – first 15 minutes.
- Push-back palatoplasty – first 40 minutes.
- Push-back plus superior pharyngeal flap pharyngoplasty – 120 minutes.

Cleft palate fistulas: A multivariate statistical analysis of prevalence, aetiology, and surgical management

Cohen SR. *Plast Reconstr Surg* 1991;**87**:1041–1047.

This is a retrospective review of 129 non-syndromic CL/P patients with an overall 23% fistula rate. The fistulae were mostly small (1–2 mm) and located in the anterior part of the hard palate.

Multivariate analysis showed that causative risk factors were: push-back palatoplasty (43% developed fistulae), Veau classification 3 and 4, and the operating surgeon.

Factors that did not seem to contribute included intravelar veloplasty and age and gender of patient although recurrent fistulae (37%) were more common in females.

Options for surgical management (with average recurrence rate of 25%) included total revision of the palate repair, local mucoperiosteal flaps, vomerine flaps, bone grafting plus soft tissue closure and tongue flaps.

- 16% large fistulae (> 5 mm), repaired early due to speech problems.
- 47% small fistulae (1–2 mm), repaired at time of lip revision, nasal surgery or bone grafting i.e. delayed.

Cleft palate closure in the neonate: preliminary report

Denk MJ. *Cleft Palate Craniofacial J* 1996;**33**:57–61.

Against

- Anaesthetic risk and technical difficulty.
- Implications for facial growth.
- Chance of missing undiagnosed anomalies.
- Hypoglycaemia and jaundice may result.

For

- Improved speech and easier feeding.
- Psychologically better for parents (especially fathers?).
- Can perform synchronous palate (Furlow's) and lip closure under one anaesthetic.

The authors report on their experience with 21 patients operated within 28 days of birth; they conclude that it is safe but do not recommend it as a standard.

Prenatal counselling for cleft lip and palate

Matthews MS. *Plast Reconstr Surg* 1998;**101**:1–5.

Cleft lip and palate may be diagnosed incidentally during routine prenatal screening at 15 weeks. Specifically looking for clefts with prenatal ultrasound has a low sensitivity but high specificity (high false-negative), low false-positive – most ultrasound diagnosed clefts are bilateral.

Although no parents included in this study (survey of nine families of patients with prenatal diagnosis) felt that termination would be an option for an isolated cleft, 30% were against having a further pregnancy. There was a high incidence of associated abnormalities and **karyotyping** is advised. The majority of parents felt prenatal counselling with the cleft team was helpful.

Currently, cleft lip and palate is not reliably diagnosed with prenatal transabdominal ultrasound until the facial soft tissues are distinct by 13–14 weeks; slightly earlier with transvaginal ultrasound. The fetal palate is best seen in the axial plane whilst the lips are best visualized in the coronal view. Associated anomalies of the limb and spine are seen in 33% of patients with prenatal diagnosis of cleft lip and palate; 24% cardiovascular.

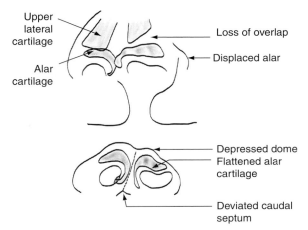

Figure 4.5 The cleft nose deformity is complex. There is loss of overlap between the upper lateral and lower lateral (alar) cartilages and the cleft side alar base is displaced laterally. The cleft side alar cartilage is flattened, buckled and hypoplastic contributing to a depressed, bifid dome. In addition, the nasal spine and causal septal cartilage is deviated to the opposite side.

V. Cleft nose

Aetiology of the cleft nose

- Intrinsic – inherited tissue defect in the cleft side traced to an ectodermal deficiency.
- Extrinsic – malposition of the nose due to developmental traction (Moss' functional matrix theory).

Unilateral cleft nose deformity

- Mild – wide alar base, but with normal alar contour and dome projection.
- Moderate – wide alar base, depressed dome or alar crease (minimal alar hypoplasia).
- Severe – wide alar base, deep alar crease, underprojecting alar dome (alar hypoplasia) with **caudal rotation** (downwards) of the alar cartilage so that the dome is **retroposed** and the nose is **lengthened** on the cleft side – normal columellar angle ~60°: cleft nose is caudally rotated (> 60°). Septum is deviated away from the cleft side – the pull of normal muscles is not counterbalanced.

Bilateral cleft nose deformity

- Short columella.
- Broad, depressed nasal tip.

In general, primary nasal correction is carried out at age 5–6 years with definitive rhinoplasty at ~16–17 years.

Primary repair of the unilateral cleft lip nose

Treatment of the unilateral cleft lip nose
McComb H. *Plast Reconstr Surg* 1975;**55**:596–601.

Primary repair of the unilateral cleft lip nasal deformity: a 10-year review

McComb H. *Plast Reconstr Surg* 1985;**75**:791–799.

Surgery for the cleft nose aims to correct caudal rotation of the alar cartilage at the time of lip repair and shorten the nose on the cleft side. The skin is mobilized off cartilage framework and the alar lift achieved with mattress sutures passing from within the vestibule of the cleft nostril and tied over a bolster at the level of the nasion.

Primary repair of the bilateral cleft lip nose: a 15-year review and a new treatment plan

McComb H. *Plast Reconstr Surg* 1990;**86**:882–886.

Following primary correction of the bilateral cleft nose by elevation of the alar cartilages and columellar lengthening using forked flaps, three undesirable features become apparent at adolescence:

- Nostrils are larger than normal.
- Broadening of the nasal tip due to separation of alar domes.
- Downward drift of the columella base.

Supposedly, it makes more embryological sense for the columella to be reconstructed from nasal tissue rather than from the prolabium that belongs to the lip, and the use of forked flaps is questioned. The nose is repaired at a first stage with repair of the lip at a second stage 1 month later – the blood supply to the pro-labium, when elevated off the premaxilla, is thus not compromised by concurrent nasal tip dissection and undermining.

Presurgical orthopaedics helps to reduce the soft tissue cleft before operation.

- Stage 1:
  - Repair of nostril floor and lip adhesion of prolabial segment to adjacent lip.
- Stage 2:
  - Open rhinoplasty approach – incisions above each alar rim meeting in the midline and mobilize alar domes with wide undermining.
  - Lip adhesions taken down and a formal lip repair performed using lateral mucomuscular flaps to the undermined prolabium.
  - Suture the displaced alar domes (now under less tension) together.
  - Close skin incisions as a V–Y to a length of 5 mm as the vertical limb in the columella.

Reverse 'U' incision for secondary repair of cleft lip nose

Tajima S. *Plast Reconstr Surg* 1977;**60**:256–261.

This technique uses an inverted 'U'-shaped inci-sion in the nasal vestibule to mobilize the dorsal nasal skin and allow suturing of the displaced alar cartilage (cleft side) to the normal side but significant under-mining is required. As the normal anatomical correc-tion of the alar cartilage is achieved, the mobilized dorsal skin is in slight excess and closure gives rise to a natural in-rolling effect.

The use of this technique has been reported in primary repairs also (Byrd HS *Plast Reconstr Surg* 2000;**106**:1276–1286).

VI. Orthodontics

Tooth development and cleft orthodontics

The alveolar cleft is usually located between the lateral incisor and the canine. The lateral incisor tooth bud may develop two incisors on either side of the cleft, may erupt into the cleft space or may be absent (10–40% of patients).

The permanent lateral incisor normally erupts at 7–8 years of age whilst the canine erupts at 11–12 years of age. Permanent teeth are generally slower to erupt around a cleft than non-cleft teeth and adjacent teeth usually have poorly formed enamel.

Stages of orthodontic treatment

- Presurgical orthopaedics (see above) can be useful in assisting the closure of the wide alveolar cleft. A prosthetic plate may also assist feeding.
- Early dental management from age 6 onwards consists of extraction of troublesome displaced deciduous teeth and correction of malocclusion of erupting permanent teeth.
- Management of permanent dentition, includes orthodontic treatment aimed at realigning teeth and correcting cross-bite, age 11 onwards. Some patients may need Le Fort I osteotomy and maxillary advancement or distraction.
  - Orthodontics relies upon bone resorption along the pressure side of a tooth and growth on the tension side.

Occlusion (Angle classification)

- Class I – Normal occlusion. The mesiobuccal cusp of the permanent maxillary first molar occludes in the buccal groove of the permanent mandibular or in other words, the first molar lower incisor contacts the middle part of the upper incisor (normal). Essentially each upper molar tooth should sit half a tooth in front of the corresponding lower tooth.
- Class II – lower incisor contacts posterior to class I e.g. Treacher Collins.
- Class III – lower incisor contacts anterior to class I e.g. Crouzon's syndrome.

Bone–base relationship

- Class I – maxilla slightly over-projects mandible (normal).
- Class II – maxilla excessively over-projects.
- Class III – mandible over-projects maxilla.

In cleft patients, the occlusion may be normal but there is often a class III occlusion. There are also variable degrees of cross-bite in the posterior teeth, some uppers biting inside the lowers – unilateral clefts tend to be associated with unilateral areas of cross-bite, bilateral clefts with bilateral cross-bite. Some teeth may be significantly displaced and need to be extracted.

Aims of alveolar cleft closure

Alveolar deformity in complete clefts can be either narrow or wide, with or without collapse. The aims of cleft closure are:

- To stabilize the maxillary arch (especially bilateral clefts) and close oronasal fistulas and anterior palatal cleft.
- To provide periodontal support for teeth to the cleft and provide a matrix into which permanent teeth may erupt.

Gingivoperiosteoplasty (closure of the alveolar cleft using periosteal flaps – Skoog) does not achieve all of these aims.

Bone grafting

Orthodontic treatment, i.e. movement of the premaxilla and maxillary segments, is impossible after bone grafting, thus it is necessary to establish good arch alignment before grafting. The eruption of permanent dentition may be needed to facilitate orthodontic treatment before bone grafting, particularly in bilateral clefts.

There is some debate regarding the timing – early (5–6 years) versus late (9–11 years); an alternate time is when 25–50% of the canine tooth is visible on the orthopantomogram (OPG). Early grafting may reduce maxillary growth and the bone graft resorbs in the absence of an erupting tooth. Late grafting deprives erupting permanent dentition of periodontal support. Conditions for surgery:

- Robust repair of the palatal cleft.
- Watertight closure of nasal lining.
- Secure lip repair.

The technique involves raising flaps of gingiva in the cleft itself and superiorly based on the alveolus to cover bone graft. The incisions should be kept further away from the gingivodental junction when raising flaps around permanent compared with deciduous teeth. Cancellous autograft from iliac crest is harvested, then packed into cleft and the gingival flaps are closed.
Complications:

- Wound dehiscence and graft exposure.
- Resorption of graft.

VII. Ear disease

Eustachian tube dysfunction

The Eustachian tube fails to open properly during swallowing; the tensor palati and levator palati that both attach to the auditory tube function abnormally. This leads to generation of negative pressure within the middle ear and collection of serous or mucoid (glue ear) effusion in the middle ear. There is usually a conductive hearing loss of 40 dB that exacerbates speech problems.

- Hearing can be tested at an early age by evoked response audiometry.
- The natural history is for the dysfunction to improve ~8 years of age: as mid-face grows the Eustachian tube begins to drain by gravity.
- Repair of the palate alone does not improve otitis media; palatoplasty often but does not always correct the dysfunction whilst adenoidectomy may also improve Eustachian tube patency. Some patients may need treatment by myringotomy and insertion of grommets before or at the time of palate repair. Grommets fall out after 6–9 months and thus benefit may be temporary; there are known complications such as damage to the tympanic membrane (4.8%), displacement into middle ear, tymanosclerosis etc.

B. Investigation and management of velopharyngeal incompetence

I. Normal speech

In the English language there are 24 consonants, 15 short vowel sounds and nine long vowel sounds.
Classification of consonants:

- Voicing of sounds.
  - Vocal folds vibrating – all vowels and B, G, D, Z.
  - Vocal folds held apart – mainly **plosive** sounds P, T, K, S.
- Place of articulation.
  - Lips – M, P, B.
  - Labiodental – F, V (lower lip and upper incisors).
  - Dental – TH (tongue plus teeth).
  - Alveolar – T, D (tongue plus alveolar ridge).
  - Palato-alveolar – SH (air passes beneath the palate).

- ○ Palatal – Y.
- ○ Velar.
- ○ Glottal.

During normal speech, the soft palate ascends to close off the nasopharynx and inadequate closure causes velopharyngeal incompetence (VPI). Symptoms include:

- Hypernasality (rhinolalia).
- Audible nasal escape – only the sounds M, N and NG **normally** allow nasal escape in the English language.
- Lack of voice projection and articulation.

Secondary symptoms of velopharyngeal incompetence

The inability to generate enough air pressure to pronounce explosive sounds (**stop plosives**) such as P, T, K, B, D and G which are substituted for by **glottal stop sounds** (compensatory articulatory method characterized by forceful adduction of vocal cords – the build-up and release of air pressure underneath the glottis results in a grunt-type sound).

- Consonants such as S, Z, SH and occasionally CH are substituted by **pharyngeal fricative sounds** (making the sound in the throat instead of the mouth).
- Unintelligible vocalization, nasal grimacing (attempting to close anterior nasal aperture), snorts (attempting to close posterior aperture) and breathlessness.

About 20% of patients require pharyngoplasty after palatoplasty which seems to be independent of the type of surgery. Velopharyngeal incompetence may result from anatomic (e.g. abnormal dentition), neuromuscular, mental disability, behavioural or a combination of disorders.

Investigation of VPI aims to define the site and size of the gap:

- Speech and hearing assessment.
- Multiview videofluoroscopy (pronouncing 'EE') – allows definition of level of closure.
- Nasendoscopy – allows visualization of closure mechanism, closure patterns include: coronal (most common, over half), circular (20%), circular with Passavant's ridge (20%), sagittal (10%). Passavant's ridge is usually 1 cm inferior to the usual level of closure.
- Magnetic resonance imaging.

II. Surgery for velopharyngeal incompetence

Indications for surgery

Nasal escape is a prominent feature and hampers the development of normal speech.

- Velopharyngeal incompetence despite adequate correction of a palatal cleft is found in approximately 20% of patients.

Surgery can be considered after accurate speech assessment and the intelligence of the patient is not unduly low.

Timing of surgery

After 5 years but before 12 years; after 12 years there is a decline in the rate of learning of new speech sounds.

Choice of procedure

- Speech assessment/therapy may be sufficient for minor VPI.
- Lengthening the palate with push-back procedures, Furlow's.
- Improving palatal movement – intravelar veloplasty (redirection of muscles).
- Narrowing the nasopharyngeal isthmus (exclude velocardiofacial syndrome – can use FISH cq22).
- Immobile soft palate (sufficient lateral wall motion): flap pharyngoplasty/pharyngeal flap.
- Mobile soft palate but inadequate lateral wall closure: sphincteroplasty.
- Nasal escape following adenoidectomy: implant (Teflon, cartilage).
  - ○ Posterior wall augmentation has been largely abandoned due to the results being rather unpredictable.
  - ○ A palatal obturator may be considered in those with very wide clefts with little movement, and with little prospect of a good surgical outcome.

Wardill technique (1928): similar to a pyloroplasty, a horizontal incision is made in the posterior pharyngeal wall at the level of Passavant's ridge (hypertrophy of palatopharyngeus and lower part of superior constrictor) and sutured vertically, creating a ledge of tissue to act as a 'valve seating for the upper surface of the soft palate'.

Sphincteroplasty

The first attempt at a sphincteroplasty was made by Wardill (1928). The modern muscle sphincteroplasty was originally described by Hynes (1951) and then modified by Orticochea (1968) and Jackson (1985). It is indicated when there is poor medial excursion of the lateral pharyngeal walls and a short anteroposterior diameter.

Pharyngoplasty by muscle transplantation

Hynes W. *Br J Plast Surg* 1951;**3**:128–133.

According to the author, a drawback of using Wardill's technique was that the ridge of tissue on the posterior pharyngeal wall may be placed too low for velopharyngeal closure if the repaired palate is short because the palate will then approach the posterior wall at a level higher than Passavant's ridge. In addition the pharyngeal wall is sutured under tension. To be effective, pharyngoplasty must:

- Reduce transverse diameter of the pharynx and reduce the anterior–posterior (A–P) diameter of the pharynx at a level higher than Passavant's ridge.
- Allow normal superior constrictor function; maintain functional muscle around the nasopharyngeal isthmus rather than inert scar.

Hynes suggested using **superiorly** based mucosal flaps from posterior tonsillar pillars including the underlying palatopharyngeus taking care to preserve branches of the vagus nerve entering the muscle at the level of the soft palate. Flaps should be 3–4 cm long and ~1.5 cm wide and then inset in the midline into a **horizontal incision** in the posterior pharyngeal wall, one above the other to form a bulky ridge and reportedly providing static and dynamic closure of the velopharynx. The donor is closed directly.

Construction of a dynamic muscle sphincter in cleft palates

Orticochea M. *Plast Reconstr Surg* 1968;**41**:323–327.

The author describes the transposition of **palatopharyngeus** myomucosal flaps towards the midline and inset into an inferiorly based **posterior pharyngeal flap**. The donor defects are left to heal by secondary intention with cicatrization which gradually closes off the lateral pharyngeal apertures.

In adults or where there is a very short palate (anteroposteriorly), there is increased risk of dehiscence of the palatopharyngeus flaps – it is often preferable to perform the surgery in two stages, one flap at a time.

Sphincter pharyngoplasty

Jackson IT. *Clin Plast Surg* 1985;**12**:711–717.

The palatopharyngeus flaps are sutured **end–end** when inset into a transverse incision on the posterior pharyngeal wall level with the upper margin of the tonsillar fossa, under a superiorly based mucosal flap.

The preferred level of inset is determined by the results of videofluoroscopy, although in practice, as high as possible above C1 arch and Passavant's ridge. Only one-third retain significant levels of muscle contraction, i.e. in most cases it is not a dynamic sphincteric procedure.

Complications of sphincter pharyngoplasty include *obstructive sleep apnea* /snoring and airway obstruction but less than pharyngeal flaps; there is a higher rate of hypernasality.

Pharyngeal flaps

These are superiorly or inferiorly based single flaps that provide static closure of velopharynx. The aim is to allow less air through lateral ports – aim for a diameter of ~0.5 cm, and over-correction will lead to mouth breathing, hyponasality and obstructive sleep apnoea.

The flap is raised in the plane of prevertebral fascia and inset into reflected flaps from the soft palate or nasal mucosa. The donor defect is partially closed or allowed to heal by secondary intention. Superiorly based flaps are usually preferred as scarring will tend to pull the soft palate upwards whilst inferiorly based flaps will tend to tether in an inferior direction.

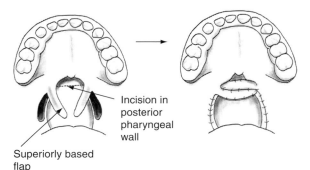

Incision in posterior pharyngeal wall

Superiorly based flap

Figure 4.6 Sphincter pharyngoplasty. Better results seem to be associated with higher level of inset.

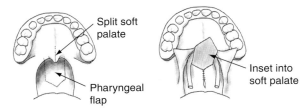

Figure 4.7 Superiorly based pharyngeal flap.

Velo-cardio-facial (Shprintzen's) syndrome

A new syndrome involving cleft palate, cardiac anomalies, typical facies and learning disabilities: Velo-cardio-facial syndrome
Shprintzen RJ. *Cleft Palate J* 1978;**15**:56–62.

Velo-cardio-facial syndrome (VCF) is the most common syndrome associated with clefts. There is inadequate development of the facial neural crest tissues, resulting in defective organogenesis of pharyngeal pouch derivatives. There is a 22q11.2 deletion that can be diagnosed by FISH test (fluorescent *in situ* hybridization) for the gene. These patients generally do badly as a group; associated abnormalities include CATCH (22):

- **Cardiac** anomalies – medially displaced anomalous carotid arteries – 25% have median carotid artery (pre-operative MRI angiography is advised), congenital heart problems, e.g. tetralogy of Fallot, coarctation of the aorta, pulmonary stenosis and ventricular septal defect (VSD) (most commonly).
- **Abnormal facies** (flat expressionless face) vertical maxillary excess, epicanthic folds, anti-Mongoloid slant, malar flattening, class II malocclusion, abundant scalp hair.
- **Thymic aplasia** (overlaps with Di George syndrome).
- **Cleft palate** (more commonly submucous) and velopharyngeal dysfunction i.e. poor movement in lateral pharyngeal wall. Magnetic resonance angiography (MRA) is recommended before surgery (usually a high wide pharyngeal flap).
- **Hypocalcaemia**.

  Also:

- Small stature.
- Abnormal dermatoglyphics.
- Mild hypotonia in early childhood.
- Spindly fingers.

- Learning difficulties and psychotic illness in adult life.

Surgical management of VPI in velo-cardio-facial syndrome

Mehendale FV. *Cleft Palate Craniofacial J* 2004;**41**:368–374.

The authors describe their experience with these cases. Their pre-surgical assessment included pre-operative intra-oral examination and lateral videofluoroscopy with or without nasendoscopy, and intra-operative assessment of velar muscular anatomy.

Surgical options were based upon assessment and included:

- Radical dissection and retropositioning of velar muscles (submucous cleft palate repair).
- Hynes pharyngoplasty.
- Palate repair followed by Hynes pharyngoplasty.

They preferred a staged approach, particularly to maximize palatal function first.

Outcomes were assessed by evaluation of resonance and nasal airflow and repeating lateral videofluoroscopy and nasendoscopy. Their results showed improvement in hypernasality in all groups.

- Staged approach showed significant improvement in nasal emission.
- Submucous CP repair resulted in increased velar length and increased velocity of closure.

An outcome evaluation of sphincter pharyngoplasty for the management of velopharyngeal insufficiency

Losken A. *Plast Reconstr Surg* 2003;**112**:1755–1761.

This is a review of 250 patients who underwent sphincter pharyngoplasty for VPI. Revision of pharyngoplasty was required in 12.8%, and was most common in the 22q11 deletion group and lowest in patients with VPI alone. Otherwise the need for further surgery is predicted by severe pre-operative hypernasal resonance and larger velopharyngeal aperture. Overall success was 99% (including those who had a single revision) and was thus judged to be an effective procedure.

Velopharyngeal surgery: a prospective randomized study of pharyngeal flaps and sphincter pharyngoplasties
Ysunza A. *Plast Reconstr Surg* 2002;**110**:1401–1407.

The incidence of residual VPI following palatal repair is commonly quoted to be between 10–20%.

The authors described a study of 50 patients with residual VPI. They were evaluated by videonasendo-scopy and multi-view videofluoroscopy and equal numbers were randomized to undergo 'customized' pharyngeal flap repair or 'customized' sphincter pharyngoplasty ('customized' means according to the operative findings). Results i.e. residual VPI were similar in each group.

C. Craniofacial anomalies

I. Craniofacial anatomy

Craniofacial growth

The facial skeleton is effectively suspended from the skull base.

Enlow's principles of facial growth: the mid-face and mandible are proportionately very small in the neonate, and these grow by:

- Displacement – whole bone mass moves.
- Remodelling – occurs behind the wave of displacement.

Moss' functional matrix principle states that osteogenic membranes such as periosteum react to the sum of functional and morphogenic processes (the functional matrix) acting on them e.g. growth of the brain; other components of the functional matrix include the muscles of mastication and their pull and developing dentition.

Embryology

The face is recognizably human by the end of week 8. The majority of craniofacial anomalies arise during the first 12 weeks of embryological development.

The face is derived from five facial prominences – the frontonasal process and paired maxillary and mandibular processes with fusion around day 46–47. Failure of fusion leads to facial clefting. The **mesodermal penetration theory** postulates that clefting occurs due to failure of migration of mesoderm into a bilaminar ectodermal membrane resulting in loss of support to the overlying epithelial seam.

Craniofacial abnormalities

Potential factors contributing to craniofacial anomalies include:

- Genetic (e.g. FGF receptor mutations).
- Radiation (associated with microcephaly).

- Maternal infection (toxoplasmosis, rubella, cytomegalovirus) or other health problems (phenylketonuria, diabetes, vitamin deficiency, smoking).

Encephalocoeles

These have a worldwide incidence of 1 in 5000 births and are herniations of cranial contents through a defect in the skull:

- Meninges (meningocoele).
- Meninges and brain (meningoencephalocoele/encephalomeningocoele).
- Meninges, brain and ventricle (meningoencephalocystocoele).

Anterior encephalocoeles are more common in Russia and south-east Asia whilst posterior encephalocoeles predominate in Western Europe, North America, Australia and Japan.

Encephalomeningocoele

These are congenital midline swellings that consist of herniation of meninges/brain tissue from the anterior cranial fossa via the foramen caecum. It is a form of neural tube defect and may be associated with metopic synostosis and hypertelorism. They can occur in occipital (most common 80%), parietal, frontal, nasal and nasopharyngeal sites. Occipital encephalocoeles are usually large and the outcome is poor; 75% die or are severely disabled.

Frontoethmoidal lesions are said to arise due to failure of regression of a dural diverticulum projecting through developing nasal and frontal bones (subtypes: nasofrontal, nasoethmoidal and naso-orbital).

Common craniofacial anomalies: facial clefts and encephaloceles

Hunt JA. *Plast Reconstr Surg* 2003;**112**:606–615.

Encephalocoeles can be investigated using skull X-ray and CT/MRI. The surgery can be performed by intra-/extra-cranial approach via bicoronal incision with the assistance of a neurosurgeon. In rare cases, only the meninges protrude i.e. meningocoele; if the herniation is only glial tissue, it can be safely excised.

- Urgent closure of open skin defects.
- Incision of sac and amputation of excess tissue beyond the limits of the skull.
- Dural closure, then reconstruction of soft tissue and bone (diploic bone graft).

Prenatal sonographic diagnosis of major craniofacial anomalies

Wong GB. *Plast Reconstr Surg* 2001;**108**:1316–1333.

Craniosynostosis – ultrasound imaging of cranial sutures is possible from week 13 though detection of single or multiple suture fusions is only possible from week 16, hence an early normal scan does not exclude later synostosis. Ultrasound findings should be combined with available genetic/molecular information.

- Head measurements indicate pattern of suture fusion (e.g. scaphocephaly vs. brachycephaly).
- Measurement of interorbital distance to diagnose hypertelorism.
- Imaging of hydrocephalus, encephalocoele and spinal defects.
- Syndromic synostoses identifiable from associated limb abnormalities; transvaginal ultrasound is useful for demonstrating hand abnormalities.

Pharyngeal and oromandibular abnormalities – imaging of the fetal maxillofacial skeleton possible from week 10.

- Craniofacial abnormalities of hemifacial microsomia can be diagnosed from week 29.

Treacher Collins syndrome can be diagnosed from 15 weeks onwards.

- Canted palpebrae, microphthalmia and hypertelorism.
- Microtia and micrognathia (also found in Pierre Robin sequence and Stickler's syndrome).

Nager syndrome (Treacher Collins phenotype with preaxial limb abnormalities).

- Proximal radioulnar synostosis, thumb hypoplasia or aplasia.

II. Craniofacial clefts

Some useful definitions:

- Malformation – intrinsic inborn area of the fetal development process.
- Dysplasia – abnormal organization of cells into tissue e.g. Stickler's.
- Disruption – normal fetus subjected to tissue injury/breakdown e.g. vascular, infection, metabolic, mechanical causes e.g. thalidomide.
- Deformation – fetus with no intrinsic problem, but abnormal external forces cause secondary distortion/deformity e.g. amniotic band.

- Syndrome – dysplasia affecting two or more sites not linked embryologically.

American Society of Cleft Lip and Palate classification of craniofacial deformities:

- Clefts and encephalocoeles.
- Synostosis – syndromal and non-syndromal.
- Hypoplastic conditions – hemifacial microsomia, hemifacial atrophy.
- Hyperplastic conditions – fibrous dysplasia.

Van der Meulen classification (most recent, European and uses 'dysplasia'):

- Cerebral craniofacial dysplasia – poor brain development usually means that these fetuses are non-viable.
- Craniofacial dysplasia – clefts and synostosis.
- Craniofacial dysplasia of other origin – i.e. miscellany, neurofibromatosis, vascular anomalies and fibrous dysplasia.

Facial clefts

The commonest facial cleft is cleft lip/palate followed by isolated cleft palate; other facial clefts are actually relatively rare in comparison (up to 5 cases per 100 000 live births). These other clefts exhibit a mixture of tissue deficiency and tissue excess. Environmental factors thought to contribute to facial clefts include influenza A2 virus and toxoplasmosis infection, also drugs such as anticonvulsants, steroids and tranquillizers. See mesodermal penetration theory above.

- The **Tessier classification**, the most commonly used is anatomical, whilst the Van der Meulen classification is embryological.

Aims and principles of reconstruction

Functional and aesthetic correction of deformities with particular attention to:

- Eyelids (to prevent corneal exposure).
- Macrostomia.
- Separate confluent oral, nasal and orbital cavities.

Surgical technique

- Excision of cleft scar tissue and abnormal elements.
- Layered soft tissue closure: provide skin cover with local skin flaps and reattach soft tissue in the correct position e.g. muscles of facial expression to reanimate the face and stimulate growth.

- Delay skeletal reconstruction until child is older. Remove abnormal bone elements and reconstruct defect with transposition of neighbouring bone or bone grafts.

Craniofacial clefts

Anatomical classification of facial, craniofacial and laterofacial clefts

Tessier P. *J Maxillofac Surg* 1976;**4**:69–92.

These are numbered 0–14; facial clefts (from orbit downwards) extend to cranial clefts (orbit upwards). The numbers relate to their position relative to the midline with cleft 8 forming the equator at the lateral angle of the eye. The facial cleft number plus cranial cleft number = **14** e.g. 0–14, 1–13, 2–12 3–11, etc. In general:

- Lateral clefts tend to have more severe bony abnormalities.
- Medial clefts have more severe soft tissue abnormalities.

Clefts do not pass through bony foraminae which are the site of neurovascular structures. Each can be considered in terms of bony and soft tissue characteristics.

- Bilateral clefts do not have to be equally severe.
- Facial clefts can be combined with craniosynostoses.

Cleft 0 (0–3 are sometimes referred to as the oronasal clefts)

- Midline facial cleft.
- Median cleft lip (**absent prolabium**), bifid nose, bifid tongue, maxillary midline cleft.

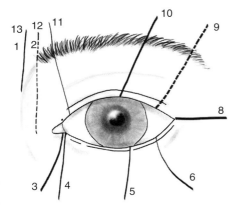

Figure 4.8 Craniofacial clefts in relation to the eye

- Extends to cleft 14 – holoprosencephaly deformities (including cyclopia) and frontonasal encephalocoele may be present, though the deformity is very variable. The crista galli is bifid.

Cleft 1

- Soft tissue cleft from Cupid's bow through alar dome and bony cleft passes between central and lateral incisors. The septum is intact but the alar dome is notched, the columella broad, with absent nasal bones. The prognosis is related to the degree of brain development.
- It extends to cleft 13 that passes medial to the inner limit of the eyebrow, producing hypertelorism; encephalocoeles. The cribriform plate is widened and the ethmoid cells are hypertrophied.

Cleft 2

- This is a rare cleft, a soft tissue cleft from Cupid's bow but lateral to alar dome which is hypoplastic and drawn upwards. Lacrimal drainage is usually normal.
- Maxillary alveolar cleft lateral to the lateral incisor.
- The cleft 12 passes through medial third of eyebrow, there is hypertelorism and telecanthus. The frontal and sphenoid sinuses are enlarged.

Cleft 3

- This is the most common Tessier cleft. It is an oblique facial cleft (oronasoocular cleft) from Cupid's bow to lacrimal punctum, with medial canthal ligament agenesis and colobomata. The lacrimal drainage system is disrupted.
- Bony cleft begins between lateral incisor and canine, passes along the nasomaxillary groove (nasolacrimal duct disruption) into the orbit. Absent medial wall of maxillary sinus produces a confluent cavity of mouth, nose, maxillary sinus and orbit. It involves the secondary hard palate – posterior to the incisive foramen.
- Surgery is directed at cleft lip and palate repair, nasal correction, bony reconstruction of orbital floor and maxilla, and transnasal medial canthopexy.
- Cleft 11 passes through the medial third of the upper lid and eyebrow, bony cleft lateral to the ethmoid, producing hypertelorism.

Cleft 4 (4–6 are oral ocular clefts that pass through cheek without disrupting nose i.e. meloschisis)

- Similar to a number 3 cleft but begins just lateral to Cupid's bow and passes more towards the eye, to the lower lid just lateral to the punctum. There is deficiency of the medial/inferior orbital wall that may cause secondary nasal deformities. It is the most disruptive and complicated cleft.
- The bony cleft passes medial to the infra-orbital foramen and there may be microphthalmos or anophthalmia.
- Cleft 10 cleft continues through the middle third of the supra-orbital rim, a fronto-orbital encephalocoele displaces the eye inferolaterally causing hypertelorism.

Cleft 5

- This is one of the rarest. The soft tissue cleft runs from around the lateral commissure to the middle third of the lower lid that draws lip and lid together.
- Bony cleft from the premolars passing lateral to the infra-orbital foramen to involve the orbit in its middle third and eye can herniate into maxillary sinus.
- Cleft 9 is the rarest cleft and passes from the supra-orbital rim into the forehead as the continuation of a number 5 cleft, with an association with encephalocoeles, facial nerve palsy and cranial base abnormalities.

Cleft 6

- Soft tissue abnormality includes lower lateral lid colobomas, hypertelorism and anti-Mongoloid slant.
- Bony cleft centred on the zygomaticomaxillary suture and lateral third of infra-orbital rim, with loss of malar prominence.
  - Cleft numbers 6, 7 and 8 – Treacher Collins syndrome.
  - Cleft number 8 with disruption of the lateral canthus (incomplete closure) is a component of Goldenhar syndrome. Isolated cleft 8 is rare; there is a cleft at the frontozygomatic suture.

Cleft 7 (7–9 are lateral facial clefts)

- Cleft number 7 is **hemifacial microsomia** and may be bilateral in 10%; commonest cleft at 1 in 3000 –

more common in males. Cases are usually sporadic; supposedly secondary to disruption of stapedial artery.

- It is centred on the line between the oral commissure and the ear and affects structures around this line.
- Soft tissue structures: macrostomia, ear defects, facial and trigeminal nerve, parotid.
- Bony structures: ascending ramus of mandible, maxilla, etc. There is an open bite on the affected side.

Clefts 10–14 are called cranial clefts. Number 30 cleft: midline cleft involving the mandible, the hyoid bone and sternum.

Amniotic band syndrome – the association between rare facial clefts and limb ring constrictions

Coady MS. *Plast Reconstr Surg* 1998;**101**:640–649.

Facial clefts that occur with limb ring constrictions are paramedian type (2–12, 3–11, 4–10) and these patients may also have truncal defects. Theories for this association include:

- Mechanical disruption due to amniotic bands.
- Disorders of fetal blood supply.
- Genetic programming error.
- Disorder of tissue morphogenesis.

Down's syndrome: identification and surgical management of obstructive sleep apnoea

Lefaivre JF. *Plast Reconstr Surg* 1997;**99**:629–637.

Obstructive sleep apnoea presents with:

- Daytime somnolence and poor school performance.
- Developmental delay, failure to thrive, enuresis.

In Down syndrome, obstructive sleep apnoea may be caused by:

- Increased upper airway secretions and infections.
- Tonsillar and adenoid hyperplasia.
- Mandibular and maxillary hypoplasia.
- Macroglossia or disproportionately sized tongue (small oral cavity).
- Hypotonia.

Treatment options include:

- CPAP at night.
- Tonsillectomy and adenoidectomy.
- Uvulopalatopharyngoplasty (UPPP/UP3).

- Septal surgery to correct deviation and inferior turbinectomy.
- Maxillary advancement (Le Fort I or III) or distraction but over-advancement can precipitate VPI.
- Genioplasty.
- Central tongue reduction.

III. Craniosynostosis

This is the premature fusion of one or more sutures with growth retarded in the plane perpendicular to the suture. Virchow's law relates to growth retardation in the direction perpendicular to the fused suture, with compensatory growth parallel to the suture.

The bones of the skull form via two mechanisms – intramembranous and endochondral ossification; calvarial growth parallels brain growth. **Moss's functional matrix theory** suggests that cranial bones enlarge **as a result** of growth of the underlying brain.

Craniosynostosis can be classified as:

- Simple vs. complex.
- Primary vs. secondary.
- Syndromic vs. non-syndromic (much more common).

Theories of suture closure.

- Cranial base – exerts abnormal tension.
- Intrinsic suture biology – secondary to osteoinductive properties of dura mater.
- Extrinsic factors – in utero compression, hydrocephalus decompression (e.g. after VP shunt), abnormal brain growth (e.g. microcephaly) or systemic pathology (e.g. hypothryoidism or rickets).

Syndromic synostosis

Syndromic synostosis accounts for ~10–20% of all synostoses; 50% are hereditary. These patients should have regular CT scans and monitoring of intracranial pressure (ICP) e.g. visual evoked potentials.

Acrocephalosyndactyly syndromes: a review
Prevel CD. *J Craniofac Surg* 1997;**8**:279–285.

- Crouzon's.
- Apert's.
- Pfeiffer's.
- Saethre–Chotzen.
- Carpenter's.

In general, most conditions have autosomal dominant ± variable penetrance except for Carpenter's syndrome

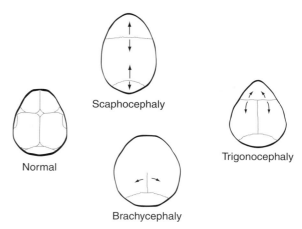

Figure 4.9 Typical skull shapes resulting from premature synostosis of cranial sutures: scaphocephaly (sagittal synostosis), trigonocephaly (metopic synostosis) and brachycephaly (bilateral coronal synostosis).

which is autosomal recessive. There are >90 reported syndromes and most have associated limb and cardiac abnormalities, and all have mid-face hypoplasia. Turribrachycephaly (turret-like) due to bicoronal synostosis is an associated feature.

Non-syndromic synostosis

These occur 0.6 in 1000 and may be due to:

- Gestational influences.
- Toxic influences.
- Sporadic congenital finding with approximate incidence of 0.05 to 0.01%.

These tend to be single suture type.
Aetiology:

- Many are associated with mutations in FGFR genes that encode tyrosine kinase receptors.
  - FGFR1 – Pfeiffer's.
  - FGFR2 – Pfeiffer's, Apert's, Crouzon's.
- Dura mater communicates with overlying cranial suture via paracrine activity of growth factors to regulate suture fusion.

Types of craniosynostoses:

- Metopic (between the frontal bones) synostosis – Trigonocephaly.
- Sagittal synostosis – Scaphocephaly.
- Unilateral coronal synostosis – Plagiocephaly.
- Bilateral coronal synostosis – Brachycephaly.
- Unilateral lambdoidal synostosis – Plagiocephaly.

Positional (deformational) plagiocephaly of the occiput is a non-synostotic deformity, otherwise known as self-correcting 'plagiocephaly without synostosis' (PWS).

Raised intracranial pressure

Raised ICP causes headache, irritability and difficulty sleeping in children. Disparity between brain growth and remodelling of overlying bone due to premature fusion of sutures may cause raised ICP (pressure >15–20 mmHg under unstressed conditions), which may cause mental impairment and optic atrophy. This is more common in those with multiple fused sutures and uncommon when only one suture is fused i.e. unilateral lambdoidal synostosis, metopic synostosis and sagittal synostosis. Clinical signs include:

- Examination: papilloedema that may lead to optic atrophy, fontanelle bulging.
- Headaches and other neurological symptoms – fits, seizures.
- X-ray shows thumb printing, copper beating or a wormian appearance as well as absence of suture line at synostosis. CT may be indicated for syndromic synostosis, as it may detect hydrocephalus/raised ICP or other brain/bone abnormalities.
- Developmental delay. The higher the ICP the lower the IQ tends to be.

Hydrocephalus is commoner in syndromic craniosynostosis and uncommon in non-syndromic craniosynostosis and is possibly due to increased venous pressure in the sagittal sinus.

Mental disability is more common where ICP is raised (multiple suture synostosis) and with hydrocephalus (syndromic synostosis). The effect of surgery on single suture synostosis and mental development remains controversial.

Intracranial pressure in single-suture craniosynostosis
Cohen SR. *Cleft Palate Craniofac J* 1998;**35**:194–196.

With single suture involvement 13% have raised ICP whilst in multiple synostosis it is 43%.

In patients resigned to undergoing corrective surgery, ICP monitoring is unnecessary whereas patients showing clinical signs of raised ICP but unwilling to undergo surgery may need ICP monitoring. Patients without signs and unwilling to undergo surgery should have close follow-up.

Mental development and learning disorders in children with single suture craniosynostosis
Kapp–Simon KA. *Cleft Palate Craniofac J* 1998;**35**: 197–203.

Children with unilateral coronal synostosis are more likely to suffer from learning disabilities than the general population but early surgery did not seem to prevent learning disability in the long term.

- All craniofacial patients should be managed by a multidisciplinary team.
- Plain skull X-ray, CT, MRI – CT may help differentiate between deformational plagiocephaly and lambdoid synostosis.

Assessment of patient with craniosynostosis

History

- Family history of craniosynostoses.
- Problems during pregnancy (including maternal drug history) or delivery, and condition at birth (Apgar scores).

Investigations

- Skull X-ray – shape and thumb printing.
- CT, with or without 3D-CT reconstruction.
- Paediatric consultation – management should ideally be multidisciplinary.

The general aim is to determine whether the patient has a deformational synostosis or true craniosynostosis – and if the latter, which one? Possible diagnoses may be suggested by specific features e.g. turribrachycephaly plus:

- No hand abnormality – Crouzon's.
- Spade, mitten or hoof hand – Apert's.
- Broad thumbs ± ankylosis of elbow – Pfeiffer's.
- Low forehead, ptosis, short stature – Saethre-Chotzen.
- Dry frizzy hair, grooved nails, bifid nasal tip – Craniofrontonasal dysplasia.
- Scaphocephaly – Carpenter's.

Treatment aims to treat deformity (create aesthetic head shape) or to prevent deformity and provide adequate volume for growing brain. Simple suture removal tends to be inadequate – the cranial shape is not immediately corrected and many have secondary deformities due to reclosure of the suture before adequate remodelling.

Modern principles of treatment of craniofacial surgery

Principles include:

- Good access.
- Rigid fixation.
  - Beware of the use of titanium miniplates during infancy as bone resorption may lead to intracranial migration; as such, absorbable plates may be preferable (also to avoid potential growth restriction).
  - Absorbable plates can be made from vicryl (polyglactic) or dexon (polyglycolic), with variable degradation rates, but generally 9–15 months by hydrolysis. The plates are thicker than metallic plates and thus more likely to be palpable and screw holes need to be tapped. They may still migrate but migration does not necessarily do harm in this case.
- Bone graft.
  - Autologous – split calvarial (parietal), split rib (hard to mould, more resorption).
  - Methylmethacrylate, hydroxyapatite – calcium phosphate, Medpor (porous polyethylene), demineralized bone.
  - Replamineform is a process to create hard porous implant material similar to coral.
- Pericranial/galeal flaps.

Timing of surgery

It is common to operate at ~**3 months**, sooner if raised ICP supervenes e.g. pan-sutural involvement. At this age, the skull bones are **malleable, heal better** and large bony defects can be reconstituted with new bone formation in children < 2 years; surgery tends to be less radical/quicker and involves less blood loss. Later surgery on the other hand reduces the need for revisional surgery. Overall, there is a 5% re-operation rate.

- The brain triples in size during the first year of life and growth (skull and brain) is ~85% complete by 3 years of age. The brain continues to grow until 6–7 years of age, continually modelling overlying bone.
- The globe triples in size between birth–adolescence: 90% of adult volume by 7 years.

While cosmesis is important, mental development is paramount. Although ICP may not be raised in Apert's (wide open fontanelles), frontal advancement in these patients in Marchac's series (vide infra) allowed better intellectual development (other surgeons have said that earlier surgery does not affect intellectual development). Parents are often reluctant to accept craniofacial surgery, and **objective measurements** such as a raised ICP help to provide stronger arguments for surgery.

Timing of treatment for craniosynostosis and facio-craniosynostosis: a 20-year experience
Marchac D. *Br J Plast Surg* 1994;**47**:211–222.

For patients with brachycephaly, frontal advancement is performed at age 2–4 months; for other craniosynostoses, correction can be performed later, between 6 and 9 months. Note that the authors suggest that there are increased re-operation rates compared with surgery performed after 9 months. This view is supported by Wall SA (*Br J Plast Surg* 1994;**47**:180–184) who go further to suggest that unless there is raised ICP or severe exorbitism, surgery should be delayed after 12 months.

Frontofacial monobloc advancement is only indicated for severe exorbitism in infancy as there is:

- Infection risk due to dead space and intracranial communication with the nasal airway (vide infra, Fearon 1997).
- Major surgery with risk of blood loss.
- If performed too early < 5 years of age, the deformity may return.
- Between 2 and 5 years supra-orbital bar advancement is complicated by the development of the frontal sinus although in these patients the frontal sinus will usually redevelop after it has been cranialized.

Thus in most cases of craniosynostosis with mid-face hypoplasia (Apert's, Crouzon's), a two- (or three-) stage approach is preferred:

- Frontal advancement first **then** facial advancement 6–12 years (Le Fort III).
- Le Fort I advancement may ultimately be required for final correction of bite at 12–18 years.

Facial bipartition can be performed to correct the hypertelorism associated with Apert's, and accompanies facial advancement.

Typical operative sequence

- Transcoronal incision and subperiosteal dissection.

- Craniotomy (with burr holes) and elevate bone off dura.
- Elevate temporalis, cut and advance frontal bar.
- Cut barrel staves and out-fracture as needed.
- Use split bone grafts as needed, moulding bone by burring, scoring or radial osteotomies.
- Replace bone flaps and fix, apply bone grafts/bone dust/exogenous e.g. hydroxyapatite.
- Close with drain.

Patients are usually kept in ICU for 24–48 hours; the haematocrit should be monitored and transfused as required (< 30).

Protection of the brain during and after intracranial surgery:

- Pre-operative antibiotics and dexamethasone (4 mg 6 hourly).
- Post-induction **drainage** of 100–120 ml CSF leads to relaxation of the brain and less retraction is needed during the operation.
- Controlled **hyperventilation** to decrease $PaCO_2$ leading to cerebral vasoconstriction and decreased brain volume.
- IV infusion of **mannitol** to decrease ICP.

Complications of surgery

Death (1–2%) due to:

- Uncontrolled intra-operative haemorrhage (disruption of dural sinuses, large areas of raw bone).
- Air embolus.
- Cerebral oedema.
- Respiratory infection or obstruction.
- CSF leak (check with intra-operative Valsava) which may lead to meningitis – use antibiotics which cross the blood–brain barrier.

Other complications:

- Optic nerve injury if bicoronal flap is reflected over the eyes for too long.
- Persistent CSF leak.
- Seizures.
- Plate migration.
- Recurrence, need for further surgery in 27% of syndromic cases, 6% for isolated synostoses.
- Infection.

Infections in craniofacial surgery

Fearon JA. *Plast Reconstr Surg* 1997;**200**:862–868.

The authors reported a 2.5% infection rate in 567 intracranial procedures. Interestingly, no patients younger than 13 months developed an infection and they suggested that this may be due to the fact that rapid brain growth obliterates dead space in such patients. Half of all infections were related to frontofacial **monobloc surgery**. The infection rates were higher in **secondary surgery**, possibly related to:

- Longer operating times.
- Scarring with decreased tissue vascularity.
- Older patients with more sinus development.

Shaving hair did not influence infection rates.

Cephalosporin prophylaxis of meningitis may have contributed to incidence of *Candida* and *Pseudomonas* infection.

Metopic synostosis (10%)

The metopic suture normally fuses ~2 years of age but metopic synostosis leads to **trigonocephaly** with flattening of the frontal bones, a midline forehead ridge and bitemporal narrowing with flaring of the parietal bones.

- Comprises < 10% of non-syndromic synostosis.
- Most occur spontaneously; autosomal dominant inheritance has been reported.
- ~4% have raised ICP and mental disability; there is an association with abnormalities of the corpus callosum.

There is also hypotelorism and Mongoloid slant; surgery can correct orbital rim hypoplasia. Note that hypotelorism is associated with metopic synostosis, Down and Binder's syndromes, most other CF syndromes have **hypertelorism**.

Surgical treatment:

- Frontoparietal advancement and remodelling with radial barrel stave osteotomies.
- Supra-orbital bar advancement.

The hypotelorism is then self-correcting without the need for orbital translocation and interorbital bone grafts.

Sagittal synostosis (50%)

This is the **most common** craniosynostosis (50%) and results in a long and narrow skull i.e. **scaphocephaly**, supposedly keel-shaped. There is reduced biparietal width with increased A–P measurement with frontal and occipital bossing which may affect anterior or posterior areas unequally. Cases are usually sporadic, though 2% have a genetic inheritance. It is four times more common in males.

Surgery aims to reduce A–P length and increase skull width.

- Sagittal strip craniectomy (sagittal sinus injury is a risk).
- Frontal, parietal and orbital bone remodelling (barrel stave).

Correction of scaphocephaly secondary to ventricular shunting

Shuster BA. *Plast Reconstr Surg* 1995;**96**:1012–1019.

Premature fusion of the sagittal suture may be precipitated by the insertion of a VP shunt (secondary synostosis) possibly due to acute reduction in intracranial volume with overriding of the sutures. However, the synostosis may also be related to the primary pathology that caused the hydrocephalus.

This affects mainly children < 6 months of age; treat by excision of the fused suture (sagittal strip craniectomy) and occipital remodelling ± frontal remodelling.

Unilateral coronal synostosis (20%)

This is rather uncommon (1 in 10 000) and results in **anterior plagiocephaly** (Greek oblique skull). There is retarded growth in an A–P direction on the affected side – the anterior cranial fossa becomes shorter, there is ipsilateral frontal flattening with contralateral parietal **bossing** (due to increased bone deposition directed away from the fused suture). It needs to be distinguished from secondary moulding deformities that may be associated with torticollis or Klippel–Feil syndrome (fusion of cervical vertebrae, a fairly rare association). Most cases of synostostic anterior plagiocephaly are females (79%).

There is compensatory growth:

- Upwards – causing a long flat forehead. The supraorbital rim is recessed and the orbit is shallow.
- Downwards – distorting the sphenoid with a loss of height of the lateral wall of the orbit, this is seen as the '**harlequin orbit**' on X-ray that is pathognomonic of coronal synostosis – 'devil's eye' that is slanted upwards with deficient lateral wall. Eyebrow is elevated on the affected side whilst the face tends to be C-shaped with chin and nose deviation away from the affected side.

There is proptosis of the globe that may lead to corneal exposure/ulceration and ultimately blindness.

Surgery restores the supra-orbital rim by advancing this segment (**bilateral fronto-orbital advancement**) along with frontal remodelling as above.

- **Unilateral frontal craniotomy and supra-orbital bar advancement** may give unsatisfactory results and bilateral surgery has been shown to give a superior appearance (Sgouros S. *J Craniofac Surg* 1996;**7**:336–340).
- Supra-orbital bar advancement may inhibit growth of the frontal sinus which then affects the projection of the glabellar region but this a theoretical complication not borne out in the series by Marchac DA (*Plast Reconstr Surg* 1995;**95**:802–811).

Bilateral coronal synostosis (20%)

Growth retardation in an A–P direction leads to **brachycephaly** which is a shortened skull or **turribrachycephaly** which is a shortened and tower-shaped skull due to compensatory growth **upwards** and laterally. X-rays may also demonstrate frontal flattening and hypoplasia of the supra-orbital rims which are recessed below a bulging forehead; bilateral harlequin orbits. This type of deformity is a feature of Apert's or Crouzon's.

- The commonest treatment is **frontal advancement** within the first year – 'floating' advancement of the frontal bone releases the synostosed suture and advances the supra-orbital bar to protect the globe.
- This is followed by **mid-face advancement** by Le Fort III osteotomy ~9–12 years of age at which time mid-face growth is complete and the patient is less likely to require secondary surgery. This was originally described by Gillies, later by Tessier.

Alternatively the whole frontal advancement and Le Fort III advancement can be done as a **monobloc** (Monasterio) but the communications between nasal and cranial cavities lead to a high infection risk and a need for bone graft.

Secondary Le Fort I osteotomy may later be required to correct occlusal problems and possibly also mandibular osteotomy (~18 years of age) with **risk of causing VPI** when significant advancement is required – this is **pertinent also to correcting malar hypoplasia associated with cleft palate**.

Bilateral coronal synostosis may lead to oxycephaly – a pointed head with recessed forehead that is tilted backwards (mesofrontal angle more than 180°);

it may follow inadequate growth after treatment of brachycephaly. It may be treated surgically.

Kleeblattschädel – clover leaf skull that results from synostosis of coronal, lambdoidal and metoptic sutures with compensatory bulging at the sagittal and squamosal sutures, leading to a trilobe-shaped skull (and brain).

- **Exorbitism** and exophthalmos, eyelids may retract behind the globe.
- **Marked hydrocephalus** and raised ICP.
- Variable degree of mid-face hypoplasia.

Treatment consists of urgent cranial vault expansion (days), and repeat/revisional procedures are usually needed.

Lambdoid synostosis

This is the **least common** synostosis and leads to synostotic **posterior plagiocephaly**:

- There is occipital flattening on the affected side but no ipsilateral frontal bossing.
- The ear is displaced inferiorly and **posteriorly (skull is trapezoid in shape)**.
- The **foramen magnum deviated** towards the fused suture on X-ray.

It is a severe progressive deformity and surgery to remodel occiput (occipital bandeau with barrel staving, or spiral osteotomy) is usually advocated.

Deformational/positional plagiocephaly (plagiocephaly without synostosis – PWS)

This occurs in up to 1 in 300 births including those with very minor plagiocephaly. In simple terms, the deformity is a **'parallelogram head'** ('p' for 'positional'

and 'parallelogram') – occipital flattening with ipsilateral frontal bossing; contralateral frontal flattening and occipital bossing. There is no radiographic synostosis and the foramen magnum is in the midline (in contrast to lambdoid synostosis, vide supra). The ear is positioned **anteriorly** on the side of occipital flattening. Five per cent have mental disability.

Occipital flattening seems to be more common on the right side probably due to decubitis position of the fetus, supine sleeping, congenital **torticollis** or abnormal vision. It may be related to restricted movement in utero; it may also be due to moulding in the birth canal and in this case resolves within 6 weeks.

The deformity is **self-correcting** in most cases and can be managed by conservative means but it must be distinguished from plagiocephaly due to unilateral coronal or lambdoidal synostosis – 3D-CT reconstruction may be helpful. Once the diagnosis of PWS is established, the deformity is treated and the underlying causes corrected:

- Head positioning; repositioning lie of baby at sleep.
- Physiotherapy for the two-thirds with torticollis.

Others have described dynamic orthotic cranioplasty – an acrylic mould with a space into which the head can grow.

Occipital plagiocephaly
David DJ. *Br J Plast Surg* 2000;**53**:367–377.

Occipital plagiocephaly may be due to lambdoidal synostosis (rare) or may be non-synostotic (PWS, majority of cases). The initial cranial asymmetry may be exacerbated by infant's preference for lying on the flattened side. Plain films (or CT if unclear) can be helpful. In addition, morphological differences can

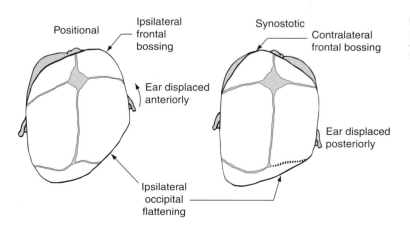

Figure 4.10 Comparison of the features of positional plagiocephaly (parallelogram head) and plagiocephaly due to unilateral lambdoid synostosis.

Table 4.1 Features of true synostosis compared to plagiocephaly without synostosis (PWS)

	True synostosis	PWS
Position of ear	Posteroinferior	Anterior
Shape of occiput	Flattened	Flattened
Shape of frontal area	No bossing	Bossing
Overall cranial shape	Trapezoid	Parallelogram

be used to differentiate between unilateral lambdoidal synostosis and PWS (see above).

True lambdoidal synostosis (or PWS failing to respond to conservative treatment) requires operative intervention to release (resection of) the fused suture – resected sutures usually show sclerosis rather than true fusion histologically, i.e. true synostosis is rare.

Crouzon's syndrome

Octave Crouzon (1874–1938), a French neurologist, described this in 1912; it occurs in 1 in 25 000 live births with autosomal dominant inheritance with variable penetrance and is associated with FGF receptor 2 (FGFR2) mutation. It is acrocephalosyndactyly type II (sometimes referred to as Apert's–Crouzon syndrome, some regard it as a variant of Apert's but it is more common). Note that there is another list of acrocephalo*poly*syndactyly syndromes. Both Crouzon's and Apert's are associated with FGFR2 gene mutations on chromosome 10.

- Usually there are no digital abnormalities.
- Mid-face hypoplasia:
  - Class III malocclusion (paradoxical retrogenia).
  - High arched palate.
  - Shallow orbits – **ocular proptosis, exorbitism** that may lead to keratitis.
  - Conductive hearing impairment.
  - Parrot beak nose.

Multiple synostoses including:

- Turribrachycephaly.
- Scaphocephaly, trigonocephaly, Kleeblattschädel.
- **Oxycephaly** – pointed skull, forehead paralleling the plane of the nasal dorsum, due to multiple suture synostoses.

There is raised ICP in two-thirds of patients that often have normal intelligence and development

(<5% learning disabled compared with Apert's, rarely normal).

Apert's syndrome

Eugene Apert (1868–1940) was a French paediatrician who described the syndrome in 1906 (it was described by Wheaton in 1894); he was a founding member of the French Eugenics society (not named after him, *eu* good, *genos* birth). It occurs in 1 in 100–160 000 live births with most cases being **sporadic** with advanced paternal age a risk factor (but autosomal dominant inheritance has been reported). An FGFR2 mutation on chromosome 10q26 has been described. It is one of the **acrocephalosyndactyly** syndromes (type I) usually with the most severe hand deformities – there is a **complex symmetrical syndactyly** of hands and feet:

- Type I – 'spade hand' – mid-digital hand mass composed of second to fourth digits.
- Type II – 'mitten' or 'spoon' hand – thumb joined to mid-digital mass by a simple syndactyly.
- Type III – 'hoof' or 'rosebud' hand – complete osseous fusion between thumb–ring finger with simple syndactyly in the fourth web space. Nail synaechia.

Types I–III will also have a short radially deviated thumb and symphalangism. The atypical type of Apert's does not have a mid-digital hand mass.

Other associated features:

- Paronychial infections during infancy.
- **Acne**.
- Vertebral fusions C5–6 (71%).
- Dysplasia of shoulder and elbow.
- Polycystic kidneys and cardiopulmonary abnormalities.
- Mid-face hypoplasia.
- Class III malocclusion with prominent mandible, high narrow arched palate; 30% have **cleft palate**.
- Orbital proptosis (exorbitism), anti-Mongoloid slant and hypertelorism.
- Flat face and short nose with a bulbous tip/beaked nose with depressed bridge.
- Low set ears and conductive hearing loss.

The cranial deformity is most commonly **turribrachycephaly** – high forehead and flat face – due to bicoronal synostosis but may have Kleeblattschädel, which is associated with a poor prognosis with profound mental disability. There is raised ICP in ~43% but mental disability is common (~50%) even in the absence of raised ICP due to primary brain abnormality and surgery does little to affect the mental disability. Ventriculoperitoneal shunting is often needed.

- Hydrocephalus.
- Agenesis of the corpus callosum.

Pfeiffer's syndrome

This was first described in a family by Rudolf Pfeiffer, a German geneticist in 1964; the family had also been studied by Noack in 1959 but was classified as Apert's. It affects approximately 1 in 100 000. Inheritance is autosomal dominant but many arise due to sporadic mutations; FGFR1 and FGFR2 mutations on chromosomes 8 and 10 respectively have been described. It is also known as acrocephalosyndactyly type V. Raised ICP is common though many have normal intelligence.

Type I 'Classic Pfeiffer'

- Craniosynostosis especially turribrachycephaly.
- **Broad thumbs** and great toes, **incomplete** syndactyly of second web space.
- Severe mid-face hypoplasia, shallow orbits/exorbitism, hypertelorism/anti-mongoloid slant.
- Cervical fusion 30%.
- Intelligence and lifespan more likely to be normal.

Type II

- As above but with ankylosis of elbows and Kleeblattschädel and mental disability.

Type III

- Ankylosis of elbows but no Kleeblattschädel and mental disability.

Types II and III are associated with FGFR2 gene mutations only.

Le Fort III advancement with gradual distraction using internal devices

Chin M. *Plast Reconstr Surg* 1997;**100**:819–830.

The authors describe results of gradual distraction in craniosynostotic patients (Crouzon's, Apert's and Pfeiffer's) between 4 and 13 years of age.

- Advancement gap of ~10 mm created by Le Fort III osteotomy before distraction was tolerated well in **children** with no non-union and increased

advancement compared with bone–plate fixation alone – eliminates latency period.
- Nasal-frontal osteotomies were grafted with cancellous bone.

The distraction devices were custom-made using computer-aided design based on cephalometric assessment in each patient and were left in place for 6 months. Conventional advancement occurs at 1 mm of advancement per day, whilst the authors describe a technique of **accelerated distraction** with the rate guided by the resistance created in the soft tissues and use of a torque wrench. This increased advancement to ~2 mm/day for ~5 days.

Their results show improvements in exorbitism, class III malocclusion and obstructive sleep apnoea post-operatively.

Maxillary distraction osteogenesis in Pfeiffer's syndrome: urgent ocular protection by gradual midfacial skeletal advancement

Britto JA. *Br J Plast Surg* 1998;**5**:343–349.

They describe a case using distraction following Le Fort III osteotomy as an adjunct to supra-orbital bar advancement in the management of ocular proptosis. These cases were advanced at a rate of 1 mm/day initially, and then increased to 2 mm/day after the first week – gradual advancement aims to avoid creating a **dead space** with the resultant danger of infection.

Distraction rate and latency: factors in the outcome of paediatric maxillary distraction

Higuera S. *J Plast Aesthet Surg* **62**:1564–1567.

The authors demonstrate the successful use of distraction osteogenesis of 7 paediatric maxillae after a 24-hour latent period, followed by a distraction rate of 2 mm/day. They suggest that Ilizarov's 'ideal' protocol of 3–5 days of latency and distraction at a rate of 2 mm/day does not apply to the paediatric facial skeleton. Some surgeons believe that the latent period allows formation of a 'bone haematoma' as a foundation for bone regeneration.

Saethre–Chotzen syndrome

This acrocephalosyndactyly type III was described by Saethre in 1931 and Chotzen in 1932. It occurs in 1 in 25–50 000. There is autosomal dominant inheritance with incomplete penetrance and has been associated with deletion or mutation of the TWIST gene on chromosome 7. Mild mental disability and schizophrenia have been reported.

- Short stature and incomplete **syndactyly**, mainly second web space.
- Craniosynostosis, mainly turribrachycephaly due to bicoronal synostosis but may be asymmetric.
- Mid-face hypoplasia including cleft palate.
- **Low set hairline**, flattened forehead and ptosis of the eyelids.
- Facial asymmetry with deviation of the nasal septum.

Carpenter's syndrome

This was described by George Carpenter, a British physician, in 1909 and is distinct from the others by exhibiting autosomal **recessive** pattern inheritance. It is defined as an acrocephalosyndactyly type II and the diagnosis is made clinically though it is often confused for Apert's. It is one of the least common of the craniosynostosis syndromes and affects 1 in 1 million live births in the USA.

- Craniosynostosis: sagittal synostosis (scaphocephaly), bicoronal synostosis and also lambdoid synostosis in some cases. There may also be acrocephaly or turribrachycephaly depending on the combination of sutures involved which is often asymmetric.
- Short hands, symbrachydactyly and preaxial **polydactyly of the feet**.

- **Congenital heart defects** in 1/3, ventricular septal defect (VSD)/arterial septal defect (ASD)

Patients have short stature, moderate obesity, umbilical herniae, cryptorchidism and decreased hip mobility; many have mental disability. Treatment aims to treat/prevent raised ICP as well as the airway and eyes.

Patau syndrome

Klaus Patau, a geneticist, identified the cytogenetic basis of the disease in 1960. The clinical picture had been described in 1656 by Thomas Bartholin (1616–1680), a Danish physician and father of Caspar Bartholin the younger (of the eponymous gland/duct).

Patients with the syndrome have **trisomy 13** and it is related to a single defect during the first 3 weeks of development of the prechordal mesoderm that leads to multiple morphological defects of the mid-face, eyes and forebrain. Patients have severe mental disability and a very poor prognosis with almost half dying by 1 month and three-quarters by 1 year. For the purposes of genetic counselling, the recurrence rate depends on the genotype.

There is microcephaly with sloping forehead, wide sagittal sutures and fontanelles and aplasia cutis congenita. There may be also be holoprosencephaly (lack of septation of the forebrain – lack of a corpus callosum).

Facial features

- Eyes – micro/anophthalmia, coloboma and retinal dysplasia.

Table 4.2 Summary of the features of the common types of craniosynostosis.

Abnormality	Calvarial deformity	Main operation	Other operations
Bicoronal synostosis Most syndromal synostoses including Crouzon's, Apert's, Pfeiffer's	Turribrachy-cephaly	Floating frontoparietal advancement and remodelling with supra-orbital bar advancement: if raised intracranial pressure/exorbitism perform early (3 months). Alternative monobloc advancement	Palatal cleft surgery ~6 months. Surgery to hands < 2 years. Le Fort III advancement aged 6–12 years. Le Fort I advancement 12–18 years
Unilateral coronal synostosis	Plagio-cephaly	Bilateral supraorbital bar advancement with frontoparietal remodelling aged 6–9 months	
Sagittal synostosis Carpenter's syndrome	Scapho-cephaly	Sagittal strip craniectomy and frontoparietal remodelling aged 6–9 months	
Unilateral lambdoidal synostosis	Plagio-cephaly	Occipital remodelling aged 6–9 months	
Metopic synostosis	Trigono-cephaly	Supra-orbital bar advancement and frontal remodelling aged 6–9 months	Hypotelorism does not need correction

- Mouth – cleft lip (60–80%)/palate.
- Ears – low set ears with abnormal helices; recurrent otitis media and deafness (sensorineural, conductive).
- Hands – camptodactyly and polydactyly of hands/feet, rocker-bottom feet.

Other features

- Coarctation, ASD, patent ductus arteriosus (PDA), VSD, dextroposition.
- Males: cryptorchidism, abnormal scrotum, ambiguous genitalia.
- Females: bicornuate uterus.
- Polycystic kidneys.

IV. Craniofacial asymmetry

Congenital:

- Hemifacial microsomia (unilateral or bilateral – still asymmetrical).
- Unilateral coronal synostosis.
- Beckwith–Wiedemann syndrome.

Acquired:

- Hemifacial atrophy.
- Lipodystrophy.
- Differential growth due to radiotherapy/surgery for childhood malignancy.
- Hypoplasia.

Parry–Romberg disease (hemifacial atrophy)

This was described by Parry in 1825 and Henoch and Romberg in 1846. It is characterized by a slowly progressive atrophy of the soft tissues of half the face that begins before 20 (5–15) years of age and eventually 'burns' itself out (2–10 years). The inheritance pattern is unclear, most are sporadic, with some suggestions of autosomal dominance with variable penetrance. It is more common in females (1.5×) and is unilateral in 95%.

The main feature is the slowly progressive hemifacial soft tissue atrophy affecting skin and subcutaneous tissues (including tongue and salivary glands) early on, then later muscle and bone. Initial changes occur above the maxilla or nasolabial fold first of all. Atrophic tissues show chronic inflammation and scarring. The cause is unknown – some believe that it may be a form of localized scleroderma, it may possibly be viral or an abnormal sympathetic system.

- 'En **coup de sabre**' deformity – distinctive subcutaneous atrophy in a line from the chin to the malar area, eyebrow and forehead.

Other features

- Neurological: seizures, contralateral Jacksonian epilepsy, trigeminal neuralgia and migraine-like headaches.
- Skin: hyperpigmentation and vitiligo.
- Hair: blanching and alopecia.
- Teeth: delayed dental eruption and malocclusion.
- Eyes: enophthalmos, refractive error and heterochromia iridis.

Reconstruction/treatment is delayed until the disease is stable for at least 6 months. Choices include:

- Fat/dermofat grafts.
- Onlay grafts or implants for skeletal abnormalities or osteotomies.
- TPF, temporalis transfer.
- Free tissue transfer e.g. groin, scapular/parascapular or omentum – over-correct to allow for atrophy.

The use of the omentum-free flap for this condition was popularized by Wallace JG (*Br J Plast Surg* 1979;**32**:15).

Microvascular free flap correction of severe hemifacial atrophy
Longaker MT. *Plast Reconstr Surg* 1995;**96**:800–809.

The average duration of disease in this series was 6.7 years.

Treatment aims to restore facial contour and in this study the authors used superficial inferior epigastric and parascapular free flaps. Advantages of the latter included a long pedicle with good vessel diameter and a good donor site scar. In addition, the fascia can be extended beyond de-epithelialized skin paddle while achieving primary closure – this can be used to 'feather' the edge of the contour augmentation.

Two-thirds of patients require revisional procedures, e.g. debulking/augmentation/recontouring, but these should only be considered after 6 months.

Hemifacial microsomia

The incidence of hemifacial microsomia (HFM) is ~1 in 5600 births; it is the commonest craniofacial anomaly. It is usually unilateral but can be bilateral (but asymmetric) in ~10%. It must be distinguished from Treacher Collins syndrome which has:

- Loss of the medial lower eyelashes.
- Deformity is **symmetrical** whereas in bilateral HFM it is still asymmetrical.
- Well-defined pattern of inheritance (autosomal dominant) but bilateral craniofacial microsomia has no inheritance pattern.
- A genetic basis on chromosome 5 with autosomal dominant inheritance whereas hemifacial microsomia has no inheritance pattern, being sporadic (possibly due to stapedial artery thrombosis) except for Goldenhars. The risk of an affected parent having an affected child is 3%.

Aetiology – theories

- 'Mesodermal insufficiency' – Stark RB. *Plast Reconstr Surg* 1962;**29**:229–239.
- Vascular insult to the arches (stapedial artery) – evidence from haemorrhage and haematoma (Poswillo D. *Oral Surg Oral Med Oral Pathol* 1973;**35**:302–328) and thalidomide-induced hemifacial-like defects in monkeys. This is currently the most favoured.

The advantage of the vascular theory is that it helps to explain how the deformity does not fit exactly the pattern of the first and second arches.

Hemifacial microsomia is the result of a Tessier number 7 facial cleft whereas Treacher Collins syndrome is a consortium of abnormalities associated with numbers 6, 7 and 8. Hemifacial microsomia plus features of a number 8 cleft (peribulbar dermoids, etc.) is usually known as **Goldenhar's syndrome**:

- **Craniofacial microsomia**: mandibular hypoplasia (with aplasia of lateral pterygoid) and microtia.
- Epibulbar dermoids.
- Preauricular appendages and sinuses.
- Abnormalities of cervical vertebrae.
  - Basilar impression – deformity of the skull base around the foramen magnum, e.g. occipitalization of the atlas.
- Elevated scapula (Sprengel deformity).
- Rib abnormalities.

The OMENS classification of hemifacial microsomia

Vento AR. *Cleft Palate Craniofac J.* 1991;**28**:68–76.
Grading system of involved structures:

- Orbital dystopia (includes maxilla, zygomatic bone hypoplasia, etc.).

- **Mandibular hypoplasia**
- Ear defects – abnormalities of inner ear bones, external ear and tympanic membrane, preauricular skin tags.
- Nerve – facial nerve deficits (muscles of facial expression with variable agenesis).
- Soft tissue abnormalities – hypoplastic muscles of mastication, hypoplastic parotid, macrostomia.

Hemifacial microsomia patients may have a variety of functional problems e.g. airway, feeding, speech, eyes and facial growth. A multidisciplinary team is important.

Isolated microtia as a marker for unsuspected hemifacial microsomia

Keogh IJ. *Arch Otolaryngol Head Neck Surg* 2007;**133**:997–1001.

The authors examined 100 patients with isolated microtia who had further examination to determine their OMENS score. They found that 40 patients fitted into the diagnosis of hemifacial microsomia (cranial nerve deficits, mandibular asymmetry and hearing loss were commonest) and suggested that isolated microtia is a marker for hemifacial microsomia, that they represent different points on a spectrum of expression of the same phenomenon.

Surgical options during childhood include:

- O – see skeletal surgery below, **cleft surgery (25% have cleft palate)**.
- M – mandibular advancement/distraction or reconstruction (if severely hypoplastic).
- E – hearing device; excision of accessory auricles; microtia reconstruction.
- N – need to import muscle and nerve with two-stage facial reanimation. Simple nerve grafting of palsied facial nerve with sural grafts most successful in first year.
- S – commissuroplasty.

There is a dilemma of sorts in that early corrective surgery may cause disordered growth in the future e.g. growth of globe/eye until about 5 years of age and growth of the mandible and maxilla continues until approximately 18 years of age and is driven primarily by the secondary dentition. Multiple surgeries increase the risks and numbers of complications. The aim is to encourage growth whilst preventing functional deformities, and to ideally correct deformities when growth is complete ~16–18 years of age.

- **Infancy** – treatment during this time usually consists of crisis intervention e.g. eye, airway, feeding and speech. Early correction of deformity may be needed or possible – e.g. remove auricular appendages, cleft correction or orbits.
- **Childhood** (time of mixed dentition)
  - Prevent secondary deformity e.g. distraction, orthodontics or costochondral grafts in Prozanky 3 (overgrowth may occur later).
  - Deformity correction e.g. distraction, orthodontics.
- **Adolescence/maturity** - definitive correction of deformity (both soft tissues and skeleton), delaying until skeletal maturity when definitive requirements are known.
- Osteotomy e.g. zygomatic.
- Distraction e.g. Le Fort I.
- Soft tissue augmentation – fat transfer, seems most effective in the younger age group.
- Onlay grafts – autologous (costochondral, calvarial) or alloplastics (Medpor, MMA, hydroxyapatite) for non-load bearing areas.

Mandibular hypoplasia is the cornerstone of the condition and in general severity of this determines the severity of associated abnormalities. There is a spectrum of abnormality and this includes simple isolated microtia. The affected structures are mostly derived from the first and second arches and pharyngeal clefts.

Prozansky classification of mandibular hypoplasia:

Type 1	All parts present but hypoplastic
Type 2a	Condyle articulates as hinge
Type 2b	No condyle
Type 3	Mandible ramus absent

Types 1 and 2a can be treated with distraction whilst the others need a costochondral graft – transfer of a growth centre is useful.

Skeletal surgery:

- Fronto-orbital advancement for frontal flattening.
- Correction of orbital dystopia.
- Le Fort III osteotomy used to correct exorbitism.
- Le Fort I maxillary advancement osteotomy to restore bite.

Skeletal surgery has significant complications:

- Airway compromise, haemorrhage.
- Nerve injury.
- Non-/malunion.
- Trauma to tooth roots.

- Velopharyngeal incompetence.
- Malocclusion.

Skeletal surgery should be allowed to settle before soft tissue reconstruction is contemplated. **Distraction osteogenesis** techniques are being increasingly used instead of vascularized bone reconstruction. The phases include corticotomy/osteotomy, latency (5–7 days, callus), distraction/activation (0.25 mm four times a day) and consolidation (8 weeks, for bone mineralization). There is also distraction histiogenesis – soft tissue elongates and there is less tendency for it to shrink back.

- Zone I – fibrous tissue or fibrous interzone in the centre, highly organized parallel collagen strands with fibroblasts.
- Zone II – extending bone formation or primary mineralization front or transitional zone, either side of zone I, with osteoblasts on bone spicules.
- Zone III – remodelling zone, with osteoclasts.
- Zone IV – mature bone, thicker spicules.

Bone formation occurs by intramembranous ossification; if there is excessive motion, chondrocytes form and fibrocartilage non-union occurs. It takes about 8 months for the new bone to be close to (90%) mature bone in structure. It is very reliable in the craniofacial skeleton but should be used with caution before the age of 18 months as the bones may be too soft.

The mandibular distraction is timed to coincide with time of rapid maxillary growth ~6 years of age (Cousley RR. *Br J Plast Surg* 1997;**50**:536–551). The goals of distraction osteogenesis are to establish a fibrovascular bridge, which becomes ossified by tension forces into new bone whilst reducing the need for bone graft. It also stretches out soft tissues i.e. coordinated augmentation of bone and soft tissues. Optimizing the rate of distraction is important as:

- Too slow leads to premature fusion.
- Too fast leads to non-union.

Distractors may be internal or external, depending on the space available for the device as well as the vectors of pull required e.g. vertical/horizontal/oblique.

Treacher Collins syndrome (mandibulofacial dysostosis)

This was described by Edward Treacher Collins (1862–1932, English ophthalmologist) in 1900. The condition is due to sporadic mutation in up to 60%; whilst it also demonstrates automosal dominant inheritance with the responsible gene (TCOF1) on chromosome 5 (same chromosome as **cri du chat**).

It affects males and females equally, with an incidence of 1 in 25 000–50 000. Patients are said to have a 'bird-like facies' due to bilateral facial cleft:

- Anti-Mongoloid slant, hypertelorism, absent lower lid lashes medially and **colobomata**.
- Low set ears/**microtia**, >95% have moderate conductive hearing loss due to stenosis of external auditory canal or ankylosis of inner ear ossicles, microtia, sensorineural hearing impairment and skin tags.
- **Micrognathia** and anterior open bite.
- **Cleft palate**.
- **Mid-face hypoplasia** – zygomatic, maxillary and mandibular hypolasia; inferolateral orbital wall deficient with downward slant of supra-orbital ridge. Hypoplastic temporalis muscle.
- Broad nasal dorsum and beaked nose, choanal atresia or stenosis.

Nager syndrome (acrofacial dysostosis) is said to be a rare variant of Treacher Collins (mode of inheritance is disputed) with similar facial features and also associated with defects of the extremities, usually with short stature.

The deformities in Treacher Collins are said to be non-progressive with age and some represent a consortium of facial clefts 6, 7, 8:

- Cleft numbers 6 and 8.
  - Lower lid colobomata (notches), hypertelorism and anti-Mongoloid slant.
  - Hypoplasia of lateral orbital wall.
- Cleft number 7.
  - Macrostomia.
  - External and internal ear defects.

Patients should be treated within a multidisciplinary team e.g. speech therapist and audiologist (external bone conduction hearing device with a head band), orthodontist. The variability of expression demands that treatment be tailored to the individual patient. Patients usually have normal mental status.

Typical Tessier treatment timing

The combination of micrognathia and choanal atresia in particular, means that the **airway** is a source of concern in neonates, 'secondary' issues including vision, feeding and hearing.

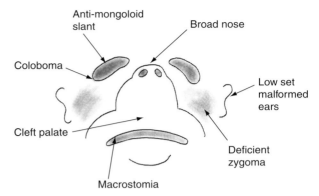

Figure 4.11 Schematic representation of the main features associated with Treacher Collins syndrome. Cleft plate is found in one-third of patients.

- 0 months – tracheostomy if needed.
- 6 months – cleft palate repair.
- 5–6 years – split calvarial onlay grafts to inferolateral orbit and zygomas that may need to be repeated due to resorption.
- 6 years – soft tissue correction:
  - Correction of colobomas (Tessier Z-plasty technique, Kuhnt–Symanowski blepharoplasty) only performed once zygomas reconstructed.
  - Ear reconstruction.
  - Commissuroplasty for macrostomia (reposition muscle).
  - Sideburns set back, abnormal hairline.
- 6–12 years – orthodontics and jaw surgery: cephalometric assessment and planning,
  - Le Fort III maxillary advancement.
  - Mandibular ramus sagittal split osteotomy and advancement or distraction.
- 12–18 years – Le Fort I advancement to finalize bite, sliding genioplasty.
- 18 years – rhinoplasty to broad nasal bridge.

Hyperplastic conditions

Fibrous dysplasia

There are monostotic (70–80%) or polyostotic forms (generally more severe and presents earlier). The aetiology is unknown.

It is related to Gs protein mutation (of alpha subunit) causing osteoblast and osteoclast activity; there is fibrous formation in the medulla of bones particularly the mandible and maxilla. The disease presents as bony swellings in < 30-year age group with some pain, whilst craniosclerosis may cause deafness. Pathological fractures may occur.

- Active fibrous dysplasia may show elevated serum alkaline phosphatase and urine hydroxyproline (indicating bone turnover). The X-ray appearance is usually distinctive enough to make the diagnosis – ground glass appearance, expansion/deformity; MRI may provide additional information including assessing for malignant change.
- **Albright's disease** is fibrous dysplasia combined with patchy skin pigmentation and precocious puberty (due to pituitary tumours). It shows autosomal dominant behaviour. Patients also have short neck, short metacarpals/metatarsals due to early epiphyseal closure.
- **Cherubism** is a familial form of polyostotic fibrous dysplasia that presents early and affects the maxilla and mandible.

It is self limiting but will not regress. The main options in treatment include curettage (20–30% recurrence) or excision and reconstruction. Bone grafts placed in areas of disease tend to become replaced by fibrous dysplasia. Nerve decompression may be needed. There is a 0.5% incidence of osteosarcoma which may be increased if there has been radiotherapy.

Medical treatment includes IV bisphosphonates (palmidronate), with calcium and phosphate supplements, vitamin D. This reduces bone pain, and may reduce bony fibrosis.

Beckwith–Wiedemann syndrome

This overgrowth disorder with unknown aetiology was described by Beckwith (US paediatric pathologist) in 1963 and Wiedemann (German geneticist) in 1964. Eighty-five per cent of cases are sporadic (slightly increased in assisted reproduction), the other are familial but with mixed patterns of inheritance. Mutations of chromosome 11p15.5 have been described. It affects about 1 in 15 000. It features variable combinations of:

- Metopic synostosis, microcephaly and large prominent eyes, **pits/grooves in earlobe**.
- **Macroglossia 90%**, gaping mouth, prognathism – it often becomes less noticeable with age, some perform reduction surgery but the optimal time is unknown.

- **Large body size** (which may affect one side of the body only) and visceromegaly, hemihypertrophy of the face may require surgery.
- **Midline abdominal wall defects**: omphalocoele, umbilical hernia or diastasis recti.
- **Neonatal hypoglycaemia** which may be profound, leading to brain damage if untreated.

Most patients do not have all these features; some suggest that two of the five common features (in bold font above) suggest the diagnosis (DeBaun MR. *Am J Hum Genet* 2002;**70**:604–611). Some patients may have plagiocephaly without synostosis (PWS) of forehead and neck.

Patients do have an increased risk of cancer; ~10% develop cancer e.g. Wilm's tumour (most common and screening with ultrasound every 3–4 months is suggested), hepatoblastoma or other malignancies. Other than this, the prognosis is very good.

Other causes of hyperplastic lesions

- **Neurofibromatosis** – 1 in 2500 that is spontaneous or autosomal dominant with variable penetrance. Type 1 is related to a mutation on chromosome 17 and type 2 with chromosome 22 respectively.
- **Gorlin's syndrome** – affects 1 in 100 000 demonstrating autosomal dominant inheritance. There are multiple basal cell carcinomas with cysts of the jaw and pits of the palm and soles. Typically these patients have hypertelorism, widened nose, frontal bossing and calcification of the falx cerebri.

Hypertelorism

This is defined as the increased distance between the bony orbits (both medial and lateral walls), whilst telecanthus is the increased intercanthal distance (where the orbit may be normal). It is a physical finding and not a syndrome by itself.

- Pseudohypertelorism is the increased distance between the medial walls but normally spaced lateral walls – this may occur with midline tumours or encephalocoeles.
- Pseudotelecanthus is the illusion of telecanthus due to a flat nasal bridge or medial epicanthal folds.

Tessier introduced the term **orbital hypertelorism** (true lateralization of whole orbit i.e. medial and lateral wall, which is usually due to failure of medialization). In contrast, there is interorbital hypertelorism (van der Meulen) in which only the medial walls are

Table 4.3 Tessier classification of orbital hypertelorism

Degree	Interocular distance (mm)	Standard deviations more than normal
1	30–34	2–4
2	35–40	4–8
3	> 40	> 8

displaced, sometimes called bony telecanthus or pseudohypertelorism.

Tan and Mulliken classification (*Plast Reconstr Surg* 1997;**99**:317–327) based on cause and anatomy.

- Frontonasal malformation (Median cleft sndrome) most common.
  - Widow's peak, short broad nose and short upper lip.
  - Symmetrical hypertelorism/telecanthus (interorbital).
  - Amblyopia and encephalocoele.
- **Craniofrontonasal dysplasia** (Cohen syndrome) second most common.
  - EFNB1 gene (ephrin-B1 protein) mutation on X chromosome; affecting females more frequently and more severely affected (unusual for an X-linked disorder).
  - Mid-face hypoplasia with high arched palate (scaphomaxillism), and/or V median cleft palate.
  - Patients have coronal synostosis, corpus callosum dysgenesis and characteristic frizzy hair.
  - Extremity deformities e.g. Sprengel deformity, syndactyly and nail pitting.
- Craniofacial clefts – especially paramedian Tessier (3–11, 2–12) – asymmetric orbital hypertelorism.
- Encephalocoeles – interorbital (usually) hypertelorism.
- Miscellaneous groups e.g. syndromic craniosynostosis (Apert's, Pfeiffer's).
  - Noonan's (1 in 1000–2500) with hypertelorism, chest deformities, short stature and cardiac disease in 50%.

Management

Medialization of orbit by surgery:

- **Facial bipartition** (removal of central bony segment) for less severe problems; it narrows the entire mid-face and rotates orbits, affects upper dental arch. In syndromic cases such as Apert's, this approach also allows mid-face advancement.
- **Box osteotomy** (rectangular osteotomy around each orbit, then remove/add bone around as needed) – allows a greater degree of medialization and can correct vertical and horizontal problems i.e. good for asymmetric anomalies. Does not affect dentition.

The ideal timing is said to be about 9–11 years, after eruption of permanent incisors and canines. This is affected by functional issues such as management of airway, eyes, clefts/encephalocoeles.

Torticollis

This can either be congenital or acquired; the sternocleidomastoid muscle contracture causes the head/chin to be tilted. The aetiology of congenital torticollis is unclear but may be damage to the sternocleidomastoid muscle due to birth trauma or intrauterine malposition in many cases. Causes such as ophthalmic (e.g. IVth nerve palsy), tumours (posterior fossa tumours), infections and drugs (antipsychotics) should be excluded.

Those with torticollis have higher incidence of positional plagiocephaly.

Treatment:

- Physiotherapy – stretching and strengthening exercises.
- Anticholinergics and baclofen.
- Botulinum toxin – neutralizing antibodies may develop with repeated treatments.
- Myoplasty for failure of medical treatment.

Miscellaneous conditions affecting the head and neck

Craniofrontonasal dysplasia

Orr DJA. *Br J Plast Surg* 1997;**50**:153–161.

This is a combination of coronal synostosis with frontonasal dysplasia.

- Mainly unilateral coronal synostosis that leads to plagiocephaly (bilateral cases cause brachycephaly).
- Frontonasal dysplasia with hypertelorism, bifid nasal tip and a broad nasal bridge.
- **Also have dry frizzy hair and long grooved nails** – disordered deposition of large keratin filaments.

The article describes ten patients treated at the Oxford craniofacial unit (all females) with forehead advancement and remodelling for synostosis within the first year. Hypertelorism was treated by facial bipartition and excision of paramedian bone and ethmoid sinuses between 4–9 years of age – it is a cosmetic procedure in principle, thus not urgent, and at this age the patient may understand the deformity and the need for surgery.

The skin is allowed to re-drape and a medial canthoplasty is performed a year later to remove any residual excess skin/epicanthic folds (Mustardé canthoplasty – jumping man). There was no subsequent impairment of mid-facial growth in these cases.

Binder's syndrome

Described by Binder in 1962 as dysostosis maxillonasalis in the original German paper.

This has an unknown aetiology but is familial in 15%. Patients have normal intelligence; there is maxillonasal dysostosis with hypoplastic mid-face, i.e. the structures around the nose are poorly formed.

- Decreased vertical height of maxilla, absent anterior nasal spine, class III malocclusion.
- Short, flat nose and **short columella**, acute nasolabial angle, perialar flatness.
- Convex upper lip with wide but shallow philtrum.
- Vertebral abnormalities in 50%.

Treatment can be difficult but usually includes nasal augmentation and Le Fort II advancement osteotomy.

Klippel–Feil sequence

Maurice Klippel (1858–1942) and Andre Feil were French neurologists who gave comprehensive but independent descriptions in 1912 of a French tailor who appeared to have no neck. This condition occurs with an incidence of about 1 in 40 000 and is due to a mutation on chromosome 8q, inherited in an autosomal dominant manner with variable penetrance. It is characterized by failure of segmentation of the cervical spine – causing cervical fusion (most commonly C2–3), a short neck with limited movement, congenital scoliosis, **Sprengel's deformity** and a low hairline in 40%.

It can be a feature of syndromes such as Goldenhar's. About one-third have hearing loss whilst one-fifth have cleft palate. Autosomal recessive inheritance has been reported with C5–6 fusion. There is a contraindication to contact sports in Feil types I and II.

Samartzis DD. *Spine* 2006;**31**:e798–804.

- Type I – a single congenitally fused cervical segment.

- Type II – multiple non-contiguous, congenitally fused segments.
- Type III – multiple contiguous, congenitally fused cervical segments.

Aplasia cutis congenita

This condition is due to an unknown cause (some have a familial component) and is usually an isolated defect though it may be multifocal in 25%. There is an absence of the midline vertex, presenting as a sharply demarcated patch usually < 2 cm in diameter. It may be associated with skull defects of variable depth with exposure of dura, sagittal sinus or brain. In certain cases, it may lead to haemorrhage or even death but in the majority it is simple, and heals spontaneously with dressings e.g. SSD to prevent desiccation.

Hurler's syndrome

Gertrude Hurler (1889–1965), a paediatrician from the then East Prussia, described this syndrome whilst training in 1919. This is a mucopolysaccharidosis (type 1H) which is related to a deficiency of alpha-L-iduronidase which is a lysosomal enzyme that degrades mucopolysaccharides, thus there is a build-up of dermatan and heparan sulphate. There is a defective IDUA gene on chromosome 4; it is autosomal recessive.

Patients are apparently healthy at birth (may have herniae) but develop signs and symptoms (coarse features/prominent forehead – **gargoylism**, skeletal deformities, corneal clouding, short stature, progressive mental disability) by 6–24 months and are usually dead by 10 years (obstructive airway disease/respiratory infections).

Enzyme replacement (IV once a week) may help in reducing pain and non-neurological symptoms. Haematopoietic stem cell transplantation (HSCT) and umbilical cord blood transplantation before deterioration have been proposed; HSCT has the best track record for treating Hurler's. Later treatment has few benefits.

V. Genioplasty

Assessment

- Medical history.
- Previous orthodontic history.
- Dentition – unerupted teeth e.g. in those under 15 years of age may be at risk during osteotomies. The elderly will have relatively poor bone stock and are poor candidates for osteotomy also.

- Occlusion (relationship between maxillary first molar mesobuccal cusp to first mandibular molar) – orthognathic surgery should be considered for those with abnormalities of occlusion.
- Rickett's E line – a line between pogonion and nose tip should lie just anterior to the lips with the upper lip approximately twice as far from the line compared with the lower lip.
- Chin–nose relationship – chin projection should touch or be 3 mm posterior to the nose–lip–chin plane (a vertical line from midpoint of RT to upper lip) in men and women respectively.
- Soft tissue.

Imaging

- Orthopantomogram.
- Cephalogram.

Cephametric landmarks of relevance

- Frankfurt plane – porion (highest part of external auditory meatus) and suborbitale (lowest part of orbit).
- Pogonion – the most forward projecting part of the chin (mandibular symphysis).
- Menton – lowest part of mandibular symphysis.
- Subspinale – deepest point on the premaxillary outer contour between the anterior nasal spine and central incisor.
- Supramentale – deepest point between pogonion and incisor.
- Nasion – nasofrontal junction or anterior point on the frontonasal suture.

Cephalometry is the measurement of the human head by imaging (Broadbent 1931) and is used to evaluate dentofacial properties and clarify the anatomic basis for problems such as malocclusion. Cephalometric radiographs use a cephalostat – a device that keeps the head in a stable horizontal position whilst the images are being acquired.

Osseus genioplasty/chin osteotomy

Preserving soft tissue attachments helps to reduce resorption.

- Sliding – for sagittal projection deficiency, inferior segment with genioglossus and geniohyoid still attached. More extensive advancement may need a stepladder genioplasty which is a two-tiered advancement.

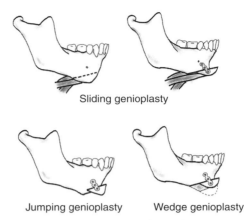

Sliding genioplasty

Jumping genioplasty   Wedge genioplasty

Figure 4.12 Common types of genioplasty.

- Jumping – the fragment is placed anterior to the symphysis as an onlay similar to an implant, it improves the sagittal projection whilst decreasing the height of the lower third.
- Wedge – for height reduction which will result in a degree of soft tissue ptosis. The segment between two parallel osteotomies is resected.
- Interpositional – with bone graft (or hydroxyapatite) to advance chin as well as increase lower face height.
- Reduction – for sagittal and vertical excess.
- Centralizing or asymmetric genioplasty – to correct asymmetry.

The average satisfaction rating for osteotomy (90–95%) is slightly higher than for implant genioplasty (85–90%).

Implant genioplasty

Implants cannot correct deficiencies of vertical height; they are generally placed over the pogonion for mild/moderate deficiencies of projection. Materials such as ivory, acrylic and precious metals are of historical interest only.

- **Synthetic** – silicone is the most popular, Medpor (porous high-density polyethylene that allows a degree of tissue ingrowth which seems to reduce infection rates, reduces capsule formation but makes removal more difficult) with newer materials such as nylon mesh or expanded PTFE (both soft) or hydroxyapatite (hard).

- **Biological** – autologous bone e.g. calvarial, rib or chondral cartilage or allogenic – irradiated cartilage etc.

According to Pitanguy (1968), the principles for implant augmentation are to position the implant at the lowest point of the mandible and it must be immobilized.

Implants can be positioned via:

- **Submental exposure** (extra-oral) which allows precise placement with less risk to the mental nerve but leaves an external scar.
- **Intra-oral route** (incision 1 cm above gingivolabial sulcus) leaves no scar and seems to have similar infection rates to extra-oral placement, however there is a tendency for less accurate placement, especially too high.

The choice between supraperiosteal or subperiosteal dissection is controversial; most agree that supraperiosteal positioning reduces bone resorption under the implant.

The implants can be fixed (screws, Mitek or sutures) or not (if the pocket is precisely made and closed).

Complications

- Haematoma (rare).
- Infection – uncommon, < 3% for osteotomies, < 5% for implants but may need removal.
  - If an implant is removed and not replaced, then either the soft tissue needs to be repositioned to reduce chin pad ptosis or an osseus genioplasty is needed to advance the bone to fill the tissue void.
- Nerve injury – usually neuropraxia of mental nerve leading to lower lip paraesthesia (and possible drooling) of 5%; it can be caused by an implant that is too large. Permanent damage is rare and usually related to damage to inferior alveolar nerve during osteotomy.
- Malposition – more common with intra-oral approach.
- Under-/over-correction or asymmetry.

A. Breast augmentation

I. Relevant anatomy and embryology

Embryology

The **milk ridge** extends from axilla to groin at 6 weeks.

- Normal development begins at 4th intercostal space.
- Accessory nipples (2%) can lie anywhere along the ridge but most commonly inframammary.

Development

Tanner staging is most commonly used.

- Stage 1 – nipple only.
- Stage 2 – nipple and small breast bud.
- Stage 3 – further enlargement.
- Stage 4 – enlargement of areola and increased pigment, double mound appearance.
- Stage 5 – final adolescent development and smooth contour.

Breast development occurs mainly at puberty at 10–12 years of age, as a result of hypothalamic gonadotrophin releasing hormones (hypothalamus–pituitary pathway) to the anterior pituitary stimulating the release of LH and FSH:

- FSH stimulates the ovaries to produce oestrogens that causes proliferation of breast ductal epithelium.
- Ovarian follicle maturation – production and release of oestrogen and progesterone that completes breast development.

Pregnancy

There are various hormones involved – oestrogen, progesterone, placental lactogen, prolactin, chorionic gonadotrophin, that cause breast ductal, lobular and alveolar growth.

- First trimester – oestrogen causes ductal sprouting and lobular growth (thus the breast enlarges) and the nipple areolar complex darkens.
- Second trimester – progestins cause lobular colostrum production/accumulation.
- Third trimester – at the time of delivery, the breast may be up to 3 times the normal size due to a combination of vascular engorgement, epithelial proliferation and colostrum accumulation.
- Delivery – withdrawal of placental lactogen and breast now predominantly influenced by prolactin.

After delivery, the nursing infant stimulates production of pituitary hormones.

- Prolactin (anterior pituitary) causes milk production and secretion.
- Oxytocin (posterior pituitary) breast contraction and milk ejection.

Involution will begin about 3 months after breastfeeding ceases with regression of extralobular stroma.

Ageing

With **menopause**, there is loss of glandular tissue that is replaced by fat.

Breast surgical anatomy

The breast gland is formed by a collection of **lobules** (functional units each with hundreds of acini) draining into 16–24 lactiferous ducts to the nipple via a central collecting duct. The breast is supported by layers of superficial fascia, whilst the ligaments of Cooper penetrate from the deeper layers of this facia into breast parenchyma and to the clavicle/clavipectoral fascia. Attenuation/degeneration of these ligaments will lead to ptosis. Sir Astley Paston Cooper (1768–1841) was an English surgeon and anatomist, working mostly at Guy's Hospital.

- Montgomery glands (12–15) are sebaceous type glands and their openings on the periphery of the areola form Montgomery tubercles (also called Morgagni tubercles – Giovanni Battista Morgagni was the first to describe the surface feature). William Featherstone Montgomery (1779–1859) was an Irish obstetrician.

The nerve supply to the nipple comes from the T4 intercostal nerves; **lateral cutaneous branch** which pierces the deep fascia at about the midaxillary level to lie in the pectoral fascia up to the midclavicular line where it runs forwards to the nipple via the parenchyma (the breast on the whole is supplied by T3–5 dermatomes, and the lower fibres of the cervical plexus/supraclavicular nerves to the upper and lateral breast).

Blood supply

- Internal thoracic – 60% – the largest perforator is the second.
- Lateral thoracic – 30%.
- Intercostal vessels – 10%.

The nipple gets its blood supply from the subdermal plexus as well as the parenchyma.

Venous drainage

Venous drainage rarely accompanies arteries, it is mostly provided by the superficial system.

- Internal mammary veins.
- Axillary vein.
- Intercostal veins.
- Superficial veins draining upwards to communicate with neck veins and medially to communicate with internal mammary veins.

Lymphatic drainage

- Predominantly to the axilla (breast-central node-apical node-supraclavicular), but 3–20% via internal mammary chain.
  - Level I – lateral to pectoralis minor which arises from 3–6th ribs to insert to coracoid process (innervated by medial pectoral nerve, which is more lateral than the lateral pectoral nerve on the chest wall).
  - Level II – beneath pectoralis minor.
  - Level III – medial to pectoralis minor (note III-II-I from superior to inferior).
  - **Rotter's nodes** – interpectoral nodes between the major and minor. Josef Rotter (1857–1924) was a German surgeon.

Rotter's node metastases. Therapeutic and prognostic considerations in early breast carcinoma
Cody HS. *Ann Surg* 1984;**199**:266–270.

In this study, the interpectoral nodes were sampled at the end of 500 consecutive magnetic resonance mammographies (MRMs) for early stage breast cancer. Nodes were found in 73%, tumour metastasis in 2.6% of all patients/4% of all with nodes sampled; 8.2% and 0.5% of axillary node positive and negative patients respectively had interpectoral metastasis.

Analysis of metastatic involvement of interpectoral (Rotter's) lymph nodes related to tumor location, size, grade, and hormone receptor status in breast cancer
Vrdoljak DV. *Tumori* 2005;**91**:177–181.

This study examined 172 breast cancer patients who had their Rotter's nodes removed as part of their surgery. Sixty-seven per cent had identifiable Rotter's nodes, with tumour in 20% of these; 30% of T3 tumours had positive Rotter's nodes. Thirty-five per cent and 4% of axillary node positive and negative patients respectively had interpectoral metastasis. The authors suggest that these nodes should be routinely removed.

II. Breast implants

- 1895 – first breast augmentation procedure carried out in Germany by Czerny – transplantation of a giant lipoma from the back into the breasts.
- 1945 – Japanese prostitutes inject liquid silicone into breasts to satisfy American servicemen clients.
- 1962 – Frank Gerow and Thomas Cronin were the first to implant what became Dow Corning's silastic mammary prosthesis. The first patient was Timmie Jean Lindsey, who still has her original implants.

Breast implants

Silicone implant controversy

- 1982 – van Nunen links silicone breast implants with connective tissue disease in three patients, but the data are largely anecdotal.
- 1984 – Stern vs. Dow Corning. Patient Maria Stern's claim that her autoimmune disease is caused by her implants is upheld by the court.
- 1988 – US Food and Drug Administration (FDA) classifies implants as Class III i.e. manufacturers need to show that they are safe and effective to keep them on the market.
- 1991 – Hopkins vs. Dow Corning. Marianne Hopkins awarded US$7.34 million for mixed connective tissue disease that the court believed was related to her ruptured implants.
  - Ramasastry SS. *Plast Reconstr Surg* 1991;**87**:1–7. Administering a chemical carcinogen caused a high cancer incidence in rats; placing an unexpanded tissue expander reduced the cancer incidence, whilst expanding the expander led to an even lower cancer incidence.
- 1992 – FDA ban on silicone implants with onus on manufacturers to prove safety despite lack of evidence that implants cause connective tissue disease. The argument was that as implants offered cosmetic advantages only, no risks would be tolerated. Only women undergoing breast reconstruction are allowed to receive silicone implants, and as part of a scientific study.
  - Dow Corning leaves silicone breast implant business along with Bristol-Myers-Squibb and Bioplasty.

- 1994 – 30 000 lawsuits filed against Dow Corning and 440 000 women register for class action settlement. Manufacturers agree to pay US$4.25 billion to women with breast implants as part of a class action settlement. Those entitled to compensation were those who had, or developed within 30 years, any of ten connective tissue diseases providing the symptoms began or worsened after the implants were placed. These ranged from scleroderma to non-specific aches and pains; even husbands were entitled to compensation for emotional suffering.
  - Medical devices agency (DoH) concludes no reason for a ban.
  - Mayo Clinic study (Gabriel SE. *New Engl J Med* 1994;**330**:1697–1702) found no link but was criticized for accepting funding from the American Society of Plastic and Reconstructive Surgery/Plastic Surgery Educational Foundation which receive contributions from Dow Corning and other implant manufacturers.
- 1995 – Dow Corning files for bankruptcy protection; Dow Chemical ordered to pay US$14.1 million to one patient by a jury in Nevada.
  - FDA recognizes body of evidence against a link to mixed connective tissue disease but maintains ban due to potential local complications.
  - Nurses' health study – no link (Sanchez-Guerrero J. *New Engl J Med* 1995;**332**:1666–1670).
  - Su C. *Plast Reconstr Surg* 1995;**96**:513–518. Placing a silicone implant and administering a chemical carcinogen in rat led to a 17% cancer incidence; without an implant, the carcinogen alone caused a 50% cancer incidence.
- 1998 – UK Independent Review Group on Silicone Gel Breast Implants (Sturrock R, Calman K) publishes review and finds no link.
- 2006 – the restriction for the USA was lifted by the FDA in November but patients had to be carefully monitored.

Assessment

The aims of the procedure seem simple enough but the patient's motivations and expectations may be very complex. The evaluation should include the psychological and relationship status – there is an excess of suicides in breast-augmentation patients.

Examination

- Skin quality: tone, elasticity and striae.
- Asymmetry: chest wall, scoliosis, intermaxillary fixation (IMF) and nipple and areola complex (NAC).
- Ptosis: severity – a degree of ptosis may be improved by augmentation (this can be gauged by asking the patient to lift their arms behind their head) but moderately severe ptosis will need a formal mastopexy.
- Breast examination – as per oncological examination, assess nipple sensation.

Measurements

- Base width.
- Sternal notch to nipple.
- Nipple to IMF.
- Pinch test – superior and inferior pole.
- Anterior pull skin stretch (APSS)
- Estimation of parenchymal fill.

General considerations

The silicone used in implants is polydimethyl siloxane, a polymer of silicon. Silicone is also found in heart valves, joint prostheses, IV cannulae/syringes and baby bottle nipples. About 100 000–150 000 women in the UK and ~1–2 million women in the USA (~1%) are estimated currently to have breast implants. It is the second most common cosmetic surgical procedure in the USA after liposuction.

The choice of implant depends on many factors:

- Preference of patient and surgeon.
- Breast characteristics – skin quality, volume required including regional deficiencies and IMF to nipple distance.

There are many different ways to estimate the volume of augmentation required; 1 cup size is approximately 125–150 ml (vide infra). Patients should be aware of the disadvantages of large augmentations:

- Unnatural appearance.
- Increased palpability and rippling.
- Breast atrophy, thinning and stretching of tissues; remodelling of rib cartilages.

Types

- **Textured vs. smooth** – a textured shell decreases the rate and degree of capsular contracture, though the effect is less pronounced than initially thought particularly when compared to smooth **saline** implants. Texturing reduces movement and is required for anatomical implants to maintain orientation. Textured implants may cause traction rippling when placed subglandularly and be more palpable due to their thicker shell. They are also more expensive.

- **Silicone vs. saline** – silicone implants tend to feel more breast-like. Saline implants can be used for limited incision surgery, including endoscopically assisted; some surgeons may overfill the implant shell to increase projection and finally, some may feel that saline implants are 'safer' and associated with a lower contracture rate. However, they do not feel like breast tissue; although the shell is thinner, underfilling will cause more rippling and earlier rupture whilst overfilling will make it firm. Some implants were given a polyurethane coating to decrease contracture, but it could break down in vivo to form a toluene derivative that was shown to cause sarcomas in rats – these were withdrawn in the UK in 1991 and then reintroduced by one manufacturer (Polytech Silimed) in 2005 with the claims of reduced contracture and movement, and that the carcinogenic risk to humans is very small and unquantifiable.

  ○ **Cohesive gel vs. liquid gel** – there is a range of cohesiveness and this has varied with different generations of implants; currently favoured implants have a thicker type of cohesive gel that does not 'run' when cut. This leads to another distinction:

  ○ **Biodimensional (anatomical) vs. non-biodimensional** – anatomical implants contain a cohesive gel to maintain shape; care is needed to avoid rotation after placement – these implants are textured to reduce rotation (another strategy is to dissect a fitting pocket i.e. avoid overdissection). They are useful in reducing the upper pole fullness which is typical of round implants, and is generally undesirable. Anatomical implants can be found in various configurations e.g. taller than wide for those with deflated upper poles, or shorter than wide for extra lower pole projection without additional height/upper pole fullness.

  ○ Hydrogel (PIP hydrogel and Novagold) and triglyceride soya oil (Trilucent) implants were removed from the UK market in 2000 and 1999 respectively.

- Profile: low, moderate and high profile.

Measurement of 2,4-toluenediamine in urine and serum samples from women with Meme or Replicon breast implants
Hester TR. *Plast Reconstr Surg* 1997;**100**:1291–1298.

This study was requested by the FDA following the reported problems with toluenediamine (TDA) release. They followed up 61 patients who had the polyurethane foam-covered implants. Levels of free TDA were measured in the serum and urine, and a risk assessment using available data provided a theoretical life time risk of 1 in a million.

Placement
Subglandular vs. submuscular

- **Subglandular placement** is suited to most cosmetic situations when the **skin envelope is sufficient** (> 2 cm). A natural breast shape is possible by filling out redundant skin envelope in the ptotic breast. However, the edges of the implant may be palpable/visible particularly at the upper pole, there is a higher contracture rate and there is more interference with mammography.
  - Subfascial plane – some surgeons have described placing implants behind the pectoralis fascia.
- **Subpectoral placement** is primarily indicated in very thin patients with insufficient soft tissue to cover the implant. In addition, there are fewer problems with capsular contracture and nipple sensation may be relatively preserved but there may be a higher rate of implant displacement and asymmetry; the implant may be subjected to unwanted superior displacement or compression with contraction of the overlying pectoralis major muscle. The lower pole shape/IMF definition tends to be less attractive; a **double bubble deformity** may develop in the very ptotic breast (consider augmentation – mastopexy in these patients). The implant may be distorted in very muscular patients.
  - **Submuscular** usually refers to having the whole implant being covered and this usually involves dissection of the serratus anterior also.
  - **Dual-plane** which aims to combine the advantages of subglandular and submuscular

methods. In addition to a subpectoral dissection, a second plane of dissection is between the breast and the muscle (up to upper level of areola) which aims to allow more soft tissue movement and redraping.

There are many different options and surgeons have their own preferences. In general, for primary cases many choose a subglandular implant as long as the soft tissue cover is sufficient (> 2 cm). The rationale for using subglandular placement and a silicone implant includes:

- More natural feel compared with a saline implant.
- Subglandular placement takes up skin envelope.
- Avoids ugly contractions of overlying pectoralis with tendency to displace laterally.

In thin patients, this may not be advisable due to the incidence of wrinkling and one may need to consider either:

- Submuscular placement to reduce wrinkling (which also increases proportion of breast tissue imaged by mammography and encourages less capsule formation) or
- Change to a smooth saline implant for subglandular placement (at the cost of slightly more capsular contracture).

Breast augmentation: choosing the optimum incision, implant and pocket plane
Hidalgo DA. *Plast Reconstr Surg* 2000;**105**:2202–2216.

A single author experience with 220 patients is discussed. The author prefers to use smooth saline-filled implants; overinflation of saline implants by 15% helps to reduce rippling.

- Axillary incision best suited to low-volume saline implant augmentation in the submuscular plane which also decreases capsular contracture risk; subpectoral placement is facilitated by inferomedial release of muscle.
- Adjustable strapping should be worn above the implants to prevent upward implant displacement.
- Implant deflation necessitated replacement in four patients within 3 years.

For secondary augmentations, the author most commonly used textured silicone gel implants (use in USA during this time was limited to secondary revisions and selected primary cases only e.g. congenital deformity).

- **Periareolar incisions** are the most versatile, being compatible with all planes and types of implant. They are considered the best choice of incision for lowering the level of the inframammary fold (but take care to avoid double bubble deformity). They provide good access for capsulectomy and submuscular pocket.
  - Also a good option in the tubular breast where concurrent circumareolar mastopexy is indicated. Avoid in the small (< 3 cm) or lightly pigmented areola; also there may be a higher risk of reduced sensation and ability to breastfeed.
- **Inframammary crease** incisions are the simplest to use and almost as versatile as the periareolar. They are ideal in those with significant breast volume beforehand and have either postpartum/weight-loss atrophy or just glandular ptosis. It is easier to change planes with this incision, and it is better for accurate subpectoral placement particularly for those with less experience. It is less useful for secondary cases requiring capsulectomy as it is at the periphery of the pocket. They should be avoided in those with a poorly defined IMF, in those with a constricted breast or a short nipple–IMF distance.
- **Axillary incisions** are more accurate when endoscopy is used but are not really suited for subglandular positioning. There is less control and a greater chance of malposition. It is a good choice in patients with low pre-operative breast volume and high breast position, as well as small areola and no inframammary crease (thus precluding the above two choices). It precludes the use of larger implants, particularly anatomical and gel types.
- Transumbilical – this is a difficult route especially to access the subpectoral plane or for gel implants. It is not FDA approved and thus off-label.

Asymmetry of nipple position is common pre-operatively and is often magnified by augmentation mammoplasty but the implants should still be placed in symmetrical pockets.

Dual plane breast augmentation

Tebbets JB. *Plast Reconstr Surg* 2001;**107**:1255–1272.

This is a paper with a great deal of detail on this technique.

Patients with a **pinch thickness of 2 cm or greater** in the upper pole of the breast are suitable for sub-glandular implant placement. Those with less than

2 cm in the upper pole require muscle coverage to avoid underfill rippling at this site. The dual plane pocket is created by:

- Using needle cautery to release the inferior insertion of pectoralis major parallel to and 1 cm above the inframammary fold (type 1) which allows the pectoralis muscle to retract 2–4 cm upwards. It is important **not to divide the muscle along the sternum** except for white tendinous insertions to avoid visible retraction of muscle along the sternum and a palpable implant edge. This is type 1 and is used in patients where the entire breast parenchyma is above the inframammary fold and there are tight attachments of parenchyma to muscle and a short nipple–inframammary fold distance of 4–6 cm under stretch.
- Additional **division of muscle–breast parenchyma attachments** to a point level with the inferior edge of the nipple–areolar complex (type 2) is used in patients where most of the breast is above the inframammary fold and there are looser attachments of breast to muscle and the nipple–inframammary fold distance is 5–6.5 cm under stretch.
- Or divided to the superior edge of the nipple–areolar complex (type 3) which is used in patients with glandular ptosis and very loose attachments (gland easily slides off pectoralis major) and markedly stretched nipple–inframammary fold distance (NAC–IMF 7–8 cm). Also suited for constricted lower pole (tuberous breast deformity, along with radial parenchyma scoring).

Incisions for access

- Inframammary vs. axillary vs. periareolar.
- Endoscopic assisted for saline implants.
- Transumbilical (implants are not approved for this route).

Complications

The re-operation rate due to implant complications is 1/4–1/3 over 5 years.

- General.
  - Infection ~2% and haematoma ~3%.
  - Scars – Medicines and Healthcare products Regulatory Agency (MHRA) quotes 1 in 20 get 'bad scars'.

- ○ Temporary change in nipple sensation reported in 15%.
- ○ Thromboembolic disorders (deep venous thrombosis (DVT)/pulmonary embolism (PE)).
- Specific.
  - ○ Capsule formation – all implants have a surrounding capsule, capsular **contracture** is the problem. Overall 25%.
  - ○ Rippling, palpable edge.
  - ○ **Rupture with cumulative risk ~2% per year.** It is important to convey to patients that lifespan of the implant cannot be guaranteed. MRI (stepladder sign) then USG are the best radiological techniques for diagnosing rupture – Ahn C. *Plast Reconstr Surg* 1994;**93**:1481–1484.
  - ○ **Gel bleed**: bleed phenomenon due to escape of silicone oil from an implant with no evidence of a hole or tear in the outer shell. It is intracapsular and asymptomatic in the majority, and may be related to lipid infiltration of the silicone elastomer.

Aesthetic complications.

- Asymmetry.
- Rippling, palpable edge.
- Final result too big or too small.

Expectations

It is important to manage patient expectations particularly during the consultation/consent process. They should be told:

- If the ribs can be felt beneath or to the side of the breast, then the implant will be palpable beneath or lateral to the breast.
- Thicker shells which are more durable may be easier to feel.
- The larger the implant, the worse it will look over time due to stretching and tissue thinning.

If the patient does not accept palpable implants, do not have augmentation.

If the patient wants a totally 'natural' breast, do not have augmentation.

Problems with pregnancy, lactation and breastfeeding

All are unaffected although oesophageal motility problems have been reported in children breastfed by mothers with silicone implants – the link is unproven.

- Patients may experience lactorrhoea post-augmentation.
- Nipple sensation is altered in ~20%.

For patients with a family of breast cancer:

- Inform them that having breast implants may delay diagnosis of breast cancer but does not affect overall survival.
- Suggest mammogram before augmentation if > 30 years old.
- Recommend submuscular placement (only 10% 'hidden' vs. 40%).
- Regular screening post-operatively.

Breast cancer and augmentation mammoplasty: the pre-operative consultation
Shons AR. *Plast Reconstr Surg* 2002;**109**:383–385.

One in 8 women in North America develop breast cancer at some point in their lives, therefore of 200 000 women who undergo augmentation each year, 25 000 will develop the disease.

Main points:

- There is no evidence to suggest that risk of induction of breast cancer after augmentation is over and above that of the general female population.
- Mammographic visualization of breast cancer may be difficult but is possible with displacement techniques (Eklund).
- Breast cancer in patients with implants have the same survival as patients without implants and detection occurs at a similar stage.

Breast augmentation: a risk factor for breast cancer?
Berkel H. *N Engl J Med* 1992;**326**:1649–1653.

In over 11 000 women with implants, the **predicted** number of patients with cancer (according to incidence in general population) should be 86 whereas the **observed** number in those with implants was much lower at 47.

Augmentation mammoplasty and breast cancer: a five-year update of the Los Angeles study
Deapen DM. *Plast Reconstr Surg* 1992;**89**:660–665.

Similarly a retrospective study of 3112 women with implants found that the observed number of breast cancers was 21 compared with the expected number of 32.

Detection of breast cancer

The fear is that delayed diagnosis may occur due to a high false-negative mammography rate. Saline implants are slightly more radiolucent than silicone but both are fairly radio-opaque, a higher dose of radiation is needed. This in addition to the microcalcification within the capsule that may **theoretically** obscure the microcalcification associated with malignancies. Overall, studies have shown no significant difference in the mammographic detection of breast cancer.

Breast cancer diagnosis and prognosis in women augmented with silicone gel-filled implants
Silverstein MJ. *Cancer* 1990;**66**:97–101.

Thirty-four of 35 patients with implants who developed cancer presented with **palpable** disease. In this group there was a 41% false-negative mammography rate (normally ~5–10%). This is similar to Carson GW (*Plast Reconstr Surg* 1993;**91**:837–40) in which 35 of 37 cases of breast cancer in augmented patients presented with palpable disease, and there was a ~50% false-negative mammography rate.

- Patients with implants are **more likely to require open biopsy** for histological diagnosis than percutaneous needle techniques but the presence of an implant does not preclude radiotherapy or FNA/Trucut biopsy.
- According to this paper, **augmented patients with breast cancer present with a higher percentage of invasive lesions and involved lymph nodes**.

In terms of imaging augmented breasts:

- Compression and displacement techniques visualize ~60% of breast if subglandular and ~90% if submuscular (Eklund). **Eklund views** (displacement techniques) should be used when obtaining mammograms in augmented patients and should be interpreted by experienced radiologists.
- Capsular contracture makes compression and displacement techniques difficult. Adjuvant radiotherapy encourages the development of a firm capsule around an implant.
- Although the presence of an implant makes radiological diagnosis **more difficult** due to false-negatives or false-positives, those women in whom breast cancer does develop tend to present at a **similar stage,** including nodal disease, and have

equivalent survival compared with non-implanted women.

The recommendations for patients at **high risk** of developing breast cancer (positive family history) are that:

- Warn patients that implants may delay diagnosis of tumours.
- A pre-operative mammogram before implant placement if > 30 years (some say 35).
- Submuscular placement is preferred as it allows greater mammographic visualization.
- Regular screening – the current recommendations for getting screening/pre-operative mammograms are no different for augmented patients. Jakubietz MG. *Plast Reconstr Surg* 2004;**113**:117e–122e.

Small breast volume and distortion of tissue due to the presence of the implant capsule may make wide local excision of the tumour difficult. Patients with implants are more likely to undergo mastectomy rather than lumpectomy. In addition, sentinel lymph node biopsy is less reliable in patients who have undergone axillary placement of their implant.

Breast cancer diagnosis and survival in women with and without breast implants
Birdsell DC. *Plast Reconstr Surg* 1993;**92**:795–800.

This study of 13 246 women with breast cancer in Alberta showed that those with breast augmentation had the same 5-year survival and same incidence of lymph node disease as non-augmented women with breast cancer. Although there was no difference in pathological stage at diagnosis, the tumours in augmented patients were **smaller** and augmented patients were ~12 years **younger** at diagnosis.

Surgical treatment of breast cancer in previously augmented patients
Karanas YL. *Plast Reconstr Surg* 2003;**111**:1078–1083.

This was a retrospective review of 58 breast-cancer patients with previous implants.

- Half were treated with a modified radical mastectomy with implant removal whilst the other half underwent breast conservation therapy (BCT) – lumpectomy, axillary lymph node dissection and radiotherapy.
- One-third initially retained their implants but half of these ultimately required complete

mastectomies with implant removal (local recurrence, residual disease and implant complications).

Breast conservation therapy with maintenance of the implant is **not** ideal for the majority of augmented patients – mastectomy with immediate reconstruction might be a more suitable choice.

Injectables for breast augmentation

It is well documented that Japanese prostitutes hoping to attract more American soldiers had their breasts injected with materials such as paraffin, sponges and liquid silicone. The last was initially called the Sakurai formula, after the first physician to perform the procedure, but it was noticed that large quantities of transformer coolant made of silicone were disappearing from Yokohama docks. This 'doctored' non-medical grade silicone was being injected directly into breasts.

- Robert Gersuny (1844–1924), an Austrian doctor, injected paraffin into breasts in 1890 which has largely overshadowed his other achievements – he was resident to Bilroth and he improved intestinal anastomotic and abdominal closure techniques.
- Symmer W St C. (*Br Med J* 1968;**3**:19–22) – a surgeon who reported on 31 cases of breasts filled with 'paraffin waxes, beeswax, silicone wax, silicone fluid, shellac, shredded oiled-silk fabric, silk tangle, glazier's putty, spun glass and epoxy resin'.

Liquid silicone was actually developed by Dow Corning during World War II, commissioned by the US government. The practice of injecting silicone passed back to the USA and the complications were so severe that the state of Nevada had to pass emergency legislation to make the injections a felony. The FDA finally banned the practice in 1965. With these events in the background, Thomas Cronin and Frank Gerow developed the first breast implants with Dow Corning.

Fat injection to the breast

(See also Fat injection)

One of the main concerns with fat injections to the breast is potential interference with oncological surveillance. Fat necrosis (fat cysts and coarse calcification) and fibrosis in particular may cause

problems, but also occur in up to 13% of breast reconstructed with flaps – the combination of targeted ultrasound and mammography is able to differentiate these from recurrence and needing biopsy for confirmation is unusual. Magnetic resonance imaging is also useful to differentiate benign post-operative changes from tumour – the former will show little uptake of contrast and will have a fatty signal intensity (often with fat-fluid levels). Pierrefeu-Lagrange AC (*Ann Chir Plast Esthet* 2006;**51**:18–28) performed multimodality imaging on 30 fat-grafted patients a year after fat injections. Four had benign calcifications, one other required biopsy of a suspicious area (turned out to be granuloma) and the rest had normal imaging.

- Fat can be injected into the various planes e.g. subcutaneous, subglandular, submuscular and intramuscular, some do not inject into the breast parenchyma whilst others have done so safely (Illouz GY. *Aesthet Plast Surg* 2009;**33**:706–715).

Fat grafting to the breast revisited: safety and efficacy

Coleman SR. *Plast Reconstr Surg* 2007;**119**:775–785.

This is a retrospective study of 17 patients who received fat injections to the breast for a variety of indications. Post-operative mammograms identified changes expected after breast surgery.

Complications after autologous fat injection to the breast

Hyakusoku H. *Plast Reconstr Surg* 2009;**123**:360–370.

This paper presented 12 patients who had fat injections to the breast with complications such as induration, pain, infection and discharge. The author made it clear that fat grafting should only be performed by trained and skilled surgeons.

Autologous fat grafting to the reconstructed breast: the management of acquired contour deformities

Kanchwala SK. *Plast Reconstr Surg* 2009;**124**:409–418.

This is a retrospective review of 110 patients who had fat injections to reconstructed breasts to correct contour deformities as well as implant rippling. The fat was harvested from the thigh and flanks using a modified Coleman technique with a gravity then Telfa pad refinement method. Median follow-up was 21 months; volume that remained after 3 months was generally 'permanent'.

Current applications and safety of autologous fat grafts: a report of the ASPS fat graft task force
Gutowski KA. *Plast Reconstr Surg* 2009;**124**:272–280.
Their recommendations were:

- Fat grafting may be considered for breast augmentation and correction of defects associated with medical conditions and previous surgeries, with the proviso that results are quite operator dependent and additional treatments may be needed.
- Fat grafting can be considered a safe method of augmentation and correction of defects. A sterile technique is necessary. Patients should be made aware of potential complications.
- Caution should be exercised in high-risk patients – those with risk factors for breast cancer: BRCA, personal or family history of breast cancer. Baseline imaging is recommended.

They found no strong evidence of interference with breast cancer detection. Radiological studies have demonstrated that current imaging (ultrasound, MMG and MRI) can differentiate between grafted fat, microcalcifications and suspicious lesions.

It was only in 1987 that the ASPS Ad-hoc Committee on New Procedures stated that 'the committee is unanimous in deploring the use of autologous fat injection in breast augmentation'.

III. Complications

Capsular contracture

The MHRA states that **1 in 10** patients will develop capsular contracture.

- Subglandular implants ~30% in 10 years.
- Subpectoral implants ~10% in 10 years.
- Smooth vs. textured – 58 vs. 11%.
- Mentor Core Study (2005) and Allergan (formerly Inamed) Core Study (2003) – studies for primary augmentation show a capsular contracture rate of 8.0% for silicone and 9% for saline.
- Capsular calcification: 0% under 10 years, 100% over 23 years; of little significance and can be removed with capsulectomy.

Baker classification of capsular contracture (1975):

- Class I – no contracture.
- Class II – palpable contracture.
- Class III – visible contracture.
- Class IV – painful contracture.

There are some theories regarding the pathogenesis of capsular contracture:

- Subclinical *Staphylococcus epidermidis* infection (betadine wash-out has been shown to reduce colonization rates).
- Fibroblastic foreign-body type reaction.

Strategies for reducing capsular contracture:

- Use of textured implants; Malata CM. *Br J Plast Surg* 1997;**50**:99; Hakelius L. *Plast Reconstr Surg* 1997;**100**:1566–1569.
  - Texturing has less effect when placed submuscularly.
- Submuscular/pectoral placement.
  - Most pronounced for smooth (saline) implants.
- Betadine/antimicrobial wash-out e.g. bacitracin 50 KU, cefazolin 1 gram, gentamicin 80 mg in 500 ml saline.

Treatment:

- Closed capsulotomy – this is not recommended due to the risk of implant rupture.
- Open capsulotomy.
- Open capsulectomy – this reduces breast parenchymal volume and there is no guarantee that recurrent capsule formation will not occur.

Calcification within the breast capsule may make interpretation of mammography difficult; it may be mistaken for malignant disease.

Textured or smooth implants for breast augmentation? A prospective controlled trial
Coleman DJ. *Br J Plast Surg* 1991;**44**:444–448.
Fifty-three patients in this prospective randomized double-blind study (usually referred to as the 'Bradford study') had subglandular smooth or textured implants and were assessed at 12 months. There was adverse capsular contracture (Baker grades 3 and 4) in 58% of breasts augmented with smooth implants compared with 8% in the textured surface implant group.

Textured or smooth implants for breast augmentation?
Malata CM. *Br J Plast Surg* 1997;**50**:99.
The 'Bradford study' was reviewed after a total of 3 years (data on 49 of the 53 patients) and adverse

capsular contracture was 59% for smooth implants and 11% for textured ones.

Eight patients (31%) with smooth prostheses underwent breast implant exchange for severe capsular contracture between the 1- and 3-year assessments compared with a revisional surgery rate of only 7.4% (2/27 patients) for the textured group.

The effect of Biocell texturing and povidone-iodine irrigation on capsular contracture around saline-inflatable breast implants
Burkhardt BR. *Plast Reconstr Surg* 1995;**96**:1317–1325.

This is a prospective, controlled, blinded 4-year trial with 60 patient volunteers, testing the effect of two independent variables (texturization and betadine irrigation) on the incidence of capsular contracture around saline-inflatable implants following subglandular augmentation.

- Textured devices irrigated with betadine – 4% contracture.
- Smooth devices irrigated with saline solution – 50% contracture.

Their conclusion was that betadine wash-out and textured implants both independently reduce contracture.

However, the FDA have recommended that implants should not come into contact with betadine due to reports of saline implant deflation possibly due to valve patch delamination affecting the adhesive. Most cases of failure stemmed from a single surgeon's practice of using the betadine intraluminally, and in vitro studies confirmed that intraluminal betadine does cause deflation. The recommendation stands despite clinical studies showing no increased deflation rates when betadine is used externally. Currently, surgeons are using antimicrobial–antiseptic mixes.

Pre-operative antibiotics and capsular contracture in augmentation mammoplasty
Gylbert L. *Plast Reconstr Surg* 1990;**86**:260–267.

This is a randomized blinded series of 76 patients undergoing subglandular augmentation with half receiving peri-operative antibiotic prophylaxis. There was no significant effect on the incidence of contracture.

Detection of subclinical infection in significant breast implant capsules
Pajkos A. *Plast Reconstr Surg* 2003;**111**:1605.

In this study, samples were obtained during explantation from 27 breasts. Swabs were all negative whilst the capsules demonstrated 17 positives in the 19 patients with significant capsules, with only one in the remaining eight with minimal or no capsules. Fourteen of the 17 yielded *Staphylococcus epidermidis*. The authors suggest that **biofilm disease** is part of the pathogenesis of contracture and suggest measures such as prophylactic antibiotics and antiseptic washing of the cavity.

Capsular contracture in subglandular breast augmentation with textured versus smooth breast implants: a systematic review
Wong CH. *Plast Reconstr Surg* 2006;**118**:1224–1236.

This review identified six randomized controlled trials comparing textured and smooth implants and found that smooth implants were associated with more contracture (III/IV) at 1 and 7 years, with relative risks of 4.16 and 2.98 respectively.

Rupture and leakage
Overall, rates of ~**1% per year** are quoted for saline implants (increased if underfilled or if intraluminal additives used) whilst there is less information for silicone.

- Leakage can be intra- or extracapsular.
- Silicone granuloma 0.1–0.5%.

Rupture of silicone-gel breast implants
Brown SL. *Lancet* 1997;**350**:1531–1537.

The strength of the silicone elastomer shell decreases with age; implant rupture can be extra- or **intracapsular** – the latter causes no change in shape or size of the breast. Causes of rupture include:

- Iatrogenic – mammography, closed capsulotomy.
- Trauma.
- Idiopathic.

Extracapsular spread of silicone has been reported in up to about one-quarter of patients, with formation of silicone granulomas in skin and nipple ducts, lymph nodes and distant sites. The authors state that ultrasound screening for implant rupture in patients without symptoms is unnecessary but that ruptured implants should be removed.

- MRI imaging of implants may detect the **linguine sign** on T2 where the implant has pulled away from the capsule, collapsing into the gel and leaving multiple parallel lines (stepladder sign on USG). MRI is most sensitive and specific.

- Snowstorm appearance and stepladder sign of ruptured implant on USG. USG has a sensitivity of 70% and a negative predictive value of 80%.

Analysis of explanted silicone implants: a report of 300 patients
Robinson OG. *Ann Plast Surg* 1995;**34**:1–7.

Five hundred and ninety-two implants (between 1 and 25 years *in situ*) that were explanted due to silicone controversy showed a 63% rupture or bleed rate irrespective of whether patients complained of symptoms or not. According to the author's calculations, only 50% of women could expect to have their prosthesis intact by 12 years and they recommend that implants should be **electively replaced at 8 years.**

Breast implant-related silicone granulomas: the literature and the litigation
Austad ED. *Plast Reconstr Surg* 2002;**109**:1724–1730.

A silicone granuloma is a foreign-body type reaction to the presence of silicone formed by aggregates of macrophages and polymorphs; it may be palpable and persists until the foreign body is degraded. Microscopic subclinical silicone granulomas may also occur.

- Granulomas are relatively rare; though the exact incidence is unknown, it is probably between **0.1 and 0.5%.** It may not always be associated with implant rupture, in some cases it may be associated with low-grade *Staphylococcus epidermidis* infection. Thus excised granulomas should be submitted for culture.
- Fragments of silicone were found in the capsules of 46 of 54 textured implants in one study. They may also occur outside the breast on the chest wall or upper limb; silicone lymphadenopathy has been reported many years after the placement of an implant or MCP joint prosthesis.

The authors conclude that there is no evidence to suggest that silicone granulomas bear any relationship to any form of systemic disease. Most silicone granulomas are excised simply to exclude malignancy.

Mixed connective tissue disease

Landmark papers

Post-mammoplasty connective tissue disease
Van Nunen SA. *Arthritis Rheum* 1982;**25**:694–697.

This was the first report of connective tissue disease (systemic lupus erythematosus (SLE), rheumatoid arthritis (RA) and a mixed connective tissue disorder) in three patients within 2.5 years of receiving silicone breast implants but none of the patients wanted to have their implants removed. Some prior reports had linked connective tissue disorder with injections of liquid paraffin into the breast.

Risk of connective-tissue diseases and other disorders after breast implantation
Gabriel SE. *N Engl J Med* 1994;**330**:1697–1702.

This Mayo Clinic study found 5/749 augmented women with connective tissue disease compared with 10/1498 controls, i.e. comparable.

Silicone breast implants and the risk of connective-tissue diseases and symptoms
Sanchez-Guerrero J. *N Engl J Med* 1995;**322**:1666–1670.

Nurses' health study – 87 501 women were evaluated of whom ~1% had implants, and there was no increased incidence of connective tissue disorders in women with implants.

Risk of connective tissue disease and related disorders among women with breast implants
Nyren O. *Br Med J* 1998;**316**:417–422.

Comparison of 7442 breast-augmentation patients with 3353 breast reduction patients found no difference in recorded first hospitalization rates for connective tissue diseases.

Absence of longitudinal changes in rheumatologic parameters after breast augmentation
Miller AS. *Plast Reconstr Surg* 1998;**102**:2299–2303.

C reactive protein (CRP), rheumatoid factor (RF), anti-nuclear Ab and anti-streptinolysin O titres were measured pre-operatively in 218 patients and post-operatively over 13 years. No increase in levels was found in women with either saline or gel-filled implants.

Background risk
There is a high incidence of rheumatoid-like symptoms in the general population – fibromyalgia ~5% and RA ~2%. Therefore by chance alone, in the women in the USA with breast implants, there should be:

- 30–50 000 with fibromyalgia.
- 10–20 000 with RA.

Conversely, studies examining patients suffering from SLE, RA and scleroderma have all found that the number with implants is no higher than the estimated percentage in the general population with implants, i.e. ~1% in the USA.

Long-term health status of Danish women with silicone breast implants
Breiting VB. *Plast Reconstr Surg* 2004;**114**:217–226.

This is a retrospective study comparing three cohorts of women: breast augmentation ($n = 190$, the majority with silicone implants in submammary pocket), breast reduction ($n = 186$) and population controls ($n = 149$). The data indicated no difference between any cohort in:

- **Incidence of breast cancer.**
- **Seropositivity for antinuclear Ab, rheumatoid factor and IgM Ab recorded in 5–10% of women in each group.** Positive autoimmune antibody tests.
- Smoking and alcohol consumption.
- Education level and marital status.
- Use of contraceptive, analgesic, anti-allergic or cardiac drugs.

The implant cohort was compared with the non-implant patients (breast reduction and population controls):

- Breast pain reported more commonly ($3 \times$) – 18% of patients reported severe pain associated with Baker IV capsular contracture.
- Higher self-reported use of antidepressant and anxiolytic drugs; **increased risk of suicide** amongst augmentation mammoplasty patients reported elsewhere (Koot VCM. *Br Med J* 2003:**326**;527–528).
- Fatigue and Raynaud-like symptoms were similar in implant and reduction cohorts, but reported more frequently than in the population control group.

Excess mortality from suicide and other causes of death among women with cosmetic breast implants
Lipworth L. *Ann Plast Surg* 2007;**59**:119–123.

This study expanded on an earlier study from the same centre. Overall there were 175 deaths amongst women with breast implants in the study population compared with the 133.4 expected from a matched general population. In the women with implants, there was an excess of deaths from alcohol and drug abuse whilst cancer deaths were comparable to the expected figure. The authors suggest that this means

that the data indicates significant psychiatric morbidity amongst these women, and that screening pre-operatively may be warranted.

Breast milk contamination and silicone implants
Semple JL. *Plast Reconstr Surg* 1998;**102**:528–533.

There is a theoretical risk of silicone breakdown products (e.g. silicon) entering breast milk in patients with implants in a submammary pocket and there have been reports of abnormal oesophageal motility in children breastfed by women with implants (Levine JJ. *JAMA* 1994;**271**:213–216).

This study measured elemental silicon (used as proxy measure for silicone) in breast milk of patients with and without implants and found them to be the same. In fact, silicon was 10 times higher in cows' milk and even higher in infant formula. Grain, rice and beer also have high levels of silicon.

Silicon analysis of breast and capsular tissue from patients with saline or silicone gel breast implants: II. Correlation with connective-tissue disease
Weinzweig J. *Plast Reconstr Surg* 1998;**101**:1836–1841.

Silicone levels in breast tissue were the same in patients with implants as those without but capsule silicone levels were significantly higher than breast tissue levels (gel implant levels higher than those with saline implants). There was no relationship between the level of capsular silicone and the incidence of connective tissue disease.

Aesthetic management of the breast following explantation: evaluation and mastopexy options
Rohrich RJ. *Plast Reconstr Surg* 1998;**101**:827–837.

This is a retrospective review of 282 patients with explantation of breast implants. Almost 50% chose not to replace the implants. Options following explantation include:

- Explantation and capsulectomy alone. The presence of microcalcification or silicone granulomas makes detection of breast cancers more difficult if the capsule is left behind. It is sometimes possible to remove the entire capsule while maintaining the implant inside.
- Re-implantation. If the plan is to replace the implant with a *saline* implant then submuscular placement is preferred to avoid rippling.
- Mastopexy – related to the degree of ptosis
  - Grade I – periareolar or vertical.

- ○ Grade II – Wise pattern.
- ○ Grade III – delayed mastopexy (3/12) especially in smokers.
- ○ Pseudoptosis – inframammary wedge excision.

Aesthetic management of the breast following explantation: evaluation and mastopexy options
Rohrich RJ. *Plast Reconstr Surg* 2007;**120**:312–315.

This is a follow-up to the study above. In the authors' current practice, the commonest choice is now implant exchange, usually a subpectoral smooth saline implant, and second is exchange with mastopexy (mostly circumareolar with vertical scar, some with Wise pattern). Fewer patients were now opting not to have another implant, which may be due to improved public confidence regarding implants.

IV. Tuberous breasts

Tuberous breast deformity: classification and treatment
von Heimburg D. *Br J Plast Surg* 1996;**49**:339–345.

Tuberous breast deformity was first described in 1976 by Rees and Aston (due to its similarity in shape to 'tubers') and is characterized by:

- A constricting ring at the base of the breast.
- Deficient horizontal and vertical development of the breast, especially lower pole.
- Herniation of the breast parenchyma toward the nipple–areolar complex.
- Areola enlargement.

'Tuberous'/'tubular'/'constricted' all describe the same deformity; there are fewer ducts and less breast tissue in the inferior quadrants. The true incidence is unknown (many mild degrees of deformity may exist and be unnoticed, though there are studies to suggest that many who present with asymmetric breast have previously unrecognized tuberous breast deformity) but it is relatively uncommon; the aetiology is also unknown.

Embryology

- Breast tissue comes from the mammary ridge, which develops from the ectoderm during the fifth week and most parts of this ridge disappear, except for a small portion in the thoracic region that persists and penetrates the underlying mesenchyme (10 to 14 weeks). No further development occurs until puberty.
  - ○ As a result of the ectodermal origin of the breast and its invagination into the underlying mesenchyme, the breast tissue is contained within a fascial envelope, the superficial and deep layers of the superficial fascia. The breast lies on the deep fascia of the pectoralis major and serratus anterior muscles.
- The breast is penetrated by fibrous attachments – suspensory ligaments of Cooper – which join the two layers of the superficial fascia and extend to the dermis of the overlying skin and the deep pectoral fascia. Critically, the superficial layer of the superficial fascia is absent in the area underneath the areola.
- There is also a constricting fibrous ring at the level of the periphery of the nipple–areola complex that inhibits the normal development of the breast.

It is distinct from a hypoplastic breast that is more easily treated. The condition may be unilateral or bilateral; asymmetry is common.

von Heimburg Classification (1996, then modified by author in 2000)

- Type 1 – hypoplasia of the inferior medial quadrant.
- Type 2 – hypoplasia of both inferior quadrants, sufficient subareolar skin.
- Type 3 – hypoplasia of both lower quadrants, subareolar skin shortage.
- Type 4 – severely constricted breast, minimal breast base.

In some modifications, von Heimburg 1 and 2 becomes I and II respectively whilst 3 and 4 is combined into III – all four quadrants deficient.

Examination

- Recline for breast cancer examination and sit up for aesthetic examination – symmetry, ptosis (Regnault classification) and degree of tubular breast deformity (Heimberg classification).
- Determine the level of the inframammary fold (IMF) on the affected side.
- Exclude Poland's syndrome.

The important features are:

- Constricted breast base – treatment needs to expand breast circumference and skin envelope of lower pole, increase volume where appropriate.
- High inframammary fold – need to lower inframammary fold.

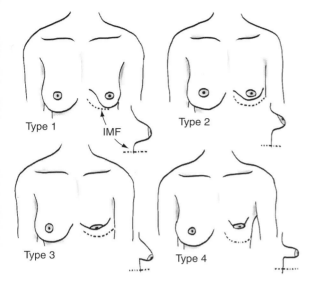

Type 1   IMF   Type 2

Type 3   Type 4

Figure 5.1 Schematic representation of the classification of tuberose breast deformity. The dotted lines represent the level of the inframammary fold (IMF).

- Breast herniation into areola – need to release constriction at edge of aerola and reduce areola.

Surgical options

- Type 1 – augmentation with a submammary implant via inframammary or infra-areolar incision, taking care to avoid a 'double bubble' deformity.
- Type 2 – augmentation plus internal flap by 'unfurling' of breast tissue on the chest wall, turned downward to augment the lower half of the breast (Puckett CL. *Aesth Plast Surg* 1990:**14**:15–19). This may be performed through an inferior circumareolar incision.
- Types 3 and 4 – augmentation plus internal flap plus skin importation to break up the constricted base at the abnormal inframammary fold which avoids 'double bubble' deformity.
  - Z-plasty across the inframammary fold – modified Maillard technique.
  - Thoraco-epigastric flap.
  - De-epithelialized epigastric flap.
  - Tissue expansion (Scheepers JH. *Br J Plast Surg* 1992;**45**:529.
  - Circumareolar mastopexy and tissue expansion.
  - Breast reduction may be considered in an adequately sized breast.

  - Consider contralateral reduction or mastopexy ± augmentation.

Aesthetic reconstruction of the tuberous breast deformity
Mandrekas AD. *Plast Reconstr Surg* 2003;**112**:1099–1108.

The authors describe their surgical approach in 11 patients, which uses a periareolar incision:

- The inferior skin flap is dissected to the chest wall and to the new inframammary fold, and also behind the breast leaving only the superior parenchyma attached to the chest wall.
- The parenchyma is exteriorized through the periareolar opening and is divided vertically down the middle.
- By dividing the constricting ring, creating two breast pillars that are allowed to redrape, there is re-arrangement of the inferior parenchyma. The breast is flatter and wider at the expense of projection.
- In cases of volume deficiency, a silicone breast implant is placed in a subglandular pocket.
- Dough-nut mastopexy to address the size of the nipple–areolar complex (NAC).

The tuberous breast revisited
Pacifico MD. *J Plast Reconstr Aesthetic Surg* 2007;**60**:455–464.

The authors suggest that there is only one major deformity in tuberous breast – that of herniation of breast tissue through the NAC, and that there is no significant skin shortage. They describe their surgical technique. A subglandular implant is placed before NAC reduction if necessary; they preferred an IMF approach but did mention that a periareolar approach was also feasible. The NAC size is agreed beforehand with the patient (3–5 cm or match contralateral side) – the position is determined by several parameters:

- IMF to inferior NAC no more than 6 cm.
- Medial NAC to midline 8–10 cm.

The NAC can be tailor tacked and the patient positioned more upright to allow adjustment to the final position. Through an incision around the 'new' areolar margin, there is circumareolar de-epithelialization up to the margins of the existing areola and further undermining outwards subdermally for 2 cm. Deep tension sutures that double-breast the dermis are then placed during wound closure.

Management of tuberous breast deformity with anatomic cohesive silicone gel breast implants
Panchapakesan V. *Aesth Plast Surg* 2009;**33**:49–53.

This paper presents results in 50 cases of tuberous breast deformity with single-stage surgery using anatomic implants with good results. For cases requiring areolar reduction, a periareolar approach is used for the implants whilst for cases with small areola/minimal herniation, the incision is at the site of the planned IMF. A subglandular position is preferred; for those with insufficient superior pole tissue, a dual plane procedure is performed. If further release of constricted tissues is required, then radial scoring with electrocautery is used up to the dermal level if necessary. Full or extra-projection implants were most often used. After the implant is in place, areolar reduction or mastopexy is performed as needed.

B. Breast reduction

I. Indications for breast reduction

The aim of breast reduction surgery is to achieve smaller breasts with aesthetic shape and volume symmetry.

It is common to refer to bra cup sizes, which is measured by the difference between the bra band size (either above the breast/below the axilla or inframammary circumference with a variable integer, usually 4–5) and chest–nipple circumference (at the fullest part of the breast). For each 2.5 cm of difference, it is an additional cup size starting from A (AA is a difference of less than 2.5 cm).

Although patients commonly refer to bra sizes for reduction and augmentations, it is close to meaningless as it does not calculate volume accurately, and patients (as well as surgeons) may have very different perceptions of what constitutes a 'full C cup' for example. **The cup size is relative to the band size** – for a 32–34-inch chest, each cup size ~ 100 g, whilst for a > 36-inch chest, one cup size ~ 180–200 g.

Reduction mammoplasty is commonly performed for:

- Bilateral macromastia.
  - Macromastia: < 2.5 kg reduction per breast.
  - Gigantomastia: > 2.5 kg reduction per breast.
  - Virginal breast hypertrophy: in pubertal and prepubertal females.
- Congenital asymmetry.

- Contralateral symmetry following cancer surgery/reconstruction.

Indications in the patient with large breasts:

- Secondary back, shoulder and neck pain.
- Difficulty with exercise.
- Poor posture.
- Low self-esteem/other psychological symptoms.
- Mastalgia.
- Difficulty with finding clothing.
- Submammary maceration and infection, intertrigo.

Symptoms and related severity experienced by women with breast hypertrophy
Sigurdson L. *Plast Reconstr Surg* 2007;**119**:481–486.

Overall, the most troublesome symptoms were the first four in the list above.

- Older women tend to complain of physical symptoms.
- Younger women tended to have more psychological symptoms.

Patients should be fully informed of the risks and complications of reduction surgery. They should also be warned about the change in breast shape with weight gain/loss, and bottoming-out and ptosis with time (especially with inferior pedicle technique). In terms of outcomes:

- 93% report improvement in symptoms and 62% increased their activity levels (Miller AP. *Plast Reconstr Surg* 1995;**95**:77–83).
- 87% overall satisfaction (Davis GM *Plast Reconstr Surg* 1995;**96**:1106–1110) despite minor complications; 93% would have the surgery again and 94% would recommend it for others.

Examination

- Cancer examination – lumps, nodes, scars, etc.
- Aesthetic examination – size, shape, symmetry, degree of ptosis (Regnault), sternal notch–nipple distance, nipple–inframammary fold distance, general body habitus.

II. Breast reduction surgery

Operative techniques are usually classified according to the type of pedicle and the type of skin markings/resection. These are independent of each other and can be combined in various ways. For example, Khan UD

(*Aesth Plast Surg* 2007;**31**:337–342) combined a verti-cal scar with a vertical bipedicle McKissock technique and Blondeel PN (*Br J Plast Surg* 2003;**56**:348–359) combined a latero-central pedicle with a Wise pattern. The most common variations in use are the inferior pedicle with an inverted T scar (ITIP) and vertical scar mammoplasty (with variety of pedicles).

- Reduce and reshape parenchyma.
- Create pedicle for NAC.
- Redrape and reduce skin.
- Reposition NAC.

Skin incisions:

- Inverted T.
- Vertical scar – Lassus/Lejour/Hall-Findlay – requires healthy skin elasticity for remodelling, high revision rate for dog ears/scar.
- B-shaped (Regnault).
- Circumareolar – generally not a useful option in breast reduction, or more than 2 cm of ptosis.

Techniques

- Liposuction alone or in combination. It has not been shown to increase calcifications in small studies.
- No pedicle (Thorek 1922) breast amputation and free nipple graft. This was conceived as a more reliable means of preventing nipple loss when previous pedicle techniques were insufficiently reliable.
- Central mound (Balch CR. Central mound technique for reduction mammaplasty. *Plast Reconstr Surg* 1981;**67**:305–311).
- Dermoglandular pedicle.
  - ○ Horizontal pedicle.
    - – Horizontal bipedicle, with inverted T scar (Strombeck JO. Report of a new technique based on the two pedicled procedure. *Br J Plast Surg* 1960;**13**:79–90).
    - – Horizontal single pedicle, with inverted T scar (Skoog T. A technique of breast reduction: transposition on a cutaneous vascular pedicle. *Acta Chir Scand* 1963;**126**:453–465).
  - ○ Lateral pedicle.
    - – Lateral pedicle and lateral scar (Duformentel C. Recent developments in mammaplasty by the lateral oblique technique. *Ann Chir Plast* 1965;**10**:227–241).
  - ○ Vertical pedicle.
    - – Bipedicle, with inverted T scar (McKissock PK. Reduction mammaplasty with a vertical dermal flap. *Plast Reconstr Surg* 1972;**49**:245–252). Most view the second (dermal) pedicle as not being strictly necessary.
    - – Superior pedicle (Weiner D. A single dermal pedicle for nipple transposition in subcutaneous mastectomy, reduction mammaplasty or mastopexy. *Plast Reconstr Surg* 1973;**51**:115–120).
    - – Superior vertical pedicle, vertical scar only (Lejour M. Reduction of mammaplasty scars: from a short inframammary scar to a vertical scar. *Ann Chir Plast Esthet* 1990;**35**:369–379).
    - – Inferior pedicle with inverted T scar (Robbins TH. A reduction mammaplasty with the areolar-nipple based on an inferior dermal pedicle. *Plast Reconstr Surg* 1977;**59**:64–67).
    - – Glanduloplasty technique, inferolateral resection, B-shaped scar (Regnault P. Breast reduction: B technique. *Plast Reconstr Surg* 1980;**65**:840–845).

Inferior pedicle with inverted T scar

This technique, often called the 'Wise' pattern (although this strictly refers to the skin incision) is one of the most popular techniques for breast reduc-tion mammoplasty. The skin incision can be marked according to a template or performed 'free-hand', e.g. an 'open' technique where the nipple position is not precut, which is more flexible in positioning (over points of maximal projection and to increase symme-try). Important landmarks/measurements are:

- Nipple areolar diameter 38–45 mm.
- Nipple position at Pitanguy's point i.e. IMF of breast.
- Sternal notch to nipple distance 21 cm.
- Nipple to IMF distance 6–8 cm.

Post-operatively, patients are usually advised to wear sports bras for 24 hours a day for up to 6 weeks.

Inferior pedicle with an inverted T scar methods are more predictable, particularly for very large reduc-tions, as they allow excision in both horizontal and vertical directions. Longer vertical limbs (> 5 cm) are prone to premature bottoming-out.

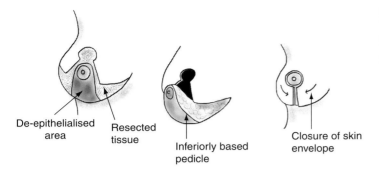

De-epithelialised area

Resected tissue

Inferiorly based pedicle

Closure of skin envelope

Figure 5.2 Inverted T inferior pedicle (ITIP) technique. The perfusion of the nipple–areolar complex is maintained by an inferiorly based parenchymal pedicle. The method largely relies on the skin envelope to maintain its shape.

Pre-operative injection using a diluted anesthetic/adrenaline solution significantly reduces blood loss in reduction mammaplasty

Wilmink H. *Plast Reconstr Surg* 1998;**102**:373–376.

Breast infiltration with adrenaline reduced operative blood loss in this series of 41 patients versus controls (29).

Routine drainage is not required in reduction mammoplasty

Wrye SW. *Plast Reconstr Surg* 2003;**111**:113–127.

This was a randomized control trial with 49 patients with ITIP reductions, with patients randomized to having a drain in either their left or right sides, and none in the other side. There was no difference in the incidence of haematomas or complications whilst patients reported that they preferred the early postoperative comfort in the side with no drain.

When to use drains in breast reduction surgery?

Ngan PG. *Ann Plast Surg* 2009;**63**:135–137.

This is a retrospective review of 182 patients with breast reductions to identify risk factors for higher output states that may require drains to be used. The authors identified age more than 50 years and reductions more than 500 g as situations where drains should be considered.

Vertical mammoplasty

The superior technique in early techniques was difficult to inset and prevented wider acceptance – the pedicle needed to be thinned to allow folding without compression/kinking but this reduces sensation and capacity for subsequent breastfeeding.

A 30-year experience with vertical mammaplasty

Lassus C. *Plast Reconstr Surg* 1996;**97**:373–380.

Lassus first described his technique in 1970 and this paper presents his experience.

Initial markings indicate position to which the nipple must move and a second point 2–4 cm above the inframammary fold defines the inferior limit of skin resection. Vertical lines are marked to connect these points after medial and lateral displacement of the breast and a keyhole pattern is incorporated to mark inset of nipple–areolar complex.

The technique uses a superior dermal pedicle that must be thin and include adequate tissue above the nipple to avoid venous congestion. After the nipple is raised on a pedicle, central breast parenchymal excision is undertaken. There is no skin undermining in this technique.

Nipple inset temporarily and the margins of resection closed; tacking ('framing') sutures are used to generate the desired breast shape and guide secondary resection. The vertical scar is closed and pleated to ensure that the scar does not descend below the inframammary fold.

Vertical mammaplasty and liposuction of the breast

Lejour M. *Plast Reconstr Surg* 1994;**94**:100–114. [The original paper in 1990 was in French.]

The technique was supposedly a modification of the Lassus technique that incorporates a vertical superior pedicle and a circumareolar and superior vertical scar that does not cross the IMF. However, there are several significant differences including fairly aggressive liposuction to model and shape the breast (the area behind the areola is not suctioned), pillar plication and relying upon substantial post-operative skin contraction and inferior breast remodelling. The contour is over-corrected to create a high, projected, narrow-based breast ('upside-down breast') that will improve with time (takes several months) for a more aesthetic final result.

Nipple numbness is not uncommon due to use of the superior pedicle (nerves enter inferolaterally). In about 10% of patients, particularly those with very large ptotic breasts, skin redundancy had to be excised from the lower part of the scar later on.

Lejour suggests that this is useful for reductions of up to 1000 g but most other surgeons would be more comfortable with a limit of 400–500 g.

'I' becomes 'L': modification of vertical mammaplasty

Pallua N. *Plast Reconstr Surg* 2003;**111**:1860–1870.

The authors propose a lateral inframammary limb to reduce the problems with the bunched-up scar of the classic Lejour i.e. wound-healing problems, whilst sparing the medial side for a 'scar-free cleavage'. They combined this with a superior pedicle in 45 patients and reported good results.

Vertical- versus Wise-pattern breast reduction: patient satisfaction, revision rates, and complications

Cruz-Korchin N. *Plast Reconstr Surg* 2003;**112**: 1573–1578.

This is a prospective, randomized study that compared the outcome of inferior pedicle/Wise pattern reduction with medial pedicle/vertical pattern reduction.

- Complications similar in both groups and overall patient satisfaction not significantly different.
- However, vertical mammoplasty was ranked significantly higher by patients in regard to scars and overall aesthetic results. Vertical scar breast reduction for moderate macromastia provides better cosmetic results but is associated with a significantly higher revision rate.

The vertical mammaplasty: a reappraisal of the technique and its complications

Berthe JV. *Plast Reconstr Surg* 2003;**111**:2192–2199.

Criticisms of the Lejour vertical mammaplasty are:

- Delayed healing on the vertical scar.
- Risk of seromas, haematoma, glandular necrosis and increased need for secondary corrections.

In this study, the results of 170 consecutive vertical mammoplasty procedures (330 breasts) were reviewed:

- Minor complications observed in 30% (minor skin edge necrosis).
- Major complications in 15% (glandular necrosis and severe infection).
- Surgical revision for scar or volume correction necessary in 28%.

The original technique was modified, decreasing the skin undermining, avoiding liposuction and primary skin excision performed in the submammary fold at the end of the operation for redundant skin. This resulted in much fewer minor and major complications but no significant change in rate of revisional surgery for secondary scar and volume corrections.

Lassus wrote a discussion piece for the article above (Lassus C. *Plast Reconstr Surg* 2003;**111**:2200–2202). He stresses that what are lumped together as 'vertical techniques' can be very different procedures, in particular he compares his technique with Lejours:

- Liposuction is part of Lejour but not Lassus.
- Skin undermining is part of Lejour but not Lassus, where the skin remains attached to the breast reducing dead-space formation.
- Lejour sutures the lateral pillars, Lassus does not.
- Lejour relies on skin contraction for scar, Lassus does not.

He comments that the modifications described by Berthe make it closer to a Lassus.

Benefits and pitfalls of vertical mammaplasty

Beer GM. *Br J Plast Surg* 2004;**57**:12–19.

This survey shows that vertical mammoplasty is more popular in Europe than the USA (12% according to a survey in 1999). Complications following vertical mammoplasty are similar to inferior pedicle inverted T scar (ITIP) breast reduction according to most studies. From their review of a modified Lassus reduction technique in 153 patients:

- Early complications in 21.6% including:
  - Haematoma 4% and infection 4%.
  - Wound dehiscence 12% especially infra-areolar area.
  - Nipple necrosis 0.7%.
- Late complications in 26%:
  - Problems with the vertical scar including scar below the new inframammary fold.
  - Major late complications required re-operation in 11.1%.

The authors suggested that the benefits over the ITIP technique, including long-lasting and enhanced projection and reduced scarring, justify its use as a standard technique.

Vertical mammaplasty

Hidalgo DA. *Plast Reconstr Surg* 2005;**115**:1179–1197.

The author reviews the evolution of vertical mammoplasty and in particular points to several key issues that improve outcomes:

- **Not using liposuction** as a major part of the procedure.
- **Not suturing the gland** to the pectoralis major (as this tends to cause distortion).
- Not undermining lower pole skin and leaving it attached to the gland.
- Creating additional pillars of adequate size and careful approximation to avoid flattening or notching. The significant parenchymal resection means that drains are more important than in ITIP methods.
- Avoiding tight closure/excessive skin resection, both of which distort the lower pole significantly.
- **Flexibility in positioning of nipple** i.e. open method where the areolar opening is not included in the pre-operative skin design – the marking along the breast meridian should be no higher than the IMF as closure of the pillars will raise the nipple slightly above the marked point. The author recommends leaving the final decision on the nipple position until the lower limbs are close and the patient is viewed sitting up.
  - An alternative is to inset the nipple into the smallest areolar opening possible that skirts the areolar when using the 'open' technique. It is inset with a temporary running suture and the patient is sat up to determine the best nipple position.
- Restricting purse-stringing vertical incision to the lower portion only.

The author suggests that surgeons taking up vertical mammoplasty should start with small volumes and minor ptosis. Not all cases are suited for this technique, particularly those with extreme problems of size and/or ptosis.

Breast reduction with a superomedial pedicle and a vertical scar (Hall-Findlay's technique)
Serra MP. *Ann Plast Surg* 2010;**64**:275–278.

A set of modifications was described by Hall-Findlay E (*Plast Reconstr Surg* 1999;**104**:748–758) with no skin undermining, no routine liposuction, no pectoralis suspension sutures in association with a superomedial pedicle. The authors present their results with this technique in 210 consecutive patients.

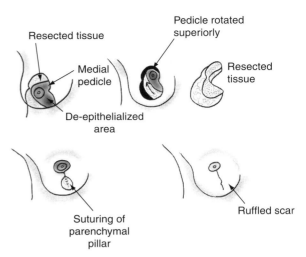

Figure 5.3 Simplified vertical mammaplasty technique based on a medial pedicle. Bringing together the parenchymal pillars cones the breast tissue and achieves a longer-lasting shape.

- The IMF is marked 2 cm below Pitanguy's point to accommodate the increased projection with this procedure.
- The lateral and medial limbs are marked by rotating the breast inwards and outwards as well as upwards; these lines are joined up in a U shape 2–6 cm above the IMF.

Most complications involved the vertical scar, more often in larger-volume reductions – in these patients, the authors suggest a short horizontal scar.

Transverse resection: a new technique of reduction mammaplasty
Piza-Katzer H. *Br J Plast Surg* 2003;**56**:365–368.

Although this is not a new technique contrary to what the authors say, it may be useful particularly when performing a 'balancing' reduction on the contralateral breast for those with reconstructed breasts after MRM.

Complications of breast reduction surgery
General

- Infection.
- Haematoma.
- Dehiscence (particularly at T-junction).
- Scarring (including hypertrophic) 4% unsatisfactory.
- DVT/PE.

Specific

- Asymmetry/under- or over-correction.
- The Pitanguy method of reduction will result in a grade I ptosis; a nipple to sternal notch distance of 12–23 cm with an inferior nipple to IMF limb of 5–7 suggested depending on the body habitus. ITIP methods tend to lower the IMF whilst vertical scar mammoplasty tends to raise it.
- **Nipple loss** – partial/complete 4–7%. Free nipple grafting is suggested for large reductions (> 1500 g) with long nipple translocations (> 25 cm), in smokers/diabetics or revisional reductions where the first pedicle used is not known. Grafts will survive better than borderline nipples on pedicles due to reduced metabolic demands. Hypopigmentation is common after grafting.
- Nipple sensation – increased/decreased up to 15%.
- **Lactation and breastfeeding** compromised (but ~70% can still lactate following inferior pedicle technique). Most larger studies suggest that successful lactation rates are similar to unoperated breasts.
- Fat necrosis.
- Revisional surgery (dog ears).
- Scar hypertrophy.

A baseline mammogram 6–12 months after surgery is recommended by some.

The effects of breast reduction on successful breastfeeding: a systematic review

Thibaudeau S. *J Plast Reconstr Aesthet Surg* 2009; doi:10.1016/j.bjps.2009.07.027

This review of 26 articles found no difference in breastfeeding capacity during the first month after delivery. With the exception of Strombeck's horizontal bipedicle technique, the majority of studies show that lactation is possible with the variety of pedicles; the limiting factor being the connection of the nipple to a significant portion of ducts and lobules – recanalization is rare. They state that **difficulties appear to be mostly explained by psychosocial issues** such as inadequate/inappropriate advice and coaching as well as other considerations. They recommend that these patients should all be encouraged to breastfeed.

III. Breast cancer and breast reduction

Pathological findings in breast reduction surgery

Incidence of breast cancer in women < 28 years of age is ~8 in 100 000; in patients < 30 years of age there is no absolute need to send tissue for histology unless there is a strong family history or the tissue appears macroscopically abnormal. Three studies suggest that sending breast reduction specimens for pathology **is** appropriate.

- ~25% of all breast reductions show abnormal pathology, although most of these are due to fibroadenosis. Titley OG. *Br J Plast Surg* 1996;**49**:447–451.
- Analysis of 5008 breast reductions by Snyderman RK. (*Plast Reconstr Surg* 1960;**25**:253–255) demonstrated 9 cancers (0.38%).
- 1998 survey of plastic surgeons in New Orleans revealed four cancers after 2576 reductions (0.16%). Jansen DA. *Plast Reconstr Surg* 1998;**101**:361–364.

It is a challenge for the pathologist to find a small clinically undetectable cancer in a large mass of breast parenchyma and fat – often the specimens are evaluated by thin slicing and selectively sending blocks for histology. Some have used specimen radiography to aid detection (Ozmen S. *Aesth Plast Surg* 2001;**25**:432–435). When sending specimens for histopathology, the surgeon must indicate the areas from which separate blocks of tissue have been removed – 60% of breast cancer occurs in the upper outer quadrant.

The role of pre-operative investigations is controversial. In the USA, it is common to:

- Recommend a baseline mammogram in those over 25 years of age (American Cancer Society (ACS) guidelines are for > 40 years). Perras C. (*Aesthetic Plast Surg* 1990;**14**:81–84) found 34 cancers by mammography in 1149 patients undergoing cosmetic breast surgery who were over 35 or had a positive family history.
- Send all specimens.
- Obtain baseline mammogram at 3–6 months after surgery.

There is evidence to suggest that breast reduction reduces cancer risk, possibly by removing either microscopic disease or simply reducing mass of potential foci i.e. breast tissue. Bilateral prophylactic mastectomy reduces the risk of breast cancer by 90%

compared with 95% reduction of risk for prophylactic contralateral mastectomy after cancer in one side.

Breast reduction surgery and breast cancer risk
Tarone RE. *Plast Reconstr Surg* 2004;**113**;2104–2110.

Five studies were reviewed and each concluded that the risk of breast cancer was less in the breast reduction patients than in the controls (relative risk, 0.2–0.7). In particular, the Scandinavian studies found almost no reduction in risk in women under 40 (at the time of breast reduction) but substantial reductions in women aged over 40.

Occult breast carcinoma in reduction mammaplasty specimens: 14-year experience
Colwell AS. *Plast Reconstr Surg* 2004;**113**:1984–1988.

- Maliniac first described the association of breast cancer and reduction mammoplasty, incriminating his free nipple graft as the source of ductal stasis and subsequent carcinoma.
- Tang C (*Plast Reconstr Surg* 1999;**103**:1682–1686) documented invasive carcinoma in 0.06% of 27 500 breast reductions from the Ontario registry whilst other studies have reported occult breast cancer in 0.06–0.4% of breast reduction specimens.

The authors of this study report six cases (0.8%) of breast cancer in 800 breast reductions performed in their institution over a 14-year period; half were invasive, the other half were ductal carcinoma *in situ* (DCIS). **The pre-operative mammography was negative in all cases.** Occult breast cancer was more common in the reconstruction group (1.2%) compared with the macromastia (0.7%) or congenital asymmetry (0%) groups.

The role of preoperative mammography in women considering reduction mammoplasty: a single insitution review of 207 patients
Campbell MJ. *Am J Surg* 2010;**199**:636–640.

This study involved 207 patients (average age 49) considering reduction mammoplasty who had recent screening mammograms. Sixteen per cent had abnormal radiographs but all were false-positives. They could not identify factors which would predict the risk of abnormal mammograms. They advise that patients should be counselled that pre-operative mammography can have significant false-positives and possible confirmatory studies may be necessary.

Screening for breast cancer post reduction mammaplasty
Muir TM. *Clin Radiol* 2010;**65**:198–205.

This study involved reviewing 4743 women who had breast screening after breast reduction; 51 cancers were detected (4.28 per 1000 screens) which was less than the controls without breast reduction (5.99 per 1000) with a relative risk of 0.71. There were no significant differences in the pathological types or anatomical location of the tumours. The authors conclude that the post-operative changes of breast reduction (skin thickening, non-anatomical retro-areolar bands that may become fibrose, fat necrosis with oil cyst calcification or calcification along suture lines) do not hinder screening.

Breast reduction and cancer in the gland remnant: a review
Palmieri B. *Breast Cancer Res Treat* 2005;**91**:283–290.

This reviewed articles from the prior 20 years. They confirm that breast reduction does decrease the risk of breast cancer and the risk reduction for patients older than 40 is related to the amount of tissue resected, thus surgery is encouraged by the authors.

Secondary breast reduction

It is uncommon for patients to present for repeated reduction surgery as the overall patient satisfaction is high. The general advice is to use the same pedicle as before. There have been mixed outcomes with transecting pedicles.

- Hudson DA. *Plast Reconstr Surg* 1999;**104**:401–408 – recommend using the same pedicle and free nipple grafting if the previous pedicle/technique is unknown. There is an increase in complications such as delayed wound healing and loss of NAC with repeat reductions.
- Losee J. *Plast Reconstr Surg* 2000;**106**:1004–1008 – Three of four patients with complications (out of a total of 10) had transected pedicles (average time from first surgery 15 years) i.e. different pedicles, but these complications all healed conservatively.

IV. Mastopexy
Ptosis is Greek for the act of 'falling'.

Regnault classification of ptosis
- First degree – nipple descends to the level of the inframammary fold.

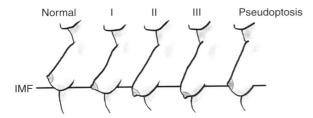

Figure 5.4 Classification of breast ptosis.

- Second degree – nipple falls below fold but remains above lowest contour of breast.
- Third degree – nipple reaches the lowest contour of the breast.
- Pseudoptosis – loose, lax breast but nipple remains at/above inframammary fold whilst majority of parenchyma falls below the level of the fold. There is an increase in the NAC–IMF distance.

Assessment

- Evaluate the patient's concerns and expectations.
- Breast history and relevant past medical history.

Examination

- Skin and parenchymal quality.
- Areolar size and shape.
- Degree of ptosis.
- Measurements: sternal notch to NAC, NAC to IMF.

The basic aims are similar to breast reduction i.e. to produce a pleasing breast shape whilst ensuring reliable NAC transposition and optimization of the scar. However, many different techniques have been described in the literature, which usually suggests the absence of a single ideal technique for mastopexy.

Mastopexy preferences: a survey of board-certified plastic surgeons
Rohrich RJ. *Plast Reconstr Surg* 2006;**118**:1631–1638.

According to this survey with 487 responses, the traditional inverted-T scar technique is the most popular technique. Satisfaction was highest with short-scar techniques e.g. short-scar periareolar inferior pedicle reduction (SPAIR by Hammond) and Hall-Findlay techniques but physician satisfaction was lowest with periareolar techniques with a higher rate of revision surgery. The three most common complications were suture splitting, excess scarring and bottoming-out (inverted T).

Basic techniques

- **Periareolar** - this is suited for mild to moderate ptosis. At its simplest, it is a simple periareolar incision with concentric de-epithelialization and closure (Bartels RJ. *Plast Reconstr Surg* 1976;**57**:687) but this tends to enlarge and flatten the areola/breast when used too aggressively. Many other variants involve parenchymal reshaping whilst permanent purse-string sutures have reduced areolar/scar widening. Contraindications to periareolar mastopexy include sternal notch to NAC distance of more than 24 cm, ptosis grade of 2 or more or implants being removed or downsized.
  - **Benelli round block technique** incorporates parenchymal moulding. The nipple is kept on a superior pedicle whilst the gland is undermined; medial and lateral parenchymal flaps are coned. The periareolar incision is closed with nylon i.e. permanent suture.
- **Vertical/short scar techniques** – these techniques, based on the vertical scar reduction mammoplasties (especially Lassus and Lejour), are useful for moderately severe forms of ptosis. These techniques, including more recent variations described by Hall-Findlay (1999) and Hammond (1999) have increased in popularity as they tend to incorporate parenchymal rearrangement and do not rely on the skin for long-term support.
  - Graf R. Breast shape: a technique for better upper pole fullness. *Aesth Plast Surg* 2000;**24**:348–352. An inferior dermoglandular flap is tunnelled superiorly under a loop of pectoralis major muscle – this is usually referred to as the **Graf/Biggs flap.**
  - Flowers RS. 'Flip-flap' mastopexy. *Aesth Plast Surg* 1998;**22**:425. The inferior parenchyma is folded under the superior pedicle and sutured to the pectoralis fascia.
  - Hall-Findlay EJ (Pedicles in vertical breast reduction and mastopexy. *Clin Plastic Surg* 2002;**29**:379–391) prefers to use a lateral pedicle for the nipple and a medial pedicle for the inferolateral breast tissue that is mobilized and rotated up as an autoaugmentation. In this paper, the author also emphasizes the point that the pedicle is independent of the skin excision pattern.
- **Inverted T inferior pedicle (ITIP)** – these may be considered in severe ptosis and severe skin excess

but the main criticisms are the scarring and the bottoming-out over the long term. The inferior parenchyma can be repositioned and sutured to the pectoralis fascia to restore some upper pole fullness.

- ○ Foustanos A. A double flap technique. *Plast Reconstr Surg* 2007;**120**:55–60. The authors use a Pitanguy skin pattern (similar to Wise, resulting in an inverted T), the nipple is carried on a superior pedicle (first flap) whilst an inferior pedicle is developed and sutured to the superior chest wall (second flap). This has been likened to a form of 'auto-augmentation'; something similar was described by Honig JF. *Aesth Plast Surg* 2009;**33**:302–307.

Overall, the complications are similar to breast reduction.

Augmentation is useful in ptosis as it restores breast volume. It can be an alternative to, or most often combined with, mastopexy; skin excision will be required for more severe degrees of ptosis in the low-volume breast with the implant filling out the remaining volume. The implant can be placed either subglandularly or submuscularly or dual plane.

Augmentation mastopexy is the most frequently litigated operation in plastic surgery in the USA. Although augmentation mastopexy can be performed in a single stage (and is a hot topic in conferences), many would suggest a two-stage procedure with the mastopexy first, particularly when > 3 cm of nipple elevation is needed. When performed together, it is preferable to only mark the new nipple position tentatively and to confirm the position after the implants are in place and the skin is tailor-tacked with the patient sitting up.

Key points in mastopexy
De Benito J. *Aesth Plast Surg* Published Online: 25 May 2010 doi: 10.1007/s00266-010-9527-5.

This article presents the authors' experiences with implants for mastopexy. They prefer **anatomical implants** because when the implant is placed 60% below the NAC, the NAC tends to move up whilst a round implant would tend to move the NAC down. Silicone gel implants have less tendency to expand or atrophy the lower pole than saline implants (Tebbetts JB. *Clin Plast Surg* 2001;**28**:501–521). The authors prefer to use a subpectoral or subfascial plane.

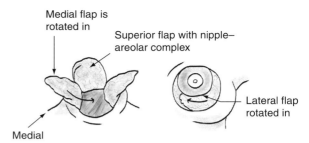

Figure 5.5 Benelli mastopexy. The nipple–areolar complex is supported by a superior flap; medial and lateral glandular flaps are developed. The medial flap is rotated in under the superior flap and sutured in; the lateral flap is rotated medially over the medial flap. The nipple–areolar complex is sutured in with a round-block permanent purse-string suture.

Augmentation/mastopexy: 'surgeon beware'
Spear SL. *Plast Reconstr Surg* 2003;**112**:905–906.

The author explains his viewpoint on combining augmentation with mastopexy. He states that individually they are simple procedures with relatively few complications, however, in combination they increase the likelihood of complications of the other. Where a mastopexy tends to reshape the breast and reduce the skin, an augmentation enlarges the breast volume and expands the skin, setting up a set of competing factors that may lead to insufficient soft tissue cover, with the implant also creating tension and reduced vascularity.

- There is an increased risk of infection and implant exposure due to the overlying soft tissue rearrangement.
- There is an increased risk of loss of nipple sensation or malposition as the mastopexy after augmentation will reposition the breast.

Conservative augmentation with periareolar mastopexy reduces complications and treats a variety of breast types
Cannon CL. *Ann Plast Surg* 2010;**64**:516–521.

This paper emphasizes the combination of a small/moderate implant and a periareolar mastopexy to reduce the incidence of complications. The authors suggest that favourable factors are implants 360 ml or less, flaccid empty breasts, nipple elevation 4 cm or less, light skin tones and absence of stretch marks.

See also breast contouring with explantation in 'Breast augmentation'.

V. Gynaecomastia

Gynaecomastia is abnormal breast development in the male that can be due to a wide variety of causes. It has an incidence of 32–65% in the male population. Very rarely, male breast cancer may masquerade as gynaecomastia; an eccentric mass should raise suspicions.

Aetiology

The aetiology is multifactorial but in many cases, a clear identifiable cause is missing.

Physiological

- Neonatal (up to 60%), pubertal and senile (up to 60%) gynaecomastia that may be due to some androgen–oestrogen imbalance.
- It affects up to 75% of pubertal males – 75% resolve within 2 years. It is possibly due to increased androgen to oestrogen conversion in the tissues.
- In the elderly, it may be due to testicular failure, increased fat levels/aromatase activity.

Pathological

- Systemic disease.
  - Liver disease (e.g. cirrhosis) and hyperthyroidism increases serum hormone binding globulin (decreases free androgens).
  - Renal disease increases luteinizing hormone (LH) and oestrogens.
  - General debility that interferes with pituitary–hypothalamic axis, e.g. burns.
- Hormone-producing tumours.
  - Seminomas, teratomas, choriocarcinomas of testis that produce human chorionic gonadotrophin (HCG).
  - Leydig, Sertoli and granulosa theca cell of testis producing oestrogen.
  - Lung, liver, kidney tumours producing gonadotrophin releasing hormone (GRH).
- Hypogonadism/testicular failure.
  - Pituitary disorders (decreased GRH).
  - Androgen insensitivity syndrome (5-α-reductase deficiency).
  - Klinefelter's syndrome, also have 20–60× increased risk of breast cancer.

Pharmacological

- Spironolactone, cimetidine (block androgen action), digoxin, metoclopramide, tricyclics, methyldopa, marijuana, steroids (adrenal suppression).
- Drugs used in the treatment of prostate cancer.
  - Luteinizing hormone releasing hormone (LHRH) analogues (e.g. Zoladex used in the treatment of prostate cancer) increases testosterone then decreases it due to negative feedback.
  - Anti-androgens (cyproterone acetate) and oestrogens (stilboestrol).

Assessment

History

- Age of onset and rate of growth.
- Psychological effects.
- Symptoms such as pain or nipple discharge.
- General state of health and drug history.
- Family history – familial forms have been described.

Examination should include examination of thyroid, abdomen (liver, kidneys) and genitalia/testes.

- Testicular asymmetry may be due to tumours (steroid producing or paraneoplastic HCG); 5% of testicular tumours present with gynaecomastia.
- Small testes may be associated with Klinefelter's syndrome (also have low testosterone).

Investigations

Routine tests are usually not required.

Extensive work-up is rarely indicated but in certain groups, selected investigations may be useful e.g. **prepubertal** gynaecomastia – testicular examination/ultrasound may yield a significant number of functional endocrine tumours; other clues include – small testicles, decreased libido/fertility, lack of male hair or eunuchoid body. Other significant features include tenderness, rapid enlargement, eccentric hard/irregular mass or lesion > 4 cm in diameter.

- Liver function test.
- Hormone screen.
  - Serum testosterone, LH/follicle-stimulating hormone (FSH) for hypogonadism.
  - HCG, oestradiol (consider CT to exclude adrenal tumour – increased substrate for oestrogen production by peripheral aromatase) and dehydroepiandrosterone (DHEA).
- Chest X-ray (CXR).
- Investigations directed towards possible aetiological factors.

- Karyotype considered if low testosterone, features of feminization with Marfanoid characteristics (to exclude Klinefelter's).

Clinical classification

Simon BE. *Plast Reconstr Surg* 1973;**51**:48–52.

- Grade I – Subareolar 'button'.
- Grade II.
  - a – Moderate enlargement, no skin excess.
  - b – Moderate enlargement with extra skin.
- Grade III – Marked enlargement with extra skin.

A new classification system based on the amount and character of breast hypertrophy and the degree of ptosis was proposed by Rohrich RJ (2003, vide infra).

- Grade I: minimal hypertrophy (< 250 g of breast tissue) without ptosis.
  - IA primarily glandular.
  - IB primarily fibrous.
- Grade II: moderate hypertrophy (between 250 and 500 g of breast tissue) without ptosis.
  - IIA primarily glandular.
  - IIB primarily fibrous.
- Grade III: moderate–severe hypertrophy (> 500 g of breast tissue) and grade I ptosis.
- Grade IV: severe hypertrophy (> 500 g of breast tissue) and grade II/III ptosis.

Cordova classification

Cordova A. *J Plast Reconstr Aesthet Surg* 2008;**61**:41–49.

- Grade I – swelling limited to areolar region, no IMF. Adenectomy via semicircular periareolar incision.
- Grade II – NAC above IMF. Suction or ultrasound-assisted liposuction (UAL) with skin-sparing adenectomy.
- Grade III – NAC at same height or less than 1 cm below IMF. Liposuction followed by periareolar skin removal. Scar wrinkling usually improves spontaneously.
- Grade IV – NAC more than 1 cm below IMF. Breast reduction with nipple repositioning usually a central pedicle.

Histological classification

There are three histological patterns with varying degrees of stromal and ductal proliferation:

- Florid pattern: increased numbers of budding ducts in a highly cellular fibroblastic stroma.

This pattern is more common in the first 4 months.
- Intermediate type: overlapping of the fibrous and florid histological patterns.
- Fibrous type: extensive stromal fibrosis with minimal ductal proliferation. Hypertrophic breast tissue becomes irreversibly fibrotic after about 12 months.

A systematic approach to surgical treatment of gynaecomastia

Fruhstorfer BH. *Br J Plast Surg* 2003;**56**:237–246.

This is a retrospective review of a single surgeon's experience with 48 breasts with gynaecomastia. Medical management has had limited success but is more effective when used during the active proliferative phase:

- Danazol, tamoxifen, clomiphene, testolactone.

Surgical treatment:

It is generally reserved for failed medical management and long-standing gynaecomastia:

- Liposuction/UAL alone or in combination with other techniques. The threshold for conversion to an open excision should be low e.g. elasticity of skin poor, according to the authors.
- Inferior semicircular areolar incision, taking care to leave 1 cm thickness in the subareolar region.
- Lejour type vertical short-scar type technique was used in a few patients.

Management

Non-surgical

- Correction of underlying causes.
- Pharmacological treatment of hormonal imbalances.
- Medication (see above). Danazol has a 60% intermediate response rate, 25% with moderate response. Tamoxifen is useful to reduce pain but seems less useful in reducing the size.

Surgical treatment

Classically, surgery for gynaecomastia depends on the grade as follows:

- Grade I – circumareolar incision, excise 'button'.
- Grade II.
  - A – Liposuction alone or in combination with excision of a disc of breast tissue via a circumareolar incision.

- B – Excision of skin using doughnut mastopexy technique, bevelled excision of breast disc and liposuction to feather the edges.
- Grade III – breast reduction. A wide range of techniques has been described and no single technique is suitable for all.
  - Inferior pedicle markings.
  - Circumareolar concentric skin reduction with subcutaneous mastectomy has been used to treat severe gynaecomastia successfully (Tashkandi M. *Ann Plast Surg* 2004;**53**:17–20) though the authors suggest free nipple grafting in some cases due to massive weight loss or tuberose breasts.
  - Horizontal skin ellipse with nipple–areolar vertical bipedicle leaving transverse scar.

Post-operative drains and compressive dressings are commonly used.

Currently, excisional techniques tend to be reserved for severe gynaecomastia with significant skin excess **after** attempted UAL.

- Suction-assisted lipectomy grade IA and grade IIA.
- **Ultrasound-assisted liposuction** is effective in **all** grades of gynaecomastia. If removal of redundant skin and/or resistant lipodystrophy is still required after UAL, excision can be delayed for 6 to 9 months to allow for maximal skin retraction and healing.

Classification and management of gynecomastia: defining the role of ultrasound-assisted liposuction Rohrich RJ. *Plast Reconstr Surg* 2003;**111**:909–923.

As surgical therapy may leave large, visible scars, UAL has emerged as a safe and effective method for the treatment of gynaecomastia with reduced external scarring.

In UAL, piezoelectric crystals placed on the ends of suction cannulae produce ultrasonic energy that emulsifies fat through cavitation whilst preserving adjacent nervous, vascular and connective tissue elements, i.e. it is selective. With higher energies, it can remove denser, fibrotic parenchymal tissue such as in gynaecomastia more efficiently than conventional liposuction. In addition, subdermal plane UAL may promote useful post-operative skin retraction.

- Subcutaneous infiltration of a wetting/tumescent solution.
- Tunnelling with UAL probe.
- Releasing the inframammary fold is important.

- Evacuation and final contouring by conventional suction-assisted lipectomy.
- The endpoints for UAL (time and loss of resistance) differ from those for standard suction-assisted lipectomy (pinch and contour).

This review of 61 patients demonstrated that UAL is effective in treating most grades of gynaecomastia and is better than conventional liposuction in addressing dense, fibrous lipodystrophy. Excision is used for skin excess after liposuction.

Some surgeons e.g. Mladick RA in his discussion of the article above, prefer to address skin excess in the same operation rather than wait for retraction. See also Vibration Amplification of Sound Energy at Resonance or VASER (a modified form of UAL).

Complications

Early:

- Haematoma.
- Infection.

Late:

- Dish-deformity and having nipple stuck to chest wall.
- Inadequate correction of gland volume or skin excess.
- Problem scarring.

C. Breast reconstruction

I. Breast cancer and screening

Epidemiology

The lifetime risk of developing breast cancer is estimated to be 12%, or one in eight (ACS data) with a median age at diagnosis of approximately 60.

About 30 000 new cases of breast cancer are diagnosed annually in the UK and half of those in the < 65-year age group require mastectomy, making around 7500 breast reconstructions per year in the UK.

Breast cancer genes

- **BRCA1 and BRCA2** genes for breast cancer (mutated tumour suppressor genes) account for 2–3% of breast-cancer cases; there are other as yet unidentified genes that may also contribute to the risk. When more than four cases of breast cancer at < 60 years of age occur within one family, there is likely to be a genetic cause; with 2–3 cases per family, it is more likely to be due to chance only.

- ○ Carriers of these genes (0.1% of women with either) are likely to develop breast cancer before 50 years of age/from age 25 onwards and have a lifetime risk of ~85%. These patients may elect to undergo subcutaneous mastectomy and reconstruction. 50% of BRCA1 carriers treated by lumpectomy and radiotherapy recur or develop a second cancer in the same breast.
- 25% of women who develop breast cancer before age 42 have a definable hereditary component.
- Tamoxifen has been shown to decrease the risk of breast cancer among BRCA1/2 mutation carriers by 50–62%.

Other factors

- Women with increased body mass index tend to have more fatty tissue and elevated peripheral oestrogen. This is associated with increased breast-cancer risk in post-menopausal (though *not pre-menopausal*) women.
- Prophylactic mastectomy is shown to decrease cancer risk by 90–100%.
- Bilateral oophorectomy before menopause reduces risk by 25–53%.
- Women screened annually by mammography have a low risk of breast cancer-related mortality, and screening remains a reasonable option for high-risk women.

Screening

Identifies approximately six cancers for every 1000 women screened.

- The pre-menopausal breast is dense and difficult to screen by mammography – hence screening is not currently offered to those < 50 years of age in the UK (it is offered every 3 years after 50 years), although some studies have indicated that this may be worthwhile and an extension for ages 47–73 is being phased in, starting in 2010 to be complete in 2012. The ACS recommends a baseline screen at 35 years, with annual screens from 40 years old onwards; those with high-risk factors should begin at 25 years of age, or 5–10 years before the age of onset in a relative with breast cancer.
  - ○ Duffy SW. *J Med Screen* 2010;**17**:25–30. The benefit of mammographic screening in terms of lives saved is greater than the harm in terms

of over-diagnosis; 2–2.5 lives are saved for every over-diagnosed case.

- ○ BRCA1-related tumours tend to be cellular rather than scirrhous, with less microcalcification and more difficult to differentiate from benign lesions on mammography, particularly in the typically younger patients.
- ○ Magnetic resonance imaging is a sensitive investigation in the premenopausal breast. A Canadian study (Warner E. *JAMA* 2004;**292**:1317–1325) demonstrated a clear superiority over mammography or ultrasound in BRCA patients though still not as good as all three modalities combined (detected 95%). A follow-up study (Bigenwald RZ. *Cancer Epidemiol Biomarkers Prev* 2008;**17**:706–711) demonstrated that MRI was still far better than mammography for older BRCA patients with less dense breasts.
- Ultrasound is good for differentiating between solid and cystic lesions and for guiding biopsies. High-resolution ultrasound can pick up some cancers and can be used to monitor tumour response to chemotherapy or radiotherapy.

Examination

- Oncological examination – site, size, chest wall fixation, skin involvement, nodes and thorough examination of the contralateral breast (breast volume, shape and ptosis).
- Donor sites e.g. abdominal/back scars, rectus diastasis, skin and soft tissue laxity.

Pathology

- 75% of breast tumours are invasive ductal carcinomas – ductal carcinoma *in situ* (DCIS) presents as microcalcification on mammograms.
- 5% invasive lobular carcinomas – lobular carcinoma *in situ* (LCIS) has no mammographic changes and is a 'coincidental' finding on biopsy; it is a marker of invasive disease rather than a precursor and tumours in such cases have the tendency to bilaterality (40%) and multifocality (60%).
- Special types generally have a better prognosis:
  - ○ Medullary (numerous lymphocytes) < 5%.
  - ○ Mucinous (bulky mucin-forming tumours) < 5%.
  - ○ Tubular (well-differentiated adenocarcinoma).

○ Phyllodes (mixed connective tissue and epithelial tumour, fern-like cellular pattern).

Staging

TNM classification – main landmarks (approximate 5-year survival %)

- Stage I – tumour < 2 cm confined to the breast (T1) (85%).
- Stage II – mobile axillary nodes (N1) (65%).
- Stage IIIa – fixed axillary nodes (N2) (40%).
- Stage IIIb – chest wall or skin involvement (T4) 25%.
- Stage IIIb – internal mammary nodes (N3).
- Stage IV – distant metastases (M1) (10%).

Tumour

- Tis – Carcinoma *in situ* or Paget's disease of the nipple with no associated tumour.
- T1 – ≤ 2 cm.
- T2 – 2–5 cm.
- T3 – > 5 cm.
- T4 – extension to chest wall or skin.

Lymph nodes

- N0 – no regional lymph node metastasis.
- N1 – mobile ipsilateral axillary lymph nodes.
- N2a – fixed ipsilateral axillary nodes.
- N2b – internal mammary nodes without evidence of axillary nodes.
- N3a – axillary and infraclavicular nodes.
- N3b – axillary and internal mammary nodes.
- N3c – supraclavicular lymph node.

Metastasis

- M0 – no distant metastasis.
- M1 – distant metastasis.

II. Mastectomy and adjuvant therapy

Tumour excision

Modified radical mastectomy (includes in-continuity axillary clearance but leaves pectoralis major) may be incorporated into a breast-reduction type marking with contralateral surgery for symmetry. Large tumours may require neo-adjuvant cyclophospha-mide, methotrexate and 5-fluorouracil (CMF) chemo-therapy, mastectomy, node clearance and adjuvant radiotherapy.

- Skin-sparing mastectomy for extensive DCIS, no node surgery/radiotherapy traditionally.

- Breast conservation surgery (BCS).
  ○ Small lump – lumpectomy + radiotherapy + node sampling or clearance, adjuvant radiotherapy.
  ○ Quadrantectomy may be treated by circumareolar-orientated mobilization of the breast mound and direct closure of the overlying skin. 'Mirror' surgery to achieve symmetry.
  ○ Thoraco-epigastric flaps (based on the superior superficial epigastric vessels) may be used for skin following lower quadrant resection whilst axillary tail transposition flap can be used for the upper outer quadrant. Inverted T breast reduction may be an option.

All patients receive tamoxifen generally.

Neo-adjuvant therapy

- Neo-adjuvant chemotherapy treats systemic disease and downstages tumour size, which may increase the chances of breast-conserving surgery. There is a significant morbidity rate associated with chemotherapy. The overall response rate to neo-adjuvant chemotherapy is about 80% with complete response in 30%, but there is no evidence of a survival advantage.
- Radiotherapy is usually used post-operatively (it has unpredictable effects on reconstructions and usually precludes use of expander implants) but neo-adjuvant radiotherapy may also be used, with the exception when local tissues are required for flap closure.

Angiosarcoma of the breast is an uncommon **complication of radiotherapy**.

Angiosarcoma of the breast

Georgiannos SN. *Br J Plast Surg* 2003;**56**:129–134.

Sarcomas account for less than 1% of all breast cancers. This article reports four cases; half were young (20 and 35 years of age, primary angiosarcoma) and the other two were older (45 and 64 years, secondary angiosarcoma) who had received radiotherapy for breast cancer. All patients were ultimately treated by mastectomy after biopsy and all were alive and disease free (3–7 years post-mastectomy). Prognosis is generally related to histological grade and excision margins; with high-grade tumours, the median disease-free survival is 15 months.

Angiosarcoma of the breast: a review of 70 cases

Hodgson NC. *Am J Clin Oncol* 2007;**30**:570–573.

Although angiosarcoma is a very rare complication of breast irradiation, it is being reported in increased numbers with the increase in BCS with irradiation after surgery. These 'secondary' types of breast angiosarcomas tend to present with more advanced disease and in an older age group.

Wide local resection may be curative; the most common site of recurrence is the contralateral breast, possibly due to lymphatic spread.

Skin-sparing mastectomy

Toth B. Modified skin incisions for mastectomy. *Plast Reconstr Surg* 1991;**87**:1048–1053.

Kroll SS. The oncologic risks of skin preservation at mastectomy when combined with immediate reconstruction of the breast. *Surg Gynecol Obstet* 1991;**172**:17–20.

Slavin SA. Skin-sparing mastectomy and immediate reconstruction. *Plast Reconstr Surg* 1998;**102**:49–62.

A skin-sparing mastectomy (SSM) removes breast, nipple–areolar complex and biopsy scar and it aims to produce a superior aesthetic result because it:

- Preserves native breast skin except for skin close to a superficial tumour.
- Preserves inframammary fold.

Classification of SSM

(Carlson GW. Skin sparing mastectomy, oncologic and reconstructive considerations. *Ann Surg* 1997;**225**:570–578.)

- Type 1 – nipple/areolar complex only (prophylactic).
- Type 2 – nipple/areolar complex + separate scar excision.
- Type 3 – nipple/areolar complex + in-continuity scar excision.
- Type 4 – nipple/areolar complex within a breast reduction (large breast, unsuitable for transverse rectus abdominis muscle (TRAM) flap and contralateral reduction planned).

A separate incision may also be needed for axillary sampling/clearance (some choose to use the same incision whilst others prefer to use a separate incision) and/or microsurgery.

Most agree that SSM seems to be a **safe treatment** for invasive cancer without compromising local control

and it has become a popular choice in early stage breast cancer where the risk of skin involvement is low. In the end, **all** forms of mastectomy leave behind **some** breast tissue and the local recurrence rate is related more to the **stage** of disease and tumour biology rather than the type of surgery. The flaps should be the same thickness as a standard mastectomy; the risk of residual tumour in the skin flaps increases when the flaps are thicker than 5 mm (Torresan RZ. *Ann Surg Oncol* 2005;**12**:1037–1044). Skin flap necrosis is a recognized complication of SSM (11%) though it does not seem to be much higher than for other types of mastectomy and can be minimized with careful patient selection (avoid smokers, diabetics, obese patients and avoiding unusually thin flaps that do not have much effect on the regional recurrence rate but do increase the rate of necrosis).

Common indications include:

- Prophylactic mastectomy.
- Stage 1 and 2 invasive breast cancer – BCS with radiotherapy is adequate treatment for these tumours and is being used more frequently.
- DCIS – this is one situation where SSM can be used and BCS is less suited.
- Multicentric tumours.
- Phyllodes tumour.
- Where immediate reconstruction is planned.

Radiotherapy is not a contraindication per se but will affect the final cosmetic outcome. The oncological risks of preserving the NAC seem to have been over-estimated in the past (Simmons RM. *Ann Plast Surg* 2003;**51**:547–551) and it may be safe as long as the tumour is not close to the nipple and frozen section assessment of the subareolar tissue is performed. A variation on this is to remove the nipple but preserve the areolar (areolar-sparing mastectomy, ASM).

The average time to local recurrence is ~2–4 years; most recurrences occur in the skin but histological examination rarely demonstrates identifiable breast tissue. Local recurrence is a marker for disseminated disease and all patients with local recurrence after total mastectomy eventually die of metastatic disease.

III. Breast reconstructive surgery

Once it had been demonstrated that immediate reconstruction of the breast was oncologically safe, it became a preferred option as the results are usually more aesthetic, it involves less psychological trauma and is cheaper than delayed reconstruction (which may be considered for inflammatory carcinomas). Adjuvant therapy is not affected by (immediate) reconstruction but adjuvant treatment may affect the quality of reconstruction – most often there is a variable volume loss. With delayed reconstruction, there is a loss of the native skin envelope, a new IMF is required, surgery involves exploration/dissection of previously operated/irradiated tissues and overall, the outcome is less aesthetic.

It is important to appreciate that breast reconstruction is a process, often involving a number of procedures, rather than a one-off operation and this needs to be clearly conveyed to patients. In addition, the contralateral breast is a major influence in the selection of the reconstruction technique e.g. for simple asymmetry after a lumpectomy, a contralateral breast reduction can be considered. Thus reconstruction can either be:

- Designed to match the contralateral breast, or
- Contralateral breast can be modified to match the reconstruction.

Reconstruction is largely dictated by the size of the contralateral breast and availability of autologous tissue.

Reconstruction of a small breast

- **Expander implants** e.g. Becker prosthesis, expandable anatomically shaped implants (see below) or expander then implant. These are useful for small/medium breast reconstruction where the patient does not accept additional scars. The implant is placed in a subpectoral pocket (which should not be made too high i.e. slightly low for smooth implants but at the correct level for textured expander implants) and slowly inflated; over-inflation 20–30% and then leaving for 3–6 months, allows some ptosis when replaced by an appropriately size implant (or by removal of some of the injected fluid).
  - ○ Capsulotomy at time of implant placement if a troublesome capsule has developed.
  - ○ Use of expander implants does not affect chemotherapy (wait 4 weeks for healing) or radiotherapy (timing or dose). Radiotherapy is given to ~20–30% of patients after mastectomy and increases the chance of capsular contracture; **half of patients with expanders treated with irradiation will need later flap salvage.**
    - ○ Use of expanders is contraindicated in the previously irradiated, or those with poor tissue quality including infection/inflammation, necrosis or tumour.
- Latissimus dorsi with implant (contralateral implant to balance size if needed).

Reconstruction of a moderate-sized breast

- Becker prosthesis or expander then implant.
- Latissimus dorsi and implant.
- Pedicled TRAM (Hartrampf) or free TRAM.
  - ○ Contralateral pedicle is generally preferred as the ipsilateral pedicle usually involves a more acute angle and may compromise venous flow, but either is possible.
- Free deep inferior epigastric perforator (DIEP) flap where only zones 1 and 2 are needed.

Reconstruction of the large breast

- Bipedicled TRAM. The donor defect is significant but it can still be used in patients with a midline scar.
- Free TRAM utilizing zones 1–3/4.
  - ○ Anastomosing end–end to the circumflex scapular vessels saves latissimus dorsi as a lifeboat.
  - ○ Anastomosing end–end to the thoracodorsal artery proximal to the serratus branch also preserves latissimus dorsi (retrograde flow from intercostal supply to serratus).
- Bipedicled DIEP.

If these are unsuitable then a contralateral breast reduction can be considered.

Reconstruction of bilateral breasts

- Bilateral pedicled TRAM flaps.
- Bilateral free TRAM/DIEP flaps.
- Bilateral latissimus dorsi and implants.

Autologous flaps for breast reconstruction

Studies have demonstrated that the long-term cost of implants is greater than for reconstruction by autologous tissue. Smoking should be stopped preoperatively: nicotine causes vasoconstriction and reduced blood flow but there is no increase in microvascular loss, carbon monoxide reduces carbon dioxide and there is also increased platelet adhesion.

Partial mastectomy

- Local rearrangement of tissues for defects up to a quarter the size of the breast. Implants tend to make the deformity worse.
- Larger and more medial defects are best treated with total MRM and autologous reconstruction in the conventional manner.

Latissimus dorsi reconstruction

Although the latissimus dorsi flap is reliable, it has traditionally been regarded as being too small to reconstruct anything other than small breasts, thus usually combined with an implant. However the size of a latissimus dorsi reconstruction can be maximized by:

- Fleur-de-lis skin paddle – but poor scar is often criticized.
- Extended latissimus dorsi – taking more fat along with the muscle.
- Orientating the skin paddle perpendicular to the pedicle axis.

The pedicle can be lengthened by:

- Dividing the tendon – the anterior fold can be reconstructed by reattaching the tendon.
- Dividing the serratus anterior branch.
- Dividing cutaneous branches to the chest wall.

In addition, the scar/seroma problems, along with the need for changing patient position, limit its use. There is no consensus currently regarding the necessity to divide the motor nerve to reduce involuntary movements, whilst preserving it may help maintain bulk; many choose to keep the nerve and divide it later if necessary later on.

TRAM reconstruction

For a unilateral breast reconstruction, the procedure of choice is usually a free flap; if the reconstruction is delayed, the internal mammary arteries are often the best choice as recipient vessels.

- TRAM flaps have a fat necrosis rate of 7–16%; zone 4 should be discarded.
- Gynaecological Pfannenstiel incisions do not usually compromise the flap as the recti are spread apart but a general surgical Pfannenstiel approach usually cuts the muscle.
- The rectus is responsible for the first 30° of flexion. The incidence of post-operative bulges is about 5–20% with hernias in 1–2%. Despite this, most are asymptomatic (though objective testing will reveal measurable weakness) except for athletes/labourers, those with pre-existing lower back pain and those with bilateral harvest. Use of a mesh if required for donor site repair does not interfere with subsequent pregnancy. The trend is to use the mesh in the retromuscular position when appropriate, where the abdominal pressures hold it against the deep surface of the muscle.

Bilateral pedicled TRAM reconstruction for bilateral mastectomy is quicker and less complicated than bilateral free TRAMs, and can also be used in the presence of a midline scar.

A call for clarity in TRAM/DIEP zones

Henry SL. *Plast Reconstr Surg* 2010;**125**:210–211e.

Zone 1 is the zone overlying the pedicle and zone 4 is the contralateral lateral zone but there is confusion over the nomenclature of zones 2 and 3 of the TRAM/DIEP flap. Initially Scheflan (1983) described the contralateral medial as zone 2 but it became clear that if one was considering the perfusion, then it was incorrect. A new scheme was proposed using Roman numerals with the contralateral medial now zone III whilst the ipsilateral lateral was zone II; this is sometimes referred to as Hartrampf zones.

Holm C. (*Plast Reconstr Surg* 2006;**117**:37–43) performed a perfusion study with indocyanine green that confirmed the Roman numeral scheme but did prompt several suggestions on renaming for 'clarity' including combining II and III as 'II' making IV now 'III'.

The authors suggest a descriptive classification – contralateral as C, medial as M and lateral as L, thus the zones would be CL, CM, IM and IL with IM as zone I etc, which seems clear and sensible enough.

TRAM flap vascular delay for high-risk breast reconstruction

Codner MA. *Plast Reconstr Surg* 1995;**96**:1615–1622.

The authors suggest that a delay procedure may be indicated for 'high risk' patients undergoing breast reconstruction with pedicled TRAMs i.e. obesity, smokers, radiation and abdominal scars (4.3% fat necrosis rate in their experience). It can be performed either open or endoscopically, 2 weeks before the definitive flap procedure. They measured blood pressure in the proximal deep inferior epigastric artery after flap transfer ('flap perfusion pressure') and it was increased from 13.3 mmHg to 40.3 mmHg.

TRAM flaps in patients with abdominal scars
Takeishi M. *Plast Reconstr Surg* 1997;**99**:713–722.

The authors present their experience with 46 TRAM breast-reconstruction patients who had pre-existing abdominal scars. Free TRAM flaps were preferred and performed wherever possible; vessel exploration was an important part of the assessment process.

- Patients with low transverse scars (Pfannenstiel) were explored and if the deep inferior epigastric artery (DIEA) flap was not intact then an ipsilateral pedicled TRAM flap or free contralateral TRAM flap was raised.
- In all patients with lower paramedian scars the vessels had been divided.
- In patients with lower midline scars, the flap was designed higher up on the abdomen so that 5–7 cm of unscarred skin formed a bridge above the umbilicus. This leaves a high, mid-abdominal, transverse scar.
- Subcostal incisions usually meant that an ipsilateral flap had to be a free flap due to possibility of division of the superior pedicle.
- Appendectomy scars do not compromise the TRAM flap.

Deep inferior epigastric perforator flap
The DIEP flap was first described by Allen in 1994 on the basis that harvesting of the muscle leads to a significant donor morbidity. Some 10–20% of patients do not return to their job/hobbies after a TRAM.

- The recti are responsible for initiating the first 35–40° of abdominal flexion and are also responsible for raising the intra-abdominal pressure.
- Sacrificing the rectus abdominis also adversely affects the function of the internal obliques as they need resistance against which to contract and this leads to a decrease in rotational strength.
- The pedicle is 7.5 cm long on average, artery and vein are 3.5 and 4 mm in diameter respectively.

When raising a DIEP flap, it is important to **preserve the segmental nerves** to keep the recti innervated, otherwise there is no point in preserving the muscle. It should be appreciated that what different surgeons report as a DIEP may involve very different levels of muscle damage and denervation, making controlled comparisons with TRAM (muscle-sparing or otherwise) difficult.

One hundred free DIEP flap breast reconstructions
Blondeel PN. *Br J Plast Surg* 1999;**52**:104–111.

The main advantage of the DIEP, according to the author, is that abdominal flexion and rotation strength is maintained when compared with TRAM.

- An **ipsilateral** flap is required if anastomosing to the internal mammary vessels.
- A **contralateral** flap is required if anastomosing to the thoracodorsal vessels.

Pre-operative duplex Doppler can be used to define perforators and create a 'road map'; the vessels at tendinous intersections are usually larger. Raising the pedicle side first, preserves the other side as a lifeboat. In this series, the majority of flaps were isolated on **one or two** perforators (more than half used only one perforator) which came from the lateral branch of the DIEA in 50% (medial and lateral branches equally dominant in 15%).

- Zone 3 may need to be discarded if the flap is nourished predominantly by lateral perforators.
- It is not necessary to dissect back to the external iliac artery as the pedicle is long enough to be divided at the lateral border of the rectus abdominis muscle (if the internal mammary vessels are used).

When raising bilateral flaps, it is advisable to dissect out the distal perforators first – if these are damaged, the flap can still be raised as a pedicled TRAM.

A 10-year retrospective review of 758 DIEP flaps for breast reconstruction
Gill PS. *Plast Reconstr Surg* 2004;**113**:1153–1160.

This is a review of 758 DIEP flaps for breast reconstruction. It demonstrated complication rates comparable to those quoted in retrospective reviews of pedicled and free TRAM flaps. Breast or abdominal complications had a significant association with smoking, hypertension and post-operative radiotherapy.

- 0.5% total flap loss, 2.5% partial flap loss and 12.9% developed fat necrosis which **increased with the number of perforators**.
- 5.9% returned to the operating theatre, 3.8% because of venous congestion (which was unrelated to the number of venous anastomoses e.g. contralateral superficial inferior epigastric vein (SIEV)).

- Post-operative abdominal hernia or bulge occurred in only five reconstructions (0.7%).

Some literature suggests that the difference in abdominal wall morbidity between DIEP and muscle-sparing TRAM flaps may not be that great (Nahabedian MY. *Plast Reconstr Surg* 2005;**115**:436–444; Bajack AK. *Plast Reconstr Surg* 2006;**117**:737–746). In part this may be due to the intramuscular dissection required for DIEP perforators particularly when they do not line up vertically along the muscle, as well as improvement in muscle-sparing TRAM (msTRAM) techniques.

One hundred fascia-sparing myocutaneous rectus abdominis flaps: an update
Rufer M. *J Plast Reconstr Aesthet Surg* 2010; online: doi:10,1016/j.bjps.2010.04.051

The authors describe their results with a fascia-sparing technique of TRAM flap harvest – the fascia was incised from perforator to perforator, then double breasted and repaired with two suture lines. The muscle was treated differently for free flaps (left intact lateral to the perforators) and pedicled flaps (all taken). Partial flap loss occured in 13, with two total losses (inferiorly pedicled). There were two early abdominal dehiscences; one patient developed an abdominal bulge (median follow-up 20 months).

The study makes some useful points but does include a heterogeneous population in terms of indications as well as flaps performed (free vs. pedicled which may be superiorly or inferiorly pedicled).

Abdominal wall following free TRAM or DIEP flap reconstruction: a meta-analysis and critical review
Man LX. *Plast Reconstr Surg* 2009;**124**:752–764.

The authors performed a meta-analysis of studies and found that DIEP patients had double the risk of flap necrosis and flap loss, but half the risk of abdominal bulge or hernia. They offer their own algorithm:

- Low-risk patients – if SIEA is greater than 1.5 mm and has a sufficient vein, then SIEA flap is used.
- Others, and those with insufficient SIE vessels.
  - Identify 1–2 large DIEP perforators close to each other for DIEP.
  - Otherwise, use a row of perforators with a small amount of anterior rectus sheath and muscle.

Mesh is usually not required but inlay polypropylene is used where necessary.

A systematic review of abdominal wall function following abdominal flaps for postmastectomy breast reconstruction
Atisha D. *Ann Plast Surg* 2009;**63**:222–230.

The authors analysed 20 studies yielded from a literature search. Objective measures did demonstrate differences:

- Isometric dynamometry – pedicled TRAM patients had up to 23% deficit in trunk flexion vs. 18% in free TRAM; DIEP patients had less flexion deficit than free TRAM patients.
- Physiotherapy measures – pedicled TRAM patients had greatest deficit in rectus and obique muscle function (53%), whilst free TRAM had minimal deficit and DIEP returned to baseline.

However, with the exception of bilateral flaps (pedicled or free TRAM), this did **not** translate to any decrease in their ability to perform ADL.

Fat necrosis in free DIEP flaps
Bozikov K. *Ann Plast Surg* 2009;**63**:138–142.

Fat necrosis is an ischaemic sequela; though it seems to be a minor complication, it can cause concern with follow-up if it cannot be adequately distinguished from tumour recurrence.

The authors examined their experience with 100 consecutive unilateral DIEP flap breast reconstructions and found that single perforator flaps, BMI ≥ 30 and revisional surgery were all significant predictors of subsequent fat necrosis.

They also found that harvesting the lateral row of perforators increased the risk of fat necrosis in the contralateral medial zone whilst harvesting the medial row increased risk in the ipsilateral medial zone.

Superficial inferior epigastric artery flap
The use of the SIEA flap in breast reconstruction was first described by Grotting in 1991 and has the potential to almost completely eliminate donor site morbidity as the fascia and musculature are not disturbed. However, it is not a common choice as the vessels are generally short and small (average 1.6 mm at the inguinal ligament) and not always 'available', being absent or hypoplastic in 35%. It cannot supply tissue across the midline.

- These vessels may have been cut in Pfannenstiel incisions.
- They are cut along with the deep inferior epigastric artery/vein (DIEA/DIEV) when delaying a pedicled TRAM.
- There is an increased seroma rate related to the inguinal dissection.

The SIEA is a direct cutaneous vessel from the common femoral artery 2–3 cm below the inguinal ligament, either by itself (17%) or from a common trunk with the superficial circumflex iliac (48%). It crosses the midpoint of the inguinal ligament deep to Scarpa's fascia, then run towards the umbilicus piercing Scarpa's to lie in the superficial subcutaneous tissue and may anastomose with periumbilical perforating arteries. The SIEA flap is an axial pattern fasciocutaneous flap not a perforator flap.

Breast reconstruction with superficial inferior epigastric artery flaps
Chevray PM. *Plast Reconstr Surg* 2004;**114**:1077–1083.

The author successfully used the SIEA flap in 14 of 47 consecutive cases of breast reconstruction; the remainder (33) were either absent or too small (a limit of 1.5 mm is used to increase reliability). The author prefers using the internal mammary artery to reduce size mismatch. There was one SIEA flap loss due to arterial thrombosis. There was an average 10% of flap volume of fat necrosis.

Other flaps
On average the TRAM (and related) flaps are not available in 25% due to previous surgery or inadequate bulk.

Superior gluteal artery perforator flap
The use of the superior gluteal artery perforator (S-GAP) flap in breast reconstruction was first described by Allen (1995). Advantages include a concealed scar and the stiff fat provides good projection in the reconstructed breast. It avoids the sciatic nerve exposure of an inferior gluteal artery perforator (I-GAP) flap (also need to sacrifice posterior cutaneous nerve of the thigh). However, the learning curve is significant; the skin paddle is relatively small, there is a moderately high risk of developing seroma, haemostasis may be difficult and the patient needs to be repositioned.

The sensate free superior gluteal artery perforator (S-GAP) flap: a valuable alternative in autologous breast reconstructions
Blondeel PN. *Br J Plast Surg* 1999;**52**:185–193.

The authors present experience with 20 free S-GAP flaps vascularized by a single perforator from the superior gluteal artery that is identified pre-operatively by Doppler. The flaps were anastomosed to the internal mammary vessels in the third intercostal space. The author proposes it as a second choice to the DIEP flap when the latter is not available e.g. due to scarring or lack of tissue. Advantages include:

- Large calibre, long vascular pedicle that avoids having to perform the difficult dissection of the (short) superior gluteal pedicle for non-perforator flaps.
- Hidden scar and no functional morbidity at donor site; leaving the muscle behind also avoids exposure of sciatic nerve.
- It can be made sensate by coaption of sensory nerves entering the flap from above (dorsal branches of lumbar segmental nerves) to the fourth intercostal nerve. The authors state that this provides early sensory recovery.

Anatomical study of the superior gluteal artery perforator (S-GAP) for free flap harvesting
Tansatit T. *J Med Assoc Thai* 2008;**91**:1244–1249.

The authors performed 30 cadaveric dissections and found that the perforators tend to be arranged in lines along the upper and lateral free border of the gluteus maximus. They suggest that the '**penetrating pedicle**' is usually found within 3 cm medial to the lateral muscle border, often in a muscle cleavage plane meaning that few muscle fibres need to be sacrificed.

Gracilis flap
This is a type II myocutaneous free flap and the pedicle comes from the ascending branch of the medial circumflex femoral artery (from the profunda femoris artery) that is only 5–6 cm long (thus the internal mammary vessels are usually the preferred site of anastomosis) and 1.6 mm diameter. It enters the proximal third of the muscle 10 cm below the inguinal ligament.

The skin paddle is orientated transversely over the upper part of the muscle in the proximal third of the medial thigh. The maximum width is 10–12 cm and in selected patients provides a moderate amount of tissue for autologous breast reconstruction. The donor-site morbidity is similar to that of a classic medial thigh lift.

It is a valuable alternative for immediate autologous breast reconstruction (Arnez ZM. *Br J Plast Surg* 2004;**57**:20–26) after skin-sparing mastectomy in patients with:

- Small and medium-sized breasts (lack of volume is main disadvantage).
- Inadequate soft-tissue bulk at the lower abdomen and gluteal region.
- Desire for no visible scar at any other donor site e.g. abdominal, back or gluteal.

The transverse myocutaneous gracilis free flap in autologous breast reconstruction
Wechselberger G. *Plast Reconstr Surg* 2004;**114**: 69–73.

Ten patients underwent autologous breast reconstruction with transverse myocutaneous gracilis free flaps **with no free-flap failure and no functional donor-site morbidity.**

Transverse myocutaneous gracilis flap: technical refinements
Fattah A. *J Reconstr Aesthet Surg* 2010;**63**:305–313.

The authors describe their experience with 19 flaps and their improved technique including recruitment of inferior fat and sparing of the long saphenous vein. The flap is usually raised as an ellipse (with the muscle more anteriorly based, and the upper border 1 cm below the actual thigh groin sulcus) that is shaped by suturing the ends together. The most common complication was minor wound dehiscence at the donor site.

Yet other flaps

- **Rubens flap** – this is based on the deep circumflex iliac artery (DCIA) flap and has a long consistent pedicle (5–6 cm long, 2–3 mm artery and 2.5–4 mm vein). However, the abdominal wall muscles must be meticulously repaired and sutured back to the iliac crest. Post-operative pain is common and there may be paraesthesia due to injury to the lateral cutaneous nerve of the thigh.
- **Thoracodorsal artery perforator** (TAP) flap. Compared with the latissimus dorsi there is sparing of the muscle and less risk of seroma, however the size is limited, and the variable

anatomy makes the learning curve moderately steep.
- **Lateral transverse thigh flap** – this uses the TFL muscle based on the lateral circumflex femoral vessels but leaves a significant contour defect and a risk to the femoral nerve.

Recipient vessel lifeboats

- Vein – external jugular, cephalic.
- Artery – thoracodorsal, thoracoacromial and circumflex scapular.

Expandable anatomical implants in breast reconstructions: a prospective study
Mahdi T. *Br J Plast Surg* 1998;**51**:425–430.

In this study, McGhan (style 150) anatomically shaped implants were inserted subpectorally using either

- A muscle-splitting approach through the mastectomy wound for immediate reconstruction.
- An inframammary approach for delayed reconstruction.

The silicone shell of the implant makes up 50% of final volume and the remaining volume in the lower pole mainly comes by expansion that begins 2 weeks post-operatively via a port in the axilla, which is designed to stay in permanently. The authors suggest dissecting at least 1 cm inferior to the inframammary fold to avoid the implant riding high.

Internal mammary vessels: a reliable recipient system for free flaps in breast reconstruction
Ninkovic M. *Br J Plast Surg* 1995;**48**:533–539.

The axilla may be scarred due to surgery or radiotherapy and thoracodorsal vessels may have been disrupted. The internal mammary artery may be used for microanastomosis – it lies 1.5 cm lateral to the lateral border of the sternum; pre-operative Doppler is used to identify their location more exactly. The third or fourth costal cartilage (a 2 cm segment 2.5 cm from the sternal edge) is removed subperichondrially to facilitate recipient vessel dissection in the third–fourth space.

Advantages include:

- A shorter pedicle is needed, and the vessels are a good size match for the DIEP vessels at 1.5 mm.
- Allows for improved positioning of the flap on the chest wall (generally placing the muscle along the

midclavicular line for maximum projection, which usually requires a pedicle of 9–10 cm to reach the thoracodorsal vessels).

- Avoids further dissection of the axilla which may worsen lymphoedema and spares latissimus dorsi as a lifeboat, and avoids use of the axilla that in cases of delayed reconstruction may have post-operative/post-radiotherapy changes. There are fewer shoulder problems overall.
- Zone IV lies lateral rather than medial; > 80% of TRAM flaps were ipsilateral.

Disadvantages include:

- Vessels can be very fragile and magnification is advisable.
- Respiratory movement and depth of vessels making anastomosis difficult.
- Compromises blood supply to sternum if the other internal mammary vessels have been used in cardiac surgery, and removes an option for future bypass grafting.
- Risk of iatrogenic pneumothorax.
- Removal of a segment of cartilage leads to visible contour deformity.

Anatomy of the internal mammary veins and their use in free TRAM flap breast reconstruction
Arnez ZM. *Br J Plast Surg* 1995;**48**:540–545.

This is an anatomical study in 34 fresh human cadavers in which they found different patterns of the internal mammary veins. The most common configuration was (type I) having a vein medial to the artery, dividing at the level of the 4th intercostal space into medial (2.7 mm mean) and lateral (1.8 mm).

Autologous free tissue breast reconstruction using the internal mammary perforators as recipient vessels
Haywood RM. *Br J Plast Surg* 2003;**56**:689–691.

The authors used **perforators** from the internal mammary vessels in the second and third intercostal spaces as recipient vessels for microsurgical breast reconstruction, thus obviating the need to remove costal cartilage to access the main vessels. Their series included DIEP, S-GAP and superficial inferior epigastric perforator (SIEP) flaps used for reconstruction and suitable recipient vessels were found in 21 of 54 cases (39%, using criteria of > 1.5 mm and good flow on release of clamps). There were no flap losses but four patients required re-exploration of anastomoses.

IV. Male breast cancer

Male breast carcinoma constitutes 1% of all breast cancers; the mean age at diagnosis is ~60 years.

- Patients with Klinefelter's syndrome have up to a 60× greater risk of developing breast cancer (incidence 1:400 to 1:1000).
- There is no increased risk for breast cancer in patients with gynaecomastia compared with the normal male population and surgical treatments (liposuction and excision) do not impair detection of male breast cancer.

Carcinoma of the male breast: an underestimated killer
Di Benedetto G. *Plast Reconstr Surg* 1998; **102**: 696–700.

The tumours are hormone dependent and the aetiology often relates to hyperoestrogenic states. The pathological types and relative incidences are the same as for female breast cancer except that invasive lobular cancer is only seen in association with Klinefelter's syndrome. However the tumours tend to be **aggressive** and although the symptoms and signs are similar as for female cancer, the diagnosis is often delayed. There is a higher incidence of positive internal mammary nodes at presentation. Reconstructive options depend on the disease stage at diagnosis; it is almost impossible to close margins after radical or modified radical mastectomy and will need some flap coverage e.g. local thoraco-epigastric fasciocutaneous flap or latissimus dorsi.

Male breast cancer: a review of clinical management
Agrawal A. *Breast Cancer Res Treat* 2007;**103**:11–21.

This is a literature review of a disease that affects about 240 men a year in the UK. The authors identify genetic risk factors such as BRCA2 families and Klinefelter's syndrome, and environmental factors such as radiation. Disease tends to present 10 years later than females as a painless mass that is subareolar in 68–90%.

Adjuvant therapies are similar to disease in women – tamoxifen is the mainstay for metastatic disease in oestrogen receptor-positive tumours; doxorubicin is used in receptor-negative tumours. Relative stage-matched survival does not seem significantly different from women.

Aesthetic subunits of the breast
Spear SL. *Plast Reconstr Surg* 2003;**112**:440–447.

Surgery for breast cancer has traditionally addressed the breast as if it were a geometric circle with associated quadrants. A subunit principle in breast reconstruction planning may significantly improve the appearance of the result by placing scars along natural lines that maximize the advantages of camouflage afforded by body contour and clothing.

The authors suggest that aesthetic lines for scar placement in breast reconstruction should incorporate the aesthetic subunits of the breast that are outlined by tissue, colour, or texture changes such as:

- Breast skin to areola.
- Areola to nipple.
- Breast skin to chest skin at the inframammary fold.
- Anterior axillary line.
- Breast to sternal skin.

The best aesthetic units are usually expanded concentric circles (expanded areolar subunits) around the nipple as the eye is accustomed to viewing a circular areola – the areolar margin is the ideal transition for this subunit in a subcutaneous mastectomy on the breast. Other suggested subunits include the entire breast and the inferior lateral subunits. In general, the advice is to avoid the upper and medial parts of the breast and to avoid 'random' patches.

Routine histological examination of the mastectomy scar at the time of breast reconstruction: important oncological surveillance?
Soldin MG. *Br J Plast Surg* 2004;**57**:143–145.

This is a review of the histology of 48 mastectomy scars in patients who underwent delayed breast reconstruction; there was no evidence of malignancy in any of scars whilst six patients had a local recurrence at the time of presentation for reconstruction (1 was clinically 'occult').

Up to 90% of local recurrence following mastectomy occurs within 3 years and since local recurrence is detectable clinically, routine histological evaluation of the mastectomy scar at the time of reconstruction is unnecessary, especially after 3 years.

This was confirmed by Munir A (Mastectomy scar histopathology of limited clinical value. *Ann Plast Surg* 2006;**57**:374–375) and Woerderman L (Routine histologica examination of 728 mastectomy scars. *Plast Reconstr Surg* 2006;**118**:1288–1292).

V. Nipple reconstruction and inverted nipple correction

Nipple reconstruction

In general, a period of at least 3 months after breast reconstruction is recommended, for the breast mound to achieve its stable shape.

Nipple sharing (tip or inferior part)

Although it is a relatively simple procedure, there are problems including scar distortion, reduced height and sensation of the donor that make it a less popular choice.

Local flaps

Many different flaps have been described and the main challenge is always to achieve longevity of projection and to reduce scarring – one should expect 50% reduction with most techniques. Some propose inserting materials such as cartilage, Alloderm, calcium hydroxyapatite to augment the results.

- **Skate flap:** the designed height is approximately twice the desired nipple height to allow for loss, the lateral wings are raised on a subdermal level whilst the central portion includes a core of fat. Typically a small FTSG is needed, attempting to close with tension will cause flattening. This technique is the most popular for large nipples. The twin flap is a variant of the skate with square flaps and islanded central flap.
- **Star flap:** this is similar in design to the skate flap but is designed with direct closure in mind and thus is more limited in its dimensions. It is a good alternative for small/medium-sized nipples.
- **S flap:** also known as the 'Double opposing tab' flap after Cronin. The flaps are raised on the subdermal level with about 10 mm of fat. Proponents of this technique say that there is less loss of projection.

Many different techniques have been described in the literature: asymmetric side flaps, arrow flaps, square side flaps with circular large flaps and C–V flaps.

Post-operative care

- Support with non-compressive bra.
- Antibiotic ointment to suture lines.
- Dressing with hole cut and covered with plastic cup or other protective device.

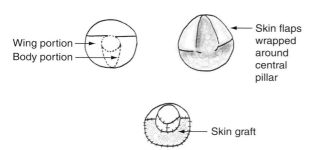

Figure 5.6 Skate flap for nipple reconstruction. The base of the flap is three times the diameter of the desired/contralateral nipple. The lateral 'wing' flaps are elevated in the subdermal level whilst the body includes some subcutaneous flap. Some variants dispense with the skin graft but this will limit the projection.

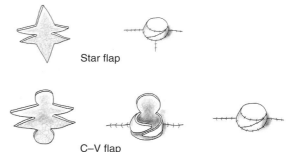

Figure 5.7 The star and C–V flaps are similar to the skate flap but do not require skin grafts.

Complications are relatively uncommon: tissue necrosis is a concern, and surgery should be avoided in smokers; flattening out is almost to be expected.

Areolar reconstruction

Areolar sharing – however, there can be a significant donor site morbidity (except if the patient is also undergoing a reduction/mastopexy to the contralateral side).

Other sites available as skin donors include labia minora FTSG, labia majora SSG, inguinal perineal skin (the donor site is easily hidden but under certain circumstances can sometimes be inconvenient) and upper inner thigh. The retroauricular area can be considered for those with light-coloured areolas.

- A technique of **'returned skin grafts'** (elevated from the same site as 'recipient' i.e. around the reconstruction nipple) has been described. Gruber used ultraviolet light to enhance graft pigmentation, but this was not popular as the results were not permanent.
- In the past, some surgeons had described **NAC banking** e.g. in the groin etc., however this practice was stopped due to several cases of cancer spread to the inguinal nodes and subsequent studies demonstrated NAC involvement in invasive and non-invasive breast cancers. Some attempt to modify the nipple to reduce the chances of 'preserving' tumour cells e.g. keep in a fridge until final histology is available, or cryopreservation, but these methods are inevitably less effective at preserving the nipple, which would lose pigment and projection.

- **Dermabrasion** to induce hyperpigmentary changes; the long-term results are unclear.
- **Tattoo** –it is common to wait 6–12 weeks after nipple reconstruction to allow for recovery of tissues, however, some suggest tattooing before nipple reconstruction as it results in a more uniform colour. Tattooing is generally safe, allergic reactions are rare but have been described. Some fading is normal and to be expected – tattooing can always be repeated.
  - The surface texture of Montgomery glands has been reproduced by placing diced cartilage under the skin.

Preserving the nipple

Instead of reconstructing the nipple after resection during mastectomy, could it actually be preserved?

Analysis of nipple/areolar involvement with mastectomy: can the areola be preserved?
Simmons RM. *Ann Surg Oncol* 2002;**9**:165–168.

This article presents data from histological evaluation of the nipple–areolar complex from 217 mastectomy patients between 1990 and 1998.

- 10.6% of patients overall had involvement of the nipple that increased to 27.3% if the tumour was central but decreased with non-central locations to 6.4%.
- Less than 1% had involvement of the areola (large tumours > 5 cm and lymphadenopathy, located centrally below the areola).

As **areolar skin does not contain ductal cells or breast parenchymal tissue**, areola-sparing mastectomy may be considered in selected patients but not preservation of the nipple.

The author followed this up with an article in 2003 reporting on areola-sparing mastectomy with immediate reconstruction in 17 breasts (12 patients) (*Ann Plast Surg* 2003;**51**:547–551).

Several groups have reported their experiences with **nipple-sparing mastectomy** and reports with larger sample sizes have demonstrated low local recurrence rates ranging from 0% at 52 months to 1 nipple recurrence in 61 patients (Sakamoto N. *Ann Surg Oncol* 2009;**16**:3406–3414; Gerber B. *Ann Surg* 2003;**238**:120–127). Patients with non-central tumours (at least 2 cm away from the nipple–areolar complex) were chosen, with intra-operative frozen sections for confirmation. Nipple necrosis occurred in 18% in the first study; some authors noted that the nipple may be insensate/non-erectile after nipple-sparing surgery.

Inverted nipple

This is a relatively common condition – up to 10% of women in some estimates. The aetiology is not fully understood (congenital deficiencies in most cases, whilst post-mastitis fibrosis may be responsible in some) but there is a reduction in subareolar soft tissue, the lactiferous ducts are shortened and fibrotic and there may be bands tethering the nipple. There are many different techniques described; extensive dissection/manipulation can cause fibrosis leading to recurrence of the inversion. As well as the cosmetic issues, it may interfere with breastfeeding.

Non-surgical management with suction devices such as the Niplette (McGeorge DD. *Br J Plast Surg* 1993;**47**:46–49) have been suggested but these are of limited use, particularly for those with established fibrosis.

Classification

Han S. (*Plast Reconstr Surg* 1999;**104**:389–395) described a classification scheme that has implications for clinical management.

- Grade I – minimal fibrosis. Easily correctable manually and maintains position without traction. Treatment with purse-string suture is usually sufficient.
- Grade II – moderate fibrosis and mildly retracted ducts. Correctable manually but position is not maintained after release after traction. Fibrosis needs to be released with blunt dissection whilst sparing the ducts, before the purse-string.

- Grade III – severe fibrosis, severely retracted ducts and insufficient soft tissue. Difficult to correct manually. Sharp release of fibrosis and ducts is required; dermal flaps may be needed e.g. star flap.

Little JW (*Plast Reconstr Surg* 1999;**104**:396–397) commented on the article in the same issue and suggested an alternative to dermal flaps in grade III inversion – that is to divide the fibrosis at a deeper level to avoid the 'empty cylinder' defect with division closer to the dermis. Then a purse-string with suture is applied.

Purse-string suture for nipple projection
Peled IJ. *Plast Reconstr Surg* 1999;**103**:1480–1482.

The author describes a simple technique for the correction of inverted nipple that can be performed under local anaesthesia.

- The nipple is everted with a skin hook and a traction suture placed at its apex.
- Fibrous bands tethering the nipple down are released using an 18-gauge needle introduced at the 6 o'clock position and swept medially and laterally in a horizontal plane.
- Through the same hole, a 4–0 clear monofilament nylon suture is placed and used to create a subcuticular purse-string around the nipple, exiting every 5 mm through the skin and reintroduced through the same hole. The purse-string tension adjusted, tied and buried at starting point.

Minimally invasive correction of inverted nipples
Kolker AR. *Ann Plast Surg* 2009;**62**:549–533.

The authors presented their experience with surgery for 58 'congenitally' inverted nipples (31 patients). After infiltration with local anaesthetic, the nipple is everted with a temporary traction suture and a 18G needle is inserted in the 6 o'clock position and used to divide the tissue (below the skin level) to allow the nipple to sit everted without traction. A monofilament (for better sliding and control of tension) purse-string suture (nylon or PDS) is inserted through the same needle hole, looping around the nipple circumference coming out every 3–5 mm and then tied with moderate tension. Two additional 5'0 catgut sutures are placed beneath the nipple. Antibiotic ointment is applied and the patient is advised not to compress them with tight clothing or otherwise for 2 weeks.

They report no recurrences in grade I nipples; the 22% recurrence rate occurred in grade II and grade III (50%). They suggest repeating the procedure for recurrences.

Dermal flaps

Many variations have been described; they create scars on the areolar skin.

- Ritz M. *Aesth Plast Surg* 2005;**29**:24–27. Two thin de-epithelialized flaps are raised pedicled at the nipple base and threaded through tunnels in the nipple.
- Kim DY. *Ann Plast Surg* 2003;**51**:636–640. Uses two triangles of areolar dermis (de-epithelialized) and tunnelled through the nipple. The tunnel is created by blunt dissection in grade II or sharp division in grade III.

Chapter 6

Hand and upper limb

A. Trauma

I. Examination

Examination follows the simple 'Look, Feel and Move' method.

Look

Start with the dorsum of hand – skin/swellings/ shrinkage/shape

- Skin – sudomotor changes, benign lesions (Garrod's pads, Heberden's nodes), malignant lesions (actinic keratoses (AKs), SCCs), pigment changes, scars, etc.
- Swellings – dorsal wrist ganglia, exostoses.
- Shrinkage, i.e. wasting – particularly dorsal interosseii.

- **'Shape' i.e. position of the hand** – e.g. ulnar claw, rheumatoid deformities; measure angles with goniometer for greatest accuracy.

Turn the hand over to look at the volar surface

- Skin – sudomotor changes, scars, palmar nodules of Dupuytren's.
- **Swellings** – volar wrist ganglion, palmar lipomata, etc.
- **Shrinkage/wasting** – thenar and hypothenar muscles.

Feel

Test for **sensation** in each of the nerve territories. It should be routine to check nerves before operating on any part of the hand, e.g. Dupuytren's where a digital nerve may be injured.

Feel the **relevant feature** to complete examination of texture, tenderness, mobility, etc. If a joint is the relevant feature then feel stability. Do not elicit pain!

Move

Passive range of movement.

Active range of movement – global and movement in an area of special interest:

- Flexor tendon division – test flexor digitorum profundis (FDP) and flexor digitorum superficialis (FDS) tendons.
- Basal joint osteoarthritis – ask patient to circumduct thumb.
- Rheumatoid arthritis – look at active wrist pronation/supination, flex/extend metacarpophalangeal joints (MCPJ).
- **Test the motor nerves to the whole hand.**

Examination for specific nerves

Median nerve

Look: wasting of the thenar musculature and sudomotor changes in the nerve distribution.
Motor:

- Median nerve at the elbow: palpate tendon of FCR with resisted **wrist flexion.**
- Anterior interosseus nerve sign: inability to make an **'O' sign** due to denervation of FDP to the index finger and flexor pollicis longus (FPL).
- **Pronation of the forearm** (quadratus) with elbow extended to neutralize pronator teres.
- Motor branch of median nerve:
  - Weakness in **abduction of the thumb** (APB).
  - **Opposition** to the little finger (true pulp to pulp – opponens pollicis).

Sensory: pulp of index

- **Moving** two-point discrimination.
- Sharp/blunt sensation.

Ulnar nerve

Look:

- Interosseus guttering and first dorsal interosseus wasting.
- Hypothenar wasting.
- Ulnar claw hand.
- Sudomotor skin changes.

Motor:

- **Froment's test** – tests adductor pollicis; may perform individual Froment's tests to the fingers – palmar interosseii.
- Resisted abduction of the index finger (first dorsal interosseus) and little finger (abductor digiti minimi, ADM).
- Flex the MCPJ of the little finger with the proximal interphalangeal joint (PIPJ) straight – flexor digiti minimi (FDM).
- Absent flexion at the distal interphalangeal joint (DIPJ) of the ulnar two fingers (ulnar-innervated FDPs).

Sensory: little finger – as above.

Radial nerve

Look:

- Sudomotor changes in the superficial branch of radial nerve distribution.
- Wasting of triceps, brachioradialis and extensor compartment.
- **Wrist drop.**

Motor:

- Above the elbow: **elbow extension** (triceps).
- At the elbow:
  - Elbow flexion, arm in mid-pronation to neutralize biceps (brachioradialis).
  - **Wrist extension** and radial deviation, fist clenched (extensor carpi radialis longus (ECRL) and extensor carpi radialis brevis (ECRB) tendons).
- Below the elbow: posterior interosseus nerve:
  - Supination with the elbow extended to neutralize biceps (supinator).
  - **Thumb extension with the palm flat (extensor pollicis longus (EPL)).**

Sensory: first web space – as above.

Specific provocation tests for nerve compression

Provocation tests aim to reproduce the symptoms of compression neuropathy.

Median nerve

- Pronator syndrome: pain with resisted pronation of the flexed forearm which pinches the median nerve between the two heads of pronator teres.

- Anterior interosseus syndrome – resisted FDS flexion of the middle finger.
- Carpal tunnel syndrome (CTS) – paraesthesia with Tinel's and Phalen's tests.

Ulnar nerve

- Cubital tunnel syndrome.
  - **Paraesthesia** with flexion of the elbow; Tinel's test unreliable.
  - Note: reduced/lack of clawing due to denervation of ulnar FDPs.
- Ulnar tunnel syndrome (Guyon's canal) – paraesthesia with pressure over Guyon's canal.

Radial nerve

- Radial tunnel syndrome.
  - **Pain** with **middle finger test** (resisted extension of the middle finger).
  - The radial nerve may be compressed by multiple structures – the medial tendinous edge of ECRB, supinator–proximal border (arcade of Frohse) or distal edge, radial recurrent vessels.
- Wartenberg's syndrome: there is dysaesthesia with compression of the superficial branch of radial nerve beneath the tendon of brachioradialis. Finkelstein test (positive in de Quervain's) may give a false-positive.

Examination for thoracic outlet syndrome

These are non-specific provocation tests and mostly examine for arterial causes.

- **Roos' test**: abduct the arms to 90° with the elbows flexed to 90° and externally rotated (palm facing forward), then open and close hands for 3 minutes. Listen for a bruit indicating subclavian artery aneurysm (most sensitive in this position) and be watchful of symptoms. This is possibly the most reliable test but some patients with CTS (and not thoracic outlet syndrome) may have symptoms limited to the median nerve distribution.
- **Wright's test**: abduct arms to 90°, hyper-extend the wrist and palpate the radial pulse as the flexed forearm is externally rotated to adopt the position of Roos' test. It is positive in 7% of normal patients.
- **Adson's test**: brace shoulders backwards raising arms to about 30 degrees of abduction and shoulder hyperextension, turn head towards the affected side, lift chin and take a deep breath in and check for diminution of the radial pulse or

paraesthesia (without similar symptoms in the contralateral limb). However this is positive in 20–25% of normal subjects; many regard this to be too high and that descriptions are for historical interest only. There are several variants of this test. The reverse Adson's positions the head away from the affected with chin down.

- **Falconer's:** brace and pull down on arms behind the patient checking for decrease in pulse.
- **Halstead brace manoeuvre:** with arms at the patient's side, move shoulders down and back with the chest out; positive result will be reduced pulsation.
- **Brachial plexus compression test** – pressure applied to the brachial plexus in the posterior triangle.
- **Costoclavicular compression test** – allow shoulders to relax, supinate forearms and apply downwards and backwards traction to both arms while palpating the radial pulse.

Also check for Horner's syndrome (involvement of the stellate ganglion), phrenic nerve (raised hemi-diaphragm CXR) and Brown–Sequard syndrome.

Examination for cervical root compression

Spurling's test: with the head turned to the affected side, downwards pressure is applied to the top of the head in an effort to compress the intervertebral foramina (hence alternative name of 'foraminal compression test'). It is positive if there is radiating pain in the upper limb. It is specific but not very sensitive in the diagnosis of acute cervical root compression.

Sensory changes

- C5 – lateral upper arm.
- C6 – lateral forearm, thumb.
- C7 – central posterior arm and forearm, middle finger.
- C8 – medial forearm, little finger.
- T1 – medial upper arm.

Motor loss

- Elbow flexion – C5, 6.
- Elbow extension – C7, 8.
- Hand intrinsics – C8, T1.

Reflexes

- Biceps – C5, 6.
- Brachioradialis – C6, 7.
- Triceps – C7, 8.

Local anaesthetics

Local anaesthetics (LA) are mostly weak bases (pKa 7.7–9.1 – at pH equivalent to the pKa, the non-ionic and ionized forms are approximately in equal proportions). Most preparations are pH 5–6 (without adrenaline) or 2–3 (with adrenaline, so these solutions tend to sting more); thus after injection, they will need to be 'buffered up' first, leading to a short delay in the onset of action before a significant amount of the non-ionized base is formed.

- Non-ionic form can travel across plasma membranes, thus pKa affects speed of onset.
- Potency is related to lipid solubility, allowing more to enter nerves (they act from the inside of membrane).
- Adrenaline – allows faster onset of and longer duration of action.

Methaemoglobinaemia may occur due to oxidation of ferric iron to the ferrous form, most commonly by prilocaine/benzocaine, and leads to cyanosis concentrations exceeding 4 g/dl; treat with methylene blue.

Allergies to LA are generally rare, though it is more common in esters (metabolized to para-aminobenzoic acid (PABA)) than in amides. In most cases, it may be due to methylparaben, a preservative/baceriostatic found in multidose vials.

Toxicity

This is related to dose and vascularity.

- Adrenaline toxicity: hypertension, tachycardia or arrhythmias.
- LA toxicity – note that the seizure threshold is lowered by hypoxia/hypercarbia and acidosis; can treat with benzodiazepines (increase threshold) and thiopental. Intralipid has also been used.
  - Central nervous system (CNS) excitation (dizzy, tinnitus, circumoral numbness/tingling, fits) before depression (respiratory, cardiorespiratory).
  - Cardiovascular – sodium channel blockage with decreased Purkinje discharge and prolonged conduction times, more ventricular arrhythmias (re-entrant).

Tourniquets

Post-operative neuritis may occur with tourniquet use, and may be related to high pressures (> 250 mmHg),

long duration (> 2 hours) or poor limb positioning/pressure protection e.g. ulnar nerve at elbow.

Digital blocks

- Dorsal approach is less painful; block dorsal and volar sides, then inject side of extensor tendons proximal to the web.
- Volar approach to common digital nerves that are proximal to bifurcations of artery – raise a wheal over flexor tendon proximal to distal palmar crease, then 2–3 ml either side of tendon. It is more painful.
- Flexor tendon sheath/intrathecal block – rapid onset.

II. Hand infections

The most common organisms involved in human hand infections are *Staphylococcus aureus* and *Streptococci*, with increased risk in diabetics, the immunosuppressed and malnourished. There is a high density of dermal lymphatics and lymphocytes in the hyponychium.

- **Cellulitis** – group A *Streptococci* (beta haemolytic), sometimes *Staphylococci* (usually less severe). Treat with dicloxacillin or cephalexin (erythromycin if penicillin-allergic). Diabetic patients may have higher risk of gram negative/polymicrobial.
- **Paronychia** is the commonest hand infection and is often associated with nail biting.
  - Acute – *Staphylococcus aureus*, occasionally anaerobes. Treat with drainage and dressings 3–4 times a day; nail plate removal may not always be needed.
  - Chronic paronychia is usually fungal (*Candida albicans*) or atypical mycobacteria. Treat initially with topical antifungals; marsupialization of eponychium (avoid damaging germinal matrix) via crescentic excision that heals by secondary intention.
- **Felon** is an abscess of the pulp space that is often secondary to a puncture; it is commonly due to *Staphylococcus aureus*. It can be drained by midvolar or high lateral incisions (avoid fishmouth-type incisions that can compromise the vascularity of the pad).
- **Herpetic whitlow** – herpes simplex virus (HSV) vesicular eruption in the fingertip that is typically preceded by burning-type pain a day before. It may

resemble a felon in appearance but the pulp itself should not be tense and the vesicles are filled with clear fluid (sometimes cloudy, may coalesce). These should only be incised if a secondary bacterial abscess has developed; otherwise the open wound is at risk of exactly this. A vesicle may be deroofed to obtain material for a Tzanck smear and viral cultures. It is usually a self-limited disease (7–10 days) but acyclovir may be used for severe infections – topical 5% to shorten disease course; oral acyclovir during prodrome to abort recurrence. It is infectious until epithelialization is complete.

Fascial spaces of the hand

Hand bursae – there are two consisting of the synovial sheaths:

- Radial bursa – encloses the FPL tendon.
- Ulnar bursa – encloses the long tendons to the little–index fingers (and is continuous with the flexor sheath to little finger).

Most people have connections between the bursae in the palm which extend into the wrist to form the space of Parona in front of pronator quadratus which can also allow the spread of infection between these spaces.
Palmar spaces: thenar, adductor (deep or dorsal to the adductor pollicis), hypothenar, mid-palmar.

- Thenar space infection – painful thumb movements.
- Mid-palm space infection – painful flexion of the three ulnar fingers.
- Web space infection – abducted fingers.

Others: dorsal subaponeurotic (deep to extensor tendons), dorsal subcutaneous, subfascial web space in the palm and interdigital area – a collar stud abscess is an infection in the subfascial palmar space pointing dorsally. The latter two are contiguous.

Flexor sheath infections

This is usually due to *Staphylococcus aureus*, less commonly due to *S. gonococcus* (haematogenous spread).
Kanavel's four cardinal signs of flexor sheath infection:

- Fusiform digital swelling (not in original description).
- Stiffness in a semiflexed position.
- Tenderness along the flexor sheath into the palm.
- Pain with passive extension.

Not all signs may be present in individual cases, particularly when seen in the early stages. The basic treatment principles of hand infections in general, are **AIDED**: antibiotics, immobilization, debridement, elevation and drainage.

Organisms in bites

- Human (2–23%) – *Staphylococcus*, *Streptococcus viridans* (alpha haemolytic), *Streptobacillus*, *Eikenella corrodens* (found in one third), anaerobes e.g. *Bacteroides*.
  - Human 'bites' (often due to punching someone in the face) may cause penetrating MCPJ injuries. Septic arthritis in general can be due to haematogenous spread (suspect gonococcal infection) or penetrating injury; gouty arthritis can mimic a septic arthritis.
- Dog (69–90%) – *Pasteurella multocida*, *Streptobacillus*, *Staphylococcus*, anaerobes.
- Cat (5–18%) – mainly *Pasteurella multocida*.
  - Cat-scratch fever is caused by *Bartonella* and not *Pasteurella*. Classically there is papule at the initial site of infection (1–2 weeks prior) along with regional lymphadenopathy and mild systemic upset. Generally it has a good prognosis and is treatable with ciproxin and doxycycline. The skin test is rarely used now as enzyme immune assay (EIA) antibody tests are available.

All respond to **Augmentin** (to a certain extent) and this is a good first-line treatment; doxycycline and metronidazole can be used in penicillin-allergic patients.

Closure of bites

Tetanus prophylaxis should be administered if needed; follow local guidelines for rabies. HIV transmission after human bites has been described though this is very rare – some recommend a 28-day course of anti-retroviral therapy if either the biter or the bitten are HIV positive.

- Human bites.
  - Acute non-infected.
    - Non-penetrative abrasion-type injuries have a lower risk of infection compared with punctures or lacerations (Stevens DL. *Clin Infect Dis* 2005;**41**:1373–1405). The latter group should have antibiotic prophylaxis e.g. Augmentin.

– Injuries that can potentially involve joints or tendons should be properly explored and irrigated, then splinted, elevated and treated with antibiotics. There is no hard evidence, but such injuries should probably be left open/loose, with secondary closure if necessary.
  ○ Infected wounds should be explored (debridement and drainage/irrigation systems may be necessary). Antibiotics should be administered intravenously.
- Animal bites.
  ○ The role of antibiotic prophylaxis is unclear, but empirically it can be given to those with puncture wounds, hand/foot/face wounds, wounds that have been closed primarily and in compromised patients e.g. diabetic, asplenic or otherwise immunosuppressed (Monteiro JA. *Eur J Int Med* 1995;**6**: 209–215).
  ○ The closure of wounds that have been thoroughly cleaned and presenting within 6 hours can probably be sutured in most cases, though antibiotics are recommended. Some recommend delayed primary closure particularly for those more than 6 hours old.

Osteomyelitis

This is usually due to *Staphylococcus aureus*, *Streptococcus pyogenes* and possibly gram-negative anaerobes. Necrotic bone should be debrided followed by antibiotics for 4–6 weeks; there is a 39% amputation rate.

Other infections

Onychomycosis – nail fungal infection that leads to a thickened, discoloured and flaking nail. Dermatophytes such as *Trichophyton rubrum* are the most common cause in temperate countries whilst *Candida* is more common in the tropics and in diabetics, and those that frequently immerse their hands in water. Laboratory confirmation is recommended before treatment; direct smear (potassium hydroxide) with histological examination, periodic acid–Schiff (PAS) staining of biopsy of nail plate.

- Debridement of nail combined with oral terbinafine (a newer antifungal that is better tolerated) is better than taking the drug alone (Potter LP. *J Dermatolog Treat* 2007;**18**:46–52). Nail avulsion can reduce the duration of oral therapy needed (Jennings MB. *J Am Podiatr Med Assoc* 2006;**96**:465–473).
- Combining oral terbinafine with amorolfine nail paint is more effective than the oral drug alone (Baran R. *Brit J Dermatol* 2007;**157**:149–157).
- Some laser-based treatments have been described.

Sporotrichosis is a fungal (*Sporothrix schenckii*) infection of the skin and subcutaneous tissues most commonly due to puncture wounds sustained during gardening, particularly rose thorns, hence 'Rose gardener's disease'. It is a chronic disease that begins as a plaque/nodule at the puncture point that then tends to ulcerate if untreated. Rarely it may spread to the lungs or become disseminated. Definitive diagnosis requires fungal culture. It is usually treated with antifungals – itraconazole, terbinafine or fluconazole – for 3–6 months (at least a month after symptoms clear). Oral saturated solution of potassium iodide (SSKI) has also been used with some efficacy in the past though its exact mechanism of action is unclear; it is cheap but poorly tolerated by most.

Atypical mycobacterial infections are relatively rare; the most common is probably *Mycobacterium marinum* which can be contracted from either fresh or salt water (except swimming pools as chlorination kills the organism). It should be suspected in those with a chronic sinus/ulcer with a compatible history; the diagnosis can be made by culturing – 8 weeks at 31°C in Lowenstein-Jensen medium, Ziehl-Nielson staining. Skin lesions generally do not need surgical debridement, and will respond to specific antibiotics e.g. doxycycline/minocycline, ciproxin as well as the combination of rifampicin and ethambutol, where possible for 2–6 months (empiric duration but most recommend at least 1 month further after resolution of lesions).

- Other water-borne infections include: *Aeromonas hydrophilia* (fresh water), *Vibrio vulnificus* (coastal sea water).

III. Flexor tendon injury

Anatomy

- Tendons are mostly made of collagen type I, with ground substance and specialized fibroblasts called tenocytes.
  ○ Endotenon is the fine covering around tendon fibres that binds them together; blood vessels, nerves and lymphatics are carried in this layer.

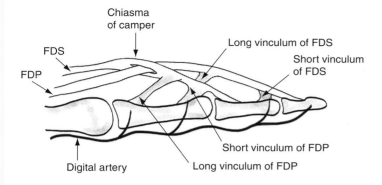

Figure 6.1 Schematic diagram of the flexor tendon arrangement of the fingers along with the vinculae derived from branches of the digital artery.

- ○ Epitenon is the fibrous outer layer of the tendon.
- ○ Paratenon is the loose adventitial layer where there is no true synovial sheath.
- Tendon nutrition.
  - ○ Direct vascularity from musculocutaneous junction (proximal end), bony junction (and Sharpey's fibres) and vincula (longum/brevis, profundus/superficialis):
    - – Short vinculum attaches FDP to neck of middle phalanx (MP).
    - – Long vinculum attaches FDP to neck of proximal phalanx (PP).
    - – The FDS also has long and short vinculae both attaching to the PP.
  - ○ Synovial fluid – diffusion.

The synovial fluid within the tendon sheath allows smooth gliding of the FDS and FDP tendons within it. There are thickened areas along the sheath that are called **pulleys.** In the fingers, there are five annular pulleys and four cruciate pulleys. They function to hold the tendons close to the bones to maximize mechanical efficiency.

- A1 – overlying MCPJ, attached to base of PP.
- A2 – overlying shaft of PP – proximal part of PP.
- A3 – overlying PIPJ, attached to base of MP.
- A4 – overlying shaft of MP – middle of MP.
- A5 – overlying DIPJ.
- C1–4 – between annular pulleys, except A1 and A2.

The crucial pulleys are A2 (proximal PP) and A4 (middle MP).

In the thumb, there are two annular pulleys and one oblique pulley:

- A1 – overlying MCPJ, attached to volar plate.
- A2 – overlying IPJ, attached to head of PP.

- Oblique – overlying shaft of PP (analogous to A2 in finger – the thumb A2 and oblique pulleys are most important).

The tendon of the adductor pollicis is attached to A1 and oblique pulleys.

Examination

When there is no active PIPJ joint flexion of the little finger, when considering the possibility of FDS injury:

- 15% of patients do not have FDS to little finger.
- 15% have a non-functioning FDS to little finger.
- Some have adhesions between FDS to ring finger and little finger preventing independent movement.

Linburg's sign: patient flexes thumb (FPL) maximally onto hypothenar eminence and actively extends index finger as far as possible. If FPL action is accompanied by limitation of DIPJ extension with pain, this is regarded as a positive sign. The cause is usually due to tendinitis at interconnection/adhesions between FPL and flexor indicis in the carpal tunnel that is seen in 10–15% of hands.

Boyes' test: this tests the extensor central slip. As the examiner holds the finger in slight extension at the PIPJ, the patient is asked to flex the DIPJ – inability/difficulty is a positive test.

Bunnel–Littler test, also known as the intrinsic-plus test: This is a passive test and aims to test the structures around the MCPJ which is held slightly extended whilst the examiner attempts to flex the PIPJ – inability to do so is a positive test which suggests capsular contracture or tight intrinsics. To differentiate between the two, flexing the MCPJ slightly should allow PIPJ flexion if the problem is intrinsic tightness, but no difference if it is due to a tight capsule.

Quadriga syndrome: results from tethering of the FDP tendon to an amputation stump which causes an active flexion deficit in uninjured fingers whilst there is still a normal passive range of movement. This is due to a failure of full excursion of the tethered tendon.

Lumbrical plus represents the opposite of quadriga. The FDP tendon is left too loose and acts via its lumbrical insertion, causing metacarpophalangeal flexion and interphalangeal extension.

Positive Bouviere's test is used to determine if the PIPJ joint capsule and extensor mechanism are working normally; if functioning normally, blocking MP joint hyperextension allows IP joint extension.

Verdan's zones

The zone of tendon injury is described as the position of the injury when the fingers and thumb are extended, rather than the site of the surface laceration.

- Fingers extended at time of injury – distal ends lie in the wound.
- Fingers flexed at time of injury – distal ends distal to the skin wound.

Fingers

- Zone 1: Insertion of the FDP to the insertion of FDS/distal to FDS insertion.
- Zone 2: Between the insertion of FDS and the A1 pulley (distal palmar crease) – 'No man's land' (Bunnell); 'critical zone' (Boyes). The FDS divides at the level of the distal palmar crease.
- Zone 3: From the A1 pulley to the distal border of the carpal tunnel.
- Zone 4: Carpal tunnel.
- Zone 5: Carpal tunnel to musculotendinous junctions of muscles.

Thumb

- Zone 1: From the A2 pulley to the insertion of FPL (distal to IPJ).
- Zone 2: A1–2 pulley (MCPJ to IPJ).
- Zone 3: A1 pulley to carpal tunnel; then as above (MCPJ to carpal tunnel).
- Zone 4: Carpal tunnel.
- Zone 5: proximal to carpal tunnel.

Flexor tendon injuries

Closed avulsion of FDP – 75% involves ring finger ('rugby jersey finger' – typically the tendon is avulsed from the distal phalanx when attempting to hold onto an opponent's collar whilst he is running away at speed).

Leddy and Packer classification (1977):

- Type I. The FDP tendon ruptures along with both vinculae but with no fracture, hence tendon retracts into the **palm** and presents as a tender lump. Early repair (within 10 days) is needed as the vincular and synovial supplies have been disrupted. It is the most severe type of avulsion injury.
- Type II. The FDP ruptures but the long vinculum remains intact and holds the distal tendon end at **PIPJ level**. There may be a small fracture fragment. Repair within 3 months. This is the commonest type of avulsion injury.
- Type III. A large fracture fragment is caught in the **A4 pulley** and the tendon is unable to retract further hence both vinculae protected. There is no specific deadline for repair and it has the best prognosis.

Boyes' classification of flexor tendon injuries

- Injury to tendon only.
- Tendon and soft tissue.
- Associated with joint contracture.
- Associated with neurovascular damage.
- Multiple digits or combinations of II–IV.

Flexor tendon repair

History

- Age, hand dominance.
- Occupation (complex reconstruction vs. pragmatic lesser option) and hobbies.
- Pre-injury hand status i.e. pre-existing hand problems.
- Mechanism of injury – laceration, crush, avulsion, etc.
- Time of injury (if long-standing may need two-stage reconstruction).
- General questions relating to factors relevant to fitness for surgery and wound healing (drugs, medical history including diabetes, smoker, etc.) and tetanus status.

Examination

- Look – perfusion, old scars, swellings, sudomotor changes, wasting, finger arcade, identify zone of injury.

Brunner   Modified brunner   V-Y flaps

Figure 6.2 Some common incisions used for exploring volar finger injuries or disease such as Dupuytren's contracture. The modified Brunner incision was described by Hettiaratchy S (*Plast Reconstr Surg* 2003;**112**:692–693).

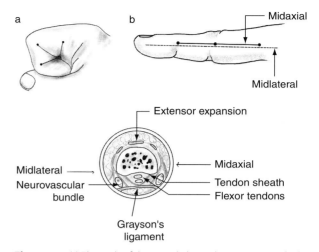

Figure 6.3 (a) The ends of the interphalangeal creases are marked with the digit fully flexed, and joining them up forms the 'midaxial' line (b). This lies slightly dorsal to the midlateral axial and the neurovascular bundle (c). A Brunner incision should touch the midaxial line.

- Feel – sensation especially distal to the injury, feel for tender mass in the palm – Leddy and Packer type I.
- Move – passive and active movement distal to the injury plus full neurological examination of the three nerves.

Investigation: AP and lateral films – to exclude fractures and foreign bodies.

Treatment

Timing

- Primary repair within 24 hours.
- Delayed primary – more than 24 hours but less than 2 weeks.
- Secondary repair.
  - Early secondary – 2–5 weeks, before significant muscle contracture occurs, thus results are similar to delayed primary.
  - Late secondary – after 5 weeks, gap between muscle and tendon means that a tendon graft is required for continuity, or a transfer to restore the 'action'.

Markings

Brunner extensions to the wound or midaxial incisions are the commonest types of incisions.

Two- or four-strand techniques

The common choice is a non-absorbable monofilament (Prolene®, easier to use but in vitro tests have shown stretching under tension leading to a tendon gap) or braided (Ticron®, braided sutures need greater attention to detail in their placement and tightening), though absorbable sutures (PDS, Maxon®) can also be satisfactory since the metabolic rate of tendon tissue is low and suture material is retained long enough to maintain tensile strength during healing.

The modified Kessler 4'0 (quadrilateral suture with small grasping bites at each corner) plus epitendinous suture 5'0 Prolene (introduced by Kleinert; some use sutures as fine as 7'0) is as good as most other techniques with the **epitendinous suture contributing 20%** to the strength of the repair. Gaps and bunching are both to be avoided.

- To maximize tendon vascularity, it is important to preserve vinculae during repair and to keep sutures volar (though studies have shown dorsally placed Kessler sutures to be stronger).

There are a variety of four-strand techniques based on the finding that the strength of the core suture is most important and is related to the number of strands crossing the tendon e.g. four-strand cruciate, MGH criss-crossing locking stitch/augmented Becker technique (Stein J. *Hand Surg Am* 1998;**23**:1043–1045 found that volarly placed sutures were as strong as dorsal). There are some six-strand techniques which are stronger than both two- and four-strand techniques.

- For tendon division up to 60%, repair with an epitendinous stitch alone.
- A second single horizontal mattress core suture can be placed, slightly dorsal (this is where most

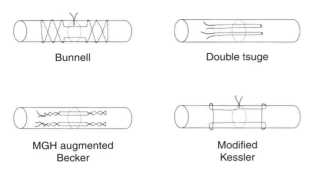

Bunnell

Double tsuge

MGH augmented
Becker

Modified
Kessler

Figure 6.4 Some methods of flexor tendon repair.

gapping occurs) in the centre to make a four-strand Kessler.

- Zone 1 injuries lead to loss of DIPJ flexion. FDP repairs may demand a reinsertion technique (Mitek anchors) as they usually need 5 mm of distal stump for suture repair. Studies have shown that direct anchoring of tendon to the bone is stronger than suturing tendons together; the FDP tendon can be advanced up to a maximum of 1 cm for direct anchoring.
- Zone 2 injuries – repair both FDS and FDP except in replants where FDP only may be repaired; **not repairing FDS** may lead to increased risk of FDP repair rupture, loss of grip strength and dexterity and late swan-neck deformity i.e. hyperextension deformity at PIPJ.
- Tendon **loss** – consider primary graft or insertion of a Hunter rod but good-quality soft tissue cover muscle must be available.

Post-operative protocol

- Extension block splint with wrist in neutral, MCPJ flexed to 70–90°, IPJ extended with a dorsal slab and no resisted flexion. Some prefer splintage in 30° wrist flexion, MCPJ 50–70° and IPJ in full extension.
- **Belfast protocol of controlled active movement** for 6 weeks under the supervision of the physiotherapists. Active mobilization every hour within splint, then passive flexion 5 times (joint mobility and reduce contracture), passive flexion and hold 5 times (maintain function of proximal muscle bellies), active flexion 10 times (to allow tendon glide to enhance intrinsic healing and reduce adhesions). It takes 3 months for tendon to achieve maximal strength.

- ○ Early active extension and passive flexion – Kleinert. Dorsal splint prevents over-extension whilst elastic bands maintain finger flexion – it allows active extension and then passive flexion by elastic recoil. It may increase risks of contracture but is associated with fewer ruptures.
- ○ Early passive mobilization – Duran.
- ○ Immobilization e.g. in a cast, may be more appropriate for children and non-compliant adults e.g. those with learning difficulties.
- Antibiotics are of debatable value in most cases.

Complications

- 5% rupture rate (more with FPL repair) – most commonly on post-operative day 10.
- Adhesions (tenolysis after 3 months if tendon inactive and there is a significant discrepancy between active and passive range of movements and no improvement with a course of physiotherapy).
- Contractures occur in up to 17% of flexor tendon repairs. Severe cases require release including capsulotomy in some cases.

The effect of partial excision of the A2 and A4 pulleys on the biomechanics of finger flexion
Tomaino M. *J Hand Surg* 1998;**23**:50–52.

This fresh-cadaver study quantified angular rotation at finger joints and the energy required for digital flexion. Venting pulleys facilitates repair in zones 1 and 2 and reduces tendon impingement on intact pulleys without significant functional sequelae. Venting may be performed without compromising pulley function up to:

- 25% A2 pulley alone (greatest effect at the DIPJ).
- 75% A4 pulley alone.
- 25% of the A2 **and** 25% of the A4 pulleys (greatest effect at the MCPJ).

A2 and A4 pulley reconstruction

- Encircling graft of extensor retinaculum of wrist (Lister).
- Encircling tendon graft (two-to-four wraps if possible).
- Tail of superficialis.

Flexor tendon grafting

Indications for tendon grafting as opposed to primary repair include:

- Primary repair not possible e.g. tendon loss or muscle contracture.
- Failed primary repair.
- Need for good soft tissue cover over potential repair site.

However all transfers/reconstruction must satisfy the following:

- Full range of passive movement with stable joints.
- Hospitable tissue planes and sensate soft tissue cover.
- Patient compliance with surgery and rehabilitation.

Tendon grafting in zone 2

A one-stage procedure is suitable for selected cases such as tendon avulsion injury with **good soft tissue cover** and tendon **sheath and pulleys** preserved. Graft options include palmaris longus (13 cm), plantaris (31 cm, found anterior and medial to the Achilles tendon), toe extensors (30 cm), FDS, extensor indicis (EI) and extensor digiti minimi (EDM) and tendon allografts.

Suture distally first, options:

- To FDP stump.
- Into bone (Bunnell).
- To pulp/nail bed (Pulvertaft).

After checking appropriate tension by tenodesis effect and matching up the cascade, connect proximally:

- Pulvertaft weave.
  - Guy Pulvertaft (1907–1986) was a renowned hand surgeon who was an inaugural member of the Hand Club and spent his last ten working years in Derby.
- Bunnell criss-cross.
  - Sterling Bunnell (1882–1957) was an American general surgeon with great expertise in hand reconstruction. He played a lead role in Army hand surgery during World War II.
- Kessler suture.

Complications:

- Tendon adhesion is the most common complication.
- Rupture of graft.
- Lumbrical plus if tendon graft too long.
- Quadriga if too short – this occurs if an FDP tendon is shortened or tethered following repair,

then the other tendons cannot shorten sufficiently to achieve full flexion.

Two-stage repair is indicated for:

- Loss/damage to sheath and pulleys.
- Late tendon reconstruction.
- Accompanying fracture or overlying skin loss.
- Nerve injury requiring nerve grafting.
- Loss of pulley system.

Stage 1: excise old tendon remnants, reconstruct pulley and insert Hunter rod which is **fixed distally only.**

Stage 2 (at least 6 months later, though a pseudo-sheath is evident by 8 weeks): harvest and insert tendon graft to replace rod – fix the distal part first (bone anchor or pull-out suture), then push through pseudosheath for proximal repair e.g. Pulvertaft weave for zone III or V. Slight over-correction of the normal cascade is aimed for.

Complications

- Intra-operative – neurovascular injury.
- Early.
  - Synovitis, infection and buckling of implant.
  - Implant extrusion or migration.
  - Pulley breakdown.
  - Skin flap necrosis.
- Late.
  - Chronic flexion deformity.
  - Complex regional pain syndrome (CRPS) type 1.

The choice of repair depends in part on whether the FDS is intact, which digit is involved and patient factors (occupation, compliance, etc.).

- **Thumb with FPL loss** (/Mannerfelt lesion): arthrodese the interphalangeal joint (usually does well) and reconstruct FPL with a two-stage tendon graft. Then transfer FDS from the ring finger.
- **Digit with loss of both FDS and FDP** – two-stage FDP graft – Pulvertaft insertion and Pulvertaft weave.
- **Digit with FDS intact** – most patients benefit from distal interphalangeal joint arthrodesis, and could consider FDP reconstruction or tenodesis of a long distal end to FDS.

Surgical treatment of the divided flexor digitorum profundus tendon in zone 2, delayed more than 6 weeks, by tendon grafting in 50 cases
Sakellarides HT. *J Hand Surg* 1996;**21**:63–66.

Tendon grafting is an alternative to DIPJ fusion or tenodesis of the distal part of the FDP (Bunnell), particularly in children and young patients.

- Must have good-quality volar skin.
- Divided FDP > 6 weeks old.

Plantaris and palmaris grafts were used and effects were improved pinch for index and middle finger and improved power for middle finger and ring finger.

Zone 3 injury

Injury is in the palm (from carpal tunnel to A1 pulley). Options include:

- Interpositional graft.
- Tenodese end to side to adjacent FDP.
- FDS transfer.

Tenolysis

It is best to wait at least 6 months before embarking on surgical tenolysis.

- The dissection can be quite difficult and using a Beaver blade (a small blade that fits into a thin cylindrical handle created to fit like a pencil in the palm, useful for delicate work in a confined space) is usually recommended, and an effort must be made to free ALL adhesions. Extensor tendon tenolysis usually is easier but may need to plan for elective skin cover. Balloon 'angioplasty' technique to expand pulleys has been described.
- Early post-operative mobilization is essential and a brachial plexus block may help. The tenolysed tendon is weak and may rupture at up to 2 months post-operation; avoid resisted movement. ADCON-L® (absorbable porcine gelatin and glycosaminoglycan) gel may inhibit further adhesion formation.
- Failed tenolysis: consider two-stage tendon grafting, arthrodesis or amputation.

IV. Extensor tendon injury

Verdan's zones

- Odd numbers overlie joints starting at zone 1 – DIPJ.
- Even numbers overlie intervening segments finishing at zone 8 – distal forearm.

Wrist compartments

There are six synovial-lined compartments at the extensor surface of the wrist.

1 Abductor pollicis longus (APL) (multiple strips to base of thumb metacarpal).
   Extensor pollicis brevis (EPB) – base of thumb proximal phalanx (PP).
2 Extensor carpi radialis longus (ECRL) – base of index metacarpal.
   Extensor carpi radialis brevis (ECRB) – base of middle metacarpal.
3 Extensor pollicis longus (EPL) – base of thumb distal phalanx (DP).
4 Extensor digitorum communis (EDC) – occasionally has two slips to ring finger, 56% have no slip to the little finger.
   Extensor indicis (EI) – is ulnar to EDC.
5 Extensor digiti minimi (EDM) – there are two slips in 80%, also ulnar to EDC – both EI and EDM have no juncture.
6 Extensor carpi ulnaris (ECU).

Extensor digitorum brevis manus is an anomalous muscle found in approximately 3% (bilateral in one-third of these) that may cause pain and a mass between the finger extensors especially 4th compartment at the wrist (often misdiagnosed as ganglion/tumour). It has variable origins from the dorsum of the radial wrist and inserts into the extensor apparatus of the fingers. It can be diagnosed pre-operatively by MRI or ultrasound, and can be excised without functional deficit (although in some cases it can be the only independent index extensor in the absence of EI).

- **IPJ extension** occurs due to intrinsic action when the MCPJ is in extension.
- IPJ extension is due to extrinsic action when the MCPJ is flexed.

Extensor tendon: anatomy, injury, and reconstruction Rockwell WB. *Plast Reconstr Surg* 2000;**106**:1592–1603.

The anatomy and function of the extensor mechanism of the hand is more complex than the flexors. The extensor apparatus is a linkage system created by

- Radial nerve-innervated extrinsic system.
- Ulnar nerve and median nerve-innervated intrinsic system.

These interconnecting components can compensate for certain deficits in function.

a

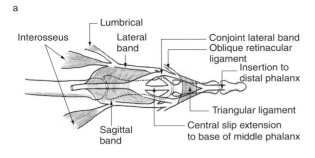

b

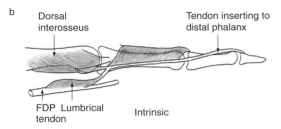

c

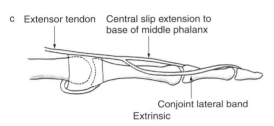

Figure 6.5 Diagram of the extensor mechanism (a) with intrinsic (b) and extrinsic (c) components isolated for clarity.

Extrinsic tendons

The muscle bellies of the extrinsic extensors arise in the forearm and enter the hand through six compartments formed by the extensor retinaculum, a fibrous band that prevents bowstringing of the tendons.

- At the wrist, the tendons are covered by a synovial sheath, but not over the dorsal hand or fingers.
- At the wrist, the extensor tendons are rounder and have sufficient bulk to hold a suture; in contrast the thin and flat tendons over the dorsum do not hold sutures well.

The four EDC tendons originate from a common muscle belly and have limited independent action. In contrast, the extensor indicis proprius (EIP) and EDM have independent muscle bellies and are common donor tendons for transfer. The EIP and EDM are usually ulnar and deep to the EDCs at the level of the MCPJ.

- The EDC to the little finger is present less than 50% of the time and when absent, it is almost always replaced by a juncturae tendinae from the ring finger to the extensor apparatus of the little finger.

The extrinsic extensor tendons have four insertions. At the MCPJ level, the extensor tendons are held in place by the intrinsic tendons and the **sagittal band** that arises from the palmar plate and the deep intermetacarpal ligament. At the PIPJ, the transverse retinacular ligament maintains the position of the extensor mechanism and limits its dorsal–palmar excursion.

- The tendon inserts into the MCPJ volar plate through the sagittal bands.
- A tenuous insertion on the PP and strong insertions on the middle and distal phalanges.
- Over the distal portion of the PP, the **central slip** trifurcates as the central slip and lateral bands (sharing fibres).
  - The central slip inserts on the base of the MP.
  - The lateral band component continues to insert on the base of the DP.

The extrinsic extensor tendons **extend**:

- The MCPJ primarily.
- The IPJ secondarily.

They contribute the **central slip** to the extensor mechanism in the finger that inserts to the base of the MP; they also contribute the lateral **bands** that join the lateral **slips** from the intrinsics to make the conjoint lateral band (these connect over the distal MP before terminating at the base of the DP).

The **intrinsic tendons** are composed of:

- Three **palmar interossei** (adductors) (PAD) and four **dorsal interossei** (abductors) (DAB) that originate from the sides of the metacarpals and run distally on both sides of the fingers except the ulnar side of the little finger. The tendons enter the finger dorsal to the intermetacarpal ligament. The tendons split into two – the superficial slip inserts onto the proximal phalanx (PP) whilst the deep tendon becomes part of the **lateral slip.**

- Four **lumbrical** muscles arise from the radial side of the FDP tendon and pass palmar to the intermetacarpal ligament.

The intrinsic muscles

- Flex the MCPJ.
- Extend the proximal and distal IPJ.

The intrinsic tendons join to form the **lateral slips (that join the lateral bands to form the conjoint lateral bands)**; the bands join the extrinsic extensor mechanism proximal to the middle of the PP and then continue distally dorsal to the axes of the IPJs. Distal to the PIPJ the conjoint lateral bands fuse to form a conjoint tendon that inserts into the base of the DP.
  Other important structures:

- The **sagittal bands** are transverse ligamentous structures passing from the extensor tendon to the MCPJ volar plate – they centralize the extensor tendon over the metacarpal head at the MCPJ as contraction of the extensor muscle pulls on the PP to flex the MCPJ. They roll proximally and distally with MCPJ extension and flexion respectively, somewhat like the visor on a motorcycle helmet. Laceration to one side of the sagittal bands causes subluxation of the extensor tendon to the other side.
- The **intermetacarpal ligament** separates the lumbrical tendon that is palmar from the interossei tendons that are dorsal.
- The **transverse retinacular ligament** stabilizes the extensor tendon at the PIPJ. It arises from volar aspect of the flexor sheath and PP to inset into the lateral bands and triangular ligament dorsal to the PIPJ axis.
- The **oblique retinacular ligament** (Landsmeer) is a component of the linkage system that helps to stabilize the lateral bands and is said to coordinate flexion and extension in the finger joints. The ligament arises from the proximal PP and the A2 pulley and inserts into the conjoint lateral band; it spirals to pass volar to the axis of the PIPJ and dorsal to the axis at the DIPJ. It is shortened in Boutonniere deformities and is said to be a reason why you cannot voluntarily flex the DIPJ with PIPJ extended.
- The **triangular ligament** connects the conjoint lateral bands over the dorsum of the middle phalanx, keeps them in close proximity and prevents them from shifting volar and so become a IPJ flexor.

The excursion of the extensor tendons over the finger is less when compared with the flexor tendons; excursion may vary from 2 to 8 mm at the PIPJ.

- The preservation of relative tendon length between the central slip and lateral bands is important and disturbance causes deformities that are progressive, making restoration of normal balance difficult.
- Overlapping linkage systems also contribute to this balance; the components of the linkage system pass palmar to one joint and dorsal to the next:
  - The intrinsic tendons create the linkage at the MCPJ and PIPJ.
  - The oblique retinacular ligaments function at the PIPJ and DIPJ.

Thus deformity at one joint may cause a reciprocal deformity at an adjacent joint.

General principles

- Repair with interrupted over-over sutures (Prolene or Ticron) in zones 1–6 and Kessler/core suture as above zones 7 and 8.
- Gutter splint injuries in zones 2–4, outrigger for zone 5–8 injuries plus night gutter splint.
- If there is loss of tendon tissue, then either graft if adequate skin cover or reconstruct with a distally based tendon flap.
- Central slip rupture/loss: reconstruct with medial portions of lateral bands.
- Repair sagittal band injuries in zones 4/5 otherwise tendon will sublux into metacarpal gutter on intact side.

Zone I injuries (mallet finger)

This deformity is due to forced flexion of the extended digit that leads to disruption of continuity of the extensor tendon over the DIPJ and can be open or closed. If left untreated, hyperextension of the PIPJ (swan-neck deformity) may also develop because of proximal retraction of the central band. It has been postulated that there is a zone of relatively poor vascularity at the site of mallet ruptures.

Doyle classification

(Doyle JR. Extensor tendons – acute injuries. In Green DP (ed). *Operative Hand Surgery*, 3rd Edn. 1993;**2**:1925–1954.)

- **Type 1** – closed, with or without small avulsion fracture. This is the most common.

- **Type 2** – open laceration at or proximal to the DIPJ with loss of tendon continuity.
- **Type 3** – open, deep laceration/abrasion with loss of skin, subcutaneous cover and tendon substance.
- **Type 4**
  - A – transepiphyseal plate fracture in children.
  - B – fracture involving 20–50% of articular surface (hyper**flexion**).
  - C – hyper**extension** injury with fracture > 50% of articular surface, with early or late volar subluxation of the distal phalanx.

Management

The management of mallet finger is still a topic for debate. In the vast majority of cases, splinting alone is sufficient. Operative treatment of a mallet injury may **downgrade** active flexion so it is preferable to treat conservatively if possible – the primary indications for surgery are large fragments that are rotated or persistent DIPJ subluxation – open reduction can be demanding.

The PIPJ is of utmost importance, and it should be kept active/free to move, to avoid a boutonnière deformity.

Type 1 (most common)

- **Stack splint for 6 weeks – continuous full-time** splinting of the DIPJ in extension (some propose slight hyperextension but no more than 5°, avoid skin blanching, inspect skin regularly) for 6 weeks, followed by 2 weeks of night splinting unless there is an occupational need for early return to work or poor patient compliance in which case consider buried K-wire. Poor skin condition is also an indication for K-wiring instead of splintage.
  - 6 weeks need to be restarted if the patient inadvertently flexes the finger.
  - Splintage is still considered for up to 6 months after the injury and will give good results in the majority.
  - For chronic injuries/failed splintage, then tenodermodesis may be considered.

Type 2

- Suture of tendon (simple figure-of-eight suture) and skin either separately or together roll-type suture (tenodermodesis/dermatotenodesis).
- Stack splint 6 weeks.

Type 3

- Primary tendon reconstruction with immediate soft tissue coverage (distally based EC flap) plus oblique K-wire to DIPJ or

- Secondary tendon reconstruction with tendon graft.

Type 4

- A – the extensor mechanism is attached to the basal epiphysis, so closed reduction (MUSA) results in correction of the deformity, followed by a Stack splint for 4 weeks.
- B–C (**fracture of distal phalanx base over 25% of the articular surface**) – open or closed reduction and K-wiring of DIPJ, maintaining reduction with pull-out suture over button on pulp; miniscrew fixation.

Other options

- Arthrodesis – comminuted intra-articular fracture, elderly.
- Amputation – severe soft tissue injury, devascularization.

Zone 2 injury (middle phalanx): if less than 50% of the tendon width is cut, routine wound care and splinting for 7 to 10 days can be followed by active motion. Injuries involving more than 50% should be repaired primarily.

Zone 3 injury (boutonnière deformity): open or closed, with or without avulsion.

- The boutonnière deformity is caused by **disruption of the central slip** at the PIPJ, which results in loss of extension at the PIPJ (often weak PIPJ flexion still possible with intact lateral bands) and hyperextension at the DIPJ. The deformity usually appears 10–14 days after the initial injury, especially after closed rupture. The initial treatment for closed injury should be splinting with the PIPJ in extension. The surgical indications for a closed boutonnière deformity are:
  - Displaced avulsion fracture at the base of the middle phalanx.
  - Instability of the PIPJ associated with loss of active or passive extension of the joint.
  - Failed non-operative treatment.

Zone 4 injuries usually involve the broad extensor mechanism but are **usually partial**, sparing the lateral bands, so that splinting the PIPJ in extension for 3–4 weeks is equivalent to repair. However, for complete lacerations, primary repair should be performed.

- Open sagittal band lacerations should be repaired to prevent extensor tendon subluxation.

- Closed sagittal band injury is suggested by pain with inability to extend the MCPJ actively, though the patient can hold the finger extended if positioned passively. There is subluxation of the tendon. Acute cases presenting within 2 weeks can be treated with splintage of MCPJ extended for 6 weeks whilst older injuries need repair.

Zone 5 injury (metacarpophalangeal joint): injuries over the MCPJ are almost always open and human bites, for example due to a punch injury, should be considered. In such cases, the joint is in flexion, so the actual tendon injury will be proximal to the level of the overlying skin wound. Primary tendon repair is indicated after thorough irrigation.

Zone 6 injuries (dorsum of hand): such injuries may be masked by adjacent extensor tendons through **the juncturae tendinae** and then diagnosis would only be made at exploration. In this zone, the tendons are thicker and more oval so repair should be performed with stronger, core-type sutures.

Zone 7 injuries (wrist) Partial release of the retinaculum is required in most cases to gain exposure to the lacerated tendons which tend to retract significantly here; some portion of the retinaculum should be preserved to prevent extensor bowstringing if at all possible. There is controversy over whether excision of part of the retinaculum over the injury site is necessary to prevent post-operative adhesions; with early dynamic splinting, adhesions are less likely.

Zone 8 injuries (forearm): multiple tendons may be injured in this area, potentially making it difficult to identify individual tendons. Additional difficulty also may be encountered with injuries at the musculotendinous junction because the fibrous septa retract into the substance of the muscles.

Dynamic splinting for extensor injuries

Early controlled motion with a dynamic extensor splint has been found to decrease adhesions and subsequent contractures, especially with more proximal injuries.

Thumb extensor tendons

The extensor mechanism of the thumb is different from that of the fingers.

- Each joint has an independent tendon for extension – the extensor pollicis longus extends the interphalangeal joint, the extensor pollicis brevis extends the MCPJ and the abductor pollicis longus extends the carpometacarpal joint.

- The abductor pollicis longus almost always has multiple tendon slips, whereas extensor pollicis brevis usually has one.

The intrinsic muscles of the thumb primarily provide rotational control whilst also contributing to MCPJ flexion and IPJ extension.

- On the radial side, the abductor pollicis brevis tendon continues to insert on the extensor pollicis longus.
- On the ulnar side, fibres of the adductor pollicis also insert on the extensor pollicis longus.

Thus these two muscles can extend the interphalangeal joint to neutral, significantly masking an extensor pollicis longus laceration.

Thumb injuries

The terminal extensor tendon of the thumb is much thicker, therefore mallet thumbs are rare (closed – splint for 6 weeks; open – repair and splint).

- Zone 3 – repair EPL and EPB and splint for 3 weeks.
- In zones 6 and 7, the abductor pollicis longus retracts significantly when divided and usually requires that the first compartment be released for successful repair.

V. Replantation and ring avulsion

Replantation

Replantation of parts offers a result that is usually superior to any other type of reconstruction. The first successful replantation of a severed limb was undertaken by Malt in Boston in 1964 (replanted the arm of a 12-year-old boy); revascularization of incompletely severed digits was performed by Kleinert and Kasdan in 1965 and the first successful digital replantation was performed by Komatsu and Tamai in Japan, in 1968.

A thorough assessment of the patient and their injury is needed to ensure that the right choice is being made.

History

- Age, occupation, hand dominance, hobbies.
- Pre-existing hand problems.
- Mechanism of injury.

- Ischaemia time and storage (ideally in a damp gauze within a plastic bag on ice).
- General health including drugs, past history, and **is the patient a smoker?**
- **Tetanus** status.

Absolute contraindications

- Life-threatening concomitant injuries.
- Multilevel injury.
- Severe premorbid chronic illness.

Relative contraindications

- **Single digit amputations** particularly at or proximal to the level of zone II (from the A1 pulley to the distal sublimis tendon insertion) are rarely indicated, with the notable exception of the thumb. Very distal amputations at the level of the nail bed are marginally indicated, as there needs to be approximately **4 mm of intact skin proximal to the nail fold** for adequate veins to be present.
- Parts of fingers that have been completely **degloved**; avulsion of tendons, nerves and vessels. Extreme **contamination** or widespread **crush.**
- Lengthy warm ischaemia time (especially larger-size replants).
  - Digit ideally under 6 hours; a warm ischaemia time of > 12 hours is usually not salvageable.
  - Forearm < 4–6 hours warm ischaemia.
- Elderly with micro-arterial disease, heavy smokers.
- Patients with severe systemic disease or trauma, severe mental disease – self harm/psychosis, intractable substance abuse, unwilling/uncooperative.

Indications

- Amputated **thumb** replantation probably offers the best functional return even with poor motion and sensation; the thumb is useful to the patient as a post for opposition.
- Replantation should be attempted with almost any part in a **child** including replantation and revascularization of the foot or lower leg.
- **Multiple digits** amputations present reconstructive difficulties that may be difficult to correct without replantation of one or all of the amputated digits.
- Partial or whole **hand.** Any hand amputation offers the chance of reasonable function after

replantation, usually superior to available prostheses.

Others:

- Replantation distal to the level of the FDP tendon insertion (zone I) usually results in good function whereas replantations of **zone II** amputations tend to have a poor outcome even after further surgery – exceptions can be made e.g. children, thumbs, musicians, certain cultures e.g. Japanese, where missing digits may be regarded as a stigmata of criminals.
- Although usually indicated, the replantation of any hand or arm proximal to the level of the mid-forearm must be carefully considered.
- The risk of complications increases and the chance of functional return decreases with amputations above the elbow.

Anatomy of digital arteries

Dominant supply:

- Ulnar digital artery – thumb, index, middle finger (radial digits).
- Radial digital artery – ring finger, little finger (ulnar digits).

The ulnar artery gives rise to the superficial palmar arch with branches distal (digital vessels) and above the flexors. All digital arteries are branches of the superficial palmar arch. The radial artery gives rise to deep palmar arch about 1 cm proximal to the superficial arch and beneath the flexors. There are some anastomoses over the dorsal carpal arch.

Arterial grafts may be needed for

- Long revascularizations (e.g. thumb replants are best revascularized using grafts where necessary, to the radial artery).
- Significant size discrepancy between proximal and distal ends.

Artery grafts can be harvested from the posterior interosseus or subscapular vessels.

Pulp, Nail, Bone (PNB) classification

PNB classification

Muneuchi G. *Ann Plast Surg* 2005;**54**:604–609.

- Zone I – distal to lunula. Volar veins can be used for repair, otherwise consider arteriovenous (AV) shunting, nail-bed bleed, leech/heparin 'chemical leech'.

- Zone II – DIPJ to lunula. Digital arteries and dorsal veins can be used.

Ring avulsion

Urbaniak classification

Microvascular management of ring avulsion injuries
Urbaniak JR. *J Hand Surg Am* 1981;**6**:25–30.

- Class I – soft tissue injury without vascular compromise i.e. circulation adequate and best treated by standard techniques.
- Class II – soft tissue injury with vascular compromise, i.e. circulation inadequate and microvascular repair required in addition to soft tissue cover:
  - A – digital arteries only.
  - B – arteries plus tendon or bone.
  - C – digital veins only.
- Class III – complete degloving/amputation, circumferential laceration. Type III injuries are unlikely to regain adequate function and amputation is usually recommended.

The authors suggest that apart from wishes of patient for replant in view of need to return to work, complications, etc. (see below) consider the status of the amputated part (sharp amputation vs. crush) and the patient (healthy vs. systemic illnesses). Assess potential for long-term function.

General principles

Examination

- Amputated part and remnant especially degree of crush/avulsion.
- Full examination to identify other pathologies, e.g. crush higher up etc. X-rays of the hand and the amputated part.
- Patient should be stabilized and exclude concomitant life-threatening injury.
- Consent for graft harvest (vein, tendon and skin) and terminalization.

Pre-surgery care

The amputated part should be gently cleansed and wrapped in a moist gauze sponge, placed in a container (either sterile bag or specimen cup), and then placed in ice.

- The warm ischaemic tolerance of digits is in the range of 12 hours (cold 24 hours), though replantation has been reported after cold ischaemia times of up to 39–94 hours.
- In more proximal amputations, the ischaemic tolerance is significantly shorter due to sensitivity of muscle to ischaemia. The absolute maximum warm ischaemic tolerance for major amputations is in the range of 4–6 hours, and cooling to the 10- to 12-hour range may prolong this.

Surgery

- General anaesthesia, tourniquet, two surgeons. A brachial plexus or axillary block may provide useful vasodilatation and post-operative analgesia.
- **Examination of the part** in the operating room before the patient is anaesthetized allows time for appropriate decision-making. Vessels must be examined under the microscope, if in doubt cut back the vessel as it is better to use grafts than unhealthy vessels. Spurt test to roughly assess pressure. Suitable nerves and vessels need to be tagged.
  - Corkscrew appearance suggests an avulsion/traction (should be excised and vein grafted).
  - 'Red line sign' bruising along the course of the digit where the neurovascular bundle runs suggests a severe avulsion injury with disruption of side branches of the digital artery and replantation may be unsuccessful.
  - A 'cobweb' sign describes the appearance with multiple laceration-like patterns on the vessel wall.
  - Measle sign – pinpoint petechiae along vessel adventitia after anastomosis due to thrombosis.
- **Shorten the bone** as needed (max 5–10 mm) – debrided minimally with a curette and managed as an open fracture osteosynthesis. Distal fixation can be placed in the amputated part. Kirschner wires, interosseous wires or plate fixation can be used.
- Repair extensor then flexor tendons (in standard manner, though some suggest placing core sutures in tendon ends before osteosynthesis).
- Digital arteries (one good artery is enough) then dorsal vein (opens up with revascularization) and nerves (some suggest nerves before veins). There should be brisk bleeding from the veins; select the two veins that are bleeding the most for venous anastomosis. Veins can usually be found on the dorsum of the hand proximal to the web spaces for

grafting to – without venous repair 80% fail. Patency can be checked with 'milking'.
- Where the digit has been avulsed with attached tendon, the carpal tunnel should be decompressed.
- Nerve gaps should be grafted in most digital replants; alternatively use conduits or vein grafts.
- Good skin/soft tissue cover with care to avoid compression of the veins by skin closure – use flaps or grafts. With volar skin loss and a problem covering the neurovascular repairs some skin overlying the vein graft may be taken with the vein graft, as a small flow-through venous flap.

Special situations
- **Multiple digital amputations** – future potential function should be considered. The finger with the highest chance of success replanted first, and not necessarily to the original finger e.g. with MF and IF amputations, if the MF is not salvageable, then the IF can be replanted onto the MF stump to avoid a gap in the rays.
- **Major limb** – reperfusion shunts can be used. Lengthy ischaemia times > 6 hours are a contraindication to replantation. Beware of reperfusion; fasciotomies are recommended along with release of nerve tunnel and intrinsic compartments. For hand amputations at the wrist level, proximal carpectomy may be needed. Monitor for hyperkalaemia and myoglobinuria.

Post-operative
- Keep patient warm, wet (hydrated) and well (pain free).
- Antibiotics e.g. first-generation cephalosporin.
- Elevation to 45° and splint in a position of function.
  - **Position of function** (also known as safe position or intrinsic-plus position): originally described by James JIP. (*Acta Ortho Scand* 1962;**32**:407–412) – 70° MCPJ flexion and full IPJ extension (most accept 45–70° and 10° respectively).
- Monitor perfusion of replant – capillary refill, temperature and turgor. Others include Doppler signal, transcutaneous oxygen, temperature probes and fluorimetry.

Drugs
- Aspirin – acetylates cyclooxygenase to reduce arachodonic acids, thromboxanes and prostaglandins to reduce platelet aggregation and vasoconstriction.
- Dextran 40 – a polysaccharide. Some suggest a test dose is needed due to risk of allergies including anaphylaxis but this is not often performed. It has antiplatelet (negative charge decreases platelet activation and inactivates vWF) and antifibrin functions, as well as providing volume expansion.
- Heparin – activates serum antithrombotic III and lowers blood viscosity. Systemic heparin is not absolutely necessary; heparin-soaked pledgets can be used on the nail bed after nail plate removal, if the venous repair is tenuous.

Outcomes
Overall success with guillotine-type amputation is 77% compared with 49% in crush injuries.

Functional outcomes
- 70% achieve < 15 mm 2-point discrimination.
- 50% achieve total active movement (TAM), 50% grip strength.
- With flexor tenolysis TAM can improve by 43%.
- Thumb replants show less improvement.

Complications
- 60% require secondary surgery especially replants proximal to the FDS (93%) vs. 11% of thumb replants.
- Neurolysis with or without grafting.
- Secondary amputation.
- 22% require open reduction and internal fixation (ORIF) for non-union.
- Cold intolerance that improves over 3 years (at least 2 years, possibly lifelong).
- CRPS.

Replantation
Pederson WC. *Plast Reconstr Surg* 2001;**107**:823–841.

Post-operative care
- Axillary infusion of marcaine may be given to provide both pain relief and a chemical sympathectomy.
- Systemic heparinization is widely used in replantation but its efficacy is difficult to prove.
- Chlorpromazine orally (25 mg 8 hourly) is a potent peripheral vasodilator and sedative.
- Aspirin 325 mg daily useful for its anti-platelet effect (given for 3 weeks).

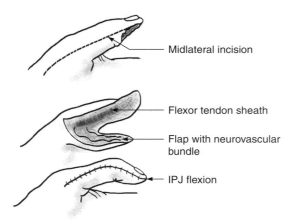

Figure 6.6 The raised volar flap should include both neurovascular bundles. Advancement to the tip of the defect requires IPJ flexion.

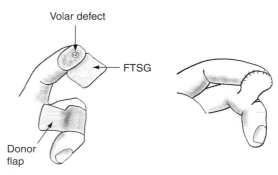

Figure 6.7 The cross finger flap can be used to cover a volar/pulp defect with exposed bone. A FTSG is first sutured along the edge nearest the donor digit (this is easier than suturing at the end). A dorsal flap is raised on the donor digit based on the side adjacent to the injury. This is sutured to the edge of the defect whilst the FTSG is sutured to the end of the donor.

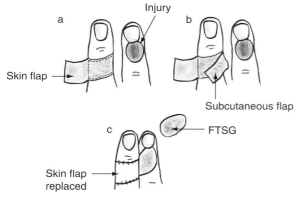

Figure 6.8 A reverse cross finger flap can be used to cover ungraftable distal dorsal defects. A skin flap (equivalent to the thickness of a thin FTSG) is elevated from the donor digit based on the edge away from the defect. A flap of subcutaneous tissue is then raised based on the other edge and is used to cover the defect (along with a thin FTSG). The donor skin flap is sutured back and a tie-over bolus dressing applied.

White finger post-replantation

- Ensure patient is warm, wet and well.
- Loosen dressings and remove sutures as needed.
- Re-explore.

Blue finger post-replantation

- Elevate limb.
- Loosen dressings (remove venous tourniquet) and remove sutures.

- Encourage venous bleeding e.g. leeches, fish-mouth incision in nail bed or heparin injections/soaks ('chemical leech').
- Re-explore.

Complications

- Intra-operative – technically impossible.
- Early post-operative – replant loss, infection.
- Late post-operative – CRPS type 1, pain, stiffness.

Thumb reconstruction

The thumb represents 40–50% of the overall hand function. It is important in key (lateral grips), pulp-to-pulp and tripod (three-point chuck) pinch as well as assisting in a power grasp. It normally reaches the middle of the proximal phalanx of the index with the web reaching the MCPJ.

Distal one-third amputation i.e. at level of IPJ is compensated fairly well leaving minimal functional impairment. For more distal amputations, and where thumb replantation is impossible, there are options for reconstruction. The general aims are:

- Restore skeletal stability.
- Provide well-padded sensory soft tissue as coverage.

Local options are often sufficient.

- Homodigital – **Moberg** volar advancement flap raised at the level of the tendon sheath can resurface defects **up to 1.5 cm** and has good sensation. Flexion contracture or stiffness may occur at the IPJ.

- Heterodigital.
  - Cross finger flaps.
  - Neurovascular flaps – cortical reintegration may be an issue.
    - Littler flap, using ulnar pad of middle finger or radial pad of ring finger. Problems with cortical reintegration and cold intolerance post-operatively have reduced its use.
    - Kite flap – first dorsal metacarpal flap – flap from radial artery just distal to EPL.
- Free pulp transfer (medial aspect of hallux) can restore a near-normal pulp and nail and offers the best functional results.

For amputations involving the **middle third** (IPJ to MCPJ) the functional impairment is related to the length of PP left but there is generally:

- Loss of fine pinch and grasp.
- Thumb index cleft is shortened/shallower.

The aim of reconstruction in this situation is to **lengthen** whilst preserving sensation, stability and mobility. Gain in actual length even of 2 cm will significantly improve the function of the thumb in proximal half amputations.

- **Phalangization** (of thumb metacarpal). For more distal amputations, the length (1.5–2 cm) may be 'gained' by deepening the web with a Z-plasty (2 or 4 flap), however the web skin must be pliable and the first metacarpal mobile. The first interossei is released and the adductor pollicis insertion is transferred which impacts on their mechanical advantage/power. It is simple but little actual functional improvement is gained whilst the resulting web looks unnatural.
  - Dorsal rotation flap into the webspace with skin graft to the donor site. Although the morbidity apart from the graft is minimal, the gain in function is also minimal.
- **Pollicization** of remaining digit – mandatory if the basal carpometacarpal joint is lost. It provides good function and cosmesis, with minimal sacrifice, but does narrow the palm.
- **Distraction osteogenesis** of the metacarpal can lengthen it by 3–3.5 cm over several weeks (1 mm/ day plus latency) but generally needs at least two-thirds of the metacarpal remaining along with good soft tissue cover which is also expanded to a certain extent. Complications include non-union and tissue necrosis. Bone grafting may be needed for bone gaps of more than 3 cm, particularly in

older patients. Web deepening may also be needed subsequently.
- **Toe–hand transfer** (if whole metacarpal preserved use hallux, if only partially preserved use second toe – metatarsal from second toe can be sacrificed but not from the first without causing a gait disturbance). The functional results are superior to other methods as well as being the only way of replacing glabrous skin, fibrous septa and a nail.
- **Osteoplastic reconstruction** – bone graft (usually iliac crest, may resorb significantly) plus neurosensory (where possible) flap (reverse radial forearm, tubed groin flap or ALT). This is usually an option only if other fingers are not available and toe transfer cannot be done. It is however multistage and the results may be neither aesthetic nor functional.

Proximal third amputations i.e. most of metacarpal missing. These require a total thumb effectively, approximately 5 cm in length or more. Options include:

- Pollicization.
- Free toe–hand – offers the best reconstruction in a single operation, providing better sensation, stability and motor control (can expect good pinch and grasp) than the above, however the patient's age, motivation and functional requirements also need to be taken into account. It can be performed secondarily or acutely, including wrap-around flap for salvage of avulsion injuries with most of the skeleton still remaining. It also has good growth potential in children.

Toe–hand transfer
Donor site
- The first dorsal metacarpal artery from the dorsalis pedis (70%, 20% from plantar metatarsal artery, 10% equal) supplies both the first and second toes and lies between the first and second metatarsals at varying levels. The EHB tendon is cut during the pedicle dissection.
- The superficial dorsal – great saphenous vein is usually used.
- Volar digital nerves from medial plantar nerve.

The function of the thenar muscles affects the functional outcome of thumb reconstructions. Donor site complications (of the hallux) may be reduced by pre-serving as much skin as possible for direct closure; the metatarsal head should be preserved along with 1 cm of the proximal phalanx for 'push off'.

Options

- **Hallux transfer** – the ipsilateral toe provides the optimal mobility, stability and strength, however on average it is more than 20% larger than the thumb and the nail is flatter and broader. The donor site cosmesis is rather poor but the effect on walking is slight. The hallux should not be harvested proximal to the MTPJ. For drivers, the non-driving foot is used.
- **Second toe is thinner** and has a shorter nail, and is narrower than the thumb. It is not as strong/stable as the hallux and skin grafts are often needed. However it offers a way of reconstructing the carpometacarpal joint (CMCJ) in more proximal injuries when the metatarsal and *metatarsal* phalangeal joint (MTPJ) is harvested (first metatarsal cannot be sacrificed). In addition, the donor site is more aesthetic and is the preferred technique for some surgeons e.g. Kay.
- **Wrap-around** (Morrison) partial toe transfer – taking soft tissue and nail from the hallux, with bone from a degloved phalanx or an iliac bone graft (thus requires a second donor site). It has relatively poor mobility (no interphalangeal joint) and may resorb but does offer a sensate thumb (pulp and glabrous skin) with very good cosmesis.
- **Trimmed toe** (Wei) – hallux is trimmed to the size of the thumb, including a longitudinal osteotomy. The result is a thumb with good sensation, strength, cosmesis and function; the disadvantage is reduced IPJ function.
- **Partial toe transfer** - from the 2nd toe – MTPJ, pulp, skin and nail.

Toe–hand transfer is an established option and it must be borne in mind during treatment of acute injuries, as it may inadvertently restrict reconstructive options.

- Skin is at a premium – local flaps cause further local scarring and skin-only free flaps use up the recipient vessels.
- If the PIPJ or MTJP can be preserved then overall functional will be much enhanced.

Fourteen per cent will require revisional surgery e.g. flexor tenolysis, joint arthrodesis or web-space deep-ening; surgery may also be required for mal/non-union.

Selection algorithm for toe transfer

- Distal to IPJ – transfer not needed.
- Proximal phalangeal stump with intact MCPJ – wrap-around gives best cosmesis whilst hallux has best strength (and has growth potential and thus is preferred in children).
- Long metacarpal – hallux is best option when harvest at MTPJ, with thenar muscle reconstruction.
- Short metacarpal – second toe is best option as the MTPJ along with some MT can be harvested, opponensplasty is often needed.
- Metacarpal missing (along with intrinsic muscles) – pollicization is the best option unless this is not possible due to finger injuries, when a second toe with MTPJ is the best option. An index metacarpal remnant can be pollicized as a base for toe transfer.

Ray amputation

Indication

- Secondary surgery following trauma, including failed replantation.
- Tumours.
- Infections.
- Congenital hand deformities.

Technique

- Index finger – subperiosteal dissection of metacarpal, osteotomize at level of metacarpal flare, transpose digital nerves into interosseus space.
- Middle finger – two main techniques:
  - **Carroll** – transposition of the index metacarpal to the base of the middle metacarpal.
  - Alternatively, suture together the intervolar plate ligaments between ring and index finger MCPJ (± closing wedge excision of the capitate).
- Ring finger – it shares hamate articulation with the little finger, allowing this to slide radially after division of the carpometacarpal ligaments. It can also be transposed to base of ring metacarpal as above.
- Little finger – preserve metacarpal base which is the site of insertion of FCU and ECU tendons.

VI. Fractures

- Finger fractures are the commonest upper limb fractures, particularly the outer rays.
- An unstable fracture is one that cannot be reduced closed or cannot be held reduced without fixation.
- Antibiotics – there is a 30% infection rate in open distal phalangeal (DP) fractures without antibiotics but 3% infection rate with antibiotics; Sloan JP. *J Br Hand Surg* 1987;**12**:123–124. A DP fracture underlying a subungual haematoma should be considered to be open.
- Healing time 4 weeks (phalangeal fractures) – 6 weeks (metacarpal fractures); note that typically radiological healing lags behind clinical healing.

Phases of fracture healing

- Inflammation (immediately to a few days) – haematoma formation and infiltration by haematopoietic cells and osteogenic precursors.
- Repair (24 hours to 3 weeks) collagen deposition and cartilaginous callus formation (it can be seen on X-ray by 3–6 months). Endochondral ossification.
- Remodelling (months to years) lamellar bone formation and repopulation of marrow. Resorption of callus.

Epiphyseal fractures

Salter–Harris classification for paediatric fractures:

- I – Shearing through the growth plate, transverse fracture (5%).
- II – Epiphysis and growth plate separate from the metaphysis, small metaphyseal fragment attached (75%).
- III – Intra-articular fracture of the epiphysis (10%).
- IV – Fracture passes through epiphysis, growth plate and metaphysis (10%).
- V – Growth plate crushed. Uncommon.

Eighty per cent of Salter–Harris fractures are type II. Some propose a 'SALTR' mnemonic – i.e. 'slipped' through growth plate, 'above' growth plate, 'lower' than growth plate, 'through' growth plate and 'rammed'.

Treatment

The method of treatment depends on a variety of factors including age, occupation and likely compliance

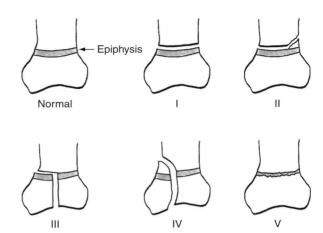

Figure 6.9 The Salter–Harris classification of paediatric fractures.

with the full treatment course. Other factors are related to the injury itself:

'Acceptable' hand fractures

- Tuft of distal phalanx.
- AP displacement of metaphyseal fractures in children.
- Metacarpal neck fractures.
  - < 15° angulation in middle finger and ring finger.
  - < 50° angulation in index finger and little finger.
- Metacarpal base fractures.
  - < 20° in adults.
  - < 40° in children.

'Unacceptable' phalangeal fractures

- Rotational angulation.
- Severe dorsal angulation.
- Lateral angulation.
- Finger scissoring.
- Open or intra-articular fractures.
- Fractures with bone loss or associated with neurovascular or tendon injury.

Generally, the indications for fixation of non-articular fractures are:

- Angulation (except modest AP angulation in children).
- Rotation.
- Shortening.

Complications of fractures

- Infection 2–11% of open fractures.
- Malunion – rotation, angulation, shortening.
- Non-union (which may require ostetomy and bone graft).
- Stiffness – loss of motion that may be due to adhesions, capsular contracture, joint injury. **Finger stiffness is the most common complication following surgical treatment of phalangeal fractures.**

Techniques of fixation

- Lag screw fixation – spiral fractures.
- Screw plus miniplate (generally only metacarpal fractures).
- Crossed K-wiring.
- Interosseus wiring/Lister loop.
- Bone tie (Sammut).
- External fixation (S-QUATTRO) – comminuted open/closed fractures.

Phalangeal fractures

- Distal phalanx – avulsion fractures associated with flexor or extensor (Mallet) injuries (see tendon injuries).
- Other phalangeal (i.e. middle or proximal) fractures.

Classification

- Unicondylar/bicondylar – tend to be unstable – displaced fractures usually need open reduction.
- Neck – closed reduction and plaster of Paris (POP) for non-displaced fractures, whilst displaced fractures require an open approach and K-wiring.
- Shaft fractures – transverse or spiral fractures are usually stable and can be treated by splintage whilst oblique fractures tend to be unstable and need fixation (closed or open). Comminuted fractures may need external fixation.
- Base – these fractures are typically impacted with apex volar angulation – up to 25° is reasonably well tolerated but greater degrees should be reduced and fixed. Fractures at the base of the MP are often associated with PIPJ dislocation (usually dorsal with avulsion of volar base of MP).

Non-union of phalangeal fractures is uncommon (except in severe soft tissue/bone injury/loss) whilst malunion is fairly common and may require corrective osteotomies.

Metacarpal fractures

Metacarpal head

These are relatively rare and are usually intra-articular. Closed fractures without joint problems (stable MCPJ on stressing) or up to 20% articular surface involvement may be managed non-operatively.

- Percutaneous K-wires with or without a circulage wire in parallel splinting to adjacent metacarpal × 2 intramedullary K-wires (neck fractures).
- Miniplate fixation via dorsal approach.
- External fixation if there is soft tissue loss or the PP is also fractured.
- MCPJ arthrodesis is a salvage procedure for a severe comminuted fracture.

Metacarpal neck

These fractures usually involve axial load to a clenched fist i.e. hitting a hard object (e.g. boxers' 5th metacarpal neck fracture) and are relatively common, comprising up to 20% of hand fractures. There is usually apex dorsal angulation since the intrinsics are volar and maintain a flexed MC head/MCPJ posture. Treatment is required in cases with:

- Angulation of more than 10–15° in the index/middle (fixed) or 30–40° ring, 50–60° (some say 40–45°) little fingers (latter have greater mobility). Less angulation is tolerated in the index/middle fingers due to the reduced CMCJ mobility.
  - There is some controversy over the 'acceptable' angulation though the more distal an injury the more angulation can be tolerated without affecting function. In general, proper reduction is advised as it improves cosmesis and avoids palmar metacarpal head deformity in the palm, which may interfere with grasping.
  - Angulations of more than 30–40° may interfere with extensor function and lead to pseudoclawing (MCPJ hyperextension with extension deficit/flexion contracture at PIPJ as the patient attempts to extend the finger).
- Rotational deformity/scissoring – every 5° rotation causes 1.5 cm digital overlap.
  - In extension, the fingers should be in parallel whilst in flexion they should point towards the scaphoid tuberosity.
- Shortening > 3 mm.

Management

- **Closed reduction should be attempted in those with angulation** (Jahss SA. *J Bone Joint Surg* 1938;**20**:178–186) – flex MCJP to 90 degrees to relax the intrinsics and tighten the collateral ligaments (and flex IPJs), then reduce the fracture with downwards (volar) pressure on the metacarpal shaft at the angulation whilst applying dorsally directed pressure at the PIPJ.
  - If it is then stable – place in POP (MCPJ flex but IPJ extended) for 2–3 weeks followed by aggressive mobilization. It may be difficult to maintain reduction with the swelling.
  - If unstable then K-wires (crossed at neck or transverse with adjacent metacarpal).
- Open reduction – dorsal approach.

Metacarpal shaft

These tend to be transverse from a direct/axial force or spiral/oblique from torsion. The border metacarpals tend to be less stable as they have less support from the intrinsics or transverse metacarpal ligament. There is usually **apex dorsal angulation** due to the action of interosseus muscles. Treat if:

- Angulation of more than 10° index, middle or 20° ring or 30° little fingers.
- Rotational deformity/scissoring.
- Shortening > 3 mm. Greater degrees of shortening are often associated with rotation.

Management

- Non-operative – closed reduction and splint with wrist 30° extension, 90° degrees MCJP and IPJ extension.
- Surgery – if unstable/multiple or open fractures via a dorsal approach – K-wires, plates or lag screws.

Metacarpal base – these are rare and usually intra-articular.

Metacarpal shaft fracture with segmental loss – stabilize and maintain length with external fixation, with immediate or delayed bone grafting; soft tissue cover may be needed.

Thumb fractures

- **Bennett's fracture** – oblique intra-articular (CMCJ) fracture of the **base** of the first metacarpal in the dorso-volar axis. It is caused by compression along a partly flexed metacarpal and is thus often sustained when punching. It is the most frequent thumb fracture and tends to be unstable.
  - The metacarpal base is subluxed dorsally, proximally and radially due to traction on the **APL tendon**. The anterior fragment of bone is attached to ulnar collateral ligament and volar plate.
  - The optimal treatment is screw fixation via a radial approach, particularly in fractures with more displacement; an alternative is a percutaneous K-wire through thumb metacarpal, trapezium and second metacarpal.
  - **Reversed Bennett's fracture** is analogous to Bennett's except that it occurs in the fifth metacarpal base. Deformation occurs due to traction by the extensor carpi ulnaris tendon and hypothenar muscles. The motor branch of ulnar nerve may be injured. It is usually treated by closed reduction and K-wire fixation to the 4th metacarpal and hamate.
- **Rolando fracture** – similar to Bennett's except that the dorsal, avulsed segment has a 'T-condylar' fracture, or Y or comminuted form. Treat by K-wiring or T-plate, except for comminuted fractures (spica cast or external fixation).

VII. Dislocation

Phalangeal dislocations

Dislocations are named in relation to the distal bone position and can be dorsal, volar or lateral. Stability should be assessed under block (wrist or ring) and compared to the contralateral digit.

- Passive stability – lateral stress to joint at full extension and 30 degrees flexion, assess collaterals.
- Active stability – active ROM, any dislocation with motion indicates an unstable joint.

Collateral ligament sprain.

- Grade I – stable with microscopic tear.
- Grade II – intact ligament but with abnormal laxity on stressing.
- Grade III – complete tear with instability.

The MCPJ has a shape likened to a box that can resist injury and dislocation with the support of intrinsic ligaments and surrounding structures e.g. sagittal bands, tendons etc. The volar plate is the floor of the joint. The shape means that with flexion there is linear stretch of the collateral ligaments and when more than 70°, the joint is laterally stable.

Metacarpophalangeal dislocation
Classification

- **Open or closed.**
- **Simple** (reduce easily) or **complex** (will not reduce due to soft tissue interposition especially volar plate interposition between metacarpal head and base of PP). In general, complex dislocations more common in 'border' digits – thumb, index and little fingers.

If closed and stable, begin movement as pain allows with buddy strap.

With the more common volar dislocations, the head of the metacarpal protrudes into the palm between lumbrical and flexor tendons and the **volar plate is in the joint space** with the flexor tendons still attached and tightened counteracting any reduction force – thus open reduction may be needed with A1 release to relax tension.

Collateral ligaments may be ruptured (ulnar collateral ligament (UCL) very rarely) particularly radial side, and may present late with persistent swelling and pain with localized tenderness as well as demonstrable instability. The joint can be immobilized in 30° flexion for 2 weeks and reassessed – persistent instability may respond to buddy strapping or may require repair, especially if more than 6 weeks.

Interphalangeal dislocation

The IPJ volar plate is confluent with the periosteum of the phalanges – it prevents hyperextension and provides lateral stability. Due to its box-like shape/configuration, dislocation usually implies disruption of at least two parts.

- DIPJ dislocations are less common and are usually dorsal. They are usually easily reduced by longitudinal traction and then should be splinted.
- PIPJ dislocations are one of the commonest ligamentous hand injuries. They commonly result in flexion contracture and permanent fusiform enlargement of the joint. **Dorsal dislocation** is more common whilst volar dislocation is rare and due to central slip avulsion after hyperextension (need K-wire for 6 weeks to allow central slip healing). There is volar plate damage in 80%.

Classification

- Type 1 – hyperextension injury with volar plate damage; there is partial articulation with the MP locked in hyperextension. These can usually be reduced without surgery and then immobilized for 2 weeks.
  - Untreated injury may lead to chronic PIPJ subluxation and swan-neck deformity. It can be distinguished from volar plate injury by asking the patient to extend the DIPJ whilst stabilizing the PIPJ in extension – extension will be normal in volar plate injury. Treatment includes FDS tenodesis (sublimis sling) with radial tendon slip passed through hole in PP in an ulnar to radial direction and then anchored to the periosteum, with the joint in about 5° of flexion.
- Type 2 – dorsal dislocation – usually a complete dislocation with volar plate avulsion. Treat as type 1.
- Type 3 – Fracture dislocation – avulsion of volar MP with the volar plate.
  - More than 40% articular surface usually means it is unstable. Large fragments need ORIF with fixation. Dynamic (Suzuki) traction is an option for comminuted fractures.
  - Stable injuries usually have less than 40% injury and are usually stable after reduction.

Management

- Simple, closed dorsal dislocations (volar plate avulsion ± small volar fragment) may be treated conservatively (mobilize plus extension-block splint).
- Complex dislocations require open reduction and volar plate removal and repair.

Collateral ligament fibrosis will follow PIPJ dislocation after about a year – it can be reduced by rehabilitation but may require excision (whilst preserving lateral band).

Thumb

The thumb MCPJ has proper and accessory collateral ligaments in addition to support by muscle insertions.

Acute UCL injury (ski thumb – associated with fall on hand with abducted thumb) is much more common than radial injury. There may be avulsion fractures of the PP – small fragments can be treated with a thumb spica whilst large displaced fragments will need ORIF and K-wire or ORIF.

- Partial tears may be treated by splintage in POP for about 4 weeks followed by active exercises. Complete ruptures generally need repair.
- **Stener lesion** is a completely torn UCL that lies superficial to the adductor expansion and will not heal without surgery.

Gamekeeper's thumb is a chronic type of UCL injury either due to progressive attenuation e.g. rheumatoid arthritis or secondary to untreated complete tears. There is a tear of the ulnar collateral ligament of the MCPJ due to hyperextension injury causing volar plate disruption. There is pain and thumb weakness.

- Reattach the ligament using an interosseus wire, suture or Mitek bone anchor and K-wire the MCPJ joint (6 weeks). Repair the UCL (may need reconstruction – PL/plantaris, FCR/APL slip), accessory ligament, volar plate and dorsal capsule as all of these will lend stability to the joint.
- Bony Gamekeeper's thumb may be treated conservatively if the fracture fragment involves < 15–20% of the articular surface.

Dorsal MCPJ dislocation is more common than volar in the thumb and is usually secondary to hyperextension injury. Reducible injuries can be splinted whilst irreducible dislocations (sesamoid bone, FPL tendon or volar plate interposition) will need surgery.

VIII. Wrist

Wrist

- All axes of wrist movement pass through the capitate.
- Two-thirds of wrist flexion occurs at the radiocarpal joint, one-third at the mid-carpal joint.
- 80% of the longitudinal force applied to the wrist is transmitted through the radiocarpal joint and 20% through the ulnocarpal articulation, but positive ulnar variance increases load through the ulna.

The insertion of the FCU tendon to the pisiform is the only direct insertion of extrinsic tendons to the carpus. The radiocarpal ligament connects the radius to the triquetral via the lunate.

In full supination, the radius and ulna lie parallel but in full pronation – they are crossed and the radius projects less distally – hence when assessing variance the forearm must be in mid-pronation: hand and wrist flat on the X-ray cassette, shoulder abducted to 90° and elbow flexed to 90°.

Distal radio-ulnar joint

The distal radio-ulnar joint (DRUJ) is a trochoid joint (rotatory joint where cylinder fits in a corresponding cavity); the triangular fibrocartilage complex (TFCC) is a major stabilizer of the joint and separates radio-carpal and radio-ulnar joints. Disease in the DRUJ such as arthritis can lead to a reduced range of movement especially supination with tenderness. The joint can be injured traumatically with fractures, subluxations or dislocations as well as TFCC tears.

The joint can be imaged with plain X-rays, MRI or arthrograms, which are the gold standard.

Carpal ligaments

The radius and carpus rotate around the free ulna and there are two types of carpal ligaments:

- **Interosseus** ligaments which are between adjacent bones and connect all four carpal bones of the distal row and individual carpal bones to forearm bones, e.g. radioscapholunate ligament of Testut.
- **Transosseus** ligaments between non-adjacent bones e.g. radioscaphocapitate (sling ligament), radiolunate (short and long), triquetrohamatocapitate (THC).

Wrist instability around the scaphoid and ligamentous laxity between proximal and distal carpal rows can be classified as dorsal or volar intercalated segment instability (DISI/VISI) and is tested for by palpating the scaphoid as the wrist is put into radial and ulnar deviation.

Wrist instability is usually due to tearing or stretching of ligaments of the carpus; the radioscapho-capitate ligament is the most important for wrist support. A common cause is a fall on an outstretched hand – which causes dorsiflexion with ulnar deviation, leading to intercarpal supination that may result in a lunate or perilunate dislocation (which are often not recognized at the time of first presentation).

- **Terry Thomas sign** – increased gap (> 3 mm) between scaphoid and lunate, named after the dental gap of the eponymous comedian (some call it the **David Letterman** sign). It suggests rupture of the scapholunate ligament (i.e. scapholunate dissociation, SLD), which can be a cause of chronic wrist pain and disability.
- An increase in the scapholunate angle beyond 60°.
- In assessing carpal height radiographically, the ratio of the distance between distal capitate and

proximal lunate to the length of the third metacarpal should be 0.54 ± 0.03.

Carpal instability patterns

- Ulnar translocation.
- DISI – relatively common. The lunate rotates into dorsiflexion whilst the capitate displaces dorsally. It occurs after SLD and scapholunate ligament tears which should be repaired.
- VISI – associated with spilled tea-cup sign.
- Non-dissociative carpal stability – lax ligaments, can shift into VISI/DISI but is correctable. There is a painful 'clunk'; X-rays and arthrogram are normal.
  - Capitolunate instability.
  - Midcarpal instability.
- Dissociative – ligament disruption, X-ray changes.
  - Scapholunate instability.
  - Lunotriquetral (LT) dissociation.

History

- Age, sex, occupation, hand dominance, hobbies.
- Site of pain.
- Duration of the pain, provoking or relieving factors.
- Functional disability.
- Any history of hand trauma/surgery, rheumatoid arthritis/osteoarthritis.
- Drugs, allergies, medical history, smoking history.

Examination of the wrist

Look

- Skin changes – scars, RSD features, wasting.
- Swellings including synovium and masses e.g. ganglia, prominent ulnar head, carpometacarpal boss.
- Shape/position of the wrist, e.g. ulnar deviation.

Feel

- Masses.
- Areas of tenderness.

Move

- Passive then active.
- Flexion/extension, supination/pronation, radial/ulnar deviation.
- Finger flexion/extension.
- Full nerve examination.

- **AP draw test** – to test mid-carpal stability – traction applied to the wrist and anteroposterior forces exerted at the mid-carpal level.
- **Pivot shift test** – supinate the hand, with a thumb behind the ulnar side of the wrist, volarly sublux the ulnar carpus and move the hand from radial to ulnar deviation. If there is excessive ligamentous laxity, the capitate will sublux volarly during this manoeuvre.

Investigations

- AP and lateral films (± Eaton views for basal joints), **Gilula's lines** for continuity of radiocarpal and mid-carpal joints.
- Look specifically for scapholunate advanced collapse pattern of arthritis (SLAC) wrist and decreased Huber index.

Differential diagnoses for wrist pain i.e. bone/joint or soft tissues

Radial wrist pain.

- Basal joint osteoarthritis (CMC axial grind test).
- Ischaemic necrosis of scaphoid.
- de Quervain's tenosynovitis (first compartment) – vide infra.
- Intersection syndrome (second compartment tenosynovitis) – vide infra.
- Wartenberg's syndrome (superficial branch of radial nerve entrapment).
- SL dissociation.
- Synovitis.

Central wrist pain.

- Kienbock's disease.
- Ganglia/metacarpal boss – a small mass of bone usually found at the base of the 2nd/3rd metacarpal bones where they meet the small bones of the wrist. Patients present with pain and lack of mobility.
- Synovitis.

Ulnar wrist pain.

- Ulnar impingement syndrome.
- Lunotriquetral dissociation/instability (ballotment test/shuck test).
- DRUJ subluxation – piano key.
- Synovitis especially flexor carpi ulnaris (FCU) tenosynovitis.

Treatment

Treatment is tailored to individual problem (see relevant sections). Rheumatoid arthritis, scaphoid necrosis and Kienbock's disease can all cause scapholunate ligament rupture and diastasis which is clinically manifested by DISI with rotatory subluxation of the scaphoid (X-rays show a SLAC wrist, decreased Huber index, Terry Thomas sign). For example:

- Primary scaphoid necrosis – treat with splint, ORIF or excision and rolled tendon spacer.
- Primary Kienbock's disease – treat with splint, ulnar lengthening/radial shortening, capitohamate fusion, excision and rolled tendon spacer.

De Quervain's disease (1895)

Musculotendinous units can become inflamed either where they pass through tunnels or at a bony attachment. De Quervain's disease is a stenosing tenovaginitis of the APL tendon within the first dorsal compartment. In 20–30% of patients there may be two separate tunnels for each tendon (APL and EPB); EPB is absent in ~5% of people. It commonly affects middle-aged women and usually presents as several months of radial wrist pain aggravated by movement and may be associated with overuse.

Signs

- Positive **Finkelstein** test (pain on ulnar deviation with the thumb clasped in the fist).
- It may co-exist with basal joint osteoarthritis, and there may be a small ganglion in the first dorsal compartment.
- It can be differentiated from the intersection syndrome where the pain is more proximally located.

Management

- Non-operative: NSAIDs, wrist immobilization and steroid injections.
- Operative: longitudinal release of the first compartment by incising extensor retinaculum through a 2-cm transverse incision just above the level of the radial styloid. In RA cases, synovectomy may also be required. It is important to preserve the superficial branch of the radial nerve.

Intersection syndrome

Pain and swelling of muscle bellies of APL and EPB at the site at which they cross (hence 'intersection') the tendons of the second dorsal compartment, ECRL and ECRB, about 4 cm proximal to the wrist. Basic pathology relates to a tenosynovitis of the second dorsal compartment. Operative treatment is by release of the second compartment in a similar fashion to De Quervain's.

Wrist dislocations

- **Lunate dislocation**: Anterior (volar) dislocation of the lunate signifies dorsal radiocarpal ligament failure and is a cause of acute CTS. Dorsal dislocations are rare.
- **Perilunate dislocation**: lunate is in the correct position but the capitate and the rest of the carpus are not.
- Mid-carpal dislocation: neither the lunate nor the capitate is in alignment with the radius.

Radiological signs: the lunate appears triangular on the AP view and the capitate does not sit in the cup of the lunate on the lateral film. In cases of perilunate dislocation, the lunate remains appropriately positioned on the radius while the rest of the carpus is displaced.

Treatment: prompt treatment with GA/muscle relaxant and traction.

- Reduce and POP (Taverners).
- Percutaneous K-wire.
- ORIF.

Scapholunate instability

This is the most common ligament injury of the wrist which, if untreated, can lead to DISI and SLAC. Scapholunate ligamentous laxity can be due to:

- Osteoarthritis, rheumatoid arthritis.
- Avascular necrosis (AVN) of the scaphoid (trauma or Presier's) or lunate (Kienbock's).

It can be classified by the Geisler staging (1–4). There is a spectrum of injury (increasing severity):

- RSS – rotatory subluxation of scaphoid.
- SLD – scapholunate dissociation/diastasis.
- DISI/VISI is due to lunotriquetral ligament disruption.
- SLAC.

X-ray signs

- Signet-ring sign on PA radiograph due to volar tilting of the scaphoid – 'double bubble' as scaphoid hyperflexes – humpback deformity.

- **Terry Thomas sign** of SLD – scapholunate interval > 2–3 mm.
- SLAC wrist with decrease in the Huber index (disease begins at the radioscaphoid joint).

Magnetic resonance arthrograms are 95% accurate for SL tears; however, arthrograms will detect SL tears in 27% of patients with no symptoms. **Arthroscopy is the definitive test**.

Treatment

- Early – closed reduction and K-wiring or open reduction and ligament repair.
- Chronic – open reduction and ligament repair (Mitek), ligament reconstruction, limited intercarpal fusion. Blatt capsulodesis or Brunelli tenodesis – split FCR is routed through drill hole in scaphoid, to stop it from flexing, and has variable results.
- RSS alone: triscaphe fusion – scaphoid, trapezium, trapezoid to provide a stable column for the radial axis.
- SLAC wrist: excision of the scaphoid and radial styloid, with 4-corner fusion of the capitate, lunate, hamate and triquetrum (CLHT) results in significant decrease in wrist range of movement. The lunate fossa and proximal articular surface of the lunate must be normal.

Surgical treatment of scapholunate advanced collapse

Krakauer JD. *J Hand Surg* 1994;**19**:751–759.

Most cases of SLAC wrist are due to scapholunate dissociation which leads to dorsal intercalated segment instability (DISI), shifting stress forces to the radioscaphoid articulation. It may also be caused by other aetiologies including rheumatoid arthritis – SLAC wrist is the most common pattern of degenerative wrist arthritis and it may have minimal symptoms.

There is sequential degeneration of:

- Radial styloid (stage 1).
- Entire scaphoid fossa of the radius (stage 2).
- Capitolunate joint (stage 3).

Surgical options:

- Scaphoid excision and silicone implant.
- Scaphoid excision and intercarpal arthrodesis – capitate, lunate, hamate, triquetrum.
- Proximal row carpectomy.

- Radiocarpal arthrodesis.
- Total wrist arthrodesis.

Ulnar abutment (impingement) syndrome

- Positive ulnar variance with degeneration of the TFCC.
- Ulnar-sided wrist pain.
- Confirmed by MRI or arthroscopy.
- Treated during arthroscopy by excision of TFCC tears (as for meniscal cartilage tears in knee arthroscopy). Salvage procedure is ulnar shortening.

Kienbock's disease

(See also Kienbock's disease. Almquist EE. *Clin Orth Rel Res* 1986;**202**:68–78.)

This is an avascular necrosis of the dorsal pole of the lunate (lunatomalacia in 1910) with collapse. It is usually idiopathic, possibly due to some primary vascular insufficiency or secondary to trauma (> 50% have a history of wrist trauma). There is a strong association with **ulnar minus/negative variant** (short ulna), which is present in 23% of normal wrists but present in 78% of Kienbock's wrists – in these patients, the lunate is subjected to greater shear stress forces potentially compromising its volar blood supply.

- Fault plate hypothesis (Watson HK. *J Hand Surg* (Br) 1997;**22**:5–7).
- Extrinsic factors e.g. lunate loading due to differential radii of curvature of lunate and capitate.
- Intrinsic factors e.g. cortical strength of lunate, trabecular pattern, vascular anatomy – the bone has many articulations and is almost completely covered by articular cartilage, with a lack of a dominant vessel.

Clinical features

It usually presents as a painful, stiff, swollen wrist in young active adults (males 4×) with decreased grip strength but there is a very variable symptomatology and rate of progression e.g. it can be asymptomatic in some. Usually the condition is unilateral, favouring the dominant wrist, and more common in manual workers or those performing repetitive tasks.

Plain radiographs may show:

- Radiolucent line indicating compression fracture.
- Demineralization surrounding a fracture line (< 3 months).

- Sclerosis of the dorsal pole (~3 months).
- Fragmentation and flattening.
- Wrist arthrosis.
- Capitate collapse (end stage).

Other methods:

- Bone scan.
- MRI/CT (shows occult fractures).

Lichtman staging (radiological)

- Stage 1: normal except possibility of linear or compression fracture.
- Stage 2: **lunate sclerosis** – density changes in lunate.
- Stage 3A: **collapse of entire lunate** without fixed scaphoid rotation.
- Stage 3B: collapse of entire lunate with fixed scaphoid rotation – in such cases, further collapse is hastened due to shifting load onto lunate shorten radius.
- Stage 4: as above with generalized degenerative changes in carpus. **Carpal arthritis**.

Modified Stahl's classification of Kienbock's disease:

- Stage 1: normal structure of the lunate, with evidence of compression fracture usually appearing as a radiodense or radiolucent line.
- Stage 2: rarification along the line of previous compression fractures, developing within the first 3 months.
- Stage 3: changes of stages 1 and 2 together with sclerosis of proximal pole, occurring at about 3 months.
- Stage 4: fragmentation or flattening of the lunate.
- Stage 5: changes of arthrosis of radial carpal and inner-carpal joints.

Treatment aims to prevent deformity and restore normal appearance and function.

Early disease

- Positive bone scan, X-ray normal – immobilization and analgesia but rarely effective even in the early stages.
- Sclerotic changes on X-ray – joint levelling procedure either radial shortening (about 2 mm) to restore neutral ulnar variance and redistributes load or some suggest ulnar lengthening (more difficult than radial shortening). This is one of the most common procedures.

- Lunate resection, fill with tendon or capito-hamate fusion to prevent capitate subluxing into proximal carpal row in the absence of the lunate. (Treatment of Kienbock's disease with capitohamate arthrodesis. Oishi SN. *Plast Reconstr Surg* 2002;**109**:1293–1300.)

Late disease

- Intercarpal fusion/limited wrist arthrodesis.
  - Scaphoid–trapezium–trapezoid fusion with excision of the radial styloid.
  - Saphoid capitate fusion.
- Revascularization procedures.
  - Pronator quadratus turnover flap.
  - Pedicled dorsal metacarpal artery buried in lunate.

Other options include:

- Wrist dennervation.
- Excision of the lunate and replacement with a silastic implant, rolled tendon graft or vascularized pisiform. (Saffar P. *Ann Chir Main* 1982;**1**:276–279.)

Ulnar variance

If a horizontal line is drawn from the junction of the distal articular surface and sigmoid notch of the radius, then neutral (ulnar head level) – normal.

- Positive variance (ulnar head above line) – may cause ulnar impingement syndrome.
- Negative variance (ulnar head below line) – may lead to **Kienbock's disease**, scapholunate dislocation.

Scaphoid fractures

The scaphoid is the most commonly fractured wrist bone – 80% of carpal bone fractures. Most are sustained by a fall on an outstretched hand – the wrist is dorsiflexed and radially deviated.

The **scaphoid series** is a PA wrist with ulnar deviation (to rotate the scaphoid away from the radius), lateral and oblique wrist. The scaphoid view i.e. ulnar deviated PA with 20–30° tube angle aims to get an *en face* view. The fracture is visible after 10–14 days, or earlier by CT or MRI – the latter is the most sensitive and specific assessment of post-traumatic avascular necrosis.

- Avascular necrosis of the proximal pole is heralded by radiological sclerosis.

- The fracture line becomes an extension of the mid-carpal joint and movement here promotes flexion of the distal row and extension of the proximal row, hence a loss of wrist extension.
- The mal/non-united scaphoid adopts a flexed attitude (apex dorsal) leading to the so-called **humpback deformity.** It is most commonly associated with DISI.
- There is a fairly predictable sequence of arthritic changes in the radioscaphoid and capitolunate joints, leading to **scapholunate advanced collapse** (SLAC wrist), rotatory subluxation of the scaphoid and a decrease in the Huber index on the X-ray.

Treatment

- **No displacement** – stable fractures can be managed conservatively by immobilization in a scaphoid plaster (**short arm thumb spica** – wrist pronated, radial deviated and moderately dorsiflexed – which should allow thumb IPJ flexion, finger MPCJ and elbow flexion); the traditional cast has its critics. 95% of waist fractures unite when fixed. Late presentation increases the rate of non-union and eventual degeneration.
  - Surgery is usually reserved for unstable fractures, very proximal fractures or mal/non-united fractures.
- **Displacement** – **unstable fractures** (displacement and angulation) and **very proximal** fractures (risk of AVN) usually need open reduction and internal fixation (Herbert screw) – with cancellous bone graft from radius to correct humpback deformity. ORIF is associated with 80% union rate.
- **Non-union without AVN** – non-vascular bone graft (Matte–Rewse) e.g. iliac.
- **Avascular necrosis** – vascularized bone graft e.g. Kuhlmann procedure with volar radial bone flap from beneath pronator quadratus on a branch from radial artery (volar carpal artery can be traced to bone surface and can be raised alone with the ulnar bone graft), or scaphoid excision and rolled tendon graft, four-corner fusion (lunate to capitate to hamate to triquetral to lunate wrist arthrodesis) may be a 'salvage' option.
- **Arthritis** – radial styloid excision, radioscaphoid fusion, proximal row carpectomy or total wrist arthrodesis (SLAC wrist).

Non-union of scaphoid
General factors

- Gap too large or separation of ends e.g. soft tissue or dead bone interposition.
- Avascularity and infection.
- Excessive interfragmentary movement.
- Poor internal fixation holding ends in distraction.
- Adverse systemic factors (anaemia, steroids, malnutrition, etc.).

Treatment

Uniting the fracture will increase function, reduce pain and reduce the risk of future degenerative disease. Surgery can be performed by either a volar approach (for waist and distal fractures) or dorsal approach (proximal pole including AVN).

Primary avascular necrosis of the scaphoid (Preiser's disease) is rare. It may be due to repetitive microtrauma or be drug-related e.g. steroids or chemotherapy, in conjunction with defective proximal pole vascularity. It presents with wrist pain at rest and with movement and decreased grip strength. It is more common in the dominant hand.

Investigations

- Radiographs, **MRI** – local decrease in intensity on T1.
- Features are similar to Kienbock's: initially cystic and sclerotic and may lead to fracture or collapse of the bone.

Hamate fractures

This injury may be incurred by falling on the outstretched hand; it is increasing in incidence due to sports particularly those played with racquets or clubs. It often presents weeks to months after with palmar pain increased with grasping, dorsoulnar deviation and flexion of 4/5th digits. It may cause ulnar nerve compression at Guyon's canal and may be associated with tendon injuries.

- Image with radiographs, CT as standard or MRI.
- The usual treatment is ORIF or excision. The traditional treatment of immobilization for 6 weeks has a high non-union rate.

Trauma-induced cold-associated symptoms (TICAS)
What is cold intolerance?
Campbell DA. *J Hand Surg* 1998;**23**:3–5.

A collection of acquired symptoms resulting in an abnormal aversion to cold:

- Pain/discomfort (93%, most troublesome) and stiffness.
- Altered sensibility.
- Colour change (least troublesome).

About half of all patients experience these symptoms from the time of injury. Approximately half experience symptoms after a lag period of ~4 months, mostly coinciding with the first cold day of winter. Patients may experience TICAS for the two winters following injury but symptoms generally improve thereafter.

IX. Nail-bed injury

Anatomy

- Hyponychium – this is the junction between the skin of the fingertip and the sterile matrix at the distal end of the nail. It has a large number of lymphocytes as an immune barrier to deal with the heavy contamination at this site.
- Eponychium – distal part of nail fold attached to surface of nail.
- Nail fold – ventral floor is the germinal matrix whilst the dorsal roof is formed from cells that impart the shiny layer to the nail surface.
- Nail plate – keratinized squamous cells attached to nail bed – strongly adherent to sterile matrix whilst it is only loosely attached to the germinal matrix. The nail acts as a counterforce to the fingertip pad to increase sensitivity; the 2-point discrimination decreases when the nail is absent.

It takes an average of 3 months for full nail growth (there is often a 3-week delay after injury); the average growth rate is 0.1 mm/day. Growth is faster in longer digits, in younger patients, nail biters and in the summer.

- The germinal matrix contributes 90% of the volume of the nail (plate).
- The sterile matrix is mainly responsible for adherence of the nail.
- The smooth surface layer is derived from the tissue at the roof of the nail fold.

Nail growth

- The germinal matrix contributes 90% of nail production. The lunula is the white arc of germinal matrix where nuclei persist in the basilar cells; as the nuclei gradually disintegrates distally, the nail plate becomes clear.
- Dorsal roof of nail fold – contributes the top layer that imparts the shine.
- Sterile matrix – this is the portion of the nail bed distal to the lunula and contributes 10% to the nail as well as providing adherence.

Injury of nail bed

Fifty per cent are associated with a fracture of the distal phalanx.

Allen classification of fingertip injuries

- I – pulp involved only – distal to nail bed. Can treat non-operatively e.g. dressing/hyphecan cap or with a skin graft.

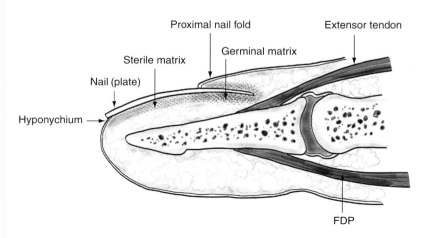

Figure 6.10 Sagittal section of a fingertip showing the structures of the nail area; the nail bed is composed of the sterile and germinal matrix.

Labels: Proximal nail fold, Germinal matrix, Extensor tendon, Sterile matrix, Nail (plate), Hyponychium, FDP

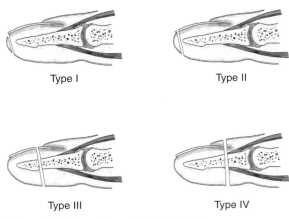

Figure 6.11 Types of fingertip/nail-bed injuries.

- II – pulp and part of nail bed but bone is not exposed. Treatment choices include non-operatively, composite graft, skin grafts or flap closure.
- III – involves distal phalanx i.e. fractured – flap/terminalization/hyphecan cap.
- IV – involves lunula as well. Replantation may be considered, flap or amputation.

Haematomas under the nail bed can be drained by trephination (using a hollow needle) if less than 50% of the area of the nail plate; larger haematomas should be formally explored with removal of the nail as there is a high risk of nail-bed injury which should be repaired.

- **Acute** treatment is preferred as secondary nail-bed repair/revisions are rarely satisfactory. Nail bed that has been detached along with a nail-plate avulsion/injury can be replaced as a free graft; large defects in the nail bed may be repaired with a split nail-bed graft from either undamaged parts of the injured finger or the hallux.
- X-rays are advised as 50% of nail-bed injuries are associated with a fracture of the distal phalanx – most are minor/non-displaced and require no treatment other than repair of the nail bed with the nail plate replaced as a splint (also important to prevent scarring/adhesions between the floor and roof of the nail fold)

Van Beek classification

- I – small (< 25%) subungual haematoma.
- II – larger (> 50%) subungual haematoma.

- III – nail-bed laceration associated with fracture of distal phalanx.
- IV – nail-bed fragmentation.
- V – nail-bed avulsion.

Classically:

- Types I and II can be treated with trephination.
- Type III – remove nail plate for exploration and repair. Splint the nail fold to prevent adhesions that may otherwise lead to ridging or other abnormalities.
- Types IV and V – secondary healing will tend to leave misshapen non-adherent nails.

In general, nail plates that are still adherent with intact nail folds should be left alone where possible whilst where the nail fold is disrupted or the plate is dislodged from the nail bed, these injuries should be explored/repaired.

Consider homodigital advancement pulp flaps (e.g. Atasoy) or heterodigital flaps with nail-bed grafts from distal amputations.

- Nail avulsion with segment of nail-bed on nail.
  ○ Remove the nail bed from the nail and use as a graft (can be placed directly on periosteum).
- Nail-bed avulsion.
  ○ For narrow (< 2 mm) avulsions, can use bipedicled advancement after wide undermining.
  ○ For wider avulsions, can use a split thickness nail-bed graft (from same digit if < 50% missing, or a toe if more) aiming to harvest 0.001 inch thickness with a 15 blade and then sewn in. Full thickness grafts e.g. lateral nail bed of hallux (close donor primarily).
  ○ Severe germinal matrix injury may require nail-bed ablation.

Fingertip injuries

The fingertip can be defined as the portion distal to the extensor and FDP tendon insertions. The skin is glabrous with a thick epidermis and deep papillary ridges that form the fingerprints. Under this, the pulp is fibrofatty tissue that has a dense network of fibrous septae from dermis to periosteum, as well as laterally by extensions from Cleland and Grayson's ligaments. Cleland ligaments are dorsal to the neurovascular bundle and attach the bone to the skin (B-C-D, bone-Cleland-dorsal); Grayson's ligaments are volar and attach the flexor to the skin.

- **Digital nerve – trifucates** at DIPJ to nail bed, distal fingertip and volar pulp.
- **Digital arteries** – trifurcate to nail fold, and two dorsal branches to volar pulp; the branches are interconnected by two anastomoses, one parallel to lunula and the other parallel to the free edge of the nail.
- Veins – predominantly via the dorsal valves that have valves even distally.

Fingertip/pulp reconstruction

Single digit replants

- Good outcome with injuries in zone I/distal to zone II.
- Poor outcome with injuries in zone II.
- Technical difficulty with venous repair if distal to an arbitrary line 4 mm proximal to the nail fold.

History

The patient assessment should include:

- Age, gender, occupation, handedness.
- Mechanism of injury and comorbidities.

Examination should concentrate on:

- Size, position and orientation of defect and its components including bone.
- State of flexor/extensor tendons.

The basic requirements of a successful reconstruction are sensate, durable padding and freedom from pain whilst preserving length and cosmesis.

There are many options including:

- **Dressings/secondary intention** – areas less than 1.5 cm^2 can heal satisfactorily by second intention.
- **Grafts**
  - Skin grafts e.g. hypothenar can be used, but there is a higher incidence of cold intolerance, post-operative tenderness and does not speed up the return to work (Holm A. *Acta Ortho Scand* 1974;**45**:382–392). Avoid use for index/thumb.
  - Composite grafts tend to work better in children under 6 years of age where replacing the fingertip at the very least works as a biological dressing.
- **Revision amputations** probably offer the quickest return to work, and should be considered in amputations proximal to the lunula or FDP/extensor tendon insertion. It is important to

prevent quadriga effect by leaving the FDP tendon untethered but it can be secured to the A4 pulley to prevent a lumbrical plus deformity (which would cause PIPJ extension and MCPJ flexion with attempted flexion due the retracting FDP pulling at the lumbrical origin). Other complications include: bone spicules, hook nail and neuroma.

- **Pedicled neurovascular island flap** – (**Foucher** flap – first dorsal metacarpal artery flap but may be of insufficient length to cover thumb pulp), **Littler** (1960) – from radial border of ring finger.
- Sensory cross-finger flap.
- **Free** neurovascular island flap from the big toe (toe–pulp transfer).

Homodigital flaps for fingertip injuries

There are many choices. In general, they can potentially provide near-normal sensation and are the method of choice for the pinch grip areas of the index and thumb.

- Kutler W. *J Am Med Assoc* 1947;**133**:29–30. (Bi) lateral V–Y advancement of distal skin.
- Hueston JT. *Plast Reconstr Surg* 1966;**37**:349–350. Volar skin transposition/advancement ± V–Y modification (Elliot) at base.
- Atasoy E. *J Bone Joint Surg* 1970;**52**:921–926. Volar V–Y advancement of distal skin, up to 1 cm.
- Macht SD. *J Hand Surg* 1980;**5**:372–376 **Moberg** flap: volar digit V–Y skin advancement for the thumb.
- Venkataswami R. *Plast Reconstr Surg* 1980;**66**:296–300. Half digit oblique volar skin advancement V–Y based on one neurovascular bundle.
- Evans 1988, Wilson 2004 (vide infra).

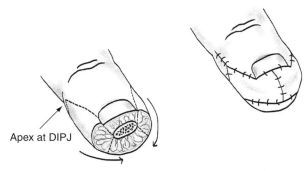

Apex at DIPJ

Figure 6.12 Kutler bilateral V–Y advancement flaps. The apex of the triangle reaches the level of the DIPJ; the triangles do not need to be equilateral. The flaps should be advanced with minimal disturbance of the subcutaneous tissue.

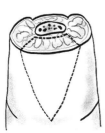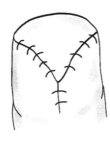

Figure 6.13 The V flap is lifted off the bone and relies on lateral attachments which should be dissected gently. Although it avoids a midline scar, the degree of advancement is often slight. A K-wire may be needed to fix the flap.

Step-advancement island flap for fingertip reconstruction

Evans DM. *Br J Plast Surg* 1988;**41**:105–111.

This technique exploits tissue laxity at the base of the finger, raising flaps down through fat to flexor sheath and under neurovascular bundle. The angles of the skin flaps get smaller proximally. This technique supposedly avoids flexion contracture occasionally seen after the Venkataswami flap. PIPJ extension can be started within 1 week.

Reverse digital artery island flap in the elderly

Wilson AD. *Injury* 2004;**35**:507–510.

This technique reconstructs the volar pulp and fingertip using an island of skin from the non-dominant border of the digit. The flap is based upon **reverse flow** in the ipsilateral digital artery via volar communicating vessels from the other side at a level 5 mm proximal to the DIP joint crease. The digital artery is ligated proximal to the flap and a segment of the dorsal nerve can be included for coaption to the distal stump of the digital nerve on the other side to render the flap sensate. A good functional outcome is possible even in elderly patients.

Heterodigital flaps

The use of non-injured digits can provide large areas of tissue but at the expense of a normal digit and reduced sensation.

- **Foucher flap** (Foucher G. *Plast Reconstr Surg* 1979;**63**:344–349) is based on the **first dorsal metacarpal artery** (DMCA). The distal skin paddle over the dorso-radial aspect of the PP of the index

finger is a random pattern extension from the dorso-radial aspect over the distal second metacarpal which must be raised with the flap. The flap is raised with a pedicle 1–2 cm in width with fascia and epimysium using a dorsal lazy-S incision, leaving paratenon for graft take; nerves are deep to veins but superficial to arteries. In 20%, there may not be a definitive vessel but there are several branches instead. The 'sink' branch at the level of the metacarpal head needs to be ligated. The superficial radial nerve can be included for protective sensation.
  - ○ It was originally described for dorsal thumb defects and may also be rotated to reconstitute dorsal ulnar defects but it is not really suitable for the thumb pulp.
- **Cross-finger flap** based upon dorsal branches of digital arteries and used mainly for volar defects of the digits – a cross-finger flap from the middle finger can be used for thumb defects. If the flap is de-epithelialized, it can be reversed for dorsal defects.
- **Littler flap** from radial border of ring finger.
- **Second DMCA flap** (Earley MI. *Br J Plast Surg* 1987;**40**:333–341) is based on the same technical principles as Foucher flap. There is a large anastomosing vessel between dorsal and palmar metacarpal arteries in the second web space which needs to be ligated (this is the vessel for Quaba flap). The second DMCA is larger than first DMCA in one-third of hands and may be used as a free flap. However, as the vein and artery lie either side of EC tendon, this does limit the arc of rotation.
- **Quaba flap** (Quaba AA. *Br J Plast Surg* 1990;**43**:24–27) is a distally based flap based on communicating vessel between second DMCA and palmar vessel which runs in second web space. There is no need to raise second DMCA beneath the skin paddle but can be raised at level of paratenon. It is useful for full-length defects of the dorsum of the finger.
- **Posterior interosseus artery flap** (Zancolli EA. *Surg Radiol Anat* 1986;**8**:209–215; Zancolli EA. *J Hand Surg* 1988;**13**:130–135). The ulnar artery gives off a common interosseus artery at the level of the neck of the radius which then divides into anterior and posterior interosseus arteries. The posterior interosseus vessels lie in the vertical septum radial to ECU and ulnar to EDM and sustains a fasciocutaneous flap with a long axis

along a line joining the ulnar head to the lateral epicondyle when the arm is pronated. When distally pedicled, the ulna head is the pivot point including around three perforators.

- **Flag flap** (Vilain R. *Plast Reconstr Surg* 1977;**52**:374–377).

Regional flaps

- Thenar flap – a reasonable choice for volar injuries of the index and middle fingers particularly in children (adults are prone to problems with contracture).
- Reversed or free radial forearm flap.

B. Upper limb nerve injuries

I. Brachial plexus anatomy

The brachial plexus has contributions from C5–T1; a plexus is termed pre-fixed or post-fixed if C4 or T2 contributes respectively.

- 'Roots' – lie behind scalenus anterior.
- Trunks – crosses the lower part of the posterior triangle.
- Divisions – lie behind the clavicle.
- Cords – embrace the axillary artery behind the pectoralis minor.
  - Lateral cord – musculocutaneous nerve.
  - Posterior cord – radial and axillary nerves.
  - Medial cord – median, ulnar and thoracodorsal nerves.

The dorsal root contains sensory afferents with cell bodies (but no synapses) in the dorsal root ganglion whilst the ventral root contains motor efferents (relay in anterior horn cells). The ventral roots combine to form the spinal nerve that splits into anterior and posterior rami. It is the **anterior rami of C5–T1** that form the 'roots' of the brachial plexus (the posterior rami become the posterior intercostal nerves and supply the erector spinae muscles).

- The serratus anterior is innervated by the long thoracic nerve – from the nerve roots of C5, 6, 7: if there is no winging of the scapula then the injury is more distal i.e. in the nerve trunks.
- Erb's point marks the convergence of the C5 and C6 roots to form the upper trunk.

Millesi classification

- I Supraganglionic.
- II Infraganglionic.

- III Trunk (or supraclavicular) – about 75% of cases.
- IV Cord (or infraclavicular) – e.g. shoulder dislocation. In general it has a better prognosis than supraclavicular injuries.

A **supraganglionic lesion** is where the disruption occurs at or proximal to the level of the dorsal root ganglion (e.g. root avulsion from cord, intradural rupture of rootlets). Such lesions are within the spinal canal hence are **not amenable to grafting** (or repair and thus usually treated by nerve transfers). As sensory nerves remain in continuity with their cell bodies in the dorsal root ganglion, sensory nerve action potentials may still be elicited. However, motor repair is not possible, as the nerves have been separated from the spinal cord.

Signs suggestive of supraganglionic injury:

- Denervation/motor paralysis of paravertebral/cervical muscles – scalenus anterior, levator scapulae and rhomboids.
- Sensory loss above shoulder/glenohumeral joint e.g. C3, 4.
- Horner's syndrome.
- Elevation of hemidiaphragm (inspiratory and expiratory CXR)
- Cervical spine fracture.
- Intractable pain.
- Lack of Tinel's at the neck.
- Sensory action potentials in anaesthetic arm with absent motor potentials.
- Negative intra-operative somatosensory evoked potentials.
- Pseudomeningocoele seen on myelography.

An **infraganglionic lesion** is where the disruption occurs in the spinal nerve distal to the dorsal root ganglion. Wallerian degeneration leads to no recordable action potentials. The paracervical muscles are intact.

Brachial plexus injuries arise largely from obstetric and (other) traumatic causes.

II. Obstetric brachial plexus injury

It occurs in about one per 1000 live births (very rare after caesarean section) and is associated with:

- Shoulder dystocia and high birth weight (maternal diabetes).
- Assisted delivery – breech presentation.

- Prolonged labour.
- Multiparity.

Diagnosis of injury is suggested by the lack of active movement with full passive mobility; Horner's syndrome (due to interruption of sympathetic outflow via the stellate ganglion, near to C8, T1) is a strong sign. Five per cent are bilateral.

Investigations

Direct diagnostic imaging is difficult:

- CXR to check for elevation of the hemidiaphragm.
- Myelography in children (needs GA) has high false-positive rate for root avulsion.
- MRI unreliable.
- EMG can be used to select muscles for transfer; in ~20% of patients with EMG showing prolonged conduction block, good recovery is possible.

Types of palsy

- **C5, 6 (+/− 7). Erb's palsy** due to downwards traction (or lateral flexion of the cervical spine or blow to the neck). It is the most common type of obstetric brachial plexus injury (Narakas type 1) (~75%).
  - Affects lateral and posterior cords (musculocutaneous, radial and axillary nerves).
  - Porter's tip position – shoulder adduction and internal rotation, elbow extension, forearm pronation, wrist flexion and finger flexion).
- **C7, 8, T1. Klumpke paralysis** is less common, and is due to traction upwards (breech delivery).
  - Affects medial cord (ulnar and median nerves).
  - Flail limb, claw hand, intrinsic muscle wasting, marbled appearance due to vasomotor changes, with or without Horner's syndrome.
- **Pan-plexus.**

Narakas classification

- Type 1 C5, 6 – Erb Duchenne (waiter's tip) (73%).
- Type 2 C5, 6, 7.
- Type 3 C5, 6, 7, 8.
- Type 4 C5, 6, 7, 8, T1 – Horner's syndrome.

Obstetric brachial palsy

Kay SP. *Br J Plast Surg* 1998;**51**:43–50.

Ninety-six per cent make a full recovery; poor recovery more likely in patients with:

- Lower root lesions, particularly those with Horner's syndrome.

- Associated fractures of clavicle, ribs, humerus.
- Avulsion injuries.

In most cases, it is advisable to wait at least 3 months for recovery of elbow flexion before exploring – most obstetric palsies will recover (there is a wide range reported for spontaneous recovery, 30–96%) but if there is no return **of biceps function by 3 months of age** then exploration is warranted. Exploration is also indicated if there is failure of recovery to progress after 9 months.

Early management consists of:

- Physiotherapy to maintain passive ROM whilst awaiting recovery and also allows spheroidal moulding of the humeral head and glenoid cavity.
- Indications for primary plexus exploration (repair, grafting):
  - Complete palsy with a flail arm.
  - C5–6 palsy with no biceps contraction at 3 months.
  - Horner's syndrome.
  - Phrenic nerve involvement.

Late management – tendon transfers, etc.

III. Traumatic brachial plexus injury

These most commonly occur in young males (15–25) particularly motorcyclists. Most are closed injuries due to traction, compression or a combination.

Causes of non-obstetric brachial plexus injury

- **Road traffic accidents** are the most common cause (70%, and 70% of these involve motorcycles). Forceful abduction of the arm overhead injures the lower trunk whilst violent bending of the neck tends to cause an upper trunk injury.
- **Open injuries** – it is important to exclude concomitant trauma to the axillary artery which may cause life- or limb-threatening haemorrhage. Sharp open injuries should be explored with immediate brachial plexus repair.
  - Low-velocity bullet injuries may cause concussive effects (neuropraxia) on the plexus and transection is rare: explore after 3 months if no recovery.
- **Iatrogenic**.
  - **Post-surgery** e.g. the lower trunk and long thoracic nerves are at risk during first rib resection in thoracic outlet syndrome.

- **Post-anaesthetic** brachial plexus palsy is usually a closed traction injury with an excellent prognosis and recovery is expected within 6 weeks. Avoiding excessive abduction of the arms or lateral neck flexion in unconscious patients may minimize these injuries. Nerve injury in the course of administering a brachial plexus block is rare but has been reported.
- **Post-radiotherapy** palsies have a poor prognosis due to the intraneural ischaemia and fibrosis. There is pain and paraesthesia that may be difficult to distinguish from tumour invasion (though this tends to be more painful and has involvement of the lower roots causing Horner's syndrome). Any nerve grafts used should be wrapped in vascularized tissue – the use of omentum has been reported.

The surgical treatment of brachial plexus injuries in adults

Terzis JK. *Plast Reconstr Surg* 2000;**106**:1097–1122.

High-velocity motor vehicle accidents account for the majority of the cases of brachial plexus injury.

History

- Age, occupation, hand dominance, hobbies and general health.
- **Time.** This is the most important determinant of the final outcome; within 6 months, there is less end organ denervation, muscle atrophy, scarring, nerve retraction etc.
- Mechanism of injury: open/closed, high/low velocity. Limb position e.g. arm hyperabducted or neck laterally flexed?
  - Nature of injury e.g.
    - **Traction** – downward force with forced neck flexion (root/trunk injury), downward force on shoulder (upper trunk) and arm hyperabduction (lower trunk).
    - Crush, direct blunt trauma to the neck and upper extremity – plexus can be crushed between the clavicle and the first rib or compressed by haematoma or adjacent injured tissue elements.
    - Direct laceration.
    - Concomitant injuries.
- Defect.
  - Immediate or delayed weakness in the arm?
  - Pre-existing neurological status.

Examination

- Thorough clinical examination, evaluation of vascularity of arm, specifically exclude Horner's syndrome and assess function of phrenic nerve.
  - Use preprinted brachial plexus diagrams that include all muscle groups of the upper extremity, sensory mapping and pain threshold to document observations.
- **Look** – attitude of the limb (including winging of scapula), wasting of muscles (delayed presentation), sudomotor changes, scars, swellings in posterior triangle (subclavian artery aneurysm).
- **Feel** – sensation C5–T1, Tinel's (distal point of nerve regeneration).
- **Move** – shoulder, elbow, wrist, fingers and thumb testing individual neuromotor units and reflexes. Passive and active range of motion of all joints. Test trapezius – spinal accessory may be used for nerve transfer.

Investigation

A priority is to classify the level of injury according to Millesi (see above).

- Complete radiological study of the cervical spine and the involved shoulder with special attention to the clavicle and scapula (more likely to be fractured in high-energy injuries).
  - **Fractures of the transverse processes** may be associated with avulsions of the corresponding roots, due to the attachments of the deep cervical fascia between the two.

Table 6.1 Summary of the actions used to screen for types of brachial plexus injury.

Levels	Action	Muscle and nerve
Roots	Retract shoulders	Rhomboids, dorsal scapular (C5)
Trunk	Abduct shoulder to horizontal	Supraspinatus, suprascapular (C5, 6)
Posterior cord	Adduct arm	Latissimus dorsi, thoracodorsal (C7)
Medial cord	Push hands against hips	Sternal head of pectoralis major, medial pectoral (C8)
Lateral cord	Push hands together at shoulder level	Clavicular head of pectoralis major, lateral pectoral (C6)

Table 6.2 Summary of the methods used to screen for the motor functions of the main peripheral nerve branches from the brachial plexus.

Peripheral nerve	Action for testing	Muscle tested
Axillary nerve (C5, 6)	Abduct shoulder above horizontal	Deltoid
Musculocutaneous (C5, 6)	Flex elbow	Biceps
Radial (C5–8)	Extend elbow	Triceps (C7)
	Extend wrist	ECRL, ECU (C7, 8)
Posterior interosseus (C8)	Extend fingers	EDC
Ulnar (C8–T1)	Cross fingers, PAD–DAB	Interossei (T1)
Median nerve (C5–T1)	Abduct thumb	Abductor pollicis (T1)
Anterior interosseus	'O' sign	

- ○ Chest X-ray – hemidiaphragm elevation.
- ○ Rib fractures may mean damage to the plexus (first two) or potential intercostal nerve donors.
- **CT/myelography** to demonstrate root avulsion particularly C8–T1: cervical myelogram is 91% predictive whilst the positive predictive value of combined CT myelography is more than 95% and is regarded as a 'gold standard' investigation. However, avulsed roots can still exist despite a normal myelogram. It is most useful to wait for at least one month after injury.
- **MRI:** this provides good visualization of the brachial plexus beyond the spinal foramen but is less useful for root avulsions, in particular lower root injuries, and with this exception is at least equivalent to CT myelography. High field strength MRI with multi planar views can easily distinguish the nerves at the distal plexus as well as defining shoulder anatomy.
  - ○ MRA can be used as an alternative to angiography in cases with suspected vascular injury.
- **Electrophysiological studies:** Wallerian degeneration results in the emergence of spontaneous electrical discharges or fibrillations. Electromyography (EMG) and nerve conduction studies should wait at least 3–6 weeks until these fibrillation potentials appear.
  - ○ **Needle electromyogram** of the paraspinal muscles, innervated by the dorsal rami of the spinal roots, should also be routinely performed; denervation of the paraspinal muscles (**fibrillation potentials**) provides strong evidence of avulsion of the corresponding roots. If these muscles are electrically intact, then the injury is most likely infra-ganglionic and the root is most likely ruptured. Serial EMGs allow monitoring; re-innervation with reduced fibrillation, nascent potentials and increased voluntary motor unit potentials.
  - ○ **Nerve conduction studies** looking at conduction velocity (m/s) which is reduced with demyelination (one of the first changes with chronic compression) whilst the amplitude is related to the number of nerve fibres present.

Treatment

Terzis states that the delay between accident and operation was prognostic for return of function but stressed the need for proper investigation rather than embarking on emergency surgery. Earlier surgery is indicated in high-velocity RTAs and in the presence of Horner's syndrome. In general:

- The best results are achieved with intervention before 6 months.
- Worse if delayed for more than a year.
- No benefit after 2 years.

Infraclavicular injuries had a better prognosis and if the injury was closed, then waiting 3–6 months for recovery before exploring was reasonable. A delay of more than 6 months woud lead to more muscular atrophy, fibrosis and joint stiffness.

- In a **flail limb,** the priorities are elbow flexion and shoulder abduction/stability, followed by hand sensibility, wrist extension/finger flexion and then wrist flexion/finger extension.
- In a **total plexus injury,** the available donor nerves are intercostals, spinal accessory and phrenic (latter two require nerve grafts).

Non-surgical treatment

- Physiotherapy to maintain joint mobility.
- Functional bracing, splintage.
- Nerve stimulation of paralysed muscles to maintain motor end plates while awaiting recovery.

- Motor re-education and strengthening exercises.
- Pain management.

Surgery **after ~3 months** (immediately if sharp injury)

- Neurolysis for neuroma in continuity.
- Nerve grafts – for discontinuous injuries.
- Nerve transfers if supraganglionic/root avulsion.
- Muscle transfers – local or free.

Exploration

Any kind of paralytics with the anaesthesia should be avoided. Explore the brachial plexus through a lymphadenectomy approach in the posterior triangle, with an incision that lies parallel to the posterior border of the sternocleidomastoid – the omohyoid and the transverse cervical vessels are identified and retracted, and the phrenic nerve is identified. The incision is extended via the deltopectoral groove to the infraclavicular area; the clavicle may have to be split though this is usually avoided (tendency to mal/non-union).

- Identify the level, type and extent of the lesion.
  - ○ **Neuromas** (in continuity or at the end of a ruptured plexus segment) are usually found between the upper roots and the trunks, but may also be present distally at the cord or peripheral nerve level. Neuromas should be excised to the level of healthy fascicles; resection and grafting provides better results than neurolysis alone.
  - ○ **Avulsed** spinal nerves: feel empty to palpation, pale in appearance and negative to electrical stimulation.
  - ○ Microneurolysis for 'hard' segments: longitudinal epineuriotomies to relieve pressure.
- **Nerve transfers and grafts:** motor and sensory donors are matched to their corresponding distal targets. Restoration of sensation particularly of median and ulnar nerves is useful.
  - ○ Intraplexus motor donors e.g. proximal stumps of ruptured roots.
  - ○ Extraplexus donors (used in multiple-root avulsions) e.g. intercostal nerves, accessory nerve and contralateral C7 root.
  - ○ External neurolysis if required and then primary repair or cable grafting (minimum of 4 cables to each cord) with sural nerve or medial cutaneous nerve of the forearm – intra-operative cortical-evoked potentials can help

determine whether there is supraganglionic injury.
  - ○ Nerve grafts can be vascularized or non-vascularized (sural nerve ~40 cm, medial cutaneous nerve of forearm ~20 cm); the former offer a faster reinnervation rate, at least in theory.
- **Restore joint movement.**
  - ○ **Shoulder abduction** – transfer to **suprascapular** and **axillary** nerves; a 'good result' is 45° of abduction.
    - – Distal spinal accessory (to suprascapular nerve).
    - – Phrenic or cervical plexus (axillary).
  - ○ **Elbow flexion** – aiming to restore innervation of biceps and brachialis (**musculocutaneous** nerve).
    - – Intraplexus donors e.g. **medial pectoral**, thoracodorsal.
    - – Extraplexus donors e.g. distal spinal accessory nerve (may need a segment of nerve graft), phrenic nerve, intercostals (3–5th, to be avoided with prior chest trauma), **contralateral C7** (a good donor of large numbers of motor nerves and up to half can be used) and vascularized ulnar graft (particularly in children). The contralateral C7 with a vascularized ulnar nerve to the median nerve is a useful way of restoring finger flexion.
    - – **Oberlin** (partial ulnar nerve, preferably FCU fascicles) transfer using 1–2 fascicles of ulnar nerve to motor branch to biceps; recovery takes 4–6 months (faster than e.g. medial pectoral nerve) as the repair is close to the muscle. The success rate is also higher (97% > M3, 94% > M4) compared with nerve transfers (71% > M3, 37% > M4).
  - ○ Hand sensation.
    - – From intercostobrachial, intercostal sensory or supraclavicular nerves.
    - – To ulnar nerve in upper arm, lateral cord to median nerve.
    - – Also transfer 4th web sensory supply to first web.
- **Muscle transfers.**
  - ○ Shoulder.
    - – Trapezius transfer (to deltoid insertion) to restore abduction. Alternative is pectoralis major.

- Advance the origins of biceps and triceps to the acromion (flexion/extension).
- Latissimus dorsi – taking the muscle around the humerus can restore external rotation (L'Episcopo).
- Alternatively, particularly with severe injury, shoulder fusion to provide a stable platform for elbow transfers to work against – 30° abduction, flexion and internal rotation.
  ○ Elbow.
  - **Pectoralis major transfer** – pedicled on clavicular head into the forearm.
  - **Latissimus dorsi transfer** (if thoracodorsal nerve spared).
  - **Triceps transfer** to the biceps insertion to provide flexion (which is more important than extension) when radial nerve (posterior cord) available but musculocutaneous nerve (lateral cord) is not. Alternative is pectoralis minor to biceps.
  - Transfer the **forearm flexor mass** (medial epicondyle) higher up on the humerus so moment for elbow flexion is increased; it does require near-normal power in these muscles (flexor-pronator) for useful elbow flexion to occur. **Steindler flexorplasty** provides less power and ROM than LD transfer.

Adjunctive procedures may be considered if the injury is more than a year old.

- Tendon transfers should be considered in older patients (> 40 years) though optimal results require have good passive ROM.
- Arthrodeses to stabilize joints if necessary, addressing shoulder, elbow, wrist (Sauvé–Kapandji procedure) and fingers in sequence.
- **Free functioning muscle transfers** e.g. gracilis, contralateral latissimus dorsi and rectus abdominis, are a useful option in total avulsions. They require an appropriate motor nerve for coaption and would need extraplexus neurotization; skin paddles can be included for soft tissue cover if needed.

In general, in terms of outcomes after brachial plexus injury/surgery:

- Better outcomes in the young.
- Better prognosis with distal lesions.

- Better outcomes for infraganglionic lesions over root avulsions.
- Motor nerve transfers are usually better than nerve grafts.

Complete traumatic brachial plexus palsy

Bentolila V. *J Bone Joint Surg* 1999;**81**:20–28.

The authors state that the priorities in complete brachial plexus injuries are restoration of (in order):

- Elbow flexion (most important) – musculocutaneous nerve (lateral cord).
- Elbow and wrist extension – radial nerve (posterior cord).
- Finger flexion for prehension – median nerve (medial cord), may need tendon transfers.
- Shoulder abduction – axillary nerve (posterior cord).

If there is no central connection for repair:

- Accessory nerve transfer to lateral cord or musculocutaneous nerve.
- Grafts from intercostal, accessory and thoracodorsal nerves (if spared) to distal stumps.

IV. Mechanisms of nerve injury

Classification of nerve injury

Wallerian degeneration is the orthograde/anterograde degeneration in the nerve **distal** to the site of division, ultimately to the end receptor. This begins at 24 hours and takes ~6 weeks, being slower in the central nervous system (CNS) compared with the peripheral nervous system (PNS).

- Axonal degeneration is followed by degradation of myelin sheath with macrophage infiltration to clear debris. The axonal disintegration is an active process and is dependent on ubiquitin and calpain proteases.
- The neurolemma remains as a hollow tube to provide pathways for regenerating axons that begin sprouting (growth cone and filopodia) after 4 days. The limiting step seems to be transportation of cytoskeletal elements along the axon; generally the rate is described as 1 mm/day plus 30 days with an apparent initial latent period. Pure motor or sensory nerves recover better than mixed nerves.

Augustus Waller observed this sequence after severing the IX/XII nerves in frogs (1850).

Table 6.3 Nerve injuries and their classification; Seddon and Sunderland compared.

Seddon	Sunderland	Insult	Prognosis
Neuropraxia	First degree	Segmental demyelination. Interruption of axon conduction whilst anatomic continuity maintained	Full recovery 1–4 months
Axonotmesis	Second degree	Axon severed, endoneurium intact	Full recovery 4–18 months
Neurotmesis	Third degree	Endoneurium (and axon) disrupted	Incomplete recovery
Neurotmesis	Fourth degree	Perineurium disrupted	Incomplete recovery
Neurotmesis	Fifth degree	Epineurium disrupted i.e. total loss of nerve continuity	No recovery
Sixth degree is combination of I–V injuries.			

Retrograde degeneration is the 'die-back' in the nerve **proximal** to the site of division back to the next most proximal branch and the cell body undergoes changes that include chromatolysis. Regenerative sprouting proceeds down the original Schwann cell myelin sheath but through new endoneural tubules.

Classification

Nerve conduction studies would be expected to yield the following results in nerve injuries:

- Neuropraxia – absent conduction over the site of the block, normal above and below.
- Incomplete lesion – prolonged **latency**, reduced **amplitude.**
- Complete lesion – no conduction.

Prognosis

Regeneration occurs at a rate of between 1 and 3 mm per day (advancing Tinel's sign). Muscles can potentially regain ~100% of function even after 1 year of denervation providing enough axons reach the motor end plates.

- Younger patient age and more distal transections do better i.e. division close to motor end plates better than proximal division.
- Sharp transection injuries usually have better recovery than avulsion injuries.

Recovery can be graded by the Medical Research Council (MRC) grading for both sensory and motor return.

Sensory recovery – MRC grading of function

- S0 no recovery.
- S1 deep **pain.**
- S1 + superficial pain.
- S2 light **touch.**
- S2 + hyperaesthesia to light touch.
- S3 2pd > 15 mm.
- S3 + 2pd 7–15 mm.
- S4 complete recovery (2pd 3–6 mm).

Innervation density tests – moving and static 2-point discrimination.

Threshold tests – Semmes–Weinstein monofilament, vibration.

Motor recovery – MRC grading of function

- M0 no contraction.
- M1 perceptible contraction, 'flicker'.
- M2 contraction with gravity eliminated.
- M3 contraction against gravity.
- M4 contraction against resistance.
- M5 full contraction.

Principles of repair

Primary repair within 10 days if at all possible is preferred.

- Aim for good **fascicular alignment** (matching size and surface vessels where possible) though clinical studies have *not* shown it to be superior to epineural repair.
  - Inverting epineural suture in purely sensory or motor nerves.
  - Fascicular (perineural) repair in mixed nerves. Motor stimulation may aid identification for the **72-hour** period that they remain responsive; sensory nerve stimulation will cause a sharp pain. Certain nerves have distinctive topographies e.g. ulnar nerve has ulnar sensory fascicles palmar, motor nerve

ventral and dorsal sensory nerve dorsal, and median nerve at carpal tunnel with motor fibres radial and palmar aspect of nerve.

- Nerve endings should be trimmed to healthy tissue and repair should be covered by vascular tissues.
- Avoid excessive tension/mobilization – gaps > 2–2.5 cm should be grafted (reversed to reduce axonal escape).
  - Suturing under tension that causes > 20% increase in the length of the nerve is likely to cause conduction impairment. Some length may be gained under certain circumstances by tranposition e.g. ulnar nerve at elbow or intratemporal dissection of facial nerve.
  - Nerve grafts can be harvested from:
    - Sural nerve (35–40 cm) found posterior to medial malleolus – numbness to lateral aspect of foot dorsum.
    - Lateral cutaneous nerve of forearm (8 cm) next to cephalic vein.
    - Medial cutaneous nerve of forearm (20 cm) next to basilic vein.
    - Posterior interosseus nerve – short segment at end of nerve.
  - Autologous nerve transplantation is nearly always possible, if not nerve **conduits** may be considered, for example:
    - Arteries and veins (vein conduit acceptable for defects up to 3 cm).
    - Bone, denatured skeletal muscle.
    - Fibronectin impregnated with growth factors, pseudosynovial sheaths.
    - Silicone and PTFE tubes.

Human nerve growth factor (NGF) and glial growth factor (GGF) may augment regeneration.

Neuroma

The diagnosis of a neuroma may be suggested by:

- Pain and exquisite tenderness.
- Pain when moving adjacent joints.
- Pressure pain.
- Dysaesthesia in the distribution of the nerve.

Common sites for upper limb neuromas include:

- Palmar cutaneous branch of the median nerve.
- Superficial branches of radial nerve or the radial digital nerves.
- Dorsal branch of the ulnar nerve.

The neuroma may be in-continuity or an end-neuroma:

- Neuroma-in-continuity.
  - Spindle – chronic irritation in an intact nerve (e.g. entrapment of lateral cutaneous nerve of thigh).
  - Lateral – develops at a site of partial nerve division or following nerve repair and is generally smaller.
- End-neuroma: often follows traumatic nerve division or amputation.

Management

Non-surgical conservative management includes:

- Desensitization exercises.
- Transcutaneous electrical **nerve stimulation** (TENS).
- Drugs – carbamazepine, etc.

Surgical management

- **Resection and coagulation** – bipolar, cryotherapy, chemical (alcohol, formaldehyde) or laser etc. Surgical strategies include:
  - Ligation or crushing; multiple sectioning may form multiple smaller neuromas.
  - Capping (silicone, vein, Histoacryl glue®) or epineural repair over the cut end.
  - Lateral neuromas can be treated by resection and repair of the disrupted perineurium of the involved fascicles only.
- **Bury** the nerve ending.
  - In nearby bone or muscle depending on the location e.g. into proximal phalanx or metacarpal in palm/digits, into pronator quadratus at wrist and into brachioradialis at forearm.
  - Implantation into nerve e.g. centro-central implantation into another nerve or implantation into the same nerve.

Nerve agents have been shown in animal experiments to destroy cell bodies of affected nerves.

V. Nerve compression syndromes
Nerve interconnections

Nerve compression and diagnosis of level of nerve injuries can be made more difficult by the presence of the following anatomical variations.

- **Martin–Gruber anastomosis** (Taams KO. *J Hand Surg Br* 1997;**22**:328–330). A branch from the median nerve joins onto the ulnar nerve in the forearm, which provides all the motor fibres to the ulnar nerve. Thus lesions to the ulnar nerve above this branch cause no motor deficit, while lesions to the median nerve cause a simian hand. This connection is present in ~23% of subjects.
- **Riche–Cannieu anastomosis.** This is similar to the Martin–Gruber anastomosis but occurs in the palm of the hand. It is more common and is found in up to 70% of subjects. It may allow for improved prognosis in low divisions of the median and ulnar nerves at the wrist
- **Nerve of Henlé** – this is a branch of the ulnar nerve in the forearm that travels with the ulnar artery to supply sensation to the distal medial forearm and proximal hypothenar eminence. It is present in ~40% of subjects and in these cases, the palmar cutaneous branch of the ulnar nerve will be absent.

Pathogenesis of nerve compression

There are a wide variety of possible causes of compression.

- Anatomical e.g. carpal tunnel.
- Postural – which may be related to occupational factors.
- Developmental – cervical rib, palmaris profundis.
- Inflammatory – tennis elbow, synovitis, scleroderma, amyloid, gout.
- Traumatic – lunate anterior dislocation, hand trauma.
- Metabolic – pregnancy, myxoedema, diabetes.
- Tumour – ganglia, neoplasms.
- Iatrogenic – trapped by plate fixation devices, inappropriate positioning on operating table.

Increased compression pressure reduces intraneural blood flow:

- 20–30 mmHg – decreased venular flow.
- 40–50 mmHg – decreased arteriolar and interfascicular blood flow.
- > 50 mmHg – no perfusion of the nerve.

Initially these changes are temporary and reversible, but long-term circulatory impairment may result from mechanical injury to intraneural blood vessels.

- Nerve conduction tests are the most sensitive tests for nerve compression with demyelination.

- Electromyography is most helpful for detecting denervation with axonal loss (fibrillation potentials after at least 3 weeks).

Compression neuropathy of the median nerve

The median nerve (C5-T1) arises from the lateral and medial cords of the brachial plexus. It runs between the intermuscular septum and the brachialis passing medial to the brachial artery. It passes below the ligament of Struthers, the bicipital aponeurosis and between the heads of pronator teres in the forearm, deep to the FDS arch and under palmaris longus at the carpal tunnel.

Anatomical sites of compression

- Pronator syndrome.
- Anterior interosseus syndrome (nerve to FPL, FDS index and middle, PQ).
- Carpal tunnel syndrome.

Pronator syndrome

There is pain in the proximal volar forearm that increases with activity and with resisted forearm pronation. It is accompanied by decreased sensation in the median nerve territory (over pronator down to thumb and index – including the palm) with nerve conduction studies showing increased latency at the elbow. Pronator syndrome deficits are sensory and motor with loss of precision pinch. It is commonly due to compression at one of four sites:

- Beneath the **ligament of Struthers** (attaches humeral head of pronator teres to the humerus above the elbow – supracondyloid process syndrome) – a relatively rare cause. Test by flexing the elbow against resistance.
    - John Struthers (1823–1899) was Professor of Anatomy at Aberdeen.
- Beneath the **lacertus fibrosus** (bicipital aponeurosis) – resisted elbow flexion with forearm supination.
- Where the nerve passes between humeral and ulnar heads of **pronator teres** (most common) – provoke with resisted pronation with extended arm.
- Under **arch of FDS** – provoke by resisted flexion of middle finger PIPJ.

Treatment

- Splint in neutral/slight pronation, wrist at 15° of dorsiflexion and elbow 90° flexion for 4–6 weeks, along with NSAIDs and activity modification. It may work in up to 50%.
- Release the nerve by dissecting it out from a point 5 cm above the elbow to below the bicipital aponeurosis, dividing the possible compressing structures above.

Comparing carpal tunnel syndrome with pronator syndrome

With pronator syndrome, there is:

- Less of a nocturnal pattern with symptoms.
- No Tinel's sign at the wrist (in proximal third of forearm instead).
- Nerve conduction may be delayed but not at the wrist; NCS can be normal as the compression may be intermittent/postural.
- However, Phalen's test is positive in 50% of patients with pronator syndrome (elbow flexion may compress the nerve in its tunnel).

Anterior interosseus syndrome

The anterior interosseus nerve is a branch of median nerve that arises 4–6 cm below the elbow and supplies flexor pollicis longus (FPL), flexor digitorum profundus (FDP) (index and middle) and pronator quadratus. There may be multiple sites of compression in the distal forearm:

- **Gantzer's muscle** (accessory head FPL).
- Muscles and fascial bands at their origins e.g. pronator, flexor digitorum superficialis (FDS), flexor carpi radialis (FCR).
- Aberrant radial artery.
- Thrombosis of ulnar collateral vessel, aberrant radial artery in forearm.
- Trauma – fractures/penetrating injury.
- HNPP (hereditary neuropathy with liability to pressure palsies) should be considered in those with multiple nerve compressions (spontaneous recovery is common); autosomal dominant – deletion/mutation in PMP22 on chromosome 17 (genetic testing is available).

The syndrome is relatively rare, making up less than 1% of all nerve compression syndromes. Patients tend to present with pain in the forearm and **weakness of pinch grip** (make an 'O' or 'OK' sign between index finger and thumb to test for FPL and index FDP, those with the syndrome tend to make a triangle). There is no sensory deficit and the presence of a Martin–Gruber anastomosis may make interpretation a little more complicated.

- Middle finger FDS flexion test.
- Nerve conduction studies (NCS) indicate latency in the upper forearm.

Treatment:

- Rest, activity modification, NSAIDs.
- Dissect out the nerve from its origin to the lower third of the forearm (may need to detach both heads of pronator teres) and divide crossing vessels.

Carpal tunnel syndrome

Anatomy

The transverse carpal ligament or flexor retinaculum attaches to the scaphoid tubercle and the trapezium on the radial side and to the hook of the hamate and the pisiform on the ulnar side. There are ten structures in the carpal tunnel: median nerve, FPL and eight finger flexors.

- The **palmar cutaneous branch** of the median nerve arises 6 cm proximal to the flexor retinaculum and passes superficial to it (occasionally this nerve may pierce it from deep to superficial and suffer from an entrapment syndrome of its own).
- The **motor branch** may follow several common variations in anatomy (Lanz U. *J Hand Surg* 1977;**2**:44–53); other variations are rare. It arises from the radiovolar aspect of the nerve; **Kaplan's line** (ulnar border of abducted thumb intersected with index–middle finger web) provides a rough approximation to the motor branch.
  - **Extraligamentous** branch, emerging distal to the carpal ligament and recurrent to thenar muscles (~50%).
  - **Subligamentous** branch, emerging beneath the carpal ligament and recurrent to thenar muscles (~30%).
  - **Transligamentous** branch, emerging beneath the carpal ligament and piercing it to reach the thenar eminence (~20%).

Causes of carpal tunnel syndrome can be either congenital or acquired but it is idiopathic in the majority of cases.

- Congenital.
  - Persistent median artery.
  - High origin of lumbrical muscles.
- Acquired.
  - Inflammatory – synovitis, RA, gout.
  - Traumatic – perilunate dislocation, Colles' fracture.
  - Fluid retention – pregnancy, renal failure, cardiac failure, myxoedema, diabetes, steroid medication.
  - Space-occupying lesions – lipoma, ganglion.
  - Effort-associated CTS may be caused by the lumbricals causing symptoms with repetitive gripping.

Compression of the median nerve within the carpal canal was first described by Paget in 1854. It affects females 6× more frequently; 40% have bilateral involvement. Patients present with

- Weakness/clumsiness – decrease in fine motor skills e.g. writing.
- Pain in the hand, occasionally referred proximally.
- Sensory disturbance (hyperaesthesia/paraesthesia) especially at night in the radial 3 and 1/2 fingers (index and thumb). Palm is spared.
- Morning stiffness and numbness.

Hand examination should focus attention on:

- Median nerve sudomotor changes.
- Muscle wasting.
- Objective assessment of sensory deficit and motor deficit.

Tests to perform include:

- Resisted pronation to exclude compression higher up.
- Ulnar nerve signs to exclude ulnar compression in Guyon's canal.
- First carpometacarpal joint tenderness to exclude basal joint osteoarthritis (Eaton stages).
- Provocation tests – Tinel's sign at carpal tunnel, median nerve compression test and Phalen's test (positive if signs < 40 s).
- Electrophysiological testing demonstrating median nerve latency > 4 ms is diagnostic, but a normal latency does not rule out CTS – 10% of NCS are false-negatives.

Diagnosis of carpal tunnel syndrome

Gunnarsson LG. *J Hand Surg* 1997;**22**:34–37.

Clinical examination by an experienced doctor is usually sufficient to diagnose typical CTS. However, atypical symptoms or signs, or a prior history of fracture in the limb, may warrant the use of nerve conduction studies.

- Numbness in median nerve distribution is the most sensitive symptom (95%) but is not very specific (26%).
- Phalen's test is more sensitive (86%) than Tinel's sign (62%) but less specific (48 vs. 57%).
- Nerve conduction studies can be used if unsure; they are highly sensitive (85%) and specific (87%) but there is a 10% false-negative rate.

Management

Non-operative treatment may be considered when entrapment of the nerve may be temporary, e.g. pregnancy.

- Activity modification and NSAIDs, latter may be more effective in those with tendonitis.
- Steroid (hydrocortisone) injections – one-third have maintained relief of symptoms at 3 months, **10–20% at 18 months**. However there is a risk of tendon/nerve injuries.
- Futuro splint at night and during provoking activities. Some patients benefit but not as much as with surgery. The optimal regime, including which is the best splint (OTC vs. custom, neutral or resting position), is not clear.
- Unclear benefit: vitamin B6, (nerve and tendon) gliding exercises and ultrasound.

Operative.

- Longitudinal release of transverse carpal ligament (Brain WR. *Lancet* 1947;**1**:277–282).
- Synovectomy where indicated.
- External neurolysis.
- Endoscopic release.

Procedure

- Local anaesthetic, tourniquet.
- Incision in line with radial border fourth ray and ulnar back-cut.
- Spread superficial palmar fascia to reveal/spare transversely orientated nerve fibres, then divide the transverse carpal ligament preserving median nerve under direct vision.

○ If concerned about motor branch look for this specifically.

○ If concerned about ulnar nerve compression then release it as well.

- Irrigate the wound and close 5/0 prolene (remove at 2 weeks).
- Post-operative splint for 3–4 days then change to a futura; however, there is some debate over splints – they do not speed up recovery and may cause more temporary pain/tender scars and a slower return to work. (Henry SL. *Plast Reconstr Surg* 2008;**122**:1095–1099).

Complications

The most common complication is a sensitive palmar scar (62%). Serious complications are rare:

- Intra-operative – injury to median nerve or deep palmar arch.
- Early – infection, haematoma, dehiscence.
- Late – inadequate release, pillar pain, flexion weakness, tender scar, CRPS.

A meta-analysis of randomized controlled trials comparing endoscopic and open carpal tunnel decompression

Thoma A. *Plast Reconstr Surg* 2004;**114**:1137–1146.

This is a meta-analysis of 13 randomized controlled clinical trials that compared endoscopic release with open release. It found that the former was associated with:

- Improved post-operative pinch and grip strength in the early post-operative phase (12 weeks) and less scar tenderness.
- Increased risk of reversible nerve injury (3 × compared with open release) – but uncommon with either technique.
- There was no difference in post-operative pain or time to return to work.

It seems that endoscopic release is a well-established technique that is effective, has some benefits (shorter scar, slightly faster recovery, slightly less early pain) but slightly higher complication and recurrence rates. Some previous proponents of endoscopic release (TJ Fischer) believe that the benefits (slightly faster recovery – few differences after 3 months) do not outweigh the risk of median nerve injury (unable to view variants of motor branch, 4.3% reversible nerve injury vs. 0.9% in open surgery). An open approach allows the surgeon to be fairly confident of complete release and allows concomitant Guyon's canal release (Jean Guyon, 1831–1920, was a French urologist; it is not clear why the canal is attributed to him). Relative contraindications for endoscopic surgery include: where contents of tunnel need exploration e.g. mass lesions, synovitis, associated with an acute fracture and cases of recurrent CTS.

Recovery

- 'Immediate' relief of pins and needles.
- Two-point discrimination – 2 weeks.
- Sensory and motor nerve latencies – 3–6 months.
- Pinch and grip strength – 6–9 months.

The more severe the symptoms and the longer the duration, the longer it takes to recover. Overall, 90% will improve significantly.

Recurrent carpal tunnel syndrome

Surgical release of CTS typically has a high success rate with up to 90% returning to their old jobs. Causes of recurrent symptoms after surgery include:

- Incomplete division of the transverse carpal ligament.
- Median nerve compressed by scar tissue.
- Flexor tenosynovitis i.e. wrong diagnosis.

Secondary carpal tunnel surgery

Tung TH. *Plast Reconstr Surg* 2001;**107**:1830–1843.

Reasons for further surgery include the following scenarios.

- **Persistent symptoms** after surgery (7–20% reported incidence) are commonly due to inadequate release (usually distally). However, it may also be due to additional undiagnosed proximal compression ('double crush') or misdiagnosis.
- **Recurrent** symptoms (i.e. previous symptoms returning after a period of initial relief).
  - ○ Post-operative scarring compressing the median nerve.
  - ○ 'Reformation' of the transverse carpal ligament with recurrent compression.
- Completely **new** symptoms.
  - ○ Neurological – tender scar due to injury to multiple small cutaneous branches (one of the most common complications), entrapment or division of the palmar cutaneous branch of the median nerve, injury to the main trunk of the median or ulnar nerves or its branches.

○ Vascular – haematoma following injury to the superficial palmar arch.

○ Wrist complaints – carpal arch alteration causing pain, pillar pain, pisotriquetral pain syndrome.

○ Tendon problems – increased incidence of triggering, thought to be due to transference of initial pulley-related forces from transverse carpal ligament to A1 pulleys, bowing or adhesions of flexor tendons.

Clinical evaluation is used to assess the possible underlying causes of symptoms and exploration is warranted for:

- Positive Phalen's test.
- Night symptoms.
- Positive NCS after 3–6 months.
  Neurophysiological testing may help identify the level of residual or recurrent compression.

Surgery

Treatment of underlying problems or exploration of alternative compression sites.

- Re-release of ligament.
- Neural surgery is controversial:
  ○ External neurolysis to separate nerve from scar tissue is standard.
  ○ Internal or interfascicular neurolysis or epineurotomy has been proposed for severe CTS but opinions differ. Curtis RM. *J Bone Joint Surg Am* 1973;**55**:733–740.
- Interpositional nerve grafts to injured segments of the median nerve.
- Revascularization of the nerve e.g. pronator quadratus turnover flap for mechanical protection of the nerve, reduction of new scar tissue and to improve local vascular support.
- Tissue interposition flaps to separate the overlying scar from the median nerve such as: pronator quadratus, abductor digiti minimi, palmaris brevis or distally based radial forearm fascial flap.

Compression neuropathy of the ulnar nerve

The ulnar nerve is the terminal branch of the medial cord. It runs medial and posterior to the brachial artery, and then pierces the middle of the medial intermuscular septum to enter the posterior compartment and then passes behind the medial epicondyle in the cubital tunnel. Distally it lies between the FDS and FDP, then radial to the FCU tendon to Guyon's canal.

It reliably innervates the 2nd and 3rd dorsal interossei and nerve dysfunction would leave the patient unable to move the middle finger side-to-side with the palm flat on a table-top.

- The dorsal branch of the ulnar nerve is at risk during excision of the ulnar head.
- The deep branch of the ulnar nerve dives down at the level of the pisiform into the hypothenar musculature.

Anatomical sites of compression

- **Arcade of Struthers.** Fibrous condensation of intermuscular septum about 8 cm proximal to the medial epicondyle, present in 70%.
- Medial intermuscular septum (between brachialis and the medial head of triceps) that is distinct from the arcade.
- Hypertrophy medial head triceps.
- Stretching caused by cubital valgus (e.g. post-supracondylar fracture).
- **Cubital tunnel.** Roof of the cubital tunnel is formed by the fascia of the flexor carpi ulnaris (FCU) and the cubital tunnel retinaculum (CTR) (also known as arcuate ligament of Osborne). The elbow capsule and medial collateral ligaments (MCL) form the floor. This is the most common site of ulnar nerve compression.
- **Guyon's canal.** Second most common.

The last muscle to be supplied by the ulnar nerve is the first dorsal interosseus – and hence it shows the earliest sign of wasting with nerve compression.

Cubital tunnel syndrome (compression of ulnar nerve at elbow)

- Passage of ulnar nerve beneath the aponeurosis joining heads of FCU.
- Trauma at the elbow; fracture, especially in children.
- Recurrent dislocation of the nerve in the ulnar groove of the medial condyle – neuritis. Asymptomatic nerve dislocation is seen in 16% of volunteers.
- Humero-ulnar osteoarthritis or rheumatoid arthritis.
- Ganglion at the humero-ulnar joint.
- Anconeus epitrochlearis.

Hyperflexion of the elbow usually provokes symptoms of cubital tunnel syndrome as it increases the distance the nerve has to travel and also tightens Osborne's ligament.

Symptoms

- Ill-defined pain in the arm.
- Numbness in the ulnar digits especially at night.
- Pain with elbow flexion.
- Weakness of pinch grip (**adductor pollicis**).

Signs

- Wasting of the **first dorsal interosseus**, other intrinsics and hypothenar eminence.
- Lack of clawing if palsy above the branch to FDP. With palsy at the wrist, the action of long flexors causes IP flexion while there is a failure of lumbrical-mediated extension at the interphalangeals and flexion at metacarpophalangeals.
- **Wartenberg's sign:** abducted little finger in the presence of an ulnar nerve injury at the wrist and an ulnar claw hand, due to insertion of the EDM tendon into the tendon of ADM (this is not Wartenberg's syndrome, which is a neuritis of the superficial radial nerve).
- Dysaesthesia in the distribution of the dorsal branch of ulnar nerve.
- Tinel's sign at the elbow (can be positive in asymptomatic patients) and Phalen's sign with elbow.
- **Positive Froment's sign** – patients with ulnar nerve palsy compensate for the lack of a working adductor pollicis by flexing the thumb IPJ (median innervated FPL).
- Test pure intrinsic function – flex MCPJ and abduct/adduct the fingers.

Nerve conduction studies will show delayed nerve conduction at the elbow in cubital tunnel syndrome; if the problem is in the neck, dysaesthesia is encountered in the C8/T1 dermatomes i.e. inner aspect of forearm and elbow. Presence of either Martin–Gruber or Riche–Cannieu anastomoses may cause confusion.

X-rays are not that helpful but some suggest:

- A–P and lateral.
- Cubital tunnel view – elbow flexed.

McGowan classification

- Mild – mild, intermittent dysaesthesia.
- Intermediate – persistent dysaesthesia, early motor loss.
- Severe – marked atrophy and weakness.

Treatment options

- Splintage to keep elbow from bending during sleep e.g. wrapping towel around elbow, soft sports knee splint.
- Medication – unclear benefits from NSAIDs, vitamin B6 and steroids.
- Surgery.
  - Decompression – division of aponeurosis connecting humeral and ulnar heads of FCU (**Osborne's ligament**) – grade I and II neuropathy.
  - Ulnar nerve transposition – subcutaneous or submuscular anterior transposition (**Learmonth's technique**) particularly for those in whom decompression has failed – grade III neuropathy, severe ulnar neuritis or persistent valgus deformity. There is a risk of nerve devascularization.
  - The medial intermuscular septum is split above the elbow where the ulnar nerve passes through to enter the volar compartment of the forearm.
  - Divide the fascia connecting the two heads of FCU.
  - Transpose the nerve anteriorly over the muscle belly of FCU (subcutaneous transposition) or beneath the humeral head of FCU (submuscular transposition).
- Medial epicondylectomy – can be performed in association with the above.

Damage to the medial cutaneous nerve of the forearm during surgery may cause formation of neuromas.

Ulnar tunnel syndrome (compression within Guyon's canal)

The ulnar nerve and artery lie on top of transverse carpal ligament and beneath the **volar/palmar carpal ligament in** Guyon's canal; nothing else traverses the canal and it does not contains any synovium, thus compression is less common compared with the carpal tunnel. Within the canal the nerve divides into the motor branch that can be rolled over the hook of the hamate and the palmar cutaneous branch.

The isolated occurrence of ulnar nerve compression within the canal is usually due to ganglia, with other causes being anomalous muscles (aberrant FCU) or an aneurysm of the ulnar artery. Masses cause up to one-third to one-half of cases of Guyon's canal compression.

Ulnar nerve signs (see above)

- Ulnar claw posture.
- Sensory, motor or mixed disturbance – some divide the canal in zones.
  - Zone I – proximal to nerve bifurcation – mixed disturbance.
  - Zone II – disto-radial, surrounds deep motor branch – pure motor.
  - Zone III – disto-ulnar, surrounds superficial sensory branch – pure sensory.
  - Typically there is motor weakness of the FDP of the ring and small fingers and the ulnar intrinsics.

If the dorsal sensory branch (arises 7 cm proximal to the pisiform) is involved (sensation to the dorsoulnar hand), then the compression cannot be in Guyon's canal – it must be proximal to it, e.g. within the cubital tunnel. Electromyography (first dorsal interosseous) will demonstrate slow conduction at the wrist.

Treatment

- Conservative.
- Surgery – release of the volar carpal ligament via a longitudinal incision radial to FCU, isolating the ulnar nerve proximal to the wrist. The volume of Guyon's canal increases after carpal tunnel release thus CTR release improves ulnar compression symptoms in one-third of patients.

Radial nerve compression

Sites of compression:

- Triangular space.
- Radial tunnel syndrome.
- Posterior interosseous nerve syndrome.
- Wartenberg's syndrome.

Radial tunnel syndrome

The radial nerve passes through triangular space formed by humerus laterally, triceps (long head) medially and teres major superiorly, to lie in the bicipital groove in the posterior compartment of the arm. It pierces the lateral intermuscular septum 10–12 cm above the lateral epicondyle and enters the radial tunnel (from radial head to distal edge of supinator) where it may become compressed.

Within the radial tunnel, within 3 cm of the elbow, the nerve gives off the motor branch (posterior interosseus nerve, third extensor compartment) and continues as a purely sensory nerve that stays close to brachioradialis. All forearm extensors are supplied by posterior interosseus nerve (C7, 8) apart from ECRL, ECRB and brachioradialis (radial nerve above the elbow). A fracture of the humerus may cause injury to the radial nerve whilst a fracture of the radius may cause injury to the posterior interosseous nerve (PIN).

There are three common constriction points (of the PIN) within the radial tunnel:

- Sharp tendinous medial border of extensor carpi radialis brevis.
- Fan of vessels from the radial recurrent artery ('**leash of Henry**') that can compress various branches of the radial nerve.
- **Arcade of Frohse** – the free aponeurotic margin of supinator under which the posterior interosseus nerve passes (thus posterior interosseus nerve syndrome). This is the most common site of radial nerve compression.

Fibrous bands around the radiohumeral joint may also cause constriction; some suggest that RTS may be a result of overuse.

Symptoms and signs

- Pain in the radial tunnel (4 cm distal to the lateral epicondyle, distinguishing it somewhat from lateral epicondylitis).
- **Sensory disturbance** radiating to the distribution of the superficial branch of radial nerve. **This is absent with compression of PIN, i.e. PIN syndrome.**
- Positive **middle finger test** – pain over radial tunnel upon extension against resistance (ECRB inserts into middle finger metacarpal and contraction causes impingement of border onto nerve). There may also be symptoms with resisted supination with elbow extended.
- Tenderness over the supinator mass, four fingerbreadths distal to the lateral epicondyle – it can be distinguished from tennis elbow/lateral epicondylitis by the tenderness over the lateral epicondyle in the latter. There is no sensory disturbance or motor loss (except due to pain) in tennis elbow (golfer's elbow = medial epicondylitis).
  - Treatment for tennis elbow includes rest, splints, anaesthetic steroid injections; surgery, including repair of tears, release of the extensor origin, partial excision of the annular ligament, may not be that successful.
- Weakness and numbness are **not** prominent features of RTS. In PIN there is weakness/paralysis

of the wrist and finger extensors (brachioradialis, ECRB, ECRL may be spared) without a sensory deficit.

Management

Electrophysiological studies are less useful for this type of nerve compression.

- Splintage, activity modification, NSAIDs.
- Treat by **nerve decompression** by exploring the radial tunnel via brachioradialis muscle-splitting or anterolateral approaches that have been described. Generally a complete release is advised (all the structures above are divided) even if no obvious evidence of compression of the nerve can be seen during surgery. There is usually a good prognosis after surgery if the symptoms can be relieved by a pre-operative nerve block.

Posterior interosseous nerve syndrome

The main features are weakness of wrist and finger extension with some forearm pain without sensory disturbance. It may be provoked by a variety of causes:

- Trauma e.g. elbow fracture/dislocation.
- Inflammation e.g. rheumatoid arthritis in the elbow.
- Swellings/masses e.g. lipoma, ganglia.
- Iatrogenic e.g. injections for tennis elbow etc.

Due to the above, investigations to clarify the cause are more valuable (than in PIN syndrome) e.g. NCS, X-ray and CT/MRI.

Treatment

Conservative as above, proceeding to surgery if the NCS is positive and there has been no recovery for 3 months. Decompression aims to treat the cause and includes release of all potential causes also.

Wartenberg's syndrome

This is neuritis of the superficial branches of the radial nerve, which may occur due to entrapment beneath the tendinous insertion of brachioradialis, anomalous fascial bands, tight jewellery and watchbands, scarring etc. It is a relatively rare cause of radial wrist pain and may resemble de Quervain's (Finkelstein's test may be positive).

- Tenderness 4 cm proximal to the wrist.
- Numbness or pain in the distribution of the superficial branch of radial nerve (reproducible by

pressure over the nerve). There is reduced two-point discrimination on testing.

Treat by surgical exploration, neurolysis and release of constricting tissues (some recommend lengthening of the brachioradialis) if conservative measures do not work.

- Robert Wartenberg (1886–1956), a Russian-born neurologist who eventually settled in California, was sometimes called the 'Rebel of Book Reviewers' due to his honest and accurate critiques.
- Wartenberg's sign is the inability to hold the little finger against the ring finger when the fingers are in extension and is due to the action of the EDM (radial innervation) being unopposed by weak palmar interossei (ulnar).

Traction neuritis

This may occur after open carpal tunnel release or ulnar nerve transposition and is manifested as chronic pain. It may be due to:

- Nerve devascularization.
- Neuroma.
- Incomplete decompression.

Re-explore if symptoms persist with internal/external neurolysis. For the ulnar nerve, submuscular transposition with or without epicondylectomy is recommended. Some cases may not improve after further intervention and this may be related to scarring.

Severe neuritis may require additional soft tissue coverage.

Thoracic outlet syndrome

The thoracic outlet is formed by the first rib inferiorly, scalenus anterior anteriorly and the scalenus medius posteriorly. In thoracic outlet syndrome (TOS), there are symptoms and signs of compression of neurovascular structures at or around this point. There is an incidence of 1 in 200, affecting those 20–50 years of age. Neurological symptomatology (i.e. 'neurogenic', 95%) is more common in **females**, whilst men tend to suffer venous involvement more frequently – arterial involvement seems equal.

Aetiology

- Cervical rib or ligamentous band, often bilateral (50%). It is present in 0.5% of the general population and 10% of patients with TOS. Rudimentary ribs, congenital fibromuscular bands; cadaver studies have shown a variety of anomalies of the scalenes.

- Swellings such as subclavian artery aneurysm, chondroma, Pancoast tumour.
- Trauma e.g. clavicular fractures, effort vein thrombosis.
- Posture – holding the shoulders excessively backwards or forwards.

Willboum classification

- Neurogenic.
  - True – relatively rare (1 in 100 000). Objective signs of chronic nerve compression are present e.g. atrophy and weakness especially C8–T1. A bony abnormality is present.
  - Disputed – 95–97%, with a wide variety of symptoms and complaints but without objective findings.
- Arterial (1–2%): half are associated with a cervical rib and are deemed 'major' if associated with a bony abnormality. Minor cases are those with intermittent compressions usually at the insertion of the pectoralis minor.
- Venous (2–3%): Paget Schroetter syndrome is a sudden effort-induced thrombosis though it may also follow poor positioning. There may be collateral vein development.

Symptoms and signs

This condition most often affects **T1 and the lower trunk** of the brachial plexus and is often bilateral.

- Pain, sensory disturbance (tingling and numbness), motor loss, vascular changes (including Raynaud's phenomenon).
  - Typically the pain is a dull ache, particularly around the shoulder and inner arm, that worsens during the day.
  - Motor loss and wasting of intrinsics and thenar muscles that are innervated by median is strongly suggestive.
- Dysaesthesia of the ulnar nerve + medial cutaneous nerve of arm + medial cutaneous nerve of forearm usually means thoracic outlet syndrome. If there is ulnar and median wasting in the hand, a thoracic outlet syndrome should also be suspected.
  - Symptoms on lateral neck flexion away from the affected side = thoracic outlet syndrome.
  - Symptoms on lateral neck flexion towards the affected side = root compression.

- Vascular signs: arterial (claudication, slow Allen's test, pallor, pulseless, reduced temperature and reduced blood pressure), venous (oedema, venous engorgement). Splinter haemorrhages may be secondary to embolism.
- Colour and temperature difference – often more obvious on the radial side of the hand.
  - Diminished pulses and lower blood pressure.
  - Thrill and bruit.

Provocation tests: none are specific (vide supra).

- Roos – probably most reliable.
- Wright's.
- Adson's – positive in 20% of 'normal' population.
- Halstead brace manoeuvre.

Imaging

- CXR: may see cervical first rib, clavicular deformity, pulmonary disease/Pancoast tumour,; loss of lordotic curve of cervical spine suggests muscle spasm.
- Duplex Doppler for vascular lesions.
- MRI may demonstrate soft tissue bands.
- Arteriograms/venograms – it is important to position the patient in the provoking posture.

Management

Non-operative

- Posture education, activity modification, weight loss.
- Physiotherapy – stretch and strengthening exercises.

Surgery

The main indications are for failure of conservative therapy, particularly for symptoms of pain. Those patients with true neurogenic and vascular symptoms are most likely to benefit.

- First rib resection (plus cervical rib if present) – via a transaxillary approach.
- Scalene release, fibromuscular bands – via supraclavicular approach.
- Neurolysis.
- Thromboendartectomy.

Specific complications include:

- Haemo-, pneumo-, chylothorax.
- Brachial plexus injury, causalgia/neuroma.

Cervical root compression (cervical radiculopathy)

Compression may be due to acute disc herniation (25% of cases, often in younger patients) or chronic impairment related to osteoarthritis, spondylitis or osteophytes (often in older patients). C6 and C7 are most commonly involved; note that C5–6 disc causes C6 root compression. Tumours are uncommon causes.

Symptoms include:

- Pain starting generally as a neck and shoulder discomfort, progressing down to forearm and hand as the radiculopathy worsens. It is exacerbated by extreme movements of the neck, as well as coughing/sneezing (possibly related to increased spinal fluid pressure).
- Radiation into occipital area (helps to distinguish it from peripheral nerve compression).
- Dysaesthesia in dermatomal pattern.
- Weakness and wasting.

Examination

- **Spurling's** foraminal compression test (vide supra) is probably the best confirmatory test for cervical radiculopathy. It is specific (93%) but not sensitive enough (30%).
- Vertebral tenderness to palpation/percussion.
- Sensory loss in dermatomal pattern.
- Motor weakness and reduced reflexes – e.g. biceps (C5–6), triceps (C7).

Investigations

- Cervical spine X-ray (lateral, A–P and oblique) is usually the first diagnostic test and may show narrowed intervertebral foramina and beaking of vertebral bodies. CT provides better visualization of the bony elements.
- MRI may demonstrate soft tissue elements (and is superior to CT with myelography). It is considered the modality of choice; it may detect abnormalities in asymptomatic patients.
- EMG can confirm nerve root dysfunction when the diagnosis is unclear. A normal EMG in a patient with typical symptoms and signs does not exclude the diagnosis.
- Selective diagnostic nerve root block with a small amount of local anaesthetic.

Polyneuropathy

- Drugs, metabolic and vitamin deficiencies.
- Connective tissue diseases including RA.

- Malignancies.
- Post-infective (Guillain–Barré).
- Hereditary (e.g. peroneal muscular atrophy i.e. Charcot–Marie–Tooth disease: champagne bottle legs).

Multiple mononeuropathy

- Diabetes.
- Leprosy, sarcoid, amyloid.
- Connective tissue diseases including systemic lupus erythematosus (SLE).
- Malignancies.

Muscle/tendon transfers for specific nerve lesions

Nerve injury is the most common indication for tendon transfer. Others include:

- Muscle/tendon injury secondary to trauma or other disease (see also rheumatoid arthritis).
- Spastic disorders (see also cerebral palsy).
- Polio – wait 6 months for any recovery.
- Leprosy – disease must be under control.

Principles of tendon transfer

The aim is to identify specific task deficits and to re-establish this function through the use of existing muscle/tendons.

Tendon transfer utilizes **existing** motor function (none is created) thus power is lost during transfer – at least one MRC grade. Therefore muscles used should have 4–5/5 power and be **expendable.** Whilst power must be adequate, over-powerful transfers may deform the joint. Transferred tendons require free passage in vascularized tissue planes with a **straight line of pull** (only change direction once). Strength is related to the cross-sectional area of the muscle whilst the length determines the excursion – wrist tendons have an excursion of 3 cm, whilst finger extensors and flexors have excursions of 5 and 7 cm respectively, meaning that when wrist tendons are used to restore finger function, correction will usually be **incomplete.**

- One function per muscle transferred.
- Full passive ROM is required before transfer; contractures should be corrected.
- Joints must be stable. Active control at the wrist is paramount for tendon transfers for the fingers.
- Restore function only to an area which is sensate (at least protective sensation). Sensory deficits limit the usefulness of tendon transfers and every effort

Table 6.4 Nerve compression syndromes and their common causes.

Neuropathy	Congenital/anatomical	Acquired
Pronator syndrome	Between heads of PT Ligament of Struthers Lacertus fibrosus (biceps)	Swellings: lipoma, ganglion
Anterior interosseus syndrome	All the above plus: Fibrous bands of FDS Ganzer's muscle (accessory head of FPL)	Swellings: lipoma, ganglion
Carpal tunnel syndrome Persistent median artery	High insertion of lumbricals	Swellings: lipoma, ganglion, bony exostoses
		Inflammatory: RA, OA
		Metabolic: pregnancy, hypothyroidism, renal failure
		Traumatic: lunate dislocation
Cubital tunnel syndrome	Anconeus epitrochlearis Two heads of FCU	Swellings: lipoma, ganglion
		Inflammatory: RA, OA
		Traumatic: cubitus valgus, supracondylar fracture
Ulnar tunnel syndrome	Accessory PL tendon High insertion of hypothenar muscles	Swellings: lipoma, ganglion
		Inflammatory: RA, OA
		Traumatic: fracture hook of hamate
Radial tunnel syndrome	Arcade of Frohse (supinator) Leash of Henry	Swellings: lipoma, ganglion
		Inflammatory: RA, OA
		Traumatic: elbow dislocation,
	Tendinous border of ECRB	Monteggia fracture
Posterior interosseus syndrome	As for radial tunnel syndrome	As for radial tunnel syndrome
Wartenberg's syndrome	Free edge of brachioradialis	Extrinsic compression by watchbands, etc.

should be made to restore function prior to tendon transfer e.g. nerve repair/graft/transfer or neurovascular island flaps.

Other considerations

- Complete division of recipient tendon burns bridges. Attachment in-continuity compromises mechanics but concept of reversibility may be important ('baby-sitting' transfers in case re-innervation of paralysed muscles occurs).
- All transfers slacken with time; use **tenodesis effect** (finger extension with wrist flexion) to get the tension right. Transfers should be within synergistic muscle groups e.g. hand opening (wrist flex/finger extend) and hand closing/grip muscles (wrist extend/finger flex). Donor muscle should be independently innervated and not act in concert with other muscles (e.g. lumbricals).

- Success requires a well-motivated patient likely to be compliant with the post-operative hand therapy. Multiple transfers may be too complicated – for the patient. Thus contraindications include:
  - Advanced age (reduce recovery/re-education and reduced demands).
  - Poor motivation/compliance.
  - Lack of a specific task deficit.
  - Local or systemic disease affecting the surgery e.g. rheumatoid arthritis must be controlled.

Timing

- Immediate – when chances of recovery are low e.g. muscle loss, advanced age, or as a interim 'baby-sitting' procedure whilst waiting for recovery e.g. in radial nerve compression, PT to ECRB.

- Delayed – if conditions (e.g. soft tissue shortage) are not ideal initially, then a delay to achieve better conditions (flap coverage) is necessary.

Low median nerve palsy

Loss of median nerve muscles (mnemonic: **L**umbricals 1 and 2, **O**pponens pollicis, **A**bductor pollicis brevis, **F**lexor pollicis brevis = LOAF muscles) and sensation, main aim is to restore **thumb opposition** i.e. APB (with contributions from opponens and FPB superficial head – deep head is usually ulnar innervated). Reliable options for **opponensplasty** include:

- Palmaris longus (PL) (Camitz, requires strip of palmar fascia).
- Flexor digitorum superficialis (FDS) ring (Bunnell, with pulley around FCU).
- Extensor indicis (EI) (Burkhalter) – probably one of the commonest; it requires no pulley or tendon graft and no loss of grasp force. The tendon is ulnar to the EDC of the index.
- Abductor digiti minimi (ADM) (Huber) – needs intact ulnar nerve. It is the classic choice in the congenital hypoplastic thumb, and also restores the bulk of the thenar eminence.

High median nerve palsy

As above with additional loss of FPL, FDP index and middle, FDS, PQ, PT and FCR.

- Opponensplasty for **thumb abduction and opposition.**
- Brachioradialis to **FPL** for **thumb flexion,** or ECRL/B.
- Suture together ulnar FDPs to median FDPs to achieve a **finger flexion** (mass action) or ECRL to FDP.
- FCU split to restore balanced **wrist flexion.**
- Re-route biceps to restore **pronation.**

Low ulnar nerve palsy (claw hand)

Loss of hypothenar muscles especially ADM, ulnar lumbricals, adductor pollicis and FPB deep head (muscle usually has dual innervation, superficial head is supplied by the median nerve), interossei and sensation. There are Froment's and Jeanne's signs (hyperflexion of IPJ and hyperextension of MCPJ respectively, with key pinch).

- Correct **clawing** (MCPJ hyperextension and inability to fully extend IPJs of ring and little

fingers – Duchenne's sign, due to absent intrinsic function). Procedures may be divided into static (e.g. tenodesis of lateral bands) or dynamic transfers.
  - FDS transfer to the radial lateral band (or A1 pulley).
  - FDS slip looped back on itself around A1 pulley (Zancolli Lasso) providing dynamic flexion movement at MCPJ.
  - Extensor carpi radialis longus (ECRL) to correct claw (Stiles–Bunnell).
  - Stitch down volar plate to flex MCPJ (static Zancolli capsulodesis) but does not add power and will stretch with time.
- Restore key pinch.
  - Brachioradialis and PL graft (Boyes, functions in both wrist flexion and extension).
  - Extensor carpi radialis brevis (ECRB) with tendon graft (Smith), strong motor donor.
  - FDS (Littler) ring or middle finger.
  - MCPJ/IPJ arthrodesis.
- Correct **Wartenberg's sign** (inability to adduct extended little finger due to unopposed EDM which is radially innervated) – re-route ulnar half of EDM to radial aspect of PP or A2 pulley of little finger.
- Enhance power grip – some recommend no treatment (Brand).
  - ECRL to lateral bands, PP and A2 – or use brachioradialis.
  - Suture together ulnar FDPs to median FDPs to achieve a finger flexion (mass action).

High ulnar nerve palsy

As above with FDP to ring and little fingers (which reduces clawing), FCU – the functional deficit is the same although **clawing may seem less obvious**.

- FCR to FCU if radial wrist deviation causes problems as ulna deviation is important for wrist flexion.

Low radial nerve palsy

Loss of ECRB, ECU, supinator and finger and thumb extensors. The loss of wrist extension (and stabilization) will reduce grip strength significantly.

- PT to **ECRB** to restore **wrist extension.**
  - Maintains some useful pronation from PT to the most central wrist extensor ECRB.
- FCR to **EDC** to restore **finger extension,** or FCU/FDS middle and ring to EDC. The FDS middle

Table 6.5 Nerve injuries, their symptoms and suitable transfers.

Injured nerve	Active deficit	Muscle functions missing	Donor muscles/tendons available
Median nerve (elbow)	Forearm pronation Wrist flexion Finger flexion	Pronator teres FCR, PL FDS (all), FDP (median)	Biceps FCU split Tenodese to ulnar FDPs
	Thumb IP flexion	FPL	Brachioradialis
	Thumb abduction	Thenar muscles	Opponensplasty using ADM or EI
Ulnar nerve (elbow)	Wrist flexion Finger flexion	FCU FDP (ulnar)	Split FCR Tenodesis to median FDPs
	Thumb adduction	AP	Brachioradialis
Ulnar nerve (wrist)	Metacarpophalangeal flexion (hyper-extended)	Lumbricals (ulnar)	FDS to radial sagittal band
Radial nerve (elbow)	Elbow flexion	Brachioradialis	Flexor mass resited higher on humerus
	Radial wrist extension	ECRB, ECRL	Pronator teres
	Finger extension	EC, EI, EDM	FCU
	Thumb extension	EPL	Palmaris longus

with its separate muscle belly, has the theoretical advantages of a straight line of pull with sufficient strength and excursion and being relatively expendable; it is usually routed through a window in the interosseus membrane of the forearm.

- PL to **EPL** to restore **thumb extension**, or FDS middle to EPL.

The first set of options is often called a **Brand transfer**, the same but FCU instead of FCR is called a FCU transfer; a Boyes' transfer (PT to ECRB, FDS middle to EDC, FDS ring to EIP and EPL, FCR to APL and EPB) can be used in patients without a palmaris longus.

With a high radial nerve palsy, there is additional loss of ECRL and brachioradialis, but treatment is essentially the same.

Post-operative care

- Splintage usually in the position of function being reconstructed, for 4–5 weeks, then night splints.
- Mobilize under supervision until strength increases at 6–8 weeks. The involvement of a good hand therapist is vital to the outcome.

There are some studies comparing results of early active motion with passive motion or immobilization by cast.

Complications include:

- Rupture.
- Adhesions.
- Incorrect tension.

VI. Complex regional pain syndromes
Stanton–Hicks definition

'A variety of painful conditions following injury ... exceeding both in magnitude and duration the expected clinical course of the inciting event.' The term 'complex regional pain syndrome (CRPS)' has been used since 1995 when it was felt that the previous terms RSD and causalgia were inadequate.

It is an abnormal pain response to injury with multifactorial causes, particularly dysfunction of the sympathetic system.

Type 1

- No predisposing event ('primary' non-nerve related CRPS) – RSD, algodystrophy.
- Increased uptake on the bone scan especially around the joints.
- Can be cited as an early and late complication of any hand surgery.

Type 2

- Identifiable primary **nerve** insult ('secondary' CRPS) – causalgia plus vasomotor, sudomotor (sweat gland) and trophic changes.
- Differential diagnosis may include **Secretan's** disease: brawny swelling and induration in the hand as a result of factitious tapping/rubbing of the hand.

Some divide it into sympathetically maintained or independent pain syndromes.

Pathogenesis

Evidence for immune system involvement in reflex sympathetic dystrophy
Calder JS. *J Hand Surg* 1998;**23**:147–150.

The authors propose that the cause is sensitization of the central nervous system to a painful stimulus following peripheral injury.

- Initiating stimulus reduces the threshold and increases the rate of firing of nociceptors which stimulates Langerhans cells.
- Langerhans cells release IL-1 and TNF-α which cause skin fibroblasts to release NGF, which is transported retrogradely to the neuronal cell body causing the release of the neuropeptides substance P (SP) and calcitonin growth-related peptide (CGRP).
- Substance P and CGRP produce oedema and inflammation, and act centrally to increase the excitability of CNS NMDA receptors in the hypothalamus.

Cytokine-mediated feedback (from the site of injury via spinothalamic tracts) to hypothalamus causes sensitization of the CNS and secondary effects mediated by sympathetic outflow from the sensitized hypothalamus.

Predisposing factors

- Surgery or trauma to hand (common after Colles' fracture) may be minor.
- Increased sympathetic activity.
- Smokers.
- Tight dressings.
- Psychological profile of patient.

Symptoms

- Pain.
- **Allodynia** – pain due to a stimulus which does not normally provoke pain (e.g. emotion, noise).

- **Hyperalgesia** – increased pain to a normally painful stimulus.
- **Hyperaesthesia** – increased sensitivity to a stimulus, e.g. light touch.
- **Hyperpathia** – excessive perception of a painful stimulus.
- **Dysaesthesia** – abnormally perceived unpleasant sensation, spontaneous or provoked.
- **Causalgia** – burning pain, allodynia and hyperpathia after traumatic nerve injury.

Signs

- Stiffness.
- Swelling/oedema.
- Discolouration – **dermographia** – triple response to a light object drawn across the skin and other skin changes such as increased hair growth, shiny skin, hyperhidrosis and atrophy of bone (osteoporosis) with reduced radiographic bone density.

Examination

- Look – observe the above features plus any other scars, swellings, sudomotor changes, wasting. Also look at the attitude of the hand, hyperhidrosis.
- Feel – hot skin, sweaty, tender.
- Move – passive and active ROM in fingers, full examination of the three nerves.

There is no single test. Diagnosis can be made if there are > 5 of the following:

- Pain out of proportion.
- Abnormal sympathetic function e.g. hyperhidrosis, (dis)colouration (white mottling/ red blue), temperature (vasomotor activity), pilomotor ('goosebumps').
- Swelling – pitting or hard/brawny particularly if well-demarcated.
- Movement disorder e.g. stiffness or dystonia.
- Changes in tissue growth (dystrophy or atrophy) e.g. altered hair growth (first coarse and then thin), shiny skin, osteoporosis – there may be osteopaenia on plain X-ray. The value of a **three-phase bone scan** is controversial.

Objective findings should be sought out aggressively (e.g. colour). Up to 80% will have a measurable temperature difference (0.6 °C on thermography), which may be dynamic depending on local temperature as well as emotional stress but can be spontaneous.

Symptoms may spread from the injury site (continuity, mirror-image or independent types) and in many cases is of long duration (but very variable).

Stages

- Acute – traumatic (1–3 months) immediate and early.
- Subacute – dystrophic (3–12 months).
- Chronic – atrophic (years).

Some would say that the concept of staging is not useful in a disease with such an unpredictable and variable course.

Stage I: Immediate.

- Inappropriate pain within 48 hours of trauma or surgery.

Stage II: Early (1 week–6 months).

- Pain – hyperpathia, hyperalgesia with reduced mobility as a consequence.
- Vasodilatation – red, sweaty, oedematous.
- Reduced bone density.

Stage II: Intermediate (6–12 months).

- Pain is constant.
- Organized oedema ('brawny').
- Discolouration and sudomotor changes – blue, cool, dry.
- Trophic changes – shiny/glossy skin, brittle nails.
- Stiffness – joint contractures.

Stage III: Late (> 12 months – 'Sudeck's atrophy').

- Intractable pain – pain at rest may decrease but pain with motion persists.
- Dry stiff atrophic skin/tissues.
- Joint stiffness/contracture that is fixed.
- Atrophic changes as above, loss of bone density (Sudeck's atrophy) with increased uptake on bone scan (osteoclastic resorption).
- Lack of shoulder movement (**shoulder–hand syndrome**) in particular.

Treatment

The aims of treatment are to relieve pain and prevent progression; psychological management/support and patient education are important. Establishing a written protocol is very useful.

Early (regular review)

- Treat primary insult.

- Physiotherapy (splintage and mobilization) ± brachial plexus block. Normal use of the limb without reinjury should be encouraged.
- Reduce pain by 'any' means possible: e.g. TENS, drugs (amitriptyline, carbamazepine, pregabalin), guanethidine block.
  - Sequential therapy to maximal doses rather than multidrug therapy from the beginning is encouraged.
  - Drugs should be tailored to the type of pain e.g. chronic pain, pain disturbing sleep, inflammatory/injury pain, paroxysmal pain, muscle cramps, sympathetically maintained pain.

Intermediate

- Steroids.
- Sympathetic blocks e.g. stellate ganglion block.

Late (difficult and often intractable)

- Sympathectomy.
- Hyperbaric oxygen – 40 sessions.
- **Ketamine coma** (5 days) described by Schwartzmann, is not approved in the USA. Pain returns in two-thirds after 6 months; sub-anaesthetic boosters may be given. Other protocols include low-dose 'awake' infusion or outpatient infusions.
- Clonidine epidural infusion (or transdermal patch).
- Implantable spinal cord stimulators – aims to replace the CRPS with a more pleasant parasthaesia. It is possible to have a trial with temporary electrodes before implanting permanent ones.

C. Diagnosis and management of congenital hand conditions

I. Relevant anatomy and embryology

About one in 600 children is born with a congenital upper limb deformity. Children cope surprisingly well with what they have and usually do not become self-conscious until they become socialized when attending school. Parents on the other hand are extremely distressed.

Swanson's classification of congenital hand deformities is based on the work of Frantz and O'Rahilly, first described in 1976 and subsequently adopted by the American Society of Surgery of the Hand as well as the International Federation of Societies of Surgery of the Hand. It is based upon prediction of an embryonic failure leading to the clinical identifying features. Some conditions have more than one anomaly and the most dominant feature is used.

- Failure of formation of parts (15%)
  - Longitudinal – radial/ulnar /central deficiencies ('club/cleft hand').
  - Transverse – amelia, brachymetacarpia.
  - Mixed – phocomelia, symbrachydactyly (terminal differentiation).
- Failure of differentiation of parts (35%)
  - Camptodactyly, clinodactyly, symphalangism, syndactyly, arthrogryposis, synostosis.
- Duplication (33%)
  - Polydactyly.
  - Mirror hand.
- Overgrowth.
  - Macrodactyly.
- Undergrowth.
  - Madelung's deformity.
- Constriction ring syndrome.
- Generalized skeletal abnormalities.

However, Swanson's classification is often regarded as being inadequate for clinical use as it is phenotypic with little relevance to treatment and prognosis; the categories are not mutually exclusive.

Overview of limb development in relation to congenital hand anomalies

Tickle A. *Ann Rev Cell Biol* 1994;**10**:121–152.
Cohn MJ. *Cell* 1995;**80**:739–746.
Tabin C. *Cell* 1995;**80**:671–674.
Robertson KE. *Br J Plast Surg* 1997:**50**:109–115.
Upper limb development occurs mainly between weeks 6–8 in the human embryo. Limb buds appear as swellings on the ventrolateral aspect of the embryo; components in the bud direct growth and differentiation.

Formation of the limb bud (area of undifferentiated mesenchyme with overlying ectoderm, day 26 approximately)

A morphogenetic field is a cluster of cells in the embryo, which undergo similar development because they lie within the same set of boundaries. *Hox* gene expression makes the limb field competent to respond to initiating factors such as FGF.

The mesoderm of the limb bud **induces** the overlying ectodermal cells to elongate, become pseudostratified and form the **apical ectodermal ridge** (AER) – both the AER and the underlying mesoderm are required for limb development – removal of the AER or loss of contact of the AER with limb bud mesoderm prevents limb development. Removing the AER early results in a severely truncated limb (e.g. formation of a humerus only), while later removal allows formation of more distal structures (e.g. radius and ulna, etc.). Cells in the limb bud mesoderm instruct the AER to develop a certain type of limb while AER cells are responsible for sustained growth and development of that limb.

Apical ectodermal ridge

The AER is required for **proximo-distal** outgrowth and patterning i.e. the interdigital necrosis to separate the fingers. Mesenchymal cells beneath the AER proliferate rapidly to form the **progress zone** (PZ). The AER actually prevents PZ cells from differentiating by releasing a factor which promotes proliferation, but once they have left the PZ and are no longer under its influence, they differentiate in a regionally specific manner.

The PZ is made of undifferentiated mesenchymal cells and expresses:

- *Msx-1* gene which encodes a transcription factor promoting proliferation and expression is stimulated by fibroblast growth factor (**FGF**) from the AER.
- *Hox* genes whose expression is dependent upon FGF and a polarizing signal (retinoic acid and/or Sonic Hedgehog *Shh*). *Hox* genes (A, B, C and D) are expressed in an overlapping series of domains in the limb bud that specify the developmental fate of groups of cells throughout the limb and thus coordinate the model for proximo-distal patterning in the PZ. Mutations in *Hox*D13 are associated with synpolydactyly.

Zone of polarizing activity

The zone of polarizing activity (ZPA) is a small block of mesoderm at the junction of the posterior part of the limb bud and the body wall. It is central to A–P axis (the thumb-to-little finger i.e. radio-ulnar axis) specification. According to the diffusible morphogen model (Wolpert 1969) a soluble morphogen (*Shh*) is released from the ZPA creating a P–A concentration gradient and cells exposed to high concentration of the morphogen form posterior side (digit 4 in chick limb bud) and those exposed to low concentration (furthest away) form anterior side (digit 2). The ZPA also maintains the AER that, in turn, is responsible for initiating and maintaining growth and development of the limb.

- *Shh* is a patterning gene that encodes a secreted factor that may act directly as the limb morphogen or, perhaps more likely, leads to transcriptional activation of the true morphogen. Downstream of *Shh* is *BMP-2*, which interacts with another group of patterning genes, the *Hox* genes.
- *Shh* is critical in regulating ZPA function but the genes involved in *Shh* signalling are under the control of other factors needed for ZPA maintenance and function, especially retinoic acid, that acts through *Hox* genes.
- **Wingless type** (WNT) is a third signalling centre in the dorsal ectoderm acting via LMX-1 for dorsal-to-ventral orientation.

There are three main sets of cell interactions:

- AER–mesenchymal (for bud outgrowth).
- Mesenchymal–mesenchymal (for axial/proximo-distal development) i.e. AER–PZ.
- Epithelial–mesenchymal (for dorsoventral and A–P development).

Congenital limb abnormalities involving either absence or duplication of parts, may be attributed to:

- Disruptions of **antero-posterior** patterning which is normally mediated by ZPA (*Shh*/*BMP-2*/*Hox* genes) leads to 'longitudinal disorders'.
  - Syndactyly – failure of apoptosis in web zones.
  - Polydactyly – anterior ectopic *Shh* expression and disruption of *Hox* gene combinatorial code.
- **Proximo-distal limb** outgrowth disorders i.e. transverse deficiencies secondary to premature failure of specification of parts by the AER via FGF.
  - Symbrachydactyly.
  - Amelia.
- Combination of AP and PD patterning.
  - Intercalated deficiencies.
  - Phocomelia.

Reconstructive considerations

- Defect.
- Availability of normal proximal structures.

- Assessment, investigation, planning and treatment within a multidisciplinary team environment.

Most surgeons will perform surgery in the subject's second year of life or before, with this 'early surgery' providing better growth potential, acceptance of the part and adaptive patterns of use which is balanced against the greater technical difficulty and anaesthetic risk.

II. Failure of formation of parts
Longitudinal arrest

The term 'deficiency' is preferred to 'club hand'.

Radial deficiency

This was commonly called 'radial club hand' with hypoplasia or absence of the radius with radial deviation of the hand. It is bilateral in up to 75% or more (depending on classification) though rarely symmetrical; in 'unilateral cases', the opposite thumb is usually hypoplastic. Mostly males are affected.

- Impaired movement in the radial digits (index and middle).
- Carpal fusion.
- Ulna is bowed and thickened and only 60% of its normal length. 25% have a duplicated median nerve which replaces an absent radial nerve.
- There is fixed extension at the elbow. Elbow stiffness may be due to ulnar dislocation caused by the fibrous anlage restricting growth.
- The humerus is shorter and almost all muscles in the affected limb are abnormal.

Frantz and O'Rahilly classification

- I – Deficient radial epiphysis – short distal radius making radius mildly shortened, with thumb hypoplasia the prominent clinical feature requiring treatment,
- II – Hypoplastic radius (rare) not requiring treatment itself like above.
- III – Partial absence distally – (most common) centralization.
- IV – Total absence distally – radial agenesis, requires centralization.

It can be associated with other anomalies i.e. syndromic radial club hand:

- Holt–Oram syndrome – association between radial club hand and cardiac septal defects.

- VATER syndrome: Vertebral abnormalities, Anal atresia, Tracheo-oesophageal fistula and Renal abnormalities; VACTERL syndrome: Vertebral anomalies, Anal atresia, Cardiovascular malformations, Tracheo-oesophageal fistula, Renal and Limb anomalies.
- **Fanconi syndrome**: pancytopenia, predisposition to malignancies. Cardiac lesions and blood dyscrasias – the anaemia tends to develop later at ~6 years and is fatal without a marrow transplant (**Fanconi's anaemia**); also TAR (thrombocytopaenia that is present at birth but tends to improve, absent radius).

All those with radial deficiencies should have Fanconi's excluded (chromosomal challenge test) to allow additional time to find a suitable marrow donor.

Assessment

Those presenting with radial deficiencies should be asked about a family history of congenital hand abnormalities with focused investigations relating to suspected associated syndromal anomalies (vide supra).

In addition to development in general, the child should be observed particularly to assess the way the hand and elbow are used, e.g. can the hand be put to the mouth? Straightening the wrist in those with inadequate elbow flexion makes feeding of themselves impossible. Examination (both sides):

- Degree of:
  - Hypoplasia of the upper limb as a whole.
  - Radial angulation of the hand.
  - Hypoplasia of the thumb (Blauth's classification).
- Movements.
  - Shoulder, elbow (joint may be extended due to humeroulnar synostosis).
  - Wrist and hand – passive and active (fingers may be stiff)

Investigations

- AP and lateral plain X-rays.

The median nerve may substitute for the radial nerve that often terminates at the elbow. Similarly the radial artery is often missing.

Management

Types I and II usually do not require specific treatment.

- Manipulation splints and physiotherapy to maximize elbow movements.
- Restore elbow flexion (physiotherapy) then
- **Centralization (Bayne's classification)**
  - Centralization of carpus on ulnar (excise lunate to create space), if there is good elbow movement.
  - Ulnar transfer of radial wrist motors release/ transfer of radial deviators – FCR, ECRB, ECRL.
  - Closing wedge osteotomy of ulna and ulnar carpus.
  - Release of radial soft tissues – Z-plasty.
  - Steinman pin through third metacarpal.
- **Buck–Gramcko: radialization** of ulnar by placing second metacarpal and radial carpus over centre of ulnar, if elbow movement is less good. There is supposedly less growth disturbance and better movement with this compared to centralization which tends to result in a stiff, short limb.
- Pollicization e.g. Buck–Gramcko technique.

Distraction lengthening has been described to treat the deformed radius.

Ulnar deficiency

Ulnar deficiency is 4–10× less common than radial deficiency, usually unilateral and shows the reverse skeletal abnormalities, though with much more variation. Some cases show autosomal dominant inheritance, other musculoskeletal abnormalities may be present whilst systemic syndromic associations are uncommon. Functionally, the wrist is good whilst the elbow tends to be worse off. Thumb and carpal anomalies are also relatively common.

Bayne's classification

- I Hypoplastic ulna.
- II Partial aplasia – most common.
- III Total aplasia.
- IV Total aplasia with radiohumeral synostosis.

Treatment

- Splinting and physiotherapy to improve passive movements.

Generally the functional status without resection of the anlage is very good, thus resection is controversial. Fusing the proximal ulna to the distal radius (thus eliminating problems with bowing of the ulnar and dislocation of the radial head) to form a one-bone forearm may create a stable forearm.

Central deficiency

There is a range of deformity from total absence of middle ray to monodactyly. The bones are absent or malpositioned, but never rudimentary. Flatt described it as a 'functional triumph and social disaster' – despite its appearance ('Lobster claw hand' is a somewhat cruel term that should be avoided), the wide central cleft allows for grasp and pinch and along with normal sensation allows good function.

There may be some confusion with **symbrachydactyly.** In contrast to symbrachydactyly, the radial side is more frequently affected and thus can be distinguished from symbrachydactyly-type of cleft hand, which is usually ulnar. In addition, in severe forms the only remaining digit is the little finger (whilst in severe symbrachydactyly, the only remaining digit is the thumb).

Barsky (after Lange) describes two types:

Typical: bilateral absence of 3rd finger creating a deep palmar cleft between the central metacarpals, with syndactyly of 1st and 4th web. There is skeletal hypertrophy adjacent to the cleft. It is usually familial and is said to show autosomal dominant inheritance and is often associated with other abnormalities including cleft lip/palate.

Atypical: unilateral deep cleft with complete/partial absence of central rays (2nd, 3rd and 4th) with short radial and ulnar digits present with a **shallow cleft**. There is hypoplasia adjacent to the cleft. It is usually sporadic and may be associated with Poland's syndrome. This is often regarded as a form of symbrachydactyly and a failure of formation, whilst the typical cleft is failure of differentiation.

Another classification is that of Cole and Manske (1–5, based on quality of thumb and first web).

Treatment

Treatment centres on cleft closure with attention to avoid limiting the first web function – not all procedures that improve appearance will improve function. Syndactyly should be separated with care, as blood supply is often tenuous.

Snow–Littler procedure ('reverse pollicization' with palmar-based interdigital flap, an alternative is Miura–Komada with a dorsal interdigital flap).

- Palmar-based flap from the cleft that is inset into first web space. The flap is often long and distal viability may be tenuous.
- Correction of syndactyly between thumb and index.
- Index metacarpal transposed ulnarly i.e. to base of third metacarpal.

The forearm is the most common level for arrest. It may be difficult to distinguish transverse arrest at the arm from constriction band syndrome which, unlike the former, tends to be unilateral. Children with unilateral problems tend to discard prostheses, and the simple cosmetic arm is more likely to be accepted than a 'functional' myoelectric prosthesis.

Phocomelia

This condition is rare. In contrast to amelia where no hand is present, a functional terminal hand is always present in phocomelia.

- Complete – hand directly attached to trunk.
- Proximal – arm absent and forearm attached to trunk.
- Distal – forearm absent, hand attaches to humerus.

Types:

- Pre-axial.
- Post-axial.
- Central.
- Intercalated defect.

Prosthetics (palmar plate or myoelectric) are the mainstay of management though extremely short limbs may make this difficult; surgery is rarely indicated.

III. Failure of differentiation of parts

This includes syndactyly, camptodactyly, clinodactyly and arthrogryposis. Other conditions that fall into category include synostoses (radio-ulnar) and carpal coalition.

Syndactyly

This condition occurs at an incidence of 1 in 2000 live births and is the second commonest congenital limb abnormality after polydactyly. It is due to failure of apoptosis in the 7th week, compared with acrosyndactyly which is a result of the constriction band syndrome. It can be associated with almost any other congenital abnormality.

Eighty per cent are sporadic. There is a family history in 10–40% (highest incidence in a small cluster in Iowa), inheritance is autosomal dominant with incomplete penetrance and variable expressivity has been described.

- 50% bilateral.
- Twice as common in males.
- 10 × more common in Whites compared with Africans.

In order of decreasing frequency, most affected web space is **3rd web space**, then 4th, 2nd and 1st (3%). In the foot, the most affected space is the 2nd.

Pathology

There is always a shortage of skin.

- There may be fascial interconnections (thickened Cleland's and Grayson's ligaments are coalesced and web-space/palmar fascia is thickened), shared flexor and extensor tendons or shared anomalous digital nerve and artery. Abnormal tendons are more common in Apert's syndrome (acrocephalosyndactyly).
- There are varying degrees of bone abnormalities.
- Individual joints commonly preserved unless there is symphalangism (more common in syndromic cases) – joints remain incompletely differentiated and progress to ankylosis.

Classification

- **Complete** (digits united as far as distal phalanx) vs. incomplete (digits united beyond mid-point of proximal phalanx but not as far as the distal phalanx).
- **Complex** (metacarpal or phalangeal synostosis) vs. simple (no synostosis). Conjoint nails are suggestive of joined bones also. Complicated syndactyly includes many forms including cases with more than simple side-to-side bony fusion e.g. polydactyly, symbrachydactyly, acrosyndactyly; these are often associated with syndromes.
- Acrosyndactyly – shortened digits that are united distally but with proximal fenestration – may be associated with congenital band syndrome (Streeter's dysplasia). It is usually isolated but may be associated with other anomalies e.g. craniofacial abnormalities and spinal dysraphism.

Contraindications to surgery

Minor degree of webbing, not cosmetically or functionally significant.

- Severe complex syndactyly, digits share common structures including digital nerves and arteries.
- Hypoplastic digits where one digit functions better than would two.
- Adjacent webs should not be released simultaneously.
- The risk of hypertrophic scarring may be increased in feet and is a relative contraindication.

Timing of surgery

Most hand movements are learned between 6 and 24 months so the argument is usually made for operating before 2 years of age (on average 18–24 months; a trend for earlier surgery at 9–12 months is quite common). Indications for early surgery (4–6 months) in syndactyly:

- Border digits.
- Length discrepancy.

Generally, one side of a digit is operated on at a time to reduce the risk of vascular insufficiency. Bilateral procedures can be performed in children less than 14 months of age but should be avoided in older children.

Surgical technique

- Dorsal and palmar zigzag incisions (or lazy-S) either to midline of digits (Cronin triangular flaps 1956) or to lateral borders (Zachariae). Mark dorsal zigzags (~60° angles) with bases over PIPJ and DIPJ of one finger, and then complementary volar flaps (a needle can be used to help plan volar flaps). Take care with the dorsal veins when raising flaps.
  - Withey techniques uses 7–8 narrower flaps, these should not be defatted – tips are tacked into place with a single stitch and raw areas heal by secondary intention.
- Web space is usually created with a proximally based dorsal flap extending from MCPJ to PIPJ or just proximal to it, and inset into the palmar surface. Web flaps should be wide to allow spread and robust to avoid skin grafts around the web spaces. Alternatively dorsal and volar inverted V flaps at the base of the web.

Separation should proceed carefully bearing in mind that the arterial bifurcation may be more distal in these patients. The level of division of the neurovascular bundle forms the limit of the web space. Defatting the flaps helps closure (Greuse), and may allow grafts

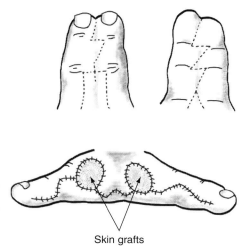

Skin grafts

Figure 6.14 Syndactyly.

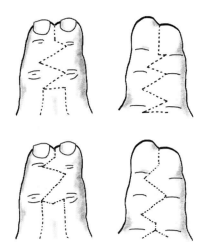

Figure 6.15 Types of incisions used for syndactyly release.

to be avoided. Where grafts are needed especially near the web, FTSG is usually preferred to SSG and may be taken from groin or instep, for example; the graft should be tied-in without tension. Techniques that use all the skin to cover one finger, and graft the other, tend to have worse results.

- Buck–Gramcko technique for division of the syndactyly nail: use matching tongue flaps at the tip of the finger curled around the raw edge of the ipsilateral nail bed.
- Deepening of web spaces (e.g. partial simple syndactyly or web creep) can be achieved by four-flap Z-plasty (120° Z-plasty provides 164% expansion compared with 75% with single Z-plasty) or jumping man flap.

Post-operative complications

Intra-operative and early

- Division of nerve or tendon.
- Circulatory compromise (grafts too tight or digital artery injury).
- Haematoma, infection, graft loss.

Late

- Destabilization of joints.
- Deformity of the digit or web.
- **Web creep**, particularly with growth spurt, may be increased with wound infections. Splints tend to be of limited use.

Camptodactyly

Camptodactyly was first described by Tamplin in 1846. It supposedly affects < 1% of the population; it is painless and is usually of no functional significance in the majority (and thus may be under-reported). It is occasionally inherited as an autosomal dominant trait; it may present in infants or in adolescence, particularly in females.

- I – congenital, isolated and unilateral. Most commonly little finger and apparent during infancy.
- II – as above but appears as a progressive flexion deformity at 7–11 years of age with female predominance.
- III – severe involvement of multiple digits and often associated with generalized conditions especially arthrogryoposis.

It is a **congenital flexion deformity** of the digit, usually involving the little finger and usually at the PIPJ. It is commonly bilateral but is rarely symmetrical. There is usually an **abnormal insertion of lumbrical or FDS**; there are secondary changes in PIPJ (X-ray may show a flattened dorsal ridge). Almost every structure around the PIPJ may be involved in the pathogenesis. The DIPJ is never involved, except if there is a secondary boutonnière deformity.

- A flexion abnormality that is reducible with MCPJ stabilization may represent MCPJ instability.
- If there is also brachydactyly ('short fingers') with a stiff PIPJ with anterior flexion/extension creases, it may be a case of symphalangism.

Options

- Conservative treatment in the form of splintage and/or stretching exercises is rarely successful except for cases with < 15° contracture that is passively correctable. Half of adolescent patients may improve with this regime.
- In cases with a normal joint, passively correctable deformity > 30°, surgery may help but may not achieve full correction.
  - Identify cause: release of anomalous intrinsic insertion or lengthen FDS.
  - Correction of soft tissue contracture (vide infra) with stepwise release of tethering structures.
  - (Philippe) Saffar procedure – subperiosteal lift, division of collateral and accessory collateral ligaments and check rein ligaments.
  - Those with severe contracture (> 90°) will need K-wires to maintain the PIPJ position.
- With a deranged joint e.g. with long-standing contractures:
  - Dorsal angulation osteotomy.
  - Arthrodesis if severely contracted.

Camptodactyly: a unifying theory

Grobbelar AO. *J Hand Surg (Am)* 1998;**23**:14–19.

Surgery should be reserved for patients with a flexion contracture of > 60°.

Tethering structures are released e.g. skin, fascia, tendon sheaths, intrinsics, collateral ligaments and volar plate. The FDS tendon is then lengthened and the central slip is plicated. All these structures have been implicated in the pathogenesis of camptodactyly but to varying degrees.

Clinodactyly

'Kliner' is Greek for 'to bend'.

Clinodactyly is curvature of a digit in a radio-ulnar plane that in most cases is usually a radial deviation at the PIPJ of the little finger and usually bilateral. It is most commonly due to an abnormally shaped phalanx (usually middle) that prevents normal longitudinal growth. The classic 'delta' phalanx (Blundell Jones, 1964) – longitudinally bracketed epiphysis – is characterized by a trapezoidal or triangular phalangeal bone with a curved 'C'-shaped epiphysis which makes angulation inevitable.

However, occasionally it is due to soft tissue problems e.g. fibrous band on the ulnar side of the digit. In some cases, the phalanx may also be shortened (brachyphalangia). The abnormal phalanx may reduce mobility; pain is not a prominent feature.

It is more common in males. It is less common in Whites (~1%) compared with up to 19.5% in non-Whites. It can be sporadic but is often inherited with an autosomal dominant pattern with variable penetrance. Marked clinodactyly may be associated with mental retardation including trisomy 21; there are many other associations including Poland's, Treacher Collins and Klinefelter's syndromes and its severity is often related to the severity of the other anomalies.

- Incidence in Down syndrome patients up to 80%.
- Incidence in general population 1–20%.

Options

Surgery is essentially cosmetic, thus leaving things alone is a choice.

- Bracket resection with horizontal growth plate preservation and fat graft to fill the defect, at 3–4 years.
- Closing wedge osteotomy (phalanx normal length but trapezoid, best to wait until skeletal maturity).
- Opening wedge osteotomy plus bone graft (if the phalanx is short).
- Reversed wedge osteotomy (wedge from long cortex turned over and inserted into shorter side).
- Vickers' procedure – rongeur of delta-phalanx epiphysis and free fat graft, useful before 6 years of age.
- The use of distraction has been reported.

Clinodactyly may be mistaken for **Kirner's deformity** (dystrophy/osteochondrosis of fifth finger, acrodysplasia), which is a volar and radial incurvature at the DIPJ.

- It is less common compared with clinodactyly and is often bilateral. There is no family history in the majority and affects young females just before puberty (7–14 years). It may be associated with Turner's syndrome.
- It starts as a painless swelling but develops into an arthrogryposis, incurved joints with the appearance of a 'windblown' hand. The distal phalanx is shortened, swollen and deflected in a volar-radial direction and a dysmorphic nail.

The exact aetiology is unknown; there is a disruption of the growth plate due to an unknown mechanism.

Treatment

- Splints (may need to be continued until school age) with variable results.
- Surgery is reserved for severe deformities e.g. soft tissue release and occasionally osteotomy with K-wire stabilization.

Symphalangism

Symphalangism (Cushing's) is the failure of segmentation of the fingers (joint is represented by a cartilaginous bar), mainly at the PIPJ and rarely at MCPJ and usually the ulnar fingers are more affected. The resultant fingers are stiff, lack flexion creases and usually more slender.

Hereditary symphalangism is an autosomal dominant trait. There may also be symbrachydactyly of the middle finger and it may be associated with hearing defects.

- True symphalangism – normal digital length.
- Brachysymphalangism – short digits.
- Syndromic e.g. Apert's and Poland's syndromes; these tend to be non-hereditary types of symphalangism.

Reconstruction tends to lead to poor results; osteotomy or arthrodesis (20°/30°/40°/50° for the digits) may be useful after skeletal maturity has been attained.

Radio-ulnar synostosis

This is fusion of the proximal radio-ulnar joint. Due to the good functional result (wrist and shoulder compensation), it is often a late/under diagnosis. It is bilateral in 60%.

Synostosis can occur at a number of other sites in the hand, e.g. metacarpal synostosis.

- **Primary** – radial head is absent.
- **Secondary** – radial head is dislocated.

There is fixed pronation deformity with compensatory hypermobility at the wrist. The radius is thickened and bowed with possible radial head agenesis or dislocation, whilst the ulnar is straight and narrow.

Options

- Minor – no treatment, there is good functional adaptation.
- Severe (fixed pronation > 45°) – de-rotational osteotomy through the synostosis with risk of injury to arteries and posterior interosseus nerve.

In bilateral cases, the limbs are placed in neutral in one and 20° pronation in the other.

Arthrogryposis

This is the presence of joint contracture affecting at least two areas which are non-progressive and are associated with (intrauterine) muscle wasting (and replacement with inelastic fibrofatty tissue). There are no flexion creases due to a lack of movement; sensation is normal. Approximately 1 in 200 are affected by arthrogryposis multiplex congenita.

Cases are usually sporadic. The cause is unknown though theories include:

- Obstruction of fetal movement – increased intrauterine pressure, oligohydramnios.
- Viral infection, chronic cyanide intoxication, exposure to paralysing agents.

It is associated with syndromes/anomalies such as:

- Klippel-Feil syndrome.
- Sprengel's deformity.
- Hypoplastic mandible, cleft palate.
- Dislocated radial head.
- Renal and cardiac anomalies.

It presents as a characteristic posture:

- Shoulder internal rotation and adduction.
- Elbow extension, forearm pronation.
- Wrist and finger flexion.
- Thumb clasped into palm.
- Lower limbs: hip dislocation, knee subluxation and club feet.

Management

A multidisciplinary team is useful.

- Splintage and stretching.
- Surgery consists mostly of a combination of skeletal reorganization and muscle transfer:
  - Shoulder – external de-rotational osteotomy of humerus.
  - Elbow – tricep release, flexion by transfer (triceps to biceps, Steindler flexorplasty, free gracilis).
  - Wrist – carpectomy (total or proximal row), osteotomies of radius and ulnar, FCU to ECRB transfer.
  - Fingers – osteotomy, FDS to extensor band transfer.
  - Thumb – thenar muscle release, 4-flap plasty.

Differential diagnoses of a flexed thumb (thumb in palm)

The newborn have flexed thumbs until approximately 3 months of age (dominant flexor innervation has been proposed).

- Fixed flexion at the IPJ due to triggering related to Notta's nodule which is a thickening of the FPL tendon. It is bilateral in 25%. It is not a true congenital abnormality as it develops in the first year or two of life. It is best to delay surgery as it may resolve spontaneously < 2 years of age (30%) but should be differentiated from a clasped thumb.
- Clasped thumb involving IPJ and MCPJ, may be due to weak or absent EPL tendon and there may also be UCL instability. Other fingers may also be involved.
- Arthrogryposis.

IV. Duplication

Polydactyly

This is the commonest congenital limb abnormality – affecting 1 in 300 Africans and 1 in 3000 Whites (and more likely to be syndromic). It may be inherited in an autosomal dominant manner. It may be radial (pre-axial), ulnar (post-axial) or central.

Stelling classification

- I – Skin only.
- II – Skeletal – part of a digit articulating with a phalanx or bifid metacarpal.
- III – Complete duplication of ray, including metacarpal (rare).

Central duplication

Types I–II

- Type II is invariably within what appears clinically to be a simple complete syndactyly.

Ulnar polydactyly

This is more common in Africans with a positive family history. It is normally unilateral, an isolated condition and it is unusual for it to be associated with other anomalies except in Whites.

Radial polydactyly i.e. duplicate thumb

This occurs 0.8 per 1000 live births; it is more common in Whites and in males (2.5×). It can be associated with other anomalies i.e. part of syndromes (e.g. Carpenter's, Holt–Oram, Wassell type VII, ASD/VSD/PDA, Fanconi anaemia) that can affect any organ system including orofacial, bone dysplasia and mental retardation. The presence of a duplicate thumb should prompt a thorough work-up.

Wassell classification (primarily a radiological classification):

- I – Bifid distal phalanx(2%), most uncommon.
- II – Duplicated distal phalanx.
- III – Bifid proximal phalanx.
- IV – Duplicated proximal phalanx (~50%), most common.
- V – Bifid metacarpal.
- VI – Duplicated metacarpal.
- VII – Partially duplicated metacarpal (also hypoplastic duplicate thumb – no skeletal elements – and **triphalangia**). Strongest familial tendency and associations with Holt–Oram and Fanconi's.

The duplicate thumb is often shorter and thinner than normal (triphalangia approaches length of fingers); there is hypoplasia of soft tissues and bone in the central portion. The eccentric insertion of tendons tends to pull the thumbs together.

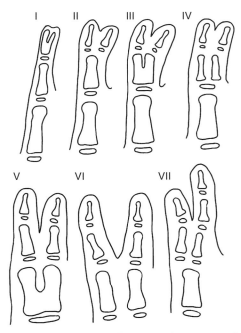

Figure 6.16 The types of thumb duplication (Wassell classification).

- Radial duplicate receives the hypothenar musculature whilst the ulnar duplicate receives adductor pollicis and the first dorsal interosseus. Absence or hypoplasia of these muscles is common.
- The anomalous insertion of FPL into the extensor expansion (Lister's tubercle) promotes abduction.

Surgery
Excision

- Appropriate where the duplicate is rudimentary (hypoplastic) without skeletal elements, e.g. pouce flottant, and also where the accessory thumb is widely separated from a normal thumb. Usually the radial digit is excised, with reattachment of the radial collateral ligament.

Combination (of parts)

This is required for all other duplications to provide optimal function and cosmesis.

- C1 (symmetric) – Bilhaut–Cloquet procedure for Wassell types I and II.
  - Excision of adjacent marginal structures with merger of bone and soft tissue in a side-to-side fashion.
- C2 (asymmetric) i.e. nearly all of one digit is retained and is augmented with tissues from the other digit, e.g. skin only and unused tissues from the 'spare-part' are excised. It is suited for Wassell type IV.
- C3 (on-top-plasty).
  - Segmental digital transposition that brings the best distal segment of one duplicate onto the best proximal segment of the other.

Revision

- Secondary surgery.
- Intrinsic transfer.
- Realignment of eccentric tendon insertions such as pollex abductus (where the FPL attaches to the EPL via an anomalous tendon that passes around the radial aspect of the thumb; it also occurs in thumb hypoplasia).

Complications

- Angulation – persistence or recurrence.
- Stiffness.
- Clinodactyly.
- Instability.

Mirror hand (ulnar dimelia)

This is a rare upper limb abnormality with duplication of the ulna and absence of the radius. There is poly-dactyly with midline symmetry and there are usually seven fingers (5–4–3–2–3–4–5) with no thumb. It has been attributed to the limb bud having an additional progress zone (PZ). Elbow mobility may be limited.

Six cases of multiple hand have been described in the literature. Usually the post-axial side is more func-tional and regarded as dominant; the accessory 4 is pollicized whilst the accessory III and V are resected (Entin procedure).

V. Overgrowth
Macrodactyly

This is defined as congenital enlargement of a digit and is rare (2 in 100 000), making up approximately 1% of all upper limb congenital anomalies. In many cases, it is probably a form of neurofibromatosis, whilst it could also be vascular malformations in others – however, it remains a heterogeneous group and can cause confusion when interpreting the literature. The most common 'true' form is related to lipofibromatous nerve enlargement. Ninety per cent are unilateral, whilst 70% involve more than one digit especially index and middle.

- Usually the metacarpals are of normal size, whilst the phalanges are enlarged.
- The tendons and blood vessels are of normal size (leading to ischaemia).

Upton's classification

- I – macrodactyly with lipomatous nerve (especially median), most common and usually sporadic.
- II – with neurofibromatosis (often bilateral) with gigantism with greater areas of upper and lower limbs.
- III – with hyperostosis i.e. multiple osseous osteochondral nodules, very rare.
- IV – with hemihypertrophy or Proteus syndrome (very rare, 1 in a million), generalized gigantism with hyperplasia of connective tissues, blood vessels and bone.

The part usually has little movement and there may be gross curvature. The deformity may be classed as:

- **Static** – born with large digit and development of the digit keeps pace with growth of the hand.

- **Progressive** – more common, more aggressive, rapid growth of a normal-sized digit at birth, increasing in size until epiphyseal closure. It is particularly debilitating.

Assessment

- Assess size discrepancy and effect on form and function.
- Investigations include X-ray of adjacent joints and angiography when vascular malformations are suspected.

Treatment

Amputation may be best option, otherwise:

- Debulking of soft tissues (best staged) and bones i.e. reduction and longitudinal osteotomy.
- Nerve stripping, in some cases; it was once thought that nerve resection would reduce further overgrowth. Tsuge regarded it as being 'nerve-driven' overgrowth.
- Epiphyseal ablation/epiphysiodesis (when digit same size as parent).

Surgical outcomes can be poor but are generally better than no treatment at all; secondary surgery is often required.

VI. Undergrowth

Hypoplasia of the thumb

This is usually an isolated anomaly though there is often a hypoplastic/absent radius. The cause is unknown but may be related to a fetal neurogenic injury, reduced fetal oxygen tension or, in some cases, due to maternal thalidomide intake. There is an association with other anomalies that should be excluded e.g. cardiac (Holt–Oram, VACTERL) and blood dyscrasias (TAR, Fanconi anaemia).

 The condition commonly requires pollicization of the index finger in the first year of life.

Buck–Gramcko modification of the Blauth classification

- I – Hypoplasia – normal skeleton and musculature but *all hypoplastic* leading to reduced gross size but normal range of motion.
- II – Hypoplasia – smaller thumb, bones narrow, reduced volume or absence of thenar muscles and first web space adduction contracture due to adductor–abductor imbalance.

- III – Hypoplasia – even smaller thumb and the absence of thenar muscles leads to severe first web space contracture. There is MCJP instability and bones/joints at base are variably affected – there may be absence of trapezium and scaphoid.
- IV – Pouce flottant – a rudimentary appendage with no metacarpal, trapezium or scaphoid (trapezoid usually normal) and absence of muscles except 2nd metacarpal origin of the first dorsal interosseus. It is attached by a small skin bridge; there may be a neurovascular pedicle within the skin bridge. Treat by amputation and pollicization.
- V – Total aplasia with no skeletal or soft tissue elements. There are compensatory changes in index finger (curvature, pulp widening, pronation and widened space between index and middle finger). Treat with pollicization.

The tendon configuration can be quite variable, including absence of intrinsic/extrinsic and anomalous connections e.g. pollex abductus, musculus lubricalis pollicis (from FPL to index causing a tight web). Blauth divided III into a and b with stable and unstable CMC joints respectively, which effectively differentiates those that can be reconstructed or require ablation/pollicization. It can be difficult to differentiate between IIIa and IIIb in a child – the latter tends to lead to a thumb that is ignored with prehension developing between index and long digits, and the index tending to pronate and rotate out.

Thumb reconstruction

Principles

- Allow opposition.
  - Distal end of a pollicized digit must reach to PIP finger crease of the middle finger when the thumb is adducted.
  - Good circumduction at carpometacarpal joint.
- The thumb must be sensate with joints stable enough to allow pinch grip.

Management

Types II–IIIa

- Opponensplasty with ring finger FDS, may need to be augmented with Huber procedure (ADM transfer).
- UCL stabilization to stabilize MCPJ.
- Four-flap Z-plasty to deepen first web.
- May also need extensor indicis to EPL.

Types III(b)–V

Pollicization (of index) is usually used. There is a rearrangement of bones, muscles (interossei) and tendons in various combinations (see variations below), in general:

- The metacarpal head assumes role of trapezium; the metacarpal is shortened.
- The thumb is dissected as an island flap pedicled on neurovascular bundles and long tendons and fixed in pronation of 160° and hyperextension at the MCPJ.
  - First dorsal interosseus assumes role of APB.
  - First palmar interosseus assumes role of adductor pollicis.
  - Extensor communis to the index becomes APL.
  - Extensor indicis becomes EPL.

Littler (Littler JW. *Plast Reconstr Surg* 1953;**12**:303–319) – this technique is suited for reconstruction of the amputated thumb.

- **Resection of the index metacarpal (and MCPJ)** and distal half of thumb metacarpal.
- Base of index PP fused to base of thumb metacarpal in 120° pronation, 10° flexion.
- Advancement of palmar and dorsal skin flaps into new first web space.
  - Transfer of first dorsal interosseus insertion to radial border of index.
  - Transfer of EPL to EDC of index.
  - Late transfer of FPL to FDP in the forearm.

Zancolli (Zancolli E. *J Bone Joint Surg Am* 1960;**42**:658–660) – this was the first pollicization technique for the congenitally absent thumb. The **index metacarpal head is fused to the trapezoid**.

- The origin of 'first' dorsal interosseus is transposed across the palm to the hypothenar eminence to cause adduction of the new thumb.
- There is no shortening of long extensors and flexors.

Carroll RE. *Clin Orthop* 1988;**220**:106–110.

- **Removal of the diaphyseal segment of the index metacarpal** and fusion in 120° pronation.
  - Shortening of extensors but not flexors.
  - Detachment of palmar and dorsal interosseii from the base of the PP and reinsertion into the base of the MP to achieve adduction and abduction.

Buck–Gramcko D. *J Bone Joint Surg Am* 1971;**53**:1605–1617.

- **Subcapital excision of the index metacarpal.** The base of the PP is hyperextended on the metacarpal head and the complex is sutured to the carpus in 160° pronation.
  - Shorten the EI tendon and use this as a permanent motor.
  - Redirect EDC volarly to act in adduction.
  - Distal advancement of interosseii as above.
  - No need to shorten flexor tendon.
  - Subsequent opponensplasty may be needed (FDS ring finger, ADM transfer).

There have been reports of microsurgical joint transfer in types IIIb and IV but results do not seem to be better than pollicization.

Options for reconstruction following trauma

- Thumb replantation.
- Finger replantation with pollicization.
- Distraction osteogenesis.
- Web-space deepening.
- Non-vascularized toe phalangeal transfer (keeping periosteum allows up to 90% growth) or other bone graft.
- Vascularized toe–hand transfer/wrap-around (first or second toes).

VII. Constriction ring syndrome

There are two main theories:

- **Extrinsic** – amniotic band (partial rupture involving only amnion layer) may encircle extremity.
- **Intrinsic** (Streeter GL. *Contributions Embryol* 1930;**22**:1–4) – internal defect in embryo leading to apoptosis. Vascular disruption relating to an intrinsic defect of the circulation. This is often used to explain the association with cleft lip/palate.

Constriction ring syndrome is usually sporadic (estimates 1 in 1200–15000) and no known prenatal risk factors have been demonstrated. There may be prenatal oligohydramnios/premature rupture and there is a strong association with clubfoot and cleft lip/palate, otherwise there is a low incidence of associated anomalies.

Patterson classification

There is a wide spectrum of anomalies. Proximal anatomy is normal.

- I – Simple constriction i.e. grooving/indentation.
- II – Constriction with distal deformity i.e. lymphoedema.
- III – Constriction with variable distal fusion i.e. acrosyndactyly.
- IV – Amputation from complete intrauterine disruption.

Urgent release may be required to reduce venous obstruction and lymphoedema e.g. multiple circumferential Z-plasty or W-plasty (though some suggest a partial 50–65% release initially to reduce vascular embarrassment), otherwise bands should be released before growth disturbances occur i.e. before 2 years. **Upton's method** – reverse skin and subcutaneous fat flaps separately transposed and closed as two layers to reduce indentation.

Acrosyndactyly

Acrosyndactyly is classified along with constriction ring syndrome and is seen in Apert's syndrome. It is attributed to the disruption after the digits have already separated, to be united by scar tissue. There may be fistulae, clefts or sinuses distal to the band and should be explored with probes.

- Deepen web spaces especially first and release small skin bridges. Staged smaller procedures are preferable to single procedures to reduce adversely affecting the vascularity.
- Amputation with delayed reconstruction may be needed.

VIII. Generalized anomalies

Arthrogryposis, achondroplasia, arachnodactyly and diastrophic dwarfism are also included in this category.

Symbrachydactyly

See the above on atypical central cleft. The cause is unknown (possibly related to deficient blood supply, like Poland's syndrome to which it has an association), it occurs in 1 in 32 000 and is not inherited.

The condition is characterized by short, stiff-webbed fingers creating a U-shaped cleft. Overall function tends to be reasonable as the condition is unilateral.

There are four types (Blauth) and affect the ulnar side more often:

- Peromelic type – digits are nubbins.
- Short finger type – short fingers, telescoped due to the action of rudimentary long tendons.
- Cleft hand type (**ulnar** side more affected).
- Monodactylous type.

Surgical options

- Distraction augmentation manoplasty.
  - Phalangeal transfer – a toe proximal phalanx usually PP of 3rd and 4th. There are potential problems with growth thus transfer is usually performed before 2 years of age when there is a better chance of growth of the transferred parts. The toes are ultimately shorter but there are few problems with mobility.
  - Distraction osteogenesis later e.g. over 7 years old, over 8–12 weeks.
  - Deepen web spaces.
- Toe–hand transfer.

Madelung's deformity

This condition with autosomal dominant inheritance is an abnormality of the radial epiphysis in ulnar anterior portion. It usually presents at ages 8–12 years.

- Radius: short, radial inclination > 20° with the horizontal.
- Ulnar: dorsal subluxation, enlarged ulnar head.
- Carpus: wedge shaped.

There is pain and decreased supination at the forearm.

Treatment options

- Excision of ulnar head (prominent).
- Wedge osteotomies of the radius.

IX. Spastic disorders of the upper limb

Aims of treatment

- Restore function.
- Relieve pressure areas and enable personal hygiene.
- Relieve pain from nerve compression.

It is usual to delay rebalancing surgery until neurological recovery is maximal, thus it is important to distinguish between reversible brain injury, non-reversible injury and chronic spasticity disorders (including cerebral palsy). Examination under regional anaesthesia may help to differentiate between spasticity and established contractures.

Non-operative treatment

- Maintain passive ROM with exercises and serial splintage.
- Protect pressure areas.
- Relieve spasm e.g. intraneural phenol injections of motor nerves and botulinum toxin injections.

Surgical treatment

- Stabilize joints.
- Tendon lengthening (partial tenotomy at musculotendinous junction).
- Nerve decompression (carpal tunnel and Guyon's canal).

The priority is to address three groups of muscles:

- Extrinsic wrist and digital extensors and flexors: forearm pronation can be relieved by pronator teres tenotomy.
- Intrinsics of the hand: release intrinsic tightness.
- Thumb and first web space: for thumb adduction, release web (four-flap Z-plasty or jumping man), release adductor pollicis from its origin on the third metacarpal and divide transverse carpal ligament (avoiding injury to the ulnar nerve).

In patients with non-functioning hands:

- Extrinsic flexor tendon contracture can be treated with FDS to FDP transfer with tenodesis to form single juncturae.
- Treat intrinsic spasticity with ulnar motor branch neurectomy at wrist if passively correctable under anaesthesia and tendon lengthening allows MCPJ extension to neutral. If passive correction is not possible then intrinsic release is performed.
- Proximal row carpectomy and wrist arthrodesis.
- Arthrodesis of subluxed MCPJ and IPJs.
- Bone block between thumb and index metacarpals.

Adult-acquired spastic hemiplegia

After a stroke (variable incidence from 20–70%), for example.

The picture is similar to that of cerebral palsy but the result of surgery (release of spastic muscles, tendon transfer) is less predictable. It is not strictly necessary to treat the spasticity just because it is there (some say that it can increase/maintain muscle tone/bulk and reduce osteoporosis), but rather to treat when it interferes with active or passive function or becomes painful.

Medication such as baclofen or dantrolene may help despite the side-effects; alternatives include nerve blocks/neurolytics with phenol or alcohol and more recently botulinum toxin. Surgery is generally reserved for those with muscle/tendon shortening who do not resort to other measures.

- Elbow (spastic) – lengthen biceps and brachialis.
- Wrist flexor (spastic) – lengthen/release FCR/FCU.
- Wrist extension (absent) – tenodesis or transfer FCU–ECRB.
- Finger flexors (spastic) – FDS–FDP transfer.
- Finger extension (absent) – brachioradialis to EDC.
- Thumb (clasped in palm) – Z-plasty web, lengthen intrinsics +/− arthrodesis IPJ.

Cerebral palsy

Cerebral palsy is not a specific disease of the brain but a congenital disorder caused by pre-, peri- or postnatal insults affecting various parts of the CNS. Clinically, it may present with a range of (non-progressive) motor and intellectual dysfunction; the hand surgeon needs to distinguish between pyramidal spastic disorders and extrapyramidal dystonic manifestations. The patient assessment should include intelligence, sensation, spontaneous use of limb (grasp and release), and motor functions (athetosis – involuntary movements vary from flaccid to spastic), tremor, ataxia and rigidity. Emotion may influence the spasticity.

The spasticity and response to stretch can be classified simply as severe, moderate and minimum. Most patients have an extrinsic type of spastic hand:

- Flexion of the elbow with forearm pronation.
- Flexion of wrist and fingers: spasticity, weakness and flexion deformity.
- Thumb in palm.
- Loss in sensation and proprioception.

The best age for surgery is 6–10 years old. Muscle imbalance and growth over time can result in fixed joint contractures and bone deformity, which are difficult to correct while maintaining function. Before 8–10 years, the upper extremity remains relatively supple. Nevertheless, skeletal maturity alone is not a contraindication to surgical reconstruction in a patient with cerebral palsy.

Voluntary control of possible muscles for transfer should be assessed; muscles active in grasp and release are not good transfers whilst stereogenesis is another good predictor of post-operative gains. Those with athetoid involuntary movements are usually too unpredictable to benefit from tendon transfer.

Most surgery is directed towards improving specific function, but may be used to improve the appearance. Most poor surgical results are due to poor selection e.g. diminishing established skills e.g. worsen finger flexion deformity by placing a flexed wrist into extension.

Zancolli classification (1968)
Classification based on wrist and fingers

- Group 1 – minimal flexion spasticity is present and full finger extension is possible with wrist neutral (or less than 20° of flexion). Spasticity mainly affects the FCU, and the deficit is a lack of complete active wrist dorsiflexion (extension) when the fingers are totally extended and a thumb deformity. Function is good and there is generally no need for surgery.
- Group 2 – active finger extension is only possible with more than 20° of wrist flexion – with subgroups depending on the wrist extensors. In group (a) the wrist extensors can actively extend the wrist with the fingers flexed, meaning that the wrist extensors are active and under voluntary control, and the spasticity is mainly in the wrist and finger flexors. In group (b) the wrist extensors are flaccid. These are generally good candidates for surgery, usually tendon transfers to extend the wrist.
- Group 3 – there is severe spasticity and deformity at the flexor-pronator mass and the wrist and finger extensors are totally paralysed. There is no finger extension even with flexed wrist. These patients usually still have poor function with surgery but may benefit in terms of cosmesis/hygiene.

Thumb classification

- Group 1 – contracture of basal joint (first dorsal interosseus and adductor pollicis).
- Group 2 – as above with MCPJ (FPB).
- Group 3 – plus IPJ (+FPL) i.e. thumb in palm deformity. This is perhaps the most crippling as the thumb accounts for 50% of the functional capacity of the hand.

Surgery

- Release of contractures – myotomy, tenotomy, neurectomy.

- Augmentation of weak muscles.
  - Lengthening of spastic muscles.
  - Transfer e.g. FCU–ECRB, ECU–ECRB, FCU–EDC, BR–ECRB.
- Skeletal stabilization.

D. Acquired conditions of the hand

I. Dupuytren's disease
General features and anatomy

This was first described by Sir Astley Cooper and Henry Cline, then by Guillame Dupuytren in 1831.

Dupuytren's disease (DD) is a benign fibroproliferative disorder characterized by abnormal thickening and contracture of the palmar fascia, affecting predominantly the longitudinal fibres and vertical fibres (of Skoog) resulting in palmar nodules and contractures of the fingers. It may be associated with other fibromatoses such as Lederhosen's and Peyronie's, also retroperitoneal fibrosis.

The disease is characterized by three phases (Luck's classification, 1959).

- Proliferative – no purposeful arrangement.
- Involutional – alignment of the myofibroblasts along lines of tension.
- Residual – the tissue becomes mostly acellular, devoid of myofibroblasts and resembles a tendon.

Pathophysiology

- Intrinsic theory (McFarlane) – perivascular fibroblasts within normal fascia are source of disease.
- Extrinsic theory (Hueston) – disease starts with proliferation of fibrous tissue *de novo* (due to say, trauma, diabetes mellitus or smoking) as nodules appear superficial to palmar fascia.
- Synthesis theory (Gosset) – combines both theories with nodules arising *de novo* and cords from pre-existing fascia.
- Murrell's hypothesis – age, environmental and genetic factors cause micro-vessel narrowing leading to local tissue ischaemia and oxygen free radical formation which stimulates fibroblasts. Subsequent increase in cell density and contracture exacerbates the ischaemia.

Dupuytren's disease: an overview
Saar JD. *Plast Reconstr Surg* 2000;**106**:125–136.

The diseased tissue possesses the biological features of benign neoplastic fibromatosis. The major collagen type of normal palmar fascia is predominantly type I, although small levels of type III are present. In DD, there is an increase in the ratio of type III to type I collagen.

- Early stage type III.
- Active stage type III and type V.
- Advanced stage type I.

Aetiology

Molecular factors: there has been a relatively large amount of literature on the subject but as yet, there is no unifying theory.

- **Myofibroblasts** (Gabiani G. *Am J Pathol* 1972;**66**:131–138).
  - Prostaglandin-F2α (PGF2α) and lysophosphatidic acid seem to promote myofibroblast contraction.
  - Expression of type VI collagen during the proliferative phase acts as a scaffold for DD fibroblasts.
  - Disturbed regulation of fibroblastic terminal differentiation (apoptosis).
- Abnormality of expression of **matrix metalloproteins.**
- **Microangiopathy**, local ischaemia and xanthine oxidase free radical production has been proposed.
- Fibrogenic cytokines (including IL-1), free radicals (via xanthine oxidase) and growth factors.
  - Increased levels of **growth factors** in the diseased palmar fascia including bFGF, PDGF and TFG-β.
  - Modulation of TGF-β receptor expression: DD fibroblasts express high-affinity type 2 receptors vs. low-affinity type 1.
  - Low levels of **interferon** in DD patients (also low in black patients with keloids).

Genetic factors

Strong family history in some patients points to a single gene defect.

- Other fibroproliferative conditions (Peyronie's, Lederhosen's) may be pleiotropic effects of the same gene.
- Possible link with trisomy 8.
- Increased relative risk 2.94 for those with HLA-DR3.

Other factors

- The commonest affected digit is IV (then little then middle); both hands are usually involved. Both sporadic and inherited disease (autosomal dominance with variable penetrance) has been described. Unilateral disease is more commonly a sporadic finding without a family history and is usually less severe.
  - Common sites for palmar nodules are base of little finger (ADM tendon), fourth ray and base of thumb and first web space.
- The disease affects mainly White men (male: female ratio ~14:1; Hueston suggests that this may be in part due to the fact that females tend to get the disease later and have a less severe form and so may not be noticed), of Celtic descent in middle to late life.
- It is more common in White races, particularly those of northern European descent thus also including North America and Australasia. Oriental races (and diabetics) tend to have palmar disease but not joint contracture and it is uncommon in pigmented races.
- Strong family history points to a single gene defect, possibly affecting the expression of γ-interferon or high-affinity TGF-β receptors on fibroblasts.
- In other patients environmental factors seem to play a role including:
  - Diabetes – twice the risk, but milder (and radial) disease and rarely need surgery – 30% risk in those with diabetes < 5 years, 80% with diabetes > 20 years. It does not seem to be related to the need for insulin; possible link is micro-angiopathy.
  - Epilepsy/anti-epilepsy drugs especially phenobarbitone – 2% of patients with DD are epileptic; incidence of DD in epileptics is 2–3 × higher.
  - Alcohol intake – studies have shown correlation with the amount of alcohol consumed though there is some controversy. This may work by affecting fatty acid oxidation.
  - Smoking – affects glycosaminoglycan concentrations.
  - Occupations involving the use of vibrating hand tools (possibly via an effect on the small vessels of the hand e.g. micro-angiopathy or oxygen free radicals).

Anatomy of the palmar fascia (McGrouther)

The palmar fascia is a complex 3-dimensional structure.

- Transverse fibres (these are usually not involved in DD).
- Vertical fibres (of Skoog) attached to the metacarpals.
- Longitudinal (horizontal) fibres of palmar fascia merge with the deep fascia of the forearm whilst distally they pass in three layers.
  - Layer 1 – inserts into skin between distal palmar crease and finger crease.
  - Layer 2 – spiral band of Gosset either side of the flexor tendon, deep to neurovascular bundle and insert to lateral digital sheet.
  - Layer 3 – deepest layer flexor tendon sheath just beyond proximal interphalangeal joint.

The natatory ligament spans the web spaces and then bifurcates at each digit to form the **lateral** band (lateral to the neurovascular bundle, intimately adherent to skin) and attach to the pretendinous band.

The spiral band passes from the pretendinous band at the base of the finger, beneath the neurovascular bundle and reattaches to the continuation of the pretendinous band, the central band, which itself attaches distally to the flexor sheath.

'Bands' are normal whilst 'cords' represent disease. It is unusual to have diseased cords on both sides of the finger.

- A **spiral cord** which causes **PIPJ contracture** is formed by the 'PLSG' – pretendinous cord, lateral digital sheet, spiral band and Grayson's ligament (on volar surface, Cleland's ligament is spared). This is important as the spiral cord can displace the neurovascular structures proximally, medially and superficially placing them at risk of injury during surgery. In the little finger the spiral cord also arises from the ADM tendon.
  - PIPJ contracture results from spiral and central cords.
- Pretendinous band becomes **pretendinous cord,** which causes **MCPJ contracture.**
- Natatory ligament becomes cord that causes **web-space/adduction contracture.**
- Lateral cord from natatory ligament to lateral digital sheet, and is rarely seen.
- Central cord has no fascial precursor and is the most common cause of PIPJ contracture.

- **Retrovascular** band of Thomine (formed by fascia just deep to the neurovascular bundle, hence the name) lies just superficial to Cleland's ligament and attaches to the periosteum of the proximal phalanx, extending to insert into the periosteum of the distal phalanx causing **DIPJ contracture** (often inadequately released).
- Nodules are independent of the fascia, and show preference for pretendinous zones e.g. base of phalanx distal to first IP crease or the area between the proximal digital crease and MCPJ. There is a high density of myofibroblasts in these nodules. Any adhesion to the aponeurosis is secondary.

Dupuytren's diathesis (Hueston)

This is an aggressive form of Dupuytren's disease.

- Young age of onset and rapid progression.
- Early recurrence as well as a greater risk of recurrence.
- Strong family history.
- Other areas of involvement:
  - Garrod's knuckle pads (PIPJ) occur in ~20% of patients, lying between skin and extensor tendon, attached to paratenon.
- Plantar fibromatosis (Lederhosen) but no flexion contracture.
- Penile curvature (Peyronie).
- Frozen shoulder.

Patient assessment

History

- Age, hand dominance, occupation or hobbies.
  - Check for Dupuytren's diathesis: age of onset of disease, family history, rate of progression of disease and other affected areas.
- Functional deficit and social history particularly if the patient lives alone, as it has implications for post-operative discharge plans.
- Drugs – aspirin/warfarin, oral hypoglycaemics, anti-epileptics.
- Smoking history (affects graft take and skin flap viability).
- Previous hand surgery.

Examination

- Look.
  - Garrod's pads (dorsum proximal interphalangeal joints).

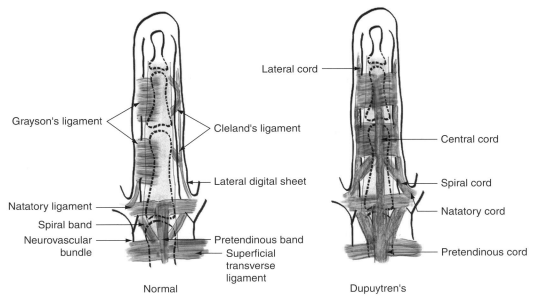

Figure 6.17 Comparison of normal structures and their analogues in a finger with Dupuytren's disease. Grayson's ligament runs from the flexor sheath to the skin and is involved in Dupuytren's disease whilst Cleland's ligament runs from bone to skin, dorsal to the neurovascular bundle but is not involved in the disease. Note that the central cord has no precursor.

- o   Scars, swellings, sudomotor changes, skin lesions, wasting, attitude of the hand.
- Feel – palmar nodules, thickening, degree of skin involvement, sensation distal to any site of proposed surgery.
- Move.
  - o   Active and passive ROM of the affected digits to quantify degree of contracture.
  - o   Examination of each of the three nerves of the hand.

Investigations

- There are no specific investigations. Plain X-rays may be used to determine degree of joint changes in long-standing patients to predict results.

Non-operative treatment

- Splintage fit with a thermoplastic night splint pending any surgery.
- Steroid injections to nodules and pads may help pain.
- Collagenase (clostridium histolyticum) injections are promising. **Xiaflex** was approved by the FDA in Februrary 2010.

Surgery is still regarded as the gold standard treatment for DD.

Indications for surgery

- Contracture of more than 30° at the metacarpophalangeal joint.
- Any contracture at the PIPJ, in practice 20°.
- Contractures of the first web space i.e. thumb adduction.
- Painful palmar nodules or Garrod's pads.
- **Hueston table-top test** – place palm on table top, if it cannot be placed flat then some would recommend surgery.

The rate of progression is probably the best indication for surgery; also it is important to consider the severity of the functional limitation and its importance to the patient.

Techniques

The fascia, skin and joint can be considered separately.

- It can be performed under general or regional brachial plexus anaesthesia.
- Make markings then inflate tourniquet. Loupes should be used.
- Variety of incisions, Brunner incisions or multiple Z-plasty; transverse wounds may be left open if short of skin and to prevent haematoma (McCash,

Dupuytren) – open palm (McCash) technique. Combination of palmar transverse incision and digital Z-plasty was first suggested by McIndoe, and modified by Skoog.

Management of the fascia

- **Fasciotomy** (Sir Astley Cooper) which only releases tension in the fascia by incising it e.g. for single band to thumb. Cline first proposed palmar fasciotomy as a surgical cure in 1787. It can be performed percutaneously i.e. **needle aponeurotomy**.
- Moermans described a **limited fasciectomy**, in which only short portions of fascia are removed – usually a limited fasciectomy of the pretendinous cord is sufficient to restore MCPJ function.
- **Regional (partial) fasciectomy is the most commonly** performed operation and entails removing all involved fascia in the palm and digit by a progressive, longitudinal dissection. It is usually via Brunner incisions with or without a joint release.
- **Extensive or radical fasciectomy** removes all involved fascia with the additional removal of uninvolved fascia to try to prevent disease progression or recurrence. This procedure is usually reserved for patients who have extensive disease or an increased diathesis.
- **Dermofasciectomy** with an FTSG (Hueston, with aim of removing dermis infiltrated by myofibroblasts) is often used to treat recurrent disease, skin involvement and diathesis patients. The **firebreak graft** aims to alter tension line to reduce recurrence of disease and inhibition of myofibroblast activity under the graft has been demonstrated in rat models.
  - John Hueston (1926–1993) was an Australian surgeon and had worked with Archibald McIndoe at East Grinstead.

Joint

- Joint release: incision of the flexor sheath, the accessory collateral ligaments and the check rein ligaments (proximal attachment of the volar plate). Release volar plate from accessory collateral ligament.
- Joint replacement: arthrodesis is a salvage procedure for severe recurrence (> 70° at PIPJ).
- Amputation is another choice for salvage.

Most extension is gained from release of metacarpo-phalangeal contracture rather than IPJ contracture. The best predictors of post-operative correction/outcome are pre-operative deformity and intra-operative correction.

Post-operative management

- A volar splint is applied at end of procedure.
- This is changed for a thermoplastic splint at ~4 days that is then kept for 2 weeks until removal of sutures. Hand exercises 1–2 hourly are initiated, under the supervision of occupational therapists and physiotherapists.
- Use splint at night only for 6 months.

Complications of surgery

Complication rates are high (McFarlane and McGrouther), as great as 17–19% overall.

- Intra-operative.
  - Division of neurovascular bundles, or over-stretching and spasm in digital arteries leading to ischaemia. Nerve and/or arterial injury in 3% of patients (McFarlane).
- Early post-operative.
  - Haematoma (mostly in the palm), skin flap necrosis or graft loss and infection.
- Late post-operative.
  - Inadequate release (inadequate fascia excision, failure to address joint contracture) or recurrent contracture (including poor compliance with physiotherapy). All patients should be advised that the disease will recur, with rates ranging from 26–80%, or more simply 50% at 5 years and 100% at more than 10 years. Dermofasciectomy should be considered for recurrent disease; arthrodesis, arthroplasty and amputation are salvage options.
  - Loss of flexion.
  - CRPS type 1 (4% of males, 8% of females) 5% of patients. The **flare response** is often regarded as a form of CRPS.
  - Scar-related problems.

Poor prognostic factors

- Early age of onset.
- Presence of Garrod's knuckle pads.
- Multiple rays involved.

- Epilepsy or alcoholism.
- Dupuytren's diathesis.

Dupuytren's disease in children

Urban M. *J Hand Surg Br* 1996;**21**:112–116.

Dupuytren's disease is very rare in children; this article presents two children with DD < 13 years of age and only seven other histologically confirmed cases of DD in this age group have ever been reported.

The authors suggest that DD in children should be treated aggressively, particularly early dermofasciectomy.

II. Hand tumours and masses

Malignant bone tumours are commonly metastases, especially bronchial carcinoma which affects the distal phalanx most frequently. The most common malignant tumour of the upper limb is SCC.

Ganglion cysts

These are mucin-filled cysts continuous with the underlying joint capsule; they are the common masses occurring in the hands. They are 3× more common in women and 70% occur in the < 40 s. There are some uncommon associations: metacarpal boss, de Quervain's disease (first extensor compartment ganglion) and Heberden's nodes (mucous cysts).

- Present due to cosmesis i.e. a 'lump', pain or wrist weakness.
- There is a history of trauma in up to 10% but there seems to be no correlation with occupation.
- They transilluminate and are thought to represent mucoid degeneration of fibrous connective tissue – histological examination demonstrates collagen without synovial or epithelial cells. The fluid contains glucosamine, albumin and hyaluronic acid.

Their pathogenesis is poorly understood (Gude W. *Curr Rev Musculoskelet Med* 2008;**1**:205–211)

- Ball valve effect.
- Metaplasia produces microcysts and fibrous metaplasia forms mucoid cells.
- Embryonic rests (ganglions may arise away from synovial joints).

It is an entirely benign condition; there have been no reported cases of malignancy. They have a tendency to subside with rest and enlarge with activity; they may also show spontaneous rupture and resolution.

Common types

Dorsal wrist ganglia (70%) lie directly over scapholunate ligament (midline) or connected to it by a pedicle; it is most often found between the 3rd and 4th metacarpals. Occult ganglions may only be identified by volar wrist flexion and may be associated with underlying scapholunate diastasis (e.g. rheumatoid arthritis). No treatment is required unless there is pain, functional disability or RSS: **60% of dorsal wrist ganglia will resolve.** Surgery involves transverse incision and exposure of the ganglion between thumb and index finger extensors (ECRL, ECRB and EPL radially and EC and EI ulnarly). Note that the rare extensor tendon ganglions are located more distally over the back of the hand.

Volar wrist ganglia (20% in adults, but most common type in children) arise mainly from the radiocarpal ligament, lying under the volar wrist crease between FCR and APL. It is important to take care to preserve the radial artery during surgery as it is often intimately attached to, or encircled by, the ganglion. Allen's test is needed before surgery; inadequate ulnar perfusion may contraindicate surgery.

Flexor sheath (seed) ganglia (~10%) are small, firm, tender masses in the palm or base of the finger and arise from the A1 pulley or occasionally more distally. They may be related to direct trauma to the flexor sheath and if excised then a small portion of the flexor sheath is taken. Aspiration or steroid injection may be temporizing measures.

Mucous cysts are ganglia of the DIPJ found on the dorsum of the finger lying to one side of the central slip insertion of the extensor tendon. The overlying skin is often taut and thin and may necrose/rupture. They can be associated with osteoarthritis (and **osteophytes** of DIPJ which need to be removed); occult cysts may exist on the other side. It is often found in older patients. There may be longitudinal grooving of the nail.

Management
Non-operative

- Aspiration and injection of steroid (small or occult dorsal ganglions).
- Extrinsic rupture ('bible' ganglions).

Operative

Operative treatment is indicated for pain, deformity or reduced function – there is a recurrence rate of up to

50% if inadequately excised. If rotatory subluxation of the scaphoid is present (clunking) then the ganglion is more likely to recur. 'Recurrence' may also be related to the presence of occult intra-osseous ganglions.

- Excision of the whole cyst with stalk and the joint surface at the point of attachment, closing the joint capsule is not essential as it may lead to prolonged immobilization and stiffness.
- Avoid injury to superficial branch of radial nerve.
- No splintage is required.

Others

- **Carpometacarpal boss.** These are palpable bony lumps (exostosis) on the dorsum of 2nd/3rd metacarpal bases that present with swelling, pain and decreased extension at the wrist. They can be confirmed by X-ray. They are twice as common in women (especially 20–30 years) and twice as common on the right hand. 30% are associated with wrist ganglion whilst many also have arthritis.
  - After excision, a cast is needed for up to 6 weeks post-operation. Recurrence may occur; rongeuring the bone after excision may help to reduce this. Recurrence may require fusion.
- **Pigmented villonodular synovitis** (giant cell tumour (GCT) of tendon sheath). This is a relatively common benign tumour that usually presents as a bossellated yellow swelling on the volar surface of finger or around a joint, particularly the radial digits. It may be confused with a ganglion but GCTs are fixed to deeper tissues, possibly eroding bone.
  - Treat by excision but typically there is a high rate of recurrence, either due to incomplete surgery or to satellite lesions.
- **Epidermoid inclusion cysts** may follow penetrating injuries that cause the deeper implantation of epidermoid cells. It presents as a firm, spherical mass on parts that are exposed to injuries i.e. fingers and palm; the contents are a mixture of protein, cholesterol and fat. These should be excised completely to avoid recurrence.

Bone tumours

Benign

Enchondromas are the commonest benign bone tumour (90% of bone tumours in the hand). They are well-demarcated swellings that are radiolucent, expansile lesions of the non-epiphyseal portions of tubular bones, usually the phalanges and metacarpals. Treat with curettage with or without cancellous bone grafts. There is a lifetime malignant risk of 10% in solitary tumours.

- Multiple enchondromas occur in Ollier's disease – a rare condition.
- Multiple enchondromas with vascular malformations is Maffucci's syndrome.
- Both can lead to chondrosarcoma (> 25% before 40 years) and should be treated by wide excision.

Osteochondroma – are relatively more common in younger patients; they appear as bony protuberances with a narrow stalk arising from the metaphyseal cortex particularly the distal end of the PP. There is a 1% risk of malignant transformation. Treatment should be wide excision.

Chondroma – benign cartilaginous tumours that often arise from an abnormal focus of cartilage.

Aneurysmal bone cysts – these consitute 5% of all benign bone tumours and occur before the closure of the epiphyseal plates in the second decade, most commonly affecting the vertebrae and knee. The aetiology is unknown – it may be related to the vascularity of the bone, some lesions are associated with pre-existing bone conditions such as GCT (19–39% of cases), fibrous dysplasia and chondro/osteo blastomas. They appear as painful radiolucent expansile locally destructive lesions particularly the metacarpals in upper limb involvement (21% of total). X-rays are usually diagnostic; MRI/CT can add detail. They can be treated by excision with bone grafting; curettage is associated with a high recurrence rate up to 60%. Lesions that cannot be resected may be treated with radiotherapy; image-guided radiofrequency ablation is another treatment option under study.

Osteoid osteoma

These lesions (10% of benign bone tumours) usually occur in young adult males (2–3 × more common than in females), are characterized by localized pain worst at night and are relieved by NSAIDs. The distal phalanx is most commonly involved. On X-ray, they show up as a radiolucent nidus with surrounding sclerosis and are 'hot spots' on a bone scan. Surgery involves curettage possibly with bone grafting – recurrences are usually associated with incomplete resection;

some cases may be treated with radiofrequency ablation.

Osteoblastomas are rare in the hand but when they do occur, they are mostly restricted to the wrist, particularly the scaphoid, presenting as painful swellings. They are poorly mineralized swellings of immature neoplastic osteoid. Surgical wide local resection is usually successful; post-operative radiotherapy may be indicated in certain cases.

Giant cell tumour of bone (osteoclastoma). These often occur around the knee rather than the hand (2–5% of total) affecting mostly middle-aged females. The cause is unknown. Most lesions are histologically benign but are locally aggressive with soft tissue involvement – some exhibit malignant-type behaviour and may metastasize to the lungs (5%) that may lead to death. However, even benign lesions may have pulmonary metastasis i.e. both the bone lesion and the metastasis are histologically benign. Giant cell tumours of the distal radius may be more aggressive than in other areas.

They are solitary lesions with a dull ache and hindrance to movement. On X-ray they are lucent/lytic lesions often near to the epiphyseal regions and their lack of sclerosis differentiates them from other bone tumours. MRI is useful to assess soft tissue and medullary involvement prior to surgery which is the preferred treatment modality (intra-lesional excision for stage I/II or en bloc with wide margin for stage III), though radiotherapy may be used for non-resectable lesions. Pathological fractures should be allowed to heal before surgery.

- Stage I – benign latent GCT with no locally aggressive activity.
- Stage II – benign active GCT; imaging demonstrates alteration of cortical structure.
- Stage III – locally aggressive; imaging demonstrates a lytic lesion and there may be tumour penetration through the cortex into the soft tissues.
- GCTs in bone are different from **GCTs of tendon sheath,** which are the second commonest in the hand. The latter are areas of localized nodular synovitis and are composed of histiocytes from flexor tendon sheath (usually volar aspect of DIPJ, bone GCTs are often found in the distal radius). They were first described by Chassaignac in 1852 who thought they were neoplasms. Their true aetiology is unknown, but probably reflect a

reactive/regenerative hyperplasia associated with an inflammatory process (Jaffe); PCR shows them to be polyclonal proliferations. There have been sporadic reports of malignancy but most are probably doubtful.

Malignant

Chondrosarcoma – this is the most common primary malignant bone tumour in the hand, often arising in an older age group (60–80 years) with an association with osteochondroma and enchondromas. It is typically a painful mass around the MCPJ with a slow clinical course and only metastasizes late on. Amputation is the mainstay of treatment but recurrence is not uncommon.

Ewing's sarcoma – this rarely affects the hand, but this subset may have a better prognosis than usual with good local control following surgery and chemotherapy with or without radiotherapy. It is typically a mass with a sclerotic reaction seen on X-ray affecting younger males (twice as common as in females).

Osteosarcoma – it is very rare in the hand (< 0.1%) but is more frequent after irradiation, in those with Paget's disease, fibrous dysplasia, GCT of bone as well as osteochondromas/enchondromas. The immature osteoid is produced by the proliferating stroma (spindle cells). The typically rapidly growing painful mass has a sunburst pattern on X-ray. Excision with wide margins and adjuvant chemotherapy results in a 70% 5-year survival in the absence of metastasis (but this decreases to 10–20% if there are metastases, which are uncommon).

Other soft tissue masses (see Soft tissue sarcomas).

- Glomus tumours.
- Peripheral nerve tumours (1–5% of hand tumours).
  - Schwannomas.
  - Neurofibromas, neurofibromatosis, malignant peripheral nerve sheath tumour.
  - Intraneural non-neural tumours (e.g. lipoma, haemangioma or lipofibromatous harmatoma. The median nerve is the most commonly affected and may be associated with macrodactyly. It is usually not possible to separate the tumour from the nerve.)
- Skin tumours.
  - Squamous cell carcinomas (SCCs) are the most common malignancy of the hand; SCCs of the hand constitute 11% of all SCCs, typically

affecting the dorsum in elderly individuals (with pre-existing actinic changes). Web-space lesions seem to have a higher risk of metastasis. Surgery is the main treatment method; recurrence ranges from 7–28% for well- to poorly differentiated lesions respectively.

- o **Basal cell carcinomas** (2% of all BCCs). Palmar and subungual lesions may be a feature of Gorlin's syndrome.
- o **Melanoma** (10–20% of all). Treat with wide excision or amputation to joint proximal to lesion.

- Sarcomas are uncommon in the hand, though 15% occur in the upper limb in younger patients. Risk factors include radiation or herbicide exposure, and disorders such as neurofibromatosis and Li–Fraumeni syndrome. There is a high incidence of lymphatic spread and regional nodal metastasis. In general, they are treated by excision with a wide (2–3cm) margin with or without adjuvant therapy radiotherapy or chemotherapy. An important determinant of the prognosis is being treated in a **Sarcoma centre**, thus it is important that referral is made for any soft tissue swelling that is:
  - o **Deep to fascia, greater than 5 cm in size, painful/hard with rapid growth.**
- Types of sarcoma include:
  - o **Epitheloid** (most common) local recurrence and distant metastasis is common.
  - o **Fibrosarcoma** – more frequent in the deep subcutaneous space. Haematogenous spread is common.
  - o **Synovial** – typically a slow-growing palm mass but the prognosis is relatively poor due to the high propensity for distant spread. Consequently treatment is usually multifactorial with surgery, radiotherapy and chemotherapy.
  - o **Clear cell** (uncommon) – typically a slow-growing deep mass that is attached to fascia and tendons. Prognosis is poor.
  - o **Malignant fibrous histiocytoma** – may be superficial or deep, multiple or solitary. There is a tendency to extend along tissue planes; it may metastasize through lymphatics or bloodstream.
  - o **Alveolar rhabdomyosarcoma** – this is a highly malignant lesion that usually affects the palm (thenar/hypothenar muscles) in children. Prognosis is poor.

- o **Kaposi's sarcoma** – these are dark blue macules (most frequently found on the lower limbs) that can be associated with AIDS/HIV. There are also:
  - – The classic type that affects elderly Mediterranean men and has no association with HIV.
  - – The endemic form associated with young Africans.
  - – The iatrogenic form related to immunosuppresion therapy.
  - – It is caused by Kaposi's sarcoma-associated herpesvirus (KSHV) infection. The HIV-associated form is $10 \times$ more common in gay males particularly in their 50s; the incidence has reduced in this subpopulation due to drugs that suppress retroviral replication. It is very variable in its clinical course – it can run a fulminant course with death within a year or be rather indolent with more than 20 years' survival. The mainstay of surgery is non-surgical i.e. radiotherapy (particularly classic non-HIV forms), chemotherapy (including intralesional vinblastine or systemic chemotherapy) or imiquimod; small localized lesions can be excised or treated with liquid nitrogen or lasers.

III. Osteoarthritis

This condition affects females more frequently and is mostly secondary to general ageing, trauma including the microtrauma of daily repetitive actions. In the hand, the most commonly affected joints are DIPJ, CMCJ, PIPJ and scaphotrapeziotrapezoid joint (STTJ) in order of decreasing frequency.

- History – in contrast to rheumatoid arthritis, there is less pain in the morning and more during the day, and it may interfere with sleep – but it is still important to formally rule out rheumatoid arthritis and its variants. The main difficulty the patient has is with movements such as opening jars or wringing out clothes.
- Examination may show point tenderness and 'grind test' (CMCJ).
  - o **Heberden's nodes** – osteophytes at the DIPJ, may be painful.
  - o **Bouchard's nodes** – osteophytes at the PIPJ.

- Radiology – typical changes are narrowed joint space, subchondral sclerosis (eburnation), cysts, osteophytes, bony exostoses etc.
  - Robert's (A–P) view of thumb with X-ray beam at 90°.
  - Eaton-Littler stress view for CMCJ.

Alnot's classification of (hand) pain (Alnot JY. *Ann Chir Main* 1985;4:11–21):

- 0 – no pain.
- I – pain during particular activities.
- II – pain during daily activities.
- III – episodes of spontaneous pain.
- IV – constant pain.

Treatment
General non-operative

- Splinting and activity modification.
- NSAIDs.
- Intra-articular steroids (may lead to ligament attenuation).

Surgery

- Basal osteotomy (wedge osteotomy, removing radial cortex to change the vector of stress forces acting on the joint).
- Trapeziectomy with FCR sling (Burton–Pellegrini) – probably the gold standard for management of late-stage CMJ osteoarthritis.
- Joint replacement.
- Arthrodesis.

Radiological staging
Distal interphalangeal joint (DIPJ)

- Mucous cysts (which may cause nail deformities) and Heberden's nodes are notable features.
- A painful DIPJ can be treated with an arthrodesis (screw, Lister loop of K-wire) via a dorsal incision (H, Y or inverted Y).

Proximal interphalangeal joint (PIPJ)

Osteoarthritis in this region is often post-traumatic and presents with pain, deformity and possibly impingement from the osteophytes (Bouchard's nodes).

- Arthrodesis is a good option particularly for the index finger to provide a stable post for pinch.
- Arthroplasty is preferred for the ring and little fingers, to accommodate the power grip but

requires reasonable bone stock. Options include Swanson's (silastic interpositional) or metal/carbon (pyocarbon) – inert with good wear characteristics. Dorsal tendon splitting, volar, lateral or Charney approaches may be used.

Thumb CMCJ/Basal joint

It is said that there is a high density of oestrogen receptors in the basal joint of the thumb (and in the hip) which have a role in degenerative changes (hence higher incidence in post-menopausal women).

Joint stability is dependent on the anterior oblique ligament (volar beak) from trapezium to volar ulnar metacarpal which limits dorsal movement of metacarpal. Traditionally, it is thought that in osteoarthritis, the ligament is attenuated/stretched, and the thumb is held adducted and hyperextended.

Symptoms include pain on the radial side of the wrist (differentials include scaphotrapeziotrapezoid (STT) osteoarthritis, de Quervain's, Wartenburg's, carpal tunnel), swelling and crepitus with a weak pinch. Positive grind test is strongly suggestive.

- Ask for Eaton views: thumbs against each other in resisted abduction, palms flat.

Eaton and Littler

(Eaton RG. *J Bone Joint Surg* 1973;55:1655–1656.)

- I < 1/3 subluxation at CMCJ.
- II 1/3 subluxation, osteophytes < 2 mm.
- III > 1/3 subluxation, > 2 mm, minor joint narrowing.
- IV Advanced. Major subluxation, joint space narrowing, sclerosis and osteophytes > 2 mm.

Revision: Eaton and Glickel classification (1987):

- **Stage I.** Mild joint narrowing or subchondral sclerosis, mild joint effusion, or ligament laxity. No subluxation or osteophyte formation are present. Treatment for this stage includes NSAIDs and immobilization, which involves splinting the thumb in abduction.
- **Stage II. Joint narrowing and small osteophytes.** Besides CMC joint narrowing and subchondral sclerosis, there may be joint debris – osteophyte formation/loose bodies (< 2 mm) at the ulnar side of the distal trapezial articular surface. Mild to moderate subluxation, with the base of the first metacarpal dislocated radially and dorsally.

Treatment: ligament reconstruction tendon interposition (LRTI).

- **Stage III Significant CMC joint destruction.** Further joint space narrowing with cystic changes and bone sclerosis. Larger joint debris > 2 mm, including prominent osteophytes at the ulnar border of the distal trapezium. The first metacarpal is moderately displaced radially and dorsally. There could be a hyperextension deformity of the CMC joint. The scaphotrapezial joint appears normal. Treat by LRTI.
- **Stage IV involvement of both CMC and ST joints.** The destruction of the CMC joint is similar to that in stage III whilst the scaphotrapezial joint has evidence of destruction with sclerosis and cysts. The CMC joint is usually immobile, and often patients have little pain. Treat by LRTI.

Indications for surgery: failure of conservative management, pain, disabling joint instability and first web contracture – **never for deformity alone**. The CMC is the most commonly reconstructed area in osteoarthritis of the upper limb.

- **Trapeziectomy** is a simple procedure (interposition with rolled-up palmaris or gel foam) and is effective in relieving pain. Disadvantages includes thumb shortening, weak pinch and reduced thumb adduction. Probably the current gold standard for late disease; by comparison, the correct management of early disease is less certain.
- **LRTI** (Burton and Pellegrini). Trapezium is excised and a distal FCR slip is tunnelled through the base of the thumb metacarpal and sutured back onto itself and anchored into the trapezial space. The Weilby technique uses the APL. The exact indications for LRTI are not well defined.
- **CMCJ fusion** – for painful instability, the thumb metacarpal is held 30–40° palmar abduction and 10–15° radial abduction. There is no evidence that arthrodesis improves strength to compensate for stiffness.
- **Metacarpal osteotomy** – particularly for stage I and II.
- **Prosthetic** (e.g. Swanson silicone trapezium implant or titanium) with possible complications of instability and prosthesis dislocation. Silastic implants are rarely used due to the high complication rate.

Scaphotrapeziotrapezoid (STT)

Scaphotrapeziotrapezoid (STT) osteoarthritis (pain and swelling at scaphoid pole in anatomical snuffbox and on wrist motion – radial grind test) should be carefully excluded as an involved joint generally excludes CMC arthroplasty. The main complication of treatment is non-union; a good outcome can be expected if union is achieved.

- Trapeziectomy for pantrapezial disease.
- For isolated STT osteoarthritis – fusion of STT with 6 weeks in plaster to decrease wrist movement, to reduce the significant non-union rate.
- Excision arthroplasty – excise distal scaphoid, 3 weeks in plaster.
- Interposition arthroplasty.

Metacarpophalangeal joint (MCPJ)

Metacarpophalangeal joint degeneration causes subluxation of the metacarpal base, and the 1st web is narrowed by metacarpal adduction deformity. There may be hyperextension deformity and instability.

The aim of treatment is to provide good pinch and stability:

- If hyperextension is greater than 30° then MCPJ arthrodesis (15° flexion and 10° pronation), volar plate capsulodesis and APL advancement.
- If hyperextension if less than 30° then K-wire.

Pisotriquetral osteoarthritis

There is typically pain over volar ulnar wrist and symptoms may be elicited by hand resting on hard surfaces e.g. writing. One-third of patients also have ulnar neuropathy.

- Provocation manoeuvre: compression with side-to-side movement that will elicit severe pain over the joint.
- Treat with steroid injection, splint wrist in slight flexion – if there is no relief after two injections then consider pisiform excision with or without minimal triquetral excision.

Carpus and wrist

The radial side is more frequently involved; involvement of the middle row is rare.

- 90% involve scaphoid.
- 50% scapholunate advanced collapse (SLAC) pattern.
- 20% STT pattern.
- 10% combination.

Scapholunate advanced collapse (SLAC) wrist

This refers to a specific pattern of osteoarthritis and subluxation resulting from untreated chronic scaphoid non-union or chronic scapholunate dissociation. There is a predictable pattern of changes in the areas of abnormal loading.

- Stage I distal radioscaphoid – attenuation of carpal ligament.
- Stage II proximal radioscaphoid – scaphoid malalignment.
- Stage III capitolunate.

Watson's scaphoid shift test assesses for SLAC – dorsally directed pressure is applied over the distal scaphoid tubercle with the examiner's thumb, if the scapholunate ligament is torn then there is pain when the scaphoid proximal pole subluxes out of the scaphoid fossa of the radius as the hand is passively moved from ulnar to radial deviation.

- SNAC (scaphoid non-union advanced collapse) wrist can be difficult to differentiate from SLAC.
- The commonest treatment is arthrodesis.

Treatment

- Denervation.
- Joint excision (scaphoid, proximal row carpectomy).
- **Arthrodesis (vide infra).**
  - Total wrist fusion – relieves pain (not always totally) whilst sacrificing function.
  - Limited carpal fusion – 4-corner fusion – if the articular surface of the proximal lunate is intact, i.e. radiolunate changes exclude the use of LCF. This is often combined with scaphoid excision.
  - Scaphoid excision and intercarpal arthrodesis.
  - Radioscaphoid, radioscapholunate.
- Arthroplasty. Numerous types of implants have been used but implant wear and loosening are common complications.

Free and island vascularized joint transfer for proximal interphalangeal reconstruction
Foucher G. *J Hand Surg Am* 1994;**19**:8–16.

Options for stiff and arthritic PIPJ are:

- Arthrodesis.
- Skoog perichondral arthroplasty.
- Silicone joint replacement (reversed Swanson's).
- Non-vascularized joint transfers (in young children).

Islanded vascularized joint transfers:

- Heterodigital joint including collateral ligaments, volar plate, extensor tendon and vascular pedicle, e.g. PIPJ or DIPJ from a non-functioning finger.
- Homodigital e.g. islanded DIPJ transfer (DIPJ contributes 15° to the flexion arc whereas the PIPJ contributes 85°), thus DIPJ transfer can be an option following complex trauma to the PIPJ. This is then followed by DIPJ arthrodesis and reinsertion of FDP.

Free vascularized joint transfer: joints harvested from a non-replantable finger, along with skin island and extensor tendon with a common example being joint transfer from the second toe.

IV. Rheumatoid arthritis

Rheumatoid arthritis (RA) is a systemic autoimmune phenomenon mediated by B and T lymphocytes affecting mainly synovial tissues within joints but also many other tissues/organs. Rheumatoid factor (RF) is a circulating macroglobulin (IgM) present in 70% of RA patients (15% of normal population); there is increased ESR, CRP and reduced haemoglobin. It affects females 4 × more frequently.

The American College of Rheumatologists state that there must be at least four of the following seven signs for at least 6 weeks.

- Morning stiffness lasting for one hour.
- Arthritis of more than three joint areas.
- Arthritis of hand joints – MCPJ, PIPJ.
- Symmetrical arthritis.
- Subcutaneous nodules (on extensor surface).
- Positive RF.
- X-ray evidence of erosions, cysts or osteopaenia, reduced joint space, carpal ankylosis.

Stages (Lister)

- Proliferative – synovial swelling, pain, restricted movement, nerve compression.
- Destructive – tendon rupture, capsular disruption, joint subluxation, bone erosion.

- Reparative – fibrosis, tendon adhesions, fibrous ankylosis, fixed deformity.

Pattern

- Moncyclic – one episode, spontaneous remission, 10%.
- Polycyclic – remissions and relapses, 45%.
- Progressive – inexorable course, 45%.

There is a mixture of soft tissue and articular changes.

Soft tissues

- Tendons. Tenosynovitis (50% in RA); synovitis is a synovial inflammation with formation of pannus and release of erosive enzymes.
  - It may manifest as tender boggy swelling dorsum of wrist and around flexor tendons in the carpal canal, leading to tendon ruptures and disruption of the stabilizing structures around joints. When a joint persistently adapts angulation, the joints either side tend to go in opposite directions due to the change in tendon mechanics i.e. Z deformities such as Swan neck or boutonnière.
  - Tenosynovitis of flexor tendons and triggering (**A1 pulley should be preserved** – release worsens volar subluxation of proximal phalanges – held by pulley to volar plate and to the head of the metacarpal, release also increases the lever arm of the tendon increasing the MCPJ flexion deformity).
  - Tendon ruptures may be due to **synovitis**, e.g. extensor communis (EDC 4/5 is sometimes known as a Vaughan–Jackson lesion) or due to **attrition** e.g. ulnar head (EDM, EDC), scaphoid tubercle (FPL, Mannerfelt lesion which is the most common flexor tendon rupture) and Lister's tubercle (EPL). The rupture of juncturae allows ulnar subluxation into metacarpal gutters. EDM rupture can be tested for with the 'horn sign', asking the patient to extend the index and little finger with the ring and middle flexed – this requires intact EI and EDM tendons.
  - The Vaughan–Jackson is the commonest tendon rupture in RA, the FPL (Mannerfelt) is the commonest *flexor* tendon rupture.
- Skin
  - **Rheumatoid nodules** (foci of fibrinoid necrosis) are the most common extra-articular manifestation (25%) and a poor prognostic factor. They are most commonly found on the subcutaneous border of the ulna.
  - Palmar erythema.
  - Vasculitic ulcers.
- Nerves
  - Nerve compression due to tenosynovitis/joint synovitis e.g. carpal tunnel syndrome, also cubital and radial tunnel.
  - Polyneuropathy.
- Muscle – atrophy of intrinsics, inflammation, myopathy (or nerve compression).
- Cardiovascular.
  - Vessels – obliterative arteritis, vasculitis and Raynaud's.
  - Cardiac – valvular, pericarditis/myocarditis.
- Respiratory – nodules, pleuritis.
- Eyes – uveitis, iritis.
- Haematological – anaemia, Felty's (splenomegaly, lymphadenopathy).

Management

Non-surgical treatment is the mainstay of RA management and usually consists of NSAIDs, steroid injections and splints.

- Drugs
  - NSAIDs are first line – aspirin, indomethacin, naproxen.
  - Corticosteroids – systemic and injections.
  - Immunomodulators – azathioprine, methotrexate, hydroquinones, cyclosporin.
  - Antimonoclonal antibody compounds – etanercept, infliximab.
- Splinting to counteract deforming forces.
- Non-weightbearing exercise programme.

The primary aims of treatment are pain relief, restore function and improve appearance of the hand. Surgery in RA is only indicated where there is pain and loss of function – **deformity alone is not an indication.**

- **Preventive** – to prevent further deformity e.g. early synovectomy if medical therapy fails after a 6-week trial with aims to reduce risk of tendon rupture, flexor tendon triggering, also decompression of median nerve.
- **Reconstructive** (to restore function i.e. stability and mobility) – tendon transfers.
- **Salvage** – e.g. pain relief, joint surgery including lower end ulna excision, replacement, fusions.

The process should be staged, addressing **proximal joints before distal ones**. It is important that cases are carefully selected, to proceed with those known to have high rates of satisfaction, for example:

- Thumb MCJP fusion.
- External synovectomy and ulnar head excision.
- Stabilize wrist.
- Flexor synovectomy.
- PIPJ fusion.
- MCJP arthroplasty.

Joints in rheumatoid arthritis

The most common joints/upper limb deformities are:

- Posterior subluxation of elbow.
- Palmar subluxation of wrist, radial deviation of wrist.
- Ulnar translocation of carpus.
- Ulnar drift of fingers (MCPJ), palmar subluxation of MCPJ.
- Swan neck and boutonnières of fingers and thumbs.
- Lateral dislocation of IPJ.

Osteoarthritis versus rheumatoid arthritis

The MCPJ and PIJP are most commonly involved in rheumatoid arthritis whilst in OA, it is the DIPJ and thumb basal joint.

Note also the neck joints, with implications for patients requiring general anaesthesia/intubation. There is a 25–50% incidence of atlanto-axial instability – screen with X-rays with flexion and extension views.

- Atlanto-axial subluxation.
- Superior migration of the odontoid peg into the foramen magnum.
- Anterior subluxation of vertebral bodies.

Elbow in rheumatoid arthritis

- Articular disease i.e. posterior subluxation – synovectomy and radial head excision for pain relief (90%); elbow arthroplasty is controversial due to the high complication rate and lack of studies.
- Extra-articular disease i.e. nodules which can be injected with steroids (risk of ulceration) whilst synovitis and bony spurs may lead to nerve compression.

Wrist in rheumatoid arthritis

The distal radio-ulnar joint (DRUJ) is the most commonly affected area in RA of the wrist; there is synovitis along with erosive changes.

The DRUJ is the area between the sigmoid notch and head of the ulnar that is responsible for the majority of forearm rotation. The TFCC (triangular fibrocartilage complex) is the most important stabilizer of this area with **an articular disc** of triangular fibrocartilage that originates from the medial border of the distal radius inserting into the base of the ulnar styloid (5 mm thick on ulnar side and 2 mm at radial side, the central 3/4 is avascular thus tears can present a healing problem) and also dorsal and volar radio-ulnar ligament, ulnocarpal ligament and ECU sheath. The TFCC also transmits about 20% of the load across the wrist.

The proximal row of carpal bones forms the **mobile intercalated segment**.

- Scaphoid becomes longitudinal/extended with ulnar deviation, whilst it is transverse/flexed with radial deviation.
- All tendons moving the wrist (except the FCU) insert beyond the carpus, therefore ligaments that connect the metacarpals to carpus and carpal bones to each other are very important.

The ulnar styloid and head are involved earliest (ulnar caput syndrome) in rheumatoid arthritis. The joint complex becomes grossly deranged.

- Supinated, radially deviated, volar subluxation of radius and carpus, dorsal subluxation of ulnar, caput ulnae.
- Unstable due to ligamentous laxity and capsular erosion e.g.
  - Scapholunate diastasis with dorsal intercalated segment instability (DISI).
  - TFCC and triquetro-lunate dissociation.

Ulna caput (head) syndrome – caput ulnae

This is seen in up to one-third of RA patients undergoing surgery. Synovitis around the ulnar head causes erosion of the triangular fibrocartilage and the ligamentous supports to the wrist. This causes pain, instability and limited wrist dorsiflexion aggravated by pronation of forearm; the wrist is the keystone of the hand.

- **Prominent ulnar head due to dorsal dislocation,** disruption of radio-ulnar ligament and DRUJ instability – which can be detected by the 'piano key test' – depress the ulnar head and release to see it spring back.

- **Supination of the carpus** on the forearm due to damage to TFCC which also causes ulnar translocation of carpus (may see as prominent ulnar head), limiting wrist dorsiflexion and supination on the forearm. This also increases risk of carpal tunnel syndrome.
- **Volar subluxation of ECU** reducing its extensor function, making it more of a wrist flexor causing radial deviation of the wrist and promoting attrition rupture of ulnar extensors over the prominent ulna head.

Radius

- Radial carpal rotation (increase in Shapiro's metacarpophalangeal angle between radius and index metacarpal, normally ~112°) due to erosion of the sling ligament (radioscaphocapitate). This causes the scaphoid to adopt a volar-flexed position with secondary loss of carpal height.
- Radial scalloping at sigmoid notch (as well as around ulnar head – both are highly indicative of DRUJ instability with increased risk of extensor tendon rupture).
  - Larsen index scoring single X-ray changes compared with Amos that looks at progression. The Wrightington system is another classification system for the rheumatoid wrist with good interobserver reliability.

Options for ulnar wrist problems in rheumatoid arthritis

Tenosynovectomy, tendon transfers (ECRL to ECU to reduce radial carpal rotation) and joint synovectomy.

Ulnar head surgery

- **Resection** by dorsal approach, taking care to preserve ECU and dorsal branches of ulnar nerve.
  - There is a limited **excision of the ulnar head** (distal 2 cm, burr edges) with synovectomy of DRUJ.
  - The distal end of the ulna is then stabilized e.g. by a distally based slip of ECU passed through a hole in the dorsal cortex of the distal end of ulna and sutured back onto itself. A turnover flap of extensor retinaculum to pass

under ECU and back on itself can stabilize the ECU.

- **Sauvé–Kapandji procedure** fuses the distal ulna to radial head after removal of a 10–15 mm segment of ulna proximal to this (the gap can be filled with pronator quadratus (PQ), effectively creating a pseudoarthrosis). It aims to allow forearm rotation for better mobility whilst preventing abnormal movements at the DRUJ as well as unloading the ulnar, allowing more force to be transmitted across the radius which is not damaged. This procedure is suited to younger patients with an arthritic painful DRUJ limiting movement. Specific complications include instability of the ulnar stump and fusion of the ends reducing mobility.
- **Darrach procedure** for relief of pain in DRUJ arthritis in the elderly with low functional demands (younger patients e.g. after Colles' malunion, will do better with distal radial osteotomy). The distal 1–2 cm of the ulna is excised (minimized to restore full motion whilst avoid instability) via a dorsal incision. If the distal ulna is unstable then it can be stabilized either by an ECU tendon strip passed through a drill hole and sutured to itself or ECU/PQ arthroplasty. Complications are more common in younger patients with instability or subluxation; also convergence (radio-ulnar impingement) that is exacerbated by power grip/ PQ contraction and is related to the amount of bone excised.

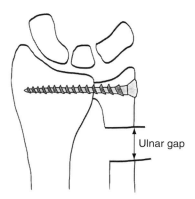

Ulnar gap

Figure 6.18 Schematic representation of a Sauvé–Kapandji procedure.

Wrist arthrodesis

Fusion may be offered to low-demand patients with advanced disease, providing predictable pain relief.

- **Limited wrist fusion** is an option for early collapse with destruction limited to radiocarpal joints. This involves synovectomy and removal of articular cartilage from affected joints, with cancellous bone graft (from distal radius or excised ulna head) and K-wires for 6 weeks.
  - Proximal row fusion – radius, scaphoid and lunate.
  - Mid-carpal fusion – all joints surrounding the capitate.
- **Total wrist fusion** may be necessary for young patients with high, long-term stresses on joints, with significant wrist deformity/instability already, poor wrist extensor function and poor bone stock.
  - The ulna head is excised and cartilage is removed from the distal radius and proximal carpal row. A Steinman pin is introduced through the third metacarpal and passed via the carpus into the radial medulla with the wrist in neutral. Alternatively two pins can be placed exiting via the second and third interosseus spaces, but these need removing after ~**4–6 months.**
  - Cancellous bone graft and arthrodesis using a plate allows for 50° dorsal angulation to be created which may be more functional than the neutral wrist position.
  - Complications include pseudoarthrosis, pin migration, nerve injury and fracture of healed fusion at ends of pin.

Wrist arthroplasty

This may be suited for high-demand patients; complications include implant failure, loosening and infection.

- Bi-axial total wrist devices (a plastic polyethylene spacer fixed to metal carpal component rocks on the flatter radial component, and can be cemented or non-cemented).
- Silicone (Swanson's) total wrist implants – for very low-demand patients with poor bone stock, who are willing to trade reduction in mobility for pain relief.

Hand in rheumatoid arthritis

Whilst the wrist is radially deviated there is ulnar deviation at MCPJs.

- Anterior subluxation of the wrist renders the flexor tendons less effective and promotes intrinsic-plus position, hence the fingers adopt a swan-neck deformity.
- First dorsal interosseus wasting, which may be masked by an adduction deformity of the thumb.

Tendons

Tenosynovitis: pain and swelling dorsum of the hand that may be accompanied by radiocarpal or radio-ulnar instability. There are fibrinoid 'rice bodies' within the tendon sheath.

The hypertrophic synovium erodes tendons (direct invasion vs. weakening); attrition rupture may occur around bony points, whilst ischaemic degeneration due to devascularization may have an additional role.

- Radial tubercle (Lister) – EPL.
- Ulnar head – EDM, EDC.

The combination of extensor tenosynovitis and tendon rupture in the digits beginning on the ulnar side (EDM, EDC) is called a Vaughan–Jackson lesion.

Extensor tenosynovitis and tendon rupture

Differential diagnosis of extensor tendon rupture i.e. failure of extension in RA.

- Dislocation of the extensor tendon into the ulnar metacarpal valley/gutters.
- Volar dislocation/subluxation of the MCPJ or other disruption.
- Paralysis of extensor musculature e.g. posterior interosseus nerve compression/radial tunnel syndrome due to synovitis at radiohumeral joint.
- Flexor synovitis and triggering.

Treatment.

- Non-surgical treatment.
- Synovitis – dorsal tenosynovectomy ± wrist joint synovectomy ± osteophyte excision. Complications include skin necrosis exposing tendons, haematoma and bowstringing if a strip of extensor retinaculum is not preserved.
- In cases of rupture, tendon transfer is needed.
  - **Isolated EPL rupture** due to hamate/radius attrition and tenosynovitis– EI to EPL transfer (tighten so that with wrist extended the thumb can still oppose to the little finger).

- or EDM transfer, APL slip transfer or interphalangeal joint arthrodesis.
  ○ **Rupture of finger extensor (little, ring then middle i.e. Vaughan–Jackson)** due to ulnar head.
    - Single tendon – 'buddy' suture to an adjacent intact extensor tendon.
    - Two tendons – suture to EDC, EI to EDM/EDC.
    - Multiple – ring finger FDS transfer (Boyes') to motor several tendons.
  ○ Normal 'rules' regarding tendon transfers do not always apply in RA patients because:
    - Hostile territory.
    - Motor tendons may be weak.
    - Full range of passive movement may not be available.

Flexor tenosynovitis and tendon rupture

The symptoms and signs of flexor tendon problems are similar to extensor as described above with the additional possibility of triggering. Common sites of attrition rupture are:

- Ridge of the trapezium – FCR.
- Hook of the hamate – FCU.
- Scaphoid bone osteophyte – FPL (Mannerfelt lesion).

Management

- Conservative treatment as above.
- Synovitis: flexor tenosynovectomy plus CTR, ± osteophyte excision.
- Rupture:
  ○ **FPL (Mannerfelt)** is most common rupture in RA due to scaphoid attrition and tenosynovitis – PL tendon graft or FDS ring/middle transfer (Bunnell).
  ○ FDP – DIPJ arthrodesis is often the best option, others include adjacent FDP transfer.
  ○ FDS and FDP rupture (usually caused by direct effects of pannus) – adjacent FDS transfer to ruptured FDP.

The metacarpophalangeal joint

The MCPJ is the key joint for finger function yet it is also the joint most commonly involved in rheumatoid arthritis. Radiologically, the metacarpophalangeal joints can be viewed with Brewerton views: MCPJ flexed to 60° with the extensor surfaces of the fingers flat on the X-ray plate. The intrinsic muscles pass volar to the axis of the joint.

The **collateral ligaments** have two main parts:

- Metacarpophalangeal part that runs between the two bones (MC and PP).
- Metacarpoglenoid part from the metacarpal head to the volar plate – the accessory collateral ligament thus effectively anchors the volar plate to the metacarpal head.

The **volar plate** has a strong attachment to the PP but is attached to the metacarpal head by only a membranous insertion and the two lateral check rein ligaments. The volar plate at the MCPJ is continuous with the transverse metacarpal ligament.

At the point of insertion of the accessory collateral ligament to the volar plate, two other structures attach:

- The sagittal bands of the extensor tendon that keep the extensor tendon in a central position and stabilize the joint.
- The proximal attachment of the flexor sheath – the A1 pulley.

Metacarpophalangeal joints in rheumatoid disease
Harrison's grading

- 1 – dislocation of extensor tendon without medial shift.
- 2 – ulnar drift and medial shift.
- 3 – reducible subluxation of MCPJ.
- 4 – irreducible subluxation of MCPJ.

Nalebuff classification

- I – synovial proliferation.
- II – recurrent synovitis without deformity.
- III – moderate articular degeneration, ulnar and palmar digital drift that is passively correctable.
- IV – severe joint destruction with fixed deformities.

Sequence of events destabilizing the MCPJ in RA

- **Ulnar drift** (ulnar rotation with ulnar shift of the phalangeal base at the MCPJ) in the fingers due to erosion and attenuation of radial sagittal bands and radial collateral ligaments.
  ○ Synovial erosion of the radial sagittal bands of the extensor tendons causing extensors to

dislocate in an ulnar direction (**the radial collateral ligaments are thinner** than the ulnar, lax collateral ligaments due to synovitis allows ulnar deviation).

- **Volar subluxation** of base of proximal phalanx.
  - ○ Weakening of dorsal capsule and **volar subluxation of extensor tendons.**
  - ○ Weakened attachment of membranous part of the volar plate to the metacarpal head due to synovial erosion and loosening of the collateral and accessory collateral ligaments. This allows the pull of the flexor tendon on the A1 pulley to be transmitted to the base of the PP (instead of to the head of the metacarpal).
  - ○ Palmar subluxation leads to telescoping.
  - ○ Joint destabilization following damage to cartilage and bone from synovitis.

Ulnar deviation is caused by normal use/anatomical predispositions:

- Thumb pressure during pinch grip.
- Ulnar inclination of metacarpal heads.
- Abductor digiti minimi action as a strong ulnar deviator.

On the other hand, **ulnar drift** describes a **pathological force** once the normal configuration/stability is lost:

- Radial wrist deviation leading to ulnar drift of MCPJ (Z-mechanism).
- Ulnar shift of extensors (extensors sublux into the intermetacarpal sulcus and thus tend to become ulnar deviators).
- Ulnar forces of flexors.
- **Intrinsic tightness** – test by attempting to flex PIPJ with MCPJ hyperextended, which is not possible with tightness of the intrinsics. This
  - ○ Reduces power grip.
  - ○ Increases ulnar drift, palmar subluxation of MCPJ and swan-neck deformity.

After an adequate trial of conservative treatment including splints and steroids, synovectomy can be offered for persistent metacarpophalangeal joint synovitis in the presence of:

- Minimal radiological changes.
- Little or no joint deformity.

It is often combined with soft tissue reconstruction, e.g. relocation of extensor tendons and intrinsic release

particularly if ulnar drift > 30°, however, there is a high incidence of recurrence.

Intrinsic muscles

These are responsible for metacarpophalangeal flexion and IP extension.

- Interosseus muscles (all supplied by ulnar nerve with occasional variant where the first dorsal interosseus is supplied by the median nerve).
  - ○ **Palmar interosseii** adduct towards the axis of the middle finger (PAD). Three small muscles serving index, ring and little fingers; adductor pollicis to the thumb. They arise from the middle finger side of their own metacarpal and insert into the same side of the extensor expansion and PP.
  - ○ **Dorsal interosseii** abduct away from the axis of the middle finger (DAB). There are four muscles serving index, middle and ring fingers; the little finger and thumb have ADM and APB respectively. They arise by two heads, one from each metacarpal bordering the interosseus space and insert into extensor expansion and PP on the side away from the middle finger. The middle finger has a dorsal interosseus on each side.
- Lumbricals arise from the radial parts of the FDP tendons and pass radial to the MCPJ and insert into the dorsum of the extensor expansion at the sagittal bands, distal to the insertion of the interosseii. They have no bony insertion.
  - ○ The lumbricals to the index and middle finger are innervated by the median nerve whilst those to ring finger and little finger are innervated by the ulnar nerve. The latter are **bicipital** i.e. arise by two heads from adjacent FDP tendons whilst median-innervated lumbricals are unicipital.

Intrinsic surgery

Intrinsic tightness can contribute to swan-neck deformity.

- **Intrinsic release** – division of the insertion of intrinsics into the ulnar sagittal band ± bony attachment. Intrinsics inserting ulnarly include dorsal interosseii to ring and middle fingers, ADM and palmar interosseus to index.
- **Crossed intrinsic transfer** – restores finger alignment with long-term correction of ulnar drift

and is usually combined with other soft tissue or joint procedures. The intrinsic insertions on the ulnar side of the ring, middle and index fingers are released and the tendons mobilized up to musculotendinous junction. The insertion is then relocated and sutured to the radial collateral ligament of the MCPJ (rather than the radial sagittal band as this may promote swan-necking).

Arthroplasty

Types of arthroplasty

- Perichondrial arthroplasty – useful for young patients, restores cartilage.
- Resection arthroplasty, e.g. basal joint of the thumb.
- Silicone joint replacement – metacarpophalangeals and interphalangeals.
- Volar plate interpositional arthroplasty – for those with poor bone stock, also known as modified Tupper (vide infra). Other materials have been used for interpositioning e.g. fascia lata, periosteum, extensor tendons and silicone.
- Vascularized joint transfer – in children, the transfer of an epiphysis allows continued growth.
- Non-vascularized bone transfer, e.g. replace metacarpal with metatarsal.

Long-term follow-up of Swanson's silastic arthroplasty of the metacarpophalangeal joints in rheumatoid arthritis

Wilson YG. *J Hand Surg* 1993;**18**:81–91.

The aims of joint surgery are:

- Painless stable joint.
- Functional range of movement ~70°.
- Better cosmesis.

The common indications for surgery are primarily pain and loss of function.

Swanson's prosthesis (1972) is essentially a dynamic joint spacer that maintains alignment. The joint is stabilized with fibrous encapsulation and relies upon a telescoping effect. Long-term follow-up shows the majority of patients have sustained improvement in pain and range of movement, though there is a gradual deterioration in range of motion with time.

- Complications include infection (1.3%), bone resorption (14%) and giant cell reactive synovitis (no patients in this study). The deformity may

recur, or the implant may fracture or dislocate thus requiring revision (3.2%) – some fractures do not impair movement and do not require revision.

Operative steps

Start with dorsal longitudinal (Swanson) or transverse incision across MCPJ taking care to preserve dorsal nerves and veins.

- Release ulnar sagittal band (intrinsic release) and longitudinal capsulotomy. The metacarpal head is excised whilst preserving the RCL on its distal attachment to the base of the PP.
- Broach and ream proximally and distally, and then the Swanson silicone joint replacement is inserted.
- Drill hole in dorsal cortex of metacarpal for reattachment of RCL.
- Close capsule and plication of radial sagittal band.
- Irrigation, Swanson's drain and skin closure.

Optional steps include division of abductor digiti minimi tendon and the ulnar intrinsics and crossed intrinsic transfer.

The metacarpophalangeal volar plate arthroplasty

Tupper JW. *J Hand Surg* 1989;**14**:371–375.

The aims of volar plate arthroplasty are to restore joint stability by tightening the ligamentous support. In addition, synovitis causing joint disease is removed and deforming forces are corrected by realignment of long flexors and interosseii. It is a useful option in patients with poor bone stock and thus unsuited for joint replacements.

- Resection arthroplasty: transverse incision, ulnar release, capsulotomy with division of the collateral ligaments (preserving RCL for later repair), followed by synovectomy and excision of the metacarpal head.
- **Vainio method**: cut the extensor tendon proximal to the MCPJ and attach the distal end to the volar plate to provide interpositional tissue whilst reinserting the cut proximal end to the dorsal surface of the extensor at the proximal edge of the PP.
- The author's criticism of the Vainio method is that the interpositional substance is not robust enough and that it also impairs extensor function as it does not correct the volar pull of the flexor on the base of the PP via the A1 pulley.

Table 6.6 Comparison of swan-neck and boutonnière deformities.

	Thumb	Fingers
Swan-neck PIPJ hyperextension, DIPJ flexion	Flexion deformity at CMC joint	Volar plate attenuation Intrinsic tightness or mallet FDS rupture
Boutonnière PIPJ hyperflexion, DIPJ hyperextension	Rupture of EPB	Rupture of central slip of EDC

- Tupper method: incise the volar plate at the proximal end at the junction between fibrocartilaginous and membranous areas, and then separate the attachment of the A1 pulley from the volar plate. The proximal end of the volar plate is reflected into the joint and attached to the dorsal edge of the cut metacarpal. The proposed advantages are that it provides thick interpositional substance, and also elevates base of PP and re-establishes anchorage of the volar plate to the metacarpal.

Thumb in rheumatoid arthritis

Swan-neck and Boutonnière deformities

Nalebuff classification of rheumatoid thumb deformity

- I – **Boutonnière**, IP joint hyperextended, rupture of EPB at the level of the metacarpophalangeal joint (i.e. MCPJ disease).
- II – Boutonnière plus metacarpal adduction (**CMC** subluxation). This is rare.
- III – **Swan-neck deformity** (extended MCPJ, flexed IPJ) volar subluxation of the thumb at the level of the carpometacarpal joint; it is often due to CMCJ synovitis.
- IV – **Gamekeeper's thumb.** Ulnar collateral ligament rupture with radial deviation of the thumb at the metacarpophalangeal joint, with adduction contracture. Treat by MCPJ fusion, ± web release.
- V – **Isolated swan neck** (MCP hyperextension with IPJ flexion) and no CMCJ subluxation. Treat with MCPJ fusion and IPJ palmar plate advancement or MP arthroplasty with IPJ fusion.
- VI – **Arthritis mutilans.**

The most common types are I and III.

Boutonnière deformity

The basic deformity is MCPJ flexion with IPJ hyperextension; most are type I (MCPJ disease) whilst type II with CMCJ disease/subluxation is rare.

Disease at the MCPJ and attrition of EPB causes loss of MCPJ extension and flexion deformity.

- The EPL tendon and adductor expansions become subluxed ulnarly, and lateral thenar expansions are displaced radially with extension at IPJ.
- Intrinsics (AP and APB) exacerbate flexion at MCPJ and extension at IP joint.

Treatment

- Stage I – supple and passively correctable.
  - Synovectomy at MCPJ.
  - Reconstruction the extensor apparatus to reposition dorsal to joint: dorsalize lateral bands and EPL re-routing to the base of the PP, silicone arthroplasty.
- Stage II – fixed MCPJ and supple IPJ. Treat with MCPJ fusion if other joints are not degenerated otherwise MCPJ arthoplasty is preferred.
- Stage III – fixed MCPJ and IPJ. Treat with IPJ fusion and MCPJ arthroplasty.

Type II boutonnière – treat with CMCJ arthroplasty and **boutonnière** reconstruction similar to above.

Swan-neck deformity

This is **more common in osteoarthritis than rheumatoid arthritis**; a 'true' swan neck does not occur at the thumb as it has one less joint.

There is disease at the trapeziometacarpal (also called carpometacarpal – CMC) joint leading to **subluxation** and **metacarpal adduction contracture**. Patient is unable to extend at the CMCJ and extension forces are transmitted to the MCPJ instead leading to **hyperextension of MCPJ and flexion of IPJ**.

- Stage I – CMCJ subluxation with no MCJP hyperextension. Treat with CMCJ arthroplasty.
- Stage II – CMCJ subluxation with MCPJ extension. If the articular surfaces are satisfactory and other joints are not damaged, then treat with CMCJ synovectomy, ligament reconstruction (FCR/ECRL) and soft tissue stablization with palmar capsulodesis/tenodesis plate, or fusion if the joint has degenerated and unstable.

- Stage III – web-space contracture. Treat as above with web release – release adductor pollicis and first dorsal interosseus. The metacarpal base may need to be resected.

Gamekeeper's thumb

Metacarpophalangeal joint disease leads to chronic UCL rupture and thus radial deviation of the thumb at the MCPJ and secondary adduction of the metacarpal.

Treatment options include:

- If the articular surfaces are intact (rare) then reconstruction of UCL with APL or a free FCR tendon graft.
- MCPJ arthrodesis ± IPJ arthrodesis if the joint surfaces are poor.
- Correction of adductors, release adductor pollicis and first dorsal interossei, ± Z-plasty web.

Fingers in rheumatoid arthritis

Swan-neck deformity – PIPJ hyperextension and DIPJ flexion secondary to imbalance of IPJ forces; it can start at either IPJ. Volar subluxation of wrist renders the flexor tendons ineffective; an intrinsic plus deformity is adopted – the intrinsics hyperextend the PIPJ via lateral bands.

It is often caused by **PIPJ synovitis**, which leads to volar plate laxity/attenuation, intrinsic tightness and loss of FDS insertion; alternatively, it may be due to DIPJ disease such as **chronic mallet**. Both lead to dorsal migration of the lateral bands, the FDP flexes the DIPJ and the volar plate stretches.

- Intrinsic and central tendon tightness with MCPJ pathology can lead to PIPJ hyperextension even before MCPJ subluxation, once the MCPJ subluxes there is a secondary PIPJ hyperextension.

Nalebuff classification

- I – **PIPJ flexible**. Treat with extension block splint to correct PIPJ hyperextension, synovectomy.
  - FDS hemitenodesis if the cartilage is not damaged. The FDS tendon is attached to the base of the MP to limit PIPJ hyperextension.
  - Dermadesis – excision of loose skin over flexor surface of PIPJ; the long-term results tend to be poor.

- Sublimis sling (Urbaniak) – FDS slip transected in palm and looped over A2 pulley to be sutured to itself; it aims to keep the PIPJ flexed/reduce hyperextension.
  - Littler (retinacular ligament reconstruction).
- II – **Limited PIPJ** flexion when MCPJ extended (intrinsic tightness). Treat with intrinsic and lateral band release ± arthroplasty if the joint has subluxed.
- III – **Limited PIPJ flexion** in all positions but joint is preserved. Treat by correcting MCPJ subluxation by arthroplasty, mobilize and release lateral bands or hemitenodesis.
- IV – **Stiff PIPJ** with poor radiographic appearance. Treat by fusion (index or middle, or if flexor tendons have ruptured) or arthroplasty (ring or little).

Boutonnière deformity – this is often due to attenuation/erosion of the central slip at the PIPJ due to synovitis and the lateral bands fall volarly, becoming fixed with the ORL and thus tend to cause flexion; there is less resistance against FDS action which flexes the PIPJ, DIPJ extension (secondary to Z mechanism) whilst the MCPJ also develops compensatory hyperextension.

Nalebuff and Millenden classification

- Stage 1 – **Mild** – 10–15° extensor lag at PIPJ which is passively correctable. Treat with Capner splint, lateral band reconstruction (relocate dorsally) or Fowler's – terminal extensor tenotomy over middle phalanx to improve DIPJ flexion (ORL extensor action at joint prevents mallet formation).
- Stage 2 – **Moderate** – 30–40° lag, passively correctable and joint space preserved. These patients often have MCPJ hyperextension. Treatment results are somewhat unpredictable: reposition lateral band with TRL release, shorten central slip – holding PIPJ in extension with a K-wire for 3 weeks.
- Stage 3 – **Severe** – fixed PIPJ deformity, tight TRL (maintains lateral bands in volar position, PIPJ flexion) and ORL (DIPJ extension and block to flexion). Treat by arthrodesis (if cartilage damaged) or arthroplasty (soft tissue attenuation makes results unpredictable) as above but only after splinting/serial casting to restore full passive extension to the PIPJ. These patients may have little functional deficit and surgery may not help.

Arthrodesis – is an option mainly for distal interphalangeal disease (or intra-articular fractures). The PIPJ is arthrodesed at angles of 20°, 30°, 40° and 50° for the index, middle, ring and little fingers respectively. In general, the PIPJ of index does better with arthrodesis than arthroplasty – a stable index can be used in pinch whilst the mobile middle can be used in grasp.

Operative steps for small joint arthrodesis:

- Dorsal incision and split extensor tendon longitudinally.
- Capsulotomy and excision of joint surfaces at appropriate angles.
- Lister loop (0.45 interosseus wire) and oblique K-wire.
- Repair extensor mechanism, irrigate and close skin.

Differential diagnoses of arthritides

Juvenile rheumatoid arthritis

This is the commonest connective tissue disorder in children. It is characterized by a proliferative synovitis that affects the knees and wrist most frequently. Diagnostic criteria include:

- Onset under 16 years of age.
- First episode lasting more than 6 weeks.
- Arthritis in more than one joint with two or more signs (joint tenderness, stiffness, pain on motion and inflammation) and other rheumatoid disease has been excluded.
- Juvenile RA patients may have non-RA features – ulnar deviation of wrist and metacarpals, radial deviation of MCPJ, abnormal ring and little finger metacarpals (secondary to accelerated maturation of epiphyses), short ulnar and narrow small tubular bones of hand.

Subtypes include:

- **Polyarticular** (40%). This form is similar to adult RA with minimal systemic involvement and tends to continue into adulthood. Those with RF tend to have a worse prognosis.
- **Monoarticular** (40%). Affects less than or equal to four joints within the first 6 months. It affects the lower limb more frequently and eye problems are common – many are RF-negative and antinuclear antibody (ANA) positive. The younger age group (< 6) tend to be female, whilst the second older age group are males.

- **Systemic onset** (Still's disease, 20%). These have intermittent pyrexia, rash, hepatosplenomegaly, lymphadenopathy, anaemia, myalgia/arthralgia and eye involvement. 25% progress to severe arthritis.

Treatment is mainly supportive with the aim of preventing deformities – upper limb deformities may result due to abnormal epiphyseal growth and anklyosis especially the wrist. Surgery may damage growth plates and is avoided unless necessary.

- Splintage, physiotherapy.
- Synovectomy for pain.

Ankylosing spondylitis

This condition is characterized by these main features:

- Back pain of insidious onset in males (10 × more frequent than females) under 40 years of age.
- Morning stiffness, and the stiffness improves with movement/exercise.
- Present for more than 3 months.

It affects the sacroiliac joints and back in particular; 20% have peripheral arthritis similar to RA but only 10% are RF positive. 90% of patients are HLA B27 positive.

Systemic lupus erythematosis

Systemic lupus erythematosis (SLE) is the commonest of the connective tissue diseases (but RA is 20 × more common). It is especially prevalent in pigmented races. On average it affects 1 in 250, mostly women (10 × more than men) 20–40 years of age.

- 90% have joint involvement although SLE arthritis affects mainly the soft tissues rather than joint surfaces. This is a non-erosive arthritis with ligamentous laxity, particularly the hands and wrists, and may lead to subluxation. In extreme cases, fusion should be considered.
- Antinuclear antibody and anti-dsDNA positive.
- Other features include:
  - Butterfly rash on face.
  - Raynaud's phenomenon.
  - Liver palms, purpuric rash in fingers.
  - Vasculitis affecting heart, lungs and kidneys.
  - May also have neurological and GI manifestations.

Psoriatic arthritis

A key feature of psoriatic arthropathy (5–30% of psoriasis sufferers) is fibrosis along with osteolytic destruction leading to phalangeal erosions and periosteal new bone formation – progressive bone loss may lead to 'pencil in a cup' (tapering of proximal bone whilst distal bone proliferates) and arthritis mutilans in 5%. It tends to begin 10 years after the skin disease manifests itself; in a minority (10–15%) the joint disease precedes the skin disease. It differs from RA in that:

- It is seronegative (HLA-B27) and asymmetric.
- Nail pits in 80% (> 20 for diagnosis in absence of typical skin involvement).
- Absence of skin nodules/rash.
- Synovitis is rare whilst stiffness is frequent; dactylitis due to inflammation of soft tissues.

Disease in the DIPJ is more likely to be psoriatic arthritis than RA – in RA, DIPJ deformity is usually secondary to PIP deformity. A subtype is often called DIP predominant (5%) and is characterized by disease localized to DIPs of fingers and toes along with marked nail changes.

Nalebuff classification

- I – spontaneous ankylosis predominates, especially at DIPJ and PIPJ.
- II – osteolytic, bone loss predominates – arthritis mutilans. Early fusion with lengthening, avoid arthroplasty.
- III – RA-like features.

Management is primarily medical: NSAIDs, steroid injections (for those with pauciarticular involvement), with second line being immunosuppression that also deals with the skin disease. More recently etanercept and infliximab (TNF alpha inhibitors) has been used for severe cases.

Surgery may be required (classically advised to wait for skin to improve, i.e. summer) including corrective osteotomies, arthrodesis (IPJ) and arthroplasty (MCPJ, PIPJ for ring and little fingers). Overall expectations are lower compared with RA with less motion and a higher infection rate; the goal is large object grasp.

Arthritis mutilans may follow RA or psoriatic arthritis, and can affect any joint. It is characterized by considerable amounts of bone loss – treatment is generally fusion with lengthening by bone graft which will tend to stop bone loss; arthroplasty is contraindicated in all but MCPJ as bone loss will continue but preserving MCPJ mobility is important.

Others

- Systemic sclerosis/scleroderma is a rare multi-organ disease, particularly in Chinese and Japanese; it is 3–6 × more common in women. There is a polyarthritis in some patients (40% of whom are RF positive). Erosive arthritis is rare but joint deformity may occur secondary to fibrous contracture. There are associations with the CREST syndrome i.e. calcinosis circumscripta, digital ischaemia etc.
- Ulcerative colitis – transient seronegative arthritis in 10% that seems to be related to ulcerative colitis disease activity.
- Behçet's syndrome – oral and genital ulcers and iritis associated with arthritis of elbow and wrist arthritis. This seems to be a form of cell-mediated autoimmunity.
- Reiter's syndrome – polyarthritis, urethritis and conjunctivitis in patients who are HLA-B27.
- Reactive arthritis – secondary to *Salmonella*, *Brucella*, *Neisseria gonorrhoeae*.

Joint contracture

Causes of flexion contracture:

- Skin/scar contracture.
- Fascia – Dupuytren's.
- Flexor tendon sheath – fibrous contracture or flexor tendon – Volkman's contracture, adhesions.
- Capsular structures – volar plate shortening.
- Block to extension – osteophytes, loose bodies, etc.

Collateral ligament shortening is *never* a cause because these are held taut in all ranges of movement at the IP joints.

Extension contracture

- Skin/scar contracture.
- Extensor tendon – shortening, adhesions.
- Intrinsic muscles – ischaemic contracture, intrinsic plus.
- Capsular structures – collateral ligament shortening (lax in extension at metacarpophalangeal joint), volar plate adhesions, dorsal capsule contracture.
- Joint surfaces – fixed extension in post-burn contracture, bony block, loose body, osteoarthritis.

- Flexor tendon – bulky tendon preventing excursion.

Bouvier's test to confirm intrinsic tightness – flexion is impossible at proximal interphalangeal and distal interphalangeal joints when the metacarpophalangeal joints are extended; shorten intrinsics by passively flexing metacarpophalangeal joints – flexion at proximal interphalangeal and distal interphalangeal joints is now possible.

Ligaments

Positions of **greatest ligamentous laxity** are assumed in the **injured hand**:

- wrist – extension.
- MPJ – extension.
- IPJ – flexion.
- Thumb – adduction.

The collateral ligament of the metacarpophalangeal joint and the volar plate of the IP joints will then shorten to create a contracture.

Trigger finger

This is a stenosing tenosynovitis of the flexor tendon which can be primary (including congenital) or secondary (usually due to RA, gout, diabetes). The ring and middle fingers are mostly frequently affected in adults (index rarely). It may co-exist with de Quervain's disease or with carpal tunnel syndrome.

Steroid injections are usually beneficial in cases of short duration but these have the tendency to recur frequently. Release of A1 pulley offers operative cure but caution is needed in RA patients as the A1 pulley attaches to the head of the metacarpal, and its release may exacerbate the tendency towards volar subluxation.

Lower limb

I. Relevant anatomy

The two tibias bear 85% of the weight.

Anatomy

Sensation

- Lateral calf – sural nerve.
- Medial calf – saphenous nerve.
- Dorsum of foot – superficial peroneal nerve.
- First web space – deep peroneal nerves.
- Sole of foot – medial and lateral plantar nerves from posterior tibial.

Dermatome testing

- L2 – lateral thigh.
- L3 – knee.
- L4 – medial calf.
- L5 – lateral calf/first web.
- S1 – lateral foot.
- S2 – posterior middle thigh.

Sole of the foot

- Layer 1: abductor hallucis, flexor digitorum brevis, abductor digiti minimi.
- Layer 2: flexor hallucis longus, flexor digitorum longus, lumbricals, flexor accessorius.
- Layer 3: flexor hallucis brevis, adductor hallucis, flexor digiti minimi brevis.
- Layer 4: interosseii.

The medial and lateral plantar nerves lie between layers 1 and 2.

General considerations

'Debridement' was described first by Pierre-Joseph Desault (French surgeon, 1744–1795) in the treatment of traumatic wounds. Advances in the management of lower limb trauma include:

- Debridement, with antibiotics/asepsis.
- Bone fixation.
- Vascular repair.
- Soft tissue coverage, flaps of choice being gracilis, rectus abdominis and latissimus dorsi.

BAPS/BOA working party report on open tibial fractures

Br J Plast Surg 1997;**50**:570–583.

This report emphasized early cooperation between senior plastic and orthopaedic surgeons.

- Half of open tibial fractures are Gustilo grades IIIA or B.
- 70% of Gustilo grade IIIB injuries require flap cover.
- 4% are Gustilo grade IV – these often proceed to amputation so rarely involve plastic surgery input.

Fractures can be classified as low- or high-energy (e.g. RTA, fall from a height and missile injuries); the latter have a poorer prognosis. Clinical signs of a high-energy injury:

- Large/multiple wounds.
- Crush or burst lacerations.
- Closed degloving.
- Signs of nerve or vascular injury.

Radiological signs of a high-energy injury:

Table 7.1 Compartments of the lower leg and their contents.

Compartment	Anterior	Lateral	Posterior superficial	Posterior deep
Muscles	EHL, EDL, tibialis anterior, peroneus tertius	Peroneus longus and brevis	Gastrocnemius, plantaris, soleus	FHL, FDL, tibialis posterior
Main function	Dorsiflexion	Eversion	Plantar flexion	
Nerve	Deep peroneal nerve	Superficial peroneal	Tibial nerve	
Artery	Anterior tibial artery	Peroneal artery	Posterior tibial artery	

EHL, extensor hallucis longus; EDL, extensor digitorum longus; FHL, flexor hallucis longus; FDL, flexor digitorum longus.

- Multiple bony fragments especially more than one fractured bone in the same limb.
- Widely spaced fragments or segmental injury.

The wound should be examined at once by the surgeon of the responsible team – digital photographs taken, and the wound dressed and left until theatre. Open tibial fractures should be closed within a maximum of 5 days:

- Wound excision and irrigation (6 litres normal saline pulsed lavage) and fracture stabilization.
  - Diaphyseal open tibial fractures – intramedullary (IM) nail.
  - Metaphyseal open tibial fractures – plate or external fixation, pin sites should avoid compromise of fasciocutaneous flaps or free flap pedicle/recipients.
- Soft tissue reconstruction ideally as soon as possible – wounds closed within 72 hours have highest success rate and lowest complication rate. However, **immediate closure is not always required** and delayed closure may enable serial debridements and compartment monitoring.

II. Classification of lower limb trauma

Gustilo and Anderson fracture classification
Prevention of infection in the treatment of 1025 open fractures of long bones
Gustilo RB. *J Bone Joint Surg Am* 1976;**58**:453–458.

The first classification had subtypes I–III for long bone fractures, which was subsequently modified and applied mostly to open tibial fractures. The classification below was published in 1990 (*J Bone Joint Surg Am* 1990;**72**:299–304) with the subtypes being an addition in 1984.

- I – clean wound < 1 cm.
- II – wound 1–5 cm but without significant tissue disruption.

- III – wound > 5 cm with significant tissue disruption.
  - IIIA local tissues provide adequate soft tissue coverage.
  - IIIB extensive soft tissue loss, contamination, periosteal stripping.
  - IIIC arterial injury requiring repair.

The classification does not actually consider the bony injury. It is widely used and relatively simple, however inter-observer reliability is not high and is best applied after wound excision.

Byrd classification (Byrd HS. *Plast Reconstr Surg* 1989;**76**:159).

- I – low energy (spiral oblique fracture with relatively clean wound, laceration < 2 cm).
- II – moderate energy (comminuted/displaced fracture with wound > 2 cm, with moderate muscle and skin contusion).
- III – high energy (severe comminution/ displacement or bony defect with extensive soft tissue injury, deviatization muscle.
- IV – extreme energy (degloving or vascular injury requiring repair).

Mangled extremity severity score (MESS; simplified)
Objective criteria accurately predict amputation following lower extremity trauma
Johanssen K. *J Trauma* 1990;**30**:568–573.

- Skeletal and soft tissue injury (1, 2, 3, 4).
  - Low/medium/high/very high energy with gross contamination.
- Limb ischaemia (1, 2, 3 – double if greater than 6 hours).
  - Pulseless but perfused.
  - Pulseless, paraesthetic with prolonged capillary refill.

○ Devascularized – cool, paraesthetic, insensate.
- Shock (0, 1, 2).
  ○ No hypotension SBP > 90 mmHg.
  ○ Transient hypotension.
  ○ Sustained hypotension.
- Age (0, 1, 2).
  ○ < 30 years.
  ○ 30–50 years.
  ○ > 50 years

The MESS is specific but not that sensitive; it may have a role in the decision of whether or not to amputate a severely traumatized leg. Score of 6 or less – salvageable limb, 7 or more salvage unlikely to be successful. However, some parts are subjective e.g. contamination in consideration of energy.

There are many more complicated systems including the AO score which has better predictive value but is rather complex, and may be most suited for audit/ data collection rather than everyday clinical use.

Arnez and Tyler classification

Classification of soft-tissue degloving in limb trauma
Arnez ZM. *Br J Plast Surg* 1999;**10**:82–86.

- Type 1 – non-circumferential degloving.
- Type 2 – abrasion but no degloving.
- Type 3 – circumferential degloving.
- Type 4 – circumferential degloving plus avulsion between deep tissue planes: intermuscular and muscle–periosteum planes.

Type 4 injuries require serial conservative debridements and delayed reconstruction as early radical debridement usually results in a functionless limb.

General management of lower limb trauma

Adhere to ATLS principles for immediate management i.e. ABC. The first priority is the airway with C-spine control – continue with the primary survey, treating life-threatening injuries, and then perform the secondary survey. Once the patient is stable, take a history and examine the limb.

- AMPLE history including 'Event' – the time and mechanism of injury, high energy vs. low energy, etc.

Investigations

- X-rays.
- Angiography if the limb is pulseless following fracture reduction.

Determining salvageability of the limb:

- Is revascularization needed or technically possible? Consider on-table angiogram for assessment.
- Is there nerve injury and does this preclude a functioning limb? The results of nerve repair and grafting in the lower limb are poor except in children.
- Is the soft tissue defect treatable with local flaps or free flaps?
- Is there any bone loss and is it reconstructable?

In assessing the patient suitability for salvage – is there any concomitant life-threatening injury and what are the needs and wishes of the patient? Patients can often return to work earlier if amputated (e.g. self-employed farmer).

Timing of soft tissue cover

- Emergency – within 24 hours (Lister G. Emergency free flaps. In Green DP (ed.) *Operative Hand Surgery*, 2nd edn. Churchill Livingstone: 1127–1149)
- Early (under 3 days) – associated with less infection and less flap failure – (Godina M. *Plast Reconstr Surg* 1986;**78**:285–292).
- Delayed – < 3/12.
- Late > 3/12 (Arnez ZM. *Clin Plast Surg* 1991;**19**:449–457).

Evidence suggests that flap success is better if performed before 3 days (Godina) or to wait for more than 3 months if early surgery is not possible for any reason (Arnez). There is a '5-day rule' that many adhere to but the evidence for this exact cut-off is lacking; according to the Standards of Management of Open Fractures of the Lower Limb (BAPRAS/ BOA 2009) microsurgery is best performed within a week before the vessels become friable or fibrosed.

Reconstructive plan

- Reduce and stabilize the fracture (this often alleviates any vasospasm).
- Restore perfusion by arterial reconstruction if necessary.
  ○ Vascular shunts may be used temporarily before fracture stabilization but definitive vascular reconstruction can become disrupted during fracture manipulation/ fixation.
- Fasciotomy for crush, reperfusion injuries.

- Debridement of all non-viable tissue and pulsed lavage under tourniquet – muscle that is dark, non-contractile and does not bleed is dead (though the converse is less reliable, i.e. a muscle that is contractile may be dead/dying).
- Soft tissue cover.

Amputation

- **Below-knee (BKA**; 6 cm below the tibial tuberosity) is vastly superior to above-knee (AKA) in terms of rehabilitation. Free flap salvage for a BKA stump may be needed and the best tissue with the best sensation is probably a pedicled fillet of sole flap or a free sole flap with nerve repair.

In general,

·	Primary closure	Gustilo I and II
·	SSG	Gustilo IIIA
·	Fasciocutaneous flap	Gustilo IIIA and B (but beware raising within a degloved area).
·	Free flap	Gustilo IIIB.

Healing by secondary intention (Papineau) – this is suitable when no local flap option exists and the patient is unsuitable for free flap surgery. The cortex can be drilled and kept moist to encourage granulation tissue formation, which is then covered by skin graft. It may take 3–4 months to heal. Some have suggested use of NPWT or Integra under similar circumstances.

The **cross-leg flap** is a poor solution as it involves immobilization (with risk of DVT, contracture) and needs a well-vascularized recipient site to support the flap after pedicle division.

III. Fracture management in compound lower limb trauma

- Intramedullary nailing.
  - ○ Reamed nails with proximal and distal locking provide very stable fixation and allows early mobilization. However, they may be difficult to use in comminuted fractures.
  - ○ Unreamed nails avoid disruption of the endosteal blood supply.
- Internal fixation – exacerbates periosteal stripping and increases infection risk.
- External fixation.

  - ○ This is often the method of choice, using Ilizarov frames that allow easy access for repeated debridement. Pins must be sited carefully to avoid compromising local flap options and track infections may occur.

Management of bone gaps

If there is no bone loss, then reduce and stabilize using either external fixator or unreamed IM nail.

- **Non-vascularized bone grafts** are suitable for small defects (< 4 cm) in well-vascularized graft beds. It is common to wait 6–12 weeks post-trauma before introducing non-vascularized bone graft into the defect.
- **Vascularized bone graft**: although it is a potentially complex reconstruction in the early post-trauma phase, use of either DCIA or free fibula can effectively reconstruct large segmental defects > 8 cm. The transferred fibula has been shown to hypertrophy with use. Good soft tissue cover is needed.

Ilizarov techniques

This is useful where the traumatic bone gap is > 4 cm, either:

- The fracture gap (4–8 cm) is compressed causing limb shortening, and is then followed by **distraction osteogenesis**, which often compensates for inadequate soft tissue for primary closure.
- For larger defects (8–12 cm), the limb can be held to length followed by **bone transport**, with a corticotomy to develop the **mobile segment** – preserving medullary and periosteal blood supply. Adequate soft tissues are needed i.e. may need a flap. This avoids the soft tissue contracture that may otherwise occur, muscle atrophy, disuse osteoporosis, joint contracture and stiffness in a shortened limb. Problems with this technique include docking non-union requiring a bone graft at the end.
  - ○ A latent period of ~5 days is needed following corticotomy before commencing distraction at one-quarter turn 4 times a day to lengthen 1 mm/day.
  - ○ The rate of distraction is monitored by serial X-rays to avoid premature fusion or the appearance of lucency indicating that distraction is too fast. When the required

length is achieved, the frame is left for ~2 months to allow for **consolidation** of the distracted segment.

- For defects > 12 cm, the bone can be held out to length with external fixator and reconstruct secondarily with vascularized bone flap (free fibula).

Complications

- Length discrepancies.
- Incomplete docking/non-union requiring secondary bone grafting.
- Pin track infections.
  - Minimize tension at the interface between pin and skin.
  - Recalcitrant infection may necessitate removal of the wire.

Physiology of distraction histogenesis

- Tension–stress effect – tissues under tension respond by forming more tissue (regeneration).
- Distracted bone regenerates by **intramembranous ossification** orchestrated by the periosteum – osteoblastic differentiation of periosteal mesenchymal cells and hence is not analogous to endochondral ossification, which would normally occur at a fracture site.
  - Patients with fibrous dysplasia cannot do this, therefore this technique cannot be used as the new bone is also dysplastic (but osteogenesis imperfecta **can** be treated in this way).

Bifocal surgery for deformity and bone loss after lower limb fractures. Comparison of bone transport and distraction-lengthening

Saleh M. *J Bone Joint Surg* 1995;**77**:429–434.

This is a retrospective review of 16 patients. Bone transport is more suited to **larger defects** in which shortening would be fairly dramatic and may have deleterious effects on soft tissues and joints. Bone transport was more complicated requiring an additional 2.2 additional operations compared with only one for compression-distraction.

- Average time to union following bone transport was 16 months, vs. 10 months for lengthening (but smaller defects in this group).
- Union at the docking site was occasionally problematic after bone transport (leading edge may be relatively avascular or obstructed by soft tissues).
- Bone transport involves the wires cutting through soft tissues – may need skin releases under LA.

Table 7.2 Comparison of distraction versus vascularized bone flaps for treatment of bone gaps.

	Ilizarov	Free fibula
Time to full mobilization	18 months	18 months
Secondary fracture	Can nail	Cannot nail
Technique	Safe, quick	Difficult, slow, flap failure
Donor site	None	Morbidity fairly high, soft tissue closure

Bifocal lengthening is distraction occurring by the movement of two ends of the bone away from the central diaphyseal segment. After distraction, some patients may need bone graft to aid consolidation.

Distraction vs. vascularized fibula flap
Chronic osteomyelitis

There is a 4.5% incidence in Gustilo III fractures but the risk can be minimized by thorough debridement.
Adult chronic osteomyelitis – an overview
Cierny G. *Orthopedics* 1984;**7**:1557–1564.

Classification

- Superficial.
- Localized.
- Diffuse.
- Medullary.

Investigations

- Plain X-rays – these still provide the best screening for acute and chronic osteomyelitis (Lazzarini J. *Bone Joint Surg Am* 2004;**86**:2305–2318). Other imaging modalities may be better for diagnosis and guiding management decisions. MRI is useful if the diagnosis is doubtful on plain radiographs, with bone scans (leucocyte for acute, technectium for chronic) if metalwork precludes the use of MRI. CT may be useful to establish surgical plans.
- Bone scan.
- Wound swab/culture.
- Arteriography.

Treatment

- Radical wound debridement (remove necrotic soft tissue and sequestrum).

Table 7.3 Comparison of fasciocutaneous flaps and muscle flaps for soft tissue reconstruction.

	Fasciocutaneous flaps	Muscle flaps
Advantages	Quick	Better in terms of providing well-vascularized tissue (greatest capillary density for tissue) that is flexible and compliant (less likely to leave a dead space) More effective against infection (Mathes SJ. *Plast Reconstr Surg* 1982:**69**:815–829)
Disadvantages	Higher complication rate (partial loss, infection, non-union) Poor donor site cosmesis Restricted by pedicle location May be compromised by external fixation	May be in zone of trauma In general may be most applicable for low-energy upper-third tibial injury (gastrocnemius)

- Bone graft the bone defect (free or vascularized) and immobilize.
- Free muscle flaps bring in a good blood supply.
- Antibiotics – local delivery systems/systemic for 2–6 weeks; consult with microbiologist.

Operative treatment includes debridement, obliteration of dead space, restoration of vascularity, adequate soft tissue cover, stabilization and reconstruction. This may not be feasible for all patients.

IV. Soft tissue coverage

Upper third

- Proximally based fasciocutaneous flap that was first described by **Ponten**.
- **Gastrocnemius muscle** (medial and or lateral).
  - Type I flap based on sural artery from the popliteal artery. The medial head is larger and suited for upper third of tibia and knee defects.
  - With the patient supine, the leg is externally rotated and the knee slightly flexed, an incision is made at the midcalf approximately 2 cm behind the medial tibial border and superiorly curves to the popliteal fossa (avoiding the saphenous vein and nerve). After raising skin flaps to expose the heads of the gastrocnemius, the plane between the medial head and the soleus is developed with blunt dissection, taking care to identify and protect the sural nerve and the muscle pedicle. Divide the distal tendon and reflect; the arc of rotation can be increased by also releasing the origin.
- Free flap.

Middle third

- Proximally/distally based fasciocutaneous flaps based on perforators of peroneal or posterior tibial arteries.
- **Soleus muscle**
  - Type II muscle flap with dual supply, medial (posterior tibial) and lateral (peroneal artery) and can be used either wholly or a single half. In a similar position as above, an incision is made from halfway between the medial malleolus and Achilles tendon superiorly 1 cm behind the medial tibial border. Raise flaps whilst taking care to preserve the saphenous vein and nerve, and then develop the plane between it and the gastrocnemius. Separate the muscle tendon from the Achilles and then reflect upwards, dividing the attachments as needed to allow rotation into the defect. Perpendicular incisions in the aponeurosis may increase the reach.
- Free flap.

Lower third

- Distally based fasciocutaneous flap based on perforators of peroneal or posterior tibial arteries that can be islanded for greater arc of rotation to reach the ankle.
  - The main perforators of the posterior tibial artery perforators are 6, 9 and 12 cm above the medial malleolus and are situated in the intermuscular septum between soleus and flexor hallucis longus (FHL) (neurovascular bundle is deep to soleus) with venous drainage via venae comitantes accompanying the

perforating arteries. Using the 12 cm perforator allows for a greater arc of rotation to reach the ankle. The skin paddle lies between the long and short saphenous veins and can be rotated through 180°.

- **Adipofascial turnover flap** which leaves a better donor defect than fasciocutaneous flaps and is particularly suited for young female patients.
- **Sural artery island flap** sacrifices the nerve and is relatively small and unreliable being based on a small artery and vein supplying the sural nerve. The pivot point (peroneal perforator) is 5 cm above the midpoint of a line joining the lateral malleolus to the Achilles tendon.
- **Free flaps** (good success rate and flexibility with a donor site remote from the trauma zone but usually a long complex procedure). Choices include:
  - Big defect – latissimus dorsi muscle flap and SSG.
  - Medium defect – rectus abdominis and SSG.
  - Smaller defect – gracilis and SSG.
  - Sole of foot – free lateral arm flap (sensate using lateral cutaneous nerve of the arm).
  - Preferred anastomosis is end–side to posterior tibial vessels within 72 hours of injury (vide infra).

A five-year review of islanded distally based fasciocutaneous flaps on the lower limbs
Erdmann MWH. *Br J Plast Surg* 1997;**50**:421–427.

Fasciocutaneous flaps replace like with like in the lower limb. In this study, flaps based on perforators of the posterior tibial artery were used preferentially in males and older females.

- Although suitable for IIIB fractures, **20% of flaps in these patients failed**.
- Three-quarters of flaps were used to close lower-third defects, but are also capable of covering Achilles/heel defects.
- Flaps raised on lateral perforators from the peroneal artery are **less reliable** because of the larger number of perforators: more must be divided to create the required arc of rotation.

These flaps are unsuitable where there has been vascular injury or degloving and heavy smokers suffered more tip loss.

Ankle/heel

- Distally based islanded fasciocutaneous flaps as above.

- **Medial plantar island** flap based on a cutaneous branch of the medial plantar artery that can be sensate.
- **Dorsalis pedis flap**, a fasciocutaneous flap based on dorsalis pedis artery used as pedicled or free flap.

Timing of free tissue transfer
Some definitions

- Emergency free flap – at the time of first debridement, within 24 hours.
- Early – 24–72 hours post-injury.
- Delayed – more than 72 hours.

The advantages of early or emergency cover of open fractures are:

- Less infection. Infection rates increase after 5 days and major complications increase after 15 days.
- Earlier mobilization.
- Fewer operations with shorter hospitalization time and lower treatment costs.

Recipient vessels

- The **posterior tibial artery** is usually well protected and is the best option for a recipient vessel (end–side, approach by Godina muscle splitting approach); by contrast the anterior tibial artery is usually compromised by the injury (vide infra).
- The geniculate vessels in the popliteal fossa are an alternative.
- Vein grafts to the superficial femoral artery (SFA) in the femoral canal.
  - Perform the proximal vein graft anastomoses before detaching the flap.
  - Leave the vein graft as a loop, then divide and anastomose to donor vessels.
- Note that the radial artery forearm flap can be used as a **flow-through flap** for revascularization of the distal extremity; the anterolateral thigh flap can be used in this way too.

Selective use of preoperative angiography in free flap reconstruction of the lower extremity
Dublin BA. *Ann Plast Surg* 1997;**38**:404–407.

In this study, 38 patients had angiography before free flaps for lower limb trauma.

- In 23 patients with normal distal pulses, there was one abnormal angiogram.

- In 15 patients with abnormal distal pulses, all had abnormal angiograms.

The authors therefore suggest that there is **no need** to perform angiography **if distal pulses are intact**.

Computed angiography in the planning of free tissue transfer in the posttraumatic setting
Duymaz A. *Plast Reconstr Surg* 2009;**124**:523–529.

This study examined 76 patients with lower extremity trauma who had computed tomography angiography (CTA) before flap reconstruction. The CTA demonstrated normal vascular anatomy in 52.6%, anatomical variants in 9.2% and atherosclerotic occlusive disease in 7.9%. The limb salvage rate was 94.7% and all four of the amputated limbs had at least single artery occlusion on pre-operative CTA.

Computed tomography angiography can provide useful information without the 1–3% risk of vessel injury (pseudoaneurysm, dissection, haematoma) associated with groin puncture for conventional angiography. There is debate over when to use either CTA (or angiography) in lower limb trauma – they do not seem to be indicated when there are two **palpable** (not just Doppler detectable – this indicates perfusion but provides no information on the actual vascular anatomy) pedal pulses (PT and DP). Others (e.g. Gonzalez MH. *Plast Reconstr Surg* 2002;**109**:592–600) use arteriograms almost routinely – over one-third of lower limb trauma patients have abnormal vessels and these have 33% risk of free-flap failure compared with 12% in those with normal arteriograms.

Preferential use of the posterior approach to blood vessels of the lower leg in microvascular surgery
Godina M. *Plast Reconstr Surg* 1991;**88**:287–291.

The authors describe a **midline muscle splitting approach** (distal extent of incision at the Achilles tendon) through the gastrocnemius and soleus that provides wide exposure of the posterior tibial artery. This facilitates end–side anastomosis, preserving blood supply to the foot. The patient can be placed in a lateral decubitus position, injured leg down.

- In addition, this avoids anastomosis at a site which is temptingly more superficial but within the zone of trauma.
- Also offers decompression of the posterior compartments. After anastomosis the muscles are approximated but fascia is not closed to avoid compartment syndrome.

- Short saphenous vein and sural nerve both lie in the midline and can be harvested as grafts if necessary.

The fate of lower extremities with failed free flaps
Benacquista T. *Plast Reconstr Surg* 1996;**98**:834–842.

In their review of patients with free flaps to the lower extremities, the failure rate in trauma patients (mainly Gustilo IIIB and C) was about 10% compared with ~7% in non-trauma patients. The commonest cause of failure was venous thrombosis, which tends to occur later and at a slower rate than arterial thrombosis, and often granulation tissue had already formed beneath the flap thus allowing for SSG as salvage.

Although vessel spasm, scarring and granulation tissue may make later reconstruction more difficult and increase need for vein grafts, the timing of surgery did not affect rate of failure in this study – results were no worse in those flaps performed on day 1 compared with later time points which contrasts with Godina (flaps before 72 h had < 1% failure whilst those performed later had a 12% failure rate).

- Overall ~80% of patients with a failed flap had their limb salvaged by other methods (SSG, local flap or a second free flap) whilst the other 20% had amputation. Culliford AT (*Ann Plast Surg* 2007;**59**:18–22) reported an 8.5% failure rate with an 18% amputation rate in these patients.
- Just under half of patients with a second free flap had another failure.
- There was a high failure rate for acute free bone flaps, thus it is recommended that the soft tissues are closed first, leaving bone reconstruction for later.

It is important to note that patients undergoing complex limb salvage, compared with primary amputation:

- Take longer to full weight bearing.
- Are less likely to return to work (salvage 25%, amputation 60%).

Lower limb salvage using parts from the contralateral amputated leg
Southern SJ. *Injury* 1997;**28**:477–479.

Large sections of skin based on septocutaneous perforators leading to the anterior and posterior tibial arteries were harvested and anastomosed to recipient vessels in the salvaged limb in two cases.

- Vein, artery, nerve, split skin and bone grafts may all be harvested as spare parts.

Cross leg free flaps for difficult cases of leg defects
Chen H. *J Trauma* 1997;**43**:486–491.

The paper describes a situation where a flap is inset into one limb but anastomosed to vessels in the other and the flap relies upon neovascularization for its blood supply. The pedicle is cross clamped for 1 hour to determine when it is safe to divide it.

This can be performed when a free flap is required but there are no suitable recipient vessels and vein grafts are inappropriate, and when cross-leg pedicle flaps may also fail to provide the right volume or tissue type. Latissimus dorsi, rectus abdominis, DCIA and parascapular free cross-leg flaps have all been reported. One of eight flaps (LD) in this series failed.

- It is really only indicated in young patients and even then only as a salvage manoeuvre.
- Average cross-leg fixation for 24 days but muscle flaps require ~4 weeks at least. No significant joint stiffness was reported on follow-up.

Reconstruction of the lower extremity after ablative resection for cancer
Walton RL. *Surg Oncol Clinics N Am* 1997;**6**:133–176.

The commonest malignancy of the lower limb in this series was skin cancer (SCC, MM). One-third of all sarcomas arise in the lower limb; malignant fibrous histiocytoma and liposarcoma are the commonest.

- Sarcomas require compartmental resection of composite tissues, and external beam radiotherapy or brachytherapy offer some benefit post-operatively.
- Prerequisites for lower limb reconstruction included:
  ○ Patient accepts multiple operations and lengthy hospitalizations.
  ○ Surgical margins must be free of tumour.
  ○ Reasonable function expected i.e. pain-free ambulation with a sensate foot (intact posterior tibial nerve), stable knee with good extension and good limb length.

The author says that with proper patient selection, the functional outcome surpasses that of the amputation group, thus justifying the issues with multiple surgeries and long stays in hospital.

The defect should be considered in terms of the tissues missing and their functional impact.

- Soft tissue defects are closed using local or distant flaps as for traumatic defects.

- Bone defects require free fibula or DCIA vascularized bone flap or a distraction technique.
- Nerve reconstruction using autologous nerve graft only considered in children or young adults.

Reconstruction in children
- If the epiphyses are still open, then there is still the potential for growth.
- Resection of a growth plate will cause progressive limb length discrepancy over time; epiphyses at lower end of femur and proximal tibia (i.e. around the knee) are responsible for ~70% of limb growth but are also common sites for sarcoma.
- Under such circumstances, transfer of vascularized bone with a growth plate would be ideal but their low availability means that distraction-lengthening or bone transport is usually used.

Lower extremity microsurgical reconstruction
Heller L. *Plast Reconstr Surg* 2001;**108**:1029–1041.

This is a CME article. According to the author, initial treatment focuses upon thorough wound debridement and bone stabilization, with the aim of soft tissue closure by day 5–7.

- Anastomoses out of the zone of injury are preferable; consider angiography for extensive injuries, especially if recipient vessels are potentially compromised.
- Bone gaps less than 6 cm can usually be managed by Ilizarov techniques; gaps greater than 6 cm may need vascularized bone grafts.
- Nerve injury does not necessarily preclude salvage if it is distal enough but patients with complex injuries with nerve damage may rehabilitate faster with an amputation.
  ○ Advanced age per se not a contraindication to free flap salvage.
  ○ Free tissue transfer in diabetics (large vessels unaffected) allows radical debridement of chronic wounds where a useful limb can be salvaged.
  ○ Compromised flaps need to be explored immediately; failed free flaps should be debrided and consideration given to a second free flap.

Ipsilateral free fibula transfer for reconstruction of a segmental femoral shaft defect
Erdmann D. *Br J Plast Surg* 2002;**55**:675–677.

The authors describe a technique for transferring a free fibula flap to a bone defect in the ipsilateral femur.

- The fibula is raised and inset into the ipsilateral bone defect, temporarily clamping the peroneal vessels after division.
- A saphenous vein graft is then harvested from the same leg and used as an interpositional vein graft loop tunnelled between the flap pedicle and the site of detachment in the lower leg – the peroneal vessels thereby become the recipient vessels and this avoids having to identify and dissect additional vessels.

A transferred fibular will hypertrophy when used as an inlay in femoral reconstruction; double-barrelled fibular flaps do not prevent stress fractures (Muramatsu K. *Br J Plast Surg* 2004;**57**:550–555); rigid stabilization in an anatomical position is most important. Muramatsu prefers to anastomose to the femoral vessels (end to side).

Long-term behaviour of the free vascularized fibula following reconstruction of large bony defects
Falder S. *Br J Plast Surg* 2003;**56**:571–584.

This is a retrospective review of 32 free fibula flaps used to reconstruct a mean bone gap of 12 cm in limb long bones following either trauma or tumour; they note a trend towards Ilizarov bone fixation. Bone union was achieved in 74%, taking a median time of 4.75 months.

- Of the 29/32 flaps that survived, flap hypertrophy (median 71%, 76.5% in the lower limb) assessed radiographically was found with periosteal vascularity and mechanical loading with greater hypertrophy in the lower limb group (more loading) and was equivalent in patients treated for trauma and tumour.
- Age is not a significant factor.

Stress fractures (21%) required plating and bone grafting in two-thirds; double-barrelled flaps were less likely to suffer stress fracture (compare with Muramatsu).

Limb salvage of lower extremity wounds using a free gracilis muscle reconstruction
Redett RJ. *Plast Reconstr Surg* 2000;**106**:1507–1513.

The authors reviewed a series of patients requiring gracilis free flap reconstruction of acute and chronic lower limb soft tissue defects:

- Gustilo IIIB (vast majority).
- Gustilo IIIC.
- Osteomyelitis or deep soft tissue infection.

Outcome was 86% successful 'limb salvage' (the authors' use of this term is a little unclear) in acute trauma setting vs. 93% in chronic wounds. Flap loss was greater in smokers and IIIC injuries. There were donor site complications in 10%, mostly infection and haematoma or seroma.

V. Compartment syndrome

This is a limb-threatening and potentially life-threatening condition: perfusion pressure falls below tissue pressure/compartment pressure, which will lead to tissue necrosis, renal failure and death if untreated. It can occur in any compartment.

- Volkman (1881) – paralytic contracture of the forearm with tight bandages. Volkman's ischaemic contracture is the final state of ischaemic necrosis and fibrosis.
- Thomas (1909) – extrinsic compression not necessarily required.
- Mubarak – compartment syndrome results from raised interstitial pressure in a closed compartment.

Classification

- Acute – recognized symptoms and signs.
- Subacute – without easily recognizable symptoms and signs but may progress to acute.
- Recurrent – found mostly in athletes.
- Chronic – unrelieved acute, ischaemia progressing to fibrosis and Volkman's.

Aetiology

Compartment syndrome can develop late (> 3 days) after injury and pressure > 40 mmHg (perfusion pressure) for > 2 hours causes irreversible necrosis. The ischaemic injury is proportional to the degree of pressure elevation and the duration. Anything that causes increased tissue volume and/or decreases compartment size can lead to compartment syndrome.

- Crush.
- Prolonged extrinsic compression including antishock trousers and POPs, prolonged lying in one position e.g. drug overdoses (head on forearm 48 mmHg, leg under the other 72 mmHg, forearm under trunk 178 mmHg).

- Vascular injury (30%) including extravasation injuries, bleeding from fractures as well as reperfusion. There is a case report of an anticoagulated patient sustaining an intracompartmental haemorrhage due to acupuncture needles. Smith DL. *West J Med* 1986;**144**:478–479.
- Swelling of soft tissue e.g. excessive exercise (increases muscle volume) or tetany/fits, electrical injury or reperfusion, virus-induced myositis, leukaemic infiltration, nephrotic syndrome (low osmolality).
- Combination e.g. burns with thick eschar and soft tissue inflammation.
- **Fractures** – there may be vascular injury, haemorrhage, soft tissue swelling and reperfusion.
  - **Gustilo grade IIIB fractures** may be complicated by compartment syndrome (6%) – the skin wound does not necessarily adequately decompress the underlying compartment(s) and other compartments may also have increased pressures. In the lower limb, the FDP and FHL are often affected first.

The basic parameters are:
  Local blood flow = Pa – Pv/resistance (Ohm's law: I = V/R)

- Reduced Pa.
  - High elevation.
  - Premorbid limb ischaemia.
- Increased Pv.
  - **High interstitial pressure**, e.g. muscle oedema, haemorrhage, external compression.
  - Limb dependency.
- Increased resistance – peripheral vascular disease.

Tissue perfusion = capillary perfusion pressure (CPP) – interstitial perfusion pressure (IPP)

- CPP and IPP are approximately 25 and 4 mmHg, respectively, as IPP rises above 30 mmHg, the capillaries will collapse.
- Anaerobic metabolism causes lactic acid accumulation and failure of sodium pump to maintain gradients that further increases oedema and compression.
- **Reperfusion** with generation of free radicals can cause additional injury.

Symptoms and signs
The five 'p's of ischaemia are not reliable.

- **Pain, especially on passive stretching, out of proportion to the injury**. Reduction of pain may herald necrosis rather than recovery. An increasing need/demand for analgesia is a classic sign.
- Tense swelling in the compartment.
- Paraesthesia/hyperaesthesia.
- Pallor and capillary refill >2 s, pulselessness (late) and poikilothermia.
- Weakness of compartment muscles (late), contracture (very late).

Investigations
- Compartment pressure measurement.
  - Tissue $P > 30$ mmHg in a normotensive patient (some cite 45 mmHg).
  - Tissue $P > 20$ mmHg in a hypotensive patient.
  - Delta-p (diastolic BP minus intracompartmental pressure) as a measure of perfusion pressure, using 30 mmHg as the cut-off and anything **below** requires decompression. (McQueen MM. *J Bone Joint Surg Br* 1996;**78**:99–104.)
- Doppler/arteriography/MRI – may be more useful for non-acute forms.
- Serum potassium, CK, clotting profile.
- Urine myoglobin.

Clinical suspicion must be followed by operative exploration of all the compartments in the area concerned.

Management
- Release any extrinsic compression and place limb at **heart level** (over-elevation may be counterproductive – it reduces mean arterial pressure (MAP) and has no effect on compartment pressure).
- Decompression by fasciotomy then splint in a position of function and elevated.
  - If compartment pressure exceeds 30 mmHg.
  - If **delta-p** (diastolic pressure – intracompartmental pressure) < 30 mmHg.
  - If high risk of progressing to compartment pressure.
- It is important to anticipate rhabdomyolyis/myoglobinuria.
  - **IV hydration** to promote urine output 1–2 ml/kg/hour to reduce myoglobin accumulation.
  - Mannitol.
- Definitive wound closure when swelling has gone down; either direct closure or skin grafting.

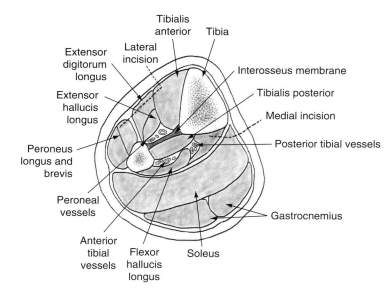

Tibialis anterior

Tibia

Extensor digitorum longus

Lateral incision

Interosseus membrane

Tibialis posterior

Extensor hallucis longus

Medial incision

Peroneus longus and brevis

Posterior tibial vessels

Peroneal vessels

Gastrocnemius

Anterior tibial vessels

Flexor hallucis longus

Soleus

Figure 7.1 A cross-sectional diagram of the lower leg demonstrating the incisions used for decompression in compartment syndrome.

Complete recovery is expected if decompression occurs within 6 hours, although this depends on the actual injury/mechanism.

- The role of HBO to protect against reperfusion injury is controversial; it is not widely available.

Consider early amputation, particularly if patient is not fit for reconstructive surgery; it avoids psychological trauma of late amputation. Use of injury severity scores to predict this:

- Prolonged ischaemia.
- Nerve injury (insensate foot).
- Multiple-level injury.

Degloved skin can be harvested as a SSG only on the day of injury and stored for later use but dead skin cannot be salvaged. Using the colour and contractility of muscle as a predictor of viability may be unreliable.

- Lower limb – fasciotomies should be placed anterior to the line of perforators both medially and laterally to preserve fasciocutaneous flap options.
  - Lateral incision – decompress anterior and lateral compartments via an incision 2 cm anterior to fibula (or halfway between fibula and tibia) and aim for the intermuscular septum going between peroneus longus, EHL/tibialis anterior. Take care to avoid the superficial peroneal nerve as it becomes superficial 10 cm above the ankle.

  - Medial incision – decompress superior and deep posterior compartment via an incision 2 cm behind the medial tibial border. Take care to avoid the long saphenous vein and nerve. Release the fascia over the gastrocnemius and soleus and then aim for the FHL in the deep compartment.
- Foot – 2 dorsal incisions along the lines of the 2nd and 4th intermetatarsal spaces, and release all compartments – interosseus, central lateral and medial.
- Thigh – medial and lateral incisions to release the medial and anterior/posterior compartments respectively.
- Upper arm.
  - Medial incision for medial compartment and lateral incision for posterior compartment.
  - Take care to avoid the ulnar and radial nerves.
- Forearm.
  - Dorsal – from epicondyle to line of middle metacarpal.
  - Volar – starting with carpal tunnel release, then proximally curve towards ulnar side before curving back radially at the elbow to avoid the ulnar nerve.
- Hands.
  - Dorsum – two incisions along 2nd and 4th intermetacarpal spaces (check release of interossei and adductor pollicis).
  - Volar – release thenar, hypothenar eminences and carpal tunnel.

Comparison of fasciotomy wound closures using traditional dressing changes and the vacuum-assisted closure device

Zannis J. *Ann Plast Surg* 2009;**62**:407–409.

This is a retrospective review of 804 fasciotomy wounds; 438 were treated exclusively with VAC, 270 saline dressings only and 96 with both. They found a shorter time for primary closure in the VAC group.

There have been many published methods for fasciotomy closure.

- Shoelace technique – Cohn BT. *Orthopedics* 1986;**9**:1243–1246.
- Vessel loop technique – Harris I. *Injury* 1993;**24**:565–566.
- Steristrips – Harrah J. *Am J Surg* 2000;**180**:55–57.
- STAR (suture tension adjustment reel). McKenney MG. *Am J Surg* 1996;**171**:275–277.
- Sure-Closure device – Narayanan K. *Injury* 1996;**27**:449–451.
- VADER (vacuum assisted dermal recruitment) – Van der Velde M. *Ann Plast Surg* 2005;**55**:660–664.

Long-term sequelae of fasciotomy wounds

Fitzgerald AM. *Br J Plast Surg* 2000;**53**:690–693.

The study demonstrates that 10% and 7% of patients have persistent pain and muscle herniation respectively.

- Altered sensation at wound edges (77%).
- Dry skin (30%) and pruritis (40%).
- Discoloured scars (30%), tethered scars (25%) and tethered tendons (7%).
- Recurrent ulceration (13%).
- Swollen limb (25%).

VI. Chronic wounds

Free flap coverage of chronic traumatic wounds of the lower leg

Gonzalez MH. *Plast Reconstr Surg* 2002;**109**:592–600.

The authors describe their results using free flaps to cover open lower leg wounds following trauma with a mean duration of 40 months (thus over half with established osteomyelitis). Flaps (latissimus dorsi) and rectus abdominis (most common) were used after an average of 2.3 debridements.

- Most underwent pre-operative angiography (36% abnormal).
- 19% (8) flap loss – 3/8 of these due to infection, 5/8 had normal angiograms and 6/8 had chronic osteomyelitis.

They conclude that diffuse chronic osteomyelitis and an abnormal angiogram increases the risk of flap failure. They recommend the use of vein grafts to ensure that anastomoses are performed outside the zone of trauma or vicinity of the chronic wound.

Diabetic foot

- There are multiple reasons that diabetic patients have problems with their feet.
- Sensory neuropathy and loss of protective sensation, derangement of joints and pressure sores over metatarsal heads.
- Increased risk of infection due to:
  - Autonomic neuropathy leading to dry, cracked skin.
  - Peripheral vascular disease causing tissue hypoxia.
  - Decreased cellular and humeral immunity.

Prevention is possible to a certain extent with effective glycaemic control and pro-active chiropody/diabetic foot-care regimes.

Management of diabetic foot wounds

- Wound debridement including bone where necessary (osteomyelitis).
- Systemic antibiotics.
- Hyperbaric oxygen (HBO) (Faglia E. *Diabetes Care* 1996;**19**;1338–1343). HBO is covered by Medicare – since April 2003 – for treatment of diabetic wounds that meet three criteria:
  - Patient has diabetes and has a lower limb wound due to diabetes.
  - Wound is Wagner grade III or higher.
  - A course of standard wound therapy has failed.
- Revascularization if the ulcer is predominantly ischaemic.

Amputation/arthrodesis:

- Amputation of non-viable toes.
  - At level of tarsometatarsal (TMT) joints (Lisfranc).
  - At level of talonavicular joint (Chopart).
  - Just above the ankle joint (Symes).
- Metatarsal phalangeal (MTP) joint arthrodesis for dorsal ulceration as a result of motor imbalance.

Soft tissue closure:

- Trial of dressings to allow healing by secondary intention.

- Granulation tissue may accept a SSG.
- Consider local flap options first, e.g. medial plantar flap or distally based FC flaps to heel defects, but significant risk of distal flap necrosis including delayed.
- Free flaps to larger defects.
  - Fasciocutaneous e.g. lateral arm flap for dorsum of foot
  - Fasciocutaneous or muscle flap plus SSG for heel/ankle (this combination is less bulky than myocutaneous flaps whilst the use of SSG provides a surface that is just as stable).

VII. Lymphoedema

Lymphoedema is the accumulation of protein-rich interstitial fluid in subcutaneous tissues; the deep muscle compartments are uninvolved. The skin becomes thick and brawny, and fissuring and ulceration result. In comparison, venous ulceration occurs in thin skin with or without varicose eczema.

Primary

- At birth – lymphoedema congenita 10% (Milroy's disease) or < 14 years.
  - Genetically determined: sex-linked cause of lymphatic aplasia.
  - Shows association with Turner's syndrome.
- Adolescence – lymphoedema praecox (14–35 years) – the most common form, 80% of all primary lymphoedema and vessels are hypoplastic.
- Later in life – lymphoedema tarda 10% (> 35 years), vessels are hyperplastic.

Secondary

- Neoplastic – malignant nodes, extrinsic compression.
- Infective – tuberculosis, *Wuchereria bancrofti*.
- Iatrogenic – lymphadenectomy, radiotherapy (lymphoedema may be delayed for a year or so after treatment).

Women are more frequently affected than men.

- Lower limb > upper limb.
- Left leg > right leg.

Pathogenesis

- Leakage of proteins into the interstitium raises the tissue oncotic pressure and disruption of Starling's equilibrium.

- The increased interstitial protein and fluid causes relative tissue hypoxia with cell death and a chronic inflammatory response.
- The accumulated fluid also acts as a medium for bacterial growth.

Clinical features

- Initially pitting then non-pitting oedema due to fibrosis of soft tissues.
- Skin ulceration.
- Pain.
- Lymphangiosarcoma may develop > 10 years following the onset of lymphoedema and carries a poor prognosis. **Stewart–Treves syndrome** is lymphangiosarcoma developing in a lymphoedematous arm following mastectomy.

Investigation of the patient with lymphoedema

Differentiate from:

- Lipoedema (lipodystrophy) – suitable for liposuction, often generally obese.
- Klippel–Trenaunay syndrome – varicose veins, limb elongation, vascular malformations, limb oedema (some have lymphatic abnormalities).
- Venous hypertension – exclude deep venous thrombosis (DVT) (Doppler/venogram).
- Oedema due to hepatic, renal or cardiac causes.

Imaging

- CT/MRI shows a honeycomb appearance of subcutaneous tissues in contrast with normal subfascial tissues.
- Lymphangiography has largely been replaced by lymphoscintigraphy (intravenous technectium).
- Image the pelvic nodes for tumours.
- Doppler US to exclude DVT.

Management of lymphoedema

Remove the precipitating cause if any. No form of treatment is curative and surgery is rarely indicated (< 10%).

Medical

- Skin care – prevention of ulceration and infections, especially fungal.
- Treatment of lymphangitis and cellulitis (common).
- Dimethylcarbazine to kill *Wuchereria bancrofti*.
- Elevation, foot pumps.

- o Complex regional physiotherapy.
- o Compression garments.

Excisional surgery

- **Charles**: excision of all soft tissue down to fascia and SSG. The aesthetic results are poor, with unstable grafts and keratotic overgrowths and so this is usually reserved for severe skin ulceration.
- **Thompson** buried dermal flap: subcutaneous tissue is excised, and a dermal flap is buried into the uninvolved muscle compartments. This creates a theoretical lymphatic communication allowing drainage of the skin via the deep compartment but this has not been substantiated and few good results have been reported. It is thus rarely performed.
- **Homans**: subcutaneous excision of lymphoedematous tissue preserving overlying skin flaps which are trimmed back later. It is usually staged i.e. medial side then lateral side whilst taking care to preserve vital structures such as the common peroneal and sural nerves. It is capable of producing good results and is consequently the most commonly performed surgery for lymphoedema.

Physiological surgery

- Pedicled omental or ileal flap.
- Ileal segment on vascular pedicle: the segment is bivalved and the mucosa is stripped off to expose lymphatic-rich submucosa. It is contraindicated following radiotherapy due to possibility of established radiation-induced endarteritis of gut vessels.
- Microsurgical lymphovenous and lympholymphatic shunts. The role of LVAs is debated; some suggest that microsurgery applies less to primary lymphoedema. The longevity of the effects is sometimes in doubt, though Koshima I (*J Reconstr Microsurg* 2003;**19**:209–215) reports persistent reductions in a series of eight patients at an average follow-up period of 3.3 years.

Use of a lymphatic bridge in the management of head and neck lymphoedema

Withey S. *Br J Plast Surg* 2001;**54**:716–719.

The main cause of lymphoedema of the head and neck is bilateral neck dissection and radiotherapy, particularly where lymphatic drainage is further compromised by repeated infections or tumour recurrence.

- The late development of lymphoedema should raise the suspicion of recurrent tumour. Lymph from the facial and scalp skin drains first to the occipital, auricular, parotid and facial nodes and then via valveless channels to the deeper cervical nodes.
- Spiral muscle system maintains orthograde lymph flow. The deep cervical chain also drains lymph from the upper aerodigestive tract.
  - o The authors describe a case of severe head and neck lymphoedema ameliorated by the inset of a tubed deltopectoral flap to act as **a lymphatic bridge**.
  - o Similar pedicled flaps have been described in the management of lymphoedema at other sites including use of a pedicled groin flap to reduce contralateral lower limb oedema.

Minimal invasive lymphaticovenular anastomosis under local anesthesia for leg lymphedema

Koshima I. *Ann Plast Surg* 2004;**53**:261–266.

This study reviewed the results of LVA under local anaesthesia in 52 patients with an average 2.1 anastomoses per patient. At a mean follow-up of 14.5 months, there was an average 41.8% reduction in leg circumference; there were effects even in stage III and IV disease.

Microsurgery for lymphedema: clinical research and long-term results

Campisi C. *Microsurgery* 2010;**30**:256–260.

This is a retrospective review from this centre in Genoa with experience totalling over 1800 patients over 30 years treated with variants of lymphatic-venous anastomosis. Their technique involves anastomosing lymphatic vessels to a collateral branch of a large vein. They report subjective improvement in 87% of patients, with objective volume improvement in 83% with an average 67% of volume, and 85% were able to discontinue conservative measures.

Supermicrosurgical lymphaticovenular anastomosis and lymphaticovenous implantation for treatment of unilateral lower extremity lymphedema

Demirtas Y. *Microsurgery* 2009;**29**:609–618.

This is a review of a 2-year experience with 42 patients (30 women) with lower limb lymphoedema. Thirty-seven patients had lymphaticovenular anastomosis with an average of 2.5 anastomoses per patient, 36 had lymphaticovenous implantations with an average of 2.4 per patient. Lymphatics larger than 0.3 mm were anastomosed to venules using supermicrosurgical techniques. The mean decrease in volume of oedema was 59% at an average follow-up of 11.8 months. In six patients the outcomes were ineffective, eight were moderate and there were 28 good outcomes.

Comparison of primary and secondary lower-extremity lymphoedema treated with supermicrosurgical lymphaticovenous anastomosis and lymphaticovenous implantation

Demirtas Y. *J Reconstr Microsurg* 2010;**26**;137–143.

This study includes 80 patients with primary lower limb lymphoedema and 21 with secondary lymphoedema. They found that the lymphatic morphology was more consistent in the latter group with at least one collector wider than 0.3 mm available in 20 of the 21, whilst in the primary group 13 of the 80 had lymphatics smaller than 0.3 mm. Reduction of swelling occurred earlier in the secondary group, but the mean final reduction in volume was comparable.

Lymphatic venous anastomosis (LVA) for treatment of secondary arm lymphedema

Damstra RJ. *Breast Cancer Res Treat* 2009;**113**:199–206.

This is a prospective study of 11 LVAs in 10 patients with lymphoedema related to breast cancer, which is estimated to occur between 7–35%. The patients were unresponsive to conservative treatment. They showed a 4.8% reduction of lymphoedema at 3 months and 2% after a year. There was a minimal improvement in the reported quality of life; non-operative treatment including elastic stockings was preferred by the patients particularly in the early stages of disease.

Intravascular stenting method for treatment of extremity lymphedema with multiconfiguration lymphaticovenous anastomosis

Narushima M. *Plast Reconstr Surg* 2010;**125**:935–943.

The authors described a novel intravascular stenting method to facilitate their lymphaticovenous microsurgical anastomosis. A segment of nylon filament two-fifths of the diameter of the vessel is inserted into the lumens of the vessels to be anastomosed with a temporary clip to prevent unwanted displacement. The sutures are then placed and the stent is removed before the final suture is tied. The authors describe using this method for fashioning 39 lymphaticovenous anastomoses of different configurations in 14 patients who had an average 11.3% reduction in limb diameter at 8.9 months mean follow-up.

Skin and soft tissue tumours

A. Overview and skin, subcutaneous and appendigeal tumours

I. Overview

A neoplasm is an abnormal mass of tissue with a growth rate which exceeds that of normal tissue. The growth is uncoordinated with that of the normal tissues and persists after cessation of the stimulus which evoked the change. According to the multistage carcinogenesis model, the following steps are involved.

- **Initiation**: a change in the genome of a cell follows exposure to a mutagen such as X-rays, ultraviolet (UV) radiation, chemical carcinogens or viruses – the cellular change does not cause significant change in the cell/tissue morphology but does confer a long-term risk of developing cancer.

- **Promotion**: the change is made permanent by cellular division. The promotion stage requires a non-mutagenic stimulus, such as chronic inflammation, which enhances cellular proliferation resulting in the formation of a localized tumour that displays self-limited non-malignant growth and may regress if the stimulant is withdrawn.

- **Progression**: further cell division to form an invasive tumour.

A malignant neoplasm is one that invades surrounding tissues and has a propensity to metastasize. Tumours may arise due to:

- Inappropriate activation of normal cellular proto-oncogenes that encode growth factors, growth factor receptors or transcription factors, to become oncogenes.

- Inactivation of other cellular genes called tumour suppressor genes e.g. p53 tumour suppressor gene is mutated in the majority of human cancers.

Ultraviolet light

Ultraviolet radiation is an important mutagenic factor – it causes mutations in cellular DNA and a failure of DNA repair.

- UVA radiation (320–400 nm) generates oxygen free radicals that damage cell membranes and nuclear DNA, contributing to erythema, photoageing and **carcinogenesis**.
- **UVB radiation (290–320 nm)** is said to be responsible for **sunburn, tanning**, local and systemic immunosuppression, photoageing, skin cancer and precancer.
- UVC is completely blocked by the ozone layer and thus is not normally a cancer risk.

Ultraviolet effects can lead to increases in production of immunosuppressive cytokines, depletion and alteration of antigen-presenting lymphocytes and systemic induction of T-suppressor cells by altered lymphocytes, inflammatory macrophages and cytokines.

Ultraviolet intensity is related to time of day and geographic factors such as elevation, latitude and cloud cover.

II. Benign skin and subcutaneous lesions

Epidermal naevi

Naevi (Latin for blemish or spot) are best defined as **cutaneous hamartomas**, usually incorporating a proliferation of sebaceous glands (sebaceous naevus), melanocytes (melanocytic naevus) or vascular tissue (vascular naevus).

- **Epidermal naevus syndromes**: association of epidermal naevi with developmental anomalies in other organ systems, especially of the CNS, eye and skeleton. Examples include:
  - Proteus syndrome – overgrowth syndrome affecting multiple sites and tumours may develop.
  - Sebaceous naevus syndrome.
  - Becker's naevus syndrome – occurrence of Becker's naevus with unilateral pectoral hypoplasia and skeletal anomalies.

Sebaceous naevus of Jadassohn (Jadassohn's disease II)

This is a hamartomatous lesion present at birth in 0.3% of neonates – histologically, there is an accumulation of mature sebaceous glands with overlying epidermal hyperplasia. The condition usually presents as flat plaques of pink colour in the scalp/head and neck. There is significant variability in appearance with some forms being particularly florid.

The lesions tend to enlarge at the time of adolescence and there is a risk of malignant transformation in < 5% (wide range quoted in literature) – classically to BCC, but also SCC, sebaceous and apocrine carcinomas. However, reviews suggest that actual risk of malignant change may be much lower and previous lesions identified as BCCs were actually trichoblastomas.

- **Sebaceous naevus syndrome** – in this rare disorder there is a large sebaceous naevus associated with other organ anomalies including neurological features such as seizures, developmental delay, palsies (cranial nerves, hemiparesis) and structural anomalies of the brain.
- Josef Jadassohn (1863–1936) was a German dermatologist who also introduced patch testing for contact dermatitis.

Treatment

Excision is a common option with the aim of preventing malignant transformation or for cosmesis. Larger lesions may need serial excision, tissue expansion or Integra and other skin/dermal substitutes.

Should naevus sebaceous be excised prophylactically? A clinical audit
Barkham MC. *J Plast Reconstr Aesthet Surg* 2007; **60**:1269–1270.

This study concluded that prophylactic excision of all lesions is not warranted and is only recommended when neoplasms are clinically suspected or for cosmetic reasons. This is agreement with several other studies.

Serial excision is a useful technique for excision of benign lesions (scars and benign naevi) when applied correctly. If a lesion is going to require more than three excisions then consider tissue expansion – the risk–benefit balance will depend on individual cases.

A user's guide for serial excision
Quaba O. *Br J Plast Surg* 2008;**61**:712–715.

- Excise early – skin elasticity is greatest and joints respond better if an enforced position is needed.
- Keep scars within the lesion and align parallel to relaxed skin tension lines if possible.

- Consider excising the periphery of scars/grafts after using a temporary pursestring type suture to estimate the 'advancement'.
- Undermine but avoid excision of subcutaneous tissue that may lead to contour defects.
- Close under moderate tension to maximize the excision as well as to recruit more skin. Sutures can be kept in longer to minimize stretching in between procedures; consider using non-absorbable buried/subcuticular sutures that do not need removal but will be excised during the next stage.

Melanocytic naevi

Melanocytes are derived from neural crest cells. Melanin is synthesized in these cells (spindle shaped with dendritic processes) from tyrosine, it accumulates and is then distributed to keratinocytes via the processes. The number of melanocytes between different races is not significantly different, rather it is the activity or melanin production per cell that differs – this is stimulated by sunlight and melanocyte-stimulating hormone (MSH) from the pituitary. Naevus cells (melanocytes leaving the epidermis to go into the dermis) are rounder and have no dendritic processes and gather in 'rests'.

Common **epidermal** melanocytoses are:

- **Freckles** – these have normal numbers of melanocytes but with increased melanin content in each. These tend to regress with reduced exposure to sunlight.
- **Lentigo** – there is an increased number of melanocytes in these lesions and they do not regress with sunlight avoidance.
- **Café au lait.**
- **Becker's naevus**/melanosis – irregular light-brown pigmentation, classically on the shoulder/torso of pubertal males that gradually enlarges, thickens and becomes hairy. It is generally regarded as an acquired condition of unknown cause (a quarter are associated with sun exposure).
  - Fehr B. *Dermatologica* 1991;**182**:77–80. Reported 9 cases of melanoma in patients with Becker's naevus but only one actually occurred in the naevus itself. Becker's naevus is regarded as a benign disease though it should be monitored; treatment is primarily cosmetic – laser hair removal is more successful than laser depigmentation, which has variable results.
  - Samuel Becker (1894–1964) was an American dermatologist.

Acquired naevi

- **Junctional naevus** – this is a melanocytic proliferation at the dermo-epidermal junction and the lesion is flat (macular) and deeply pigmented. They are found at any site, but benign acral or mucosal lesions are usually junctional naevi. Junctional naevi appear during childhood or adolescence with the tendency to progress to compound or intradermal naevus with age.
- **Compound naevus** – these are maculopapular pigmented lesions that appear in adolescence due to junctional proliferation of melanocytes forming nests and columns of dermal melanocytes.
- **Intradermal naevus** – cessation of junctional proliferation and clusters of dermal melanocytes. These are papular faintly pigmented lesions found in adults.

Congenital naevus (congenital hairy melanocytic naevus)

Congenital melanocytic naevi (CMN) are histologically similar to a compound naevus and are large, pigmented, hairy and verrucous. There is an arbitrary definition of what constitutes '**giant**' but this is usually taken to be 2% or 20 cm in the largest diameter (in adult or 'predicted' size). There are widely varying rates of malignant transformation in the literature but probably are close to 4–5% or less, mainly within first 5 years of life. Lesions overlying sacrum may be associated with meningocoele or spina bifida.

Congenital melanocytic nevi – when to worry and how to treat: facts and controversies
Price HN. *Clin Dermatol* 2010;**28**:293–302.

- Risk of melanoma in small and medium size CMN is low, and is nearly zero before puberty.
- Risk of melanoma in giant CMN is ~5%, with half in the first few years of life.
- Melanoma and neurocutaneous melanosis is most likely when size or predicted size > 40 cm, numerous satellites and truncal lesions.

It can be difficult what to advise patients/parents but in most cases if feasible, then lesions are excised, often serial excision, tissue expansion or use of dermal substitutes such as Integra can be considered. Alternatives including curettage, dermabrasion and laser are less commonly used – with the latter there is a theoretical concern that non-lethal laser energy may lead to cellular changes in surviving melanocytes.

Neurocutaneous melanosis (found in about one-third, with one-third becoming symptomatic) seems to be more common in giant naevi with **many satellites** (> 20) or in the mid-line. Some suggest MRI at the age of 4–6 months before normal brain myelination obscures small lesions.

- Symptoms include raised ICP, hydrocephalus, development delay or space-occupying lesion; the development of symptomatic disease is grave as most die within 2–3 years.
- The management of **asymptomatic** neurocutaneous melanosis remains controversial and the role of MRI screening is also debatable, except perhaps before major surgery.

Special types of naevi

Spitz naevus – this is **a benign melanocytic tumour** with cellular atypia occurring predominantly in childhood (3–13 years old) but has been reported as congenital and also occurring > 70 years of age (i.e. wide age range). It is uncommon and accounts for less than 1% of melanocytic naevi in children. Typically, these are solitary reddish-brown nodules, occasionally deeply pigmented, found on the face and legs most commonly. There is rapid initial growth before remaining static. Bleeding after minor trauma is not uncommon. It resembles a compound naevus with spindle-shaped or epithelioid cells at the dermo-epidermal junction – there are multinucleated giant cells, abundant melanin, acanthosis and atypia and it may be difficult to differentiate from melanoma on histopathological examination. These were previously called **juvenile melanomas** but this is a misnomer and the lesions are generally regarded as benign and are managed more conservatively – either a biopsy or conservative excision.

- Sophie Spitz (1910–1956) was the pathologist that described the condition (as juvenile melanoma) in 1948.

Dysplastic naevus – this is an irregular proliferation of atypical melanocytes around the basal layer that is found in 2–5% of the population. Clinically, they are nodules > 5 mm in diameter with variegated pigmentation and irregular border, usually occurring in sun-exposed areas. If there are multiple lesions, then it may be part of a **dysplastic naevus syndrome** which has

familial inheritance with a 5–10% risk of malignant change to SSM type of melanoma.

Spindle cell naevus – these are typically dense black lesions occurring most commonly on the thigh particularly of females. There are spindle cell aggregates and atypical melanocytes at the dermo-epidermal junction. Their malignant potential is unclear. It is sometimes regarded as a variant of Spitz naevus.

Dermal melanocytosis

Mongolian spot – macular pigmentation (a blue–grey patch up to 10 cm diameter) present at birth on the sacral area of > 90% of Mongoloid (East Asians, Polynesians, Indonesians and Micronesians) and ~1% of White neonates. Histologically, there are ribbon-like melanocytes around the neurovascular bundles of the dermis with a lack of melanophages. The pigmentation increases after birth but regresses by the age of 4–7 years and no treatment is required. Some 'persistent' Mongolian spots may be larger and persist for longer.

Blue naevus – nodular benign blue–black pigmentation due to a collection of **dermal** melanocytes gathered around dermal appendages which is said to represent arrested migration of melanocytes bound for the dermo-epidermal junction. The presence of melanophages distinguishes it from Mongolian spots. They are found on the extremities, buttocks and face, with 80% occurring in females and 60% present during infancy. They can be excised but malignant transformation into melanoma is very rare.

Naevus of Ota – are commonest in the Japanese and Chinese. They are blue–brown patches of pigmentation due to dermal melanocytosis of the sclera or skin adjacent to the eye (**glaucoma** is a rare association) especially, in the distribution of the ophthalmic and maxillary divisions of the fifth cranial nerve. Histologically the lesions demonstrate similar features to Mongolian spots. They are not usually present at birth; they darken during childhood and persist in adult life. The development of malignant melanoma is very rare. Q-switched laser is the treatment of choice.

- Naevus of Ito is a similar lesion distribution on the shoulder/upper arm.

Benign epithelial tumours
Seborrhoeic keratosis (basal cell papilloma, seborrhoeic or senile wart)

These are very common lesions from the fifth decade onwards with equal sex distribution. They have a warty appearance but no viruses have been isolated from them – the cause is unknown but it may run in some families (autosomal dominance has been described), and is sometimes associated with pregnancy or oestrogen therapy.

They seem to represent an accumulation of immature keratinocytes between basal and keratinizing layers – despite the name, they are **not** really caused by sebaceous glands nor limited to seborrhoeic distribution; also, they are **not** strongly associated with ultraviolet light exposure. Malignant transformation has been reported but is extremely rare.

- They are verrucous plaques with fissures and/or horn pearls, and a **'stuck on'** appearance due to the edge being slightly elevated and not attached to skin.
- They may be heavily pigmented (but this is very variable) – the proliferating keratinocytes produce melanocyte-stimulating cytokines.
- Multiple lesions are typical on the face, hands and upper trunk; lesions can be itchy, may bleed and become inflamed.

Treatment

- Shave, excision or curettage (alone or in conjunction with electrodesiccation).
- Cryotherapy, ablative laser.
- Chemical peels e.g. trichloroacetic acid or 70% glycolic acid.
- Combinations e.g. cryotherapy or glycolic acid before curettage.

Variants include:

- **Stucco keratosis** – non- or lightly pigmented flat keratosis more often found on the distal parts of the limbs.
- **Dermatosis papulosa nigra** – multiple facial lesions, usually pigmented tags, that are histologically similar to seborrhoeic keratosis (minimal keratotic content), found in darker-skinned races. They have earlier age of onset. The cause is unknown (but there is a family history in half) and they are harmless.
  - This is not the same as **Leser-Trélat sign** which is a sudden explosion of multiple inflammatory itchy seborrhoeic keratoses that may be associated with visceral malignancies (gastrointestinal, breast, lung, urinary tract etc.) and may coexist with acanthosis nigricans.

It is very rare. A sudden crop may also occur with inflammatory dermatoses such as sunburn or eczema.

Keratoacanthoma (*Molluscum sebaceum*)

This is a rapidly evolving tumour that is composed of keratinizing squamous cells originating in pilosebaceous follicles and classically resolves if left untreated. There has been a recent change in viewing it as pseudo-malignant to pseudo-benign – i.e. a cancer that resembles a benign lesion, and some have suggested a name of SCC-KA type. Similarly, some view it as a malignancy that rarely progresses, however 2% show no regression and can become invasive.

- Weedon D. (*ANZ J Surg* 2010;**80**:129–130) disputes the view that they are variants of SCC and suggests that they are distinct lesions that can be separated morphologically, specifically by their pattern of keratinization. A small number of cases of metastases from KA have been reported in the immunocompromised; in other patients, this phenomenon may arise due to SCC arising within the KA which may occur in up to 10% of KAs occurring in the over 80s.

Typical lesions are smooth and globular with a central keratin plug or horn, and are most common on the face and dorsum of hand. It grows rapidly and then stops after about 6 weeks, with a variable plateau period before it regresses over several months – however, it often **heals with scarring**. Histopathologically, there are rapidly dividing squamous cells derived from skin appendages with atypical mitoses and loss of polarity; keratin-filled crypts are another feature.

Lesions on face and hands may grow to a significant size before necrosing to leave a significant defect. Variants are less likely to regress.

- Giant (> 2–3 cm).
- Multiple lesions are rare (2%).
- **Grzybowski's eruptive keratoacanthomas**, hundreds to thousands of very itchy lesions on mucosa as well as skin, which generally do not involute.
- **Ferguson-Smith familial keratoacanthoma** that can be rather large ulcerated lesions that are ultimately self-healing. Lesions start appearing in early adulthood; more common in men.

- **Keratoacanthoma marginatum centrifugum** is an uncommon variant with central healing whilst the periphery continues to grow. It can reach large sizes and be difficult to treat.

In Whites, it is 3× less common than SCC and is 3× more common in males. The aetiology is mostly unknown although there may be some similarities to SCC and Bowen's disease e.g. role for sun exposure from epidemiological studies, and other carcinogens such as coal, tar and carcinogenic hydrocarbons (which tend to cause multiple lesions).

- Some cases involve sites of previous trauma including skin graft donor sites, excisional scars and previous cryotherapy sites.
- Human papilloma virus (HPV) has been isolated in some cases and virus DNA sequences have been detected by PCR (Forslund O. *J Cutan Pathol* 2003;**30**:423–429) but no types/subtypes predominated. The role of HPV is controversial.
- Up to one-third have chromosomal defects but their significance is unclear.
- Immunocompromise and deficient cell-mediated immunity may be factors.

Keratoacanthoma may be a marker for **Muir–Torre syndrome**: multiple internal malignancies, and sebaceous adenomas, but the association of keratoacanthomas themselves with other malignancies is more controversial. It is a rare autosomal dominant condition associated with a defect in the DNA mismatch repair (MMR) gene. Screening for internal malignancies especially colonoscopy is recommended.

Treatment

The current standard of care for suspected keratoacanthomas is active treatment; they should not be left to regress spontaneously and it is a myth that spontaneous resolution does not leave unsightly scars.

Generally, it is good practice to excise the lesions to provide a good histological specimen – shaving often produces only non-diagnostic keratin fragments. Without information regarding invasion, it cannot be distinguished from frank SCC.

5-Fluorouracil and radiotherapy (radiosensitive) may shorten time to resolution, but radiation in young people may leave poor results in the long term as the radiation damage worsens with time. Alternatives include cryotherapy for small lesions, curettage and cautery for thicker lesions, leaving scabs that come off several weeks later to leave a slightly depressed scar. In particular, healing on the lower limbs can be delayed.

There have been some (essentially anecdotal) reports for intralesional methotrexate, bleomycin, interferons, topical imiquimod and oral retinoids.

Digital fibrokeratoma

This is an uncommon benign tumour of fibrous tissue that presents as a papillary or keratotic outgrowth in the region of a finger joint found in adults (more commonly males) and may follow trauma. The cause is unknown and though trauma has been implicated, there is little evidence to support this view. Histologically, there is hyperkeratosis and acanthosis (thickening of the epidermis, specifically the stratum spinosum). Its fleshy colour and finger-like appearance on occasion, means that it should be distinguished from supernumerary digits. It is treated by excision.

III. Hair follicle tumours

Trichoepithelioma

This is a relatively rare benign epithelial tumour differentiating towards hair follicle cells. Macroscopically they are pinkish nodules found most commonly around the nose i.e. cheeks, eyelids and nasolabial folds. Typically they appear at puberty and can occur in non-familial solitary forms and familial (autosomal dominant) multiple forms; a third variant is the desmoplastic trichoepithelioma. The tumour suppressor gene associated with the familial form has been located at 9p21 whilst the sporadic form has been associated with deletions at 9q22.3.

Solitary forms are typically larger and they are often diagnosed as BCC, whilst pigmented lesions are mistaken for melanoma. There have been reported cases of malignant change into BCCs in those with the multiple-familial form.

Histologically there are rounded masses of fusiform cells and lacunae filled with keratin; tumour islands may connect with hair follicles. Immunohistochemistry may be needed to distinguish it from BCCs. They are treated by excision.

Tricholemmoma

A tricholemmoma is a hair-follicle tumour often misdiagnosed clinically as BCC; it is relatively common though the true incidence is difficult to determine. The cells of origin come from the outer root sheath, and histologically there are plaques of squamous cells containing glycogen.

The lesions occur on the face as smooth asymptomatic papules in the middle-aged/elderly with equal sex distribution. The cause is unknown although multiple lesions may be associated with Cowden disease (multiple harmatoma syndrome with increased incidence of breast and thyroid carcinoma, autosomal dominant type inheritance and more common in women) but this is rare. Confirmed lesions can be treated with shave biopsy or laser ablation.

Pilomatrixoma (benign calcifying epithelioma of Malherbe 1880)

Pilomatrixoma is a benign appendigeal tumour that most probably arises from hair matrix cells. Part of it is composed of dead calcified cells (this calcification may be demonstrated by ultrasound or X-ray) and presents as a dermal/subcutaneous tumour with stony hard consistency and often with an angulated shape – the 'tent sign'– due to stretching of overlying skin. It is most common in the head, neck and upper extremity.

Histologically, it is a well-circumscribed tumour in the lower dermis and subcutaneous layer, composed mainly of basophilic cells along the periphery of tumour nests and ghost cells, lacking basophilic granules and nucleus. Calcium deposits are found in 75%.

It is uncommon but probably more common than previously thought, particularly in adults (bimodal incidence, first peak at 5–15 years and a second peak at 50–65 years) and slightly more common in females. The cause is unknown. An association with myotonic dystrophy has been reported, whilst one study shows positive immunostaining of bcl-2, a proto-oncogene that suppresses apoptosis in tumours. Another study demonstrated CTNNB1 mutations in 75% but the significance of this is unknown.

Lesions grow slowly but may grow to a large size in some cases and in very rare cases, malignant change has been reported. Excision is the commonest treatment; recurrences are rare and if they do occur may indicate a malignant variant.

Trichilemmal cyst (pilar cyst)

These keratin-filled cysts arise from the outer root sheath of the deeper hair follicle. They occur in areas of high follicle concentration and thus most are situated on the scalp, of the middle aged. They are more common in women than men; they are often multiple (70%) and in such cases may be familial (autosomal dominant) but the responsible genes have not been found. They are often erroneously referred to as 'sebaceous cysts' but unlike these cysts, there is **no punctum**.

The cyst wall has follicular cells and thus can be histologically distinguished from epidermoid (sebaceous cyst) by presence of a granular layer in lining epithelium of the latter. Rupture causes cell proliferation and occasionally malignant change – neoplastic change (malignant or benign) is very rare. Areas of proliferation in a cyst may occur to form so-called proliferating trichilemmal cysts or pilar tumours, which may become large and ulcerated but are histologically benign. In very rare cases, malignant transformation with metastasis may occur and clinically this is the only way to distinguish a benign or malignant lesion.

Treat trichilemmal cysts by excision in a similar fashion to epidermoid cysts – either by complete excision with an ellipse or a more conservative approach, first decompressing the cyst with a punch biopsy, evacuating the contents and then pulling out the wall – larger cysts with thicker walls are more amenable to this type of treatment that leaves a shorter scar.

Trichofolliculoma

This is an uncommon harmatoma arising from hair follicles with a dilated primary follicle which may be connected to the epidermis – the cause is unknown but may be due to abortive hair-follicle differentiation. It is not associated with other disorders.

There is a flesh-coloured or white papule found mainly on the face particularly around the nose, classically with a central pore or dot from which white vellus hairs may emerge.

IV. Sebaceous and sweat gland tumours

Tumours of sebaceous glands

Benign sebaceous tumours are uncommon and difficult to classify. The following are generally **not** considered as true tumours:

- Sebaceous hyperplasia which is sebaceous gland proliferation.
- Sebaceous naevus which is a congenital harmatoma.
- Fordyce spot which is the occurrence of ectopic sebaceous structures in lesions other than hair follicles.

Sebaceous adenoma

This is a benign tumour affecting the face (including eyelid) or scalp, most frequently composed of incompletely differentiated sebaceous cells; it is rare and affects mainly the elderly with equal sex incidence. Grossly, these are small, shiny, yellowish multilobular tumours of the upper dermis and histologically, there are small basophilic sebaceous matrix germinative cells in the periphery and more numerous, larger sebocytes with a foamy, bubbly appearance. Excision or other ablative modalities is the commonest treatment; incomplete excision generally leads to recurrence.

- Some patients who have multiple sebaceous adenomas (or epitheliomas or carcinomas) may have an associated visceral malignancy (**Muir–Torre syndrome**, autosomal dominant), particularly proximal colonic carcinomas. In about one-third, the skin tumour precedes or is synchronous with the internal malignancy. Thus screening of gastrointestinal and genitourinary systems in those with sebaceous gland tumours is suggested.

Sebaceous carcinoma

Sebaceous carcinomas are malignant tumours differentiating towards sebaceous epithelium and are rare (slightly more common in women). They comprise only 0.2% of skin cancers, though they are more common in Asians, particularly Chinese, being the second most common periocular cancer after BCC with HPV being implicated. They tend to be aggressive with tendency for recurrence and metastasis. The aetiology is mostly unknown but some cases may follow radiodermatitis.

They present usually as yellowish nodules anywhere where sebaceous glands are distributed e.g. scalp and face, whilst 75% are periocular (half said to arise from Meibomian glands of the tarsal plate). Tumours tend to deeply set in dermis, with the epidermis usually uninvolved but Pagetoid spread is possible (clinically invisible involvement of adjacent epidermis beyond obvious tumour). They are often mistaken for benign lesions clinically; histologically, they differ from adenoma by the presence of dermal aggregates of poorly differentiated tumour cells with central necrosis.

Evaluation for Muir–Torre syndrome is suggested. The skin lesions are excised with 5 mm of normal tissue; exenteration may be needed if the orbit is involved. Up to one-third will recur and thus some propose Mohs micrographic surgery. Radiotherapy is usually viewed as non-curative and is reserved for palliation.

Epidermoid cyst ('sebaceous cyst' but are not of sebaceous origin)

The term encompasses inclusion cysts due to implantation of epidermis into the dermis as well as infundibular cysts that originate from proliferation of epidermal cells from infundibulum of hair follicle.

- Milia are minature epidermoid cysts.
- Dermoid cysts occur in lines of cleavage and are distinct.

Epidermoid cysts are most common in young and middle-aged adults whilst those associated with Gardner syndrome present earlier, often with multiple lesions and before the polyps in over half. The actual aetiological mechanism is unclear, though proposals include embryonic sequestration (lip, genital) or acquired occlusion of hair follicle unit or implantation (post-injury or surgery). Some speculate on a role for HPV especially for lesions of palms and soles.

Clinically, they present as spherical cysts in the dermis and tethered to the epidermis at the **punctum**. Histologically, the cyst is lined by stratified squamous epithelium and filled with birefringent keratin, often laminar and breakdown products. They enlarge slowly but may become infected/inflamed secondarily (often colonized with *Staphylococcus epidermidis* and *Proprionibacteria*) and suppurate through the punctum. Malignant change is a very rare occurrence (to BCC, SCC, Bowen's disease) and recent studies show malignancies in 0.01% rather than 1–4% from earlier smaller studies.

They are excised with an elliptical incision designed around the punctum. Some authors suggest mini incisions or punch biopsy to allow drainage of the contents followed by removal of the lining – this technique is associated with a recurrence rate of 4–9% and scarred lesions are more difficult to remove in this way. Cysts in certain areas, especially genital and umbilical, may extend deeply; intracranial intraosseus lesions have been described especially around the fontanelle regions.

Pilar cysts occur on the scalp (tricholemmal cysts or wen) and tend to have thicker walls, and have less fat/more keratin.

Sweat gland tumours

Sweat glands function mainly by eccrine secretion with some apocrine secretion.

Types of sweat glands

- **Apocrine glands** release lipid secretions in membrane-bound vesicles by decapitation, where apical portions of cytoplasm pinch off (e.g. fat secretion in breast). Apocrine sweat glands are found in the axilla, pubic and perineal areas, labia major and around the nipples. The coiled gland lies in the deep dermis or at the junction with the hypodermis and the ducts terminate in upper part (or isthmus) of **hair follicles**. The lumen is much bigger than in eccrine glands; the secretions are more viscous and less copious than the latter. They are functional from puberty onwards with the hormonal changes but their exact function is unclear; they secrete sialomucin, which is initially odourless but may become transformed by bacteria. Special variants include Moll's glands of eyelids, cerumen of ear, **milk of breast**. Apocrine glands are affected in **hidradenitis suppurativa**.
- **Eccrine glands** release secretions by exocytosis into ducts; this is also called merocrine secretion. Eccrine sweat glands have long tubular extensions from epidermis into dermis or hypodermis – the ducts open directly onto the skin surface (unlike apocrine). They are found in highest density in the palms, soles and axilla. The initially isotonic secretions are modified by active NaCl and HCO_3 reabsorption in the ducts (which patients with cystic fibrosis are unable to do). Their primary function is **thermoregulation** with cholinergic innervation; emotional stressors tend to induce sweating in the palms/soles.
- **Holocrine glands** discharge whole cells which then disintegrate to release secretions e.g. sebaceous glands of skin and meibomian glands.
- **Hybrid type apoeccrine** glands in the axilla may have a role in hyperhidrosis, being present in large numbers in those affected. They also respond to cholinergic stimuli, open directly onto the skin but have 10× the sweat production of eccrine glands.

By contrast, **sebaceous glands** are responsible for **holocrine secretion of sebum**. They are pear-shaped glands lying in superficial dermis that empty into the upper portion of hair follicles though some exist independent of hair follicles e.g. in the lips, eyelids, glans, labia minora and nipple.

Benign eccrine sweat gland tumours

The commonest examples are syringoma, acrospiroma and cylindroma.

Syringoma (papillary eccrine adenoma)

Syrinx is Greek for 'pipe' or 'tube', reflecting the characteristic appearance of convoluted ducts in the upper dermis. A syringoma is a benign tumour of eccrine sweat gland origin and is uncommon. They affect females more often with onset during adolescence.

They appear as small, yellowish dermal papules on the chest, face and neck, usually < 3 mm. They may appear cystic and injury may cause release of a small amount of clear fluid. Each lesion is generally small but they may **erupt in crops** typically on the chest to lower abdomen; this form is more common in Asians/darker skins. Eruptive forms may not be true neoplasms, but rather dermatitis-type responses to inflammation/fibrosis e.g. scalp lesions.

- Multiple tumours may be associated with Down syndrome.
- They must be differentiated from BCCs and trichoepitheliomas.

Although benign, they are a cosmetic concern, particularly on the lower eyelids.

- Excision is best for small isolated lesions (which may be left to heal secondarily).
- Electrocautery (with needle).
- Alternatives include electrodesiccation or laser ablation, cryotherapy, dermabrasion or trichloroacetic acid (TCA) peel.

Eccrine acrospiroma (hidradenoma)

This is a benign tumour derived from eccrine sweat duct epithelium from distal parts of the gland. Their appearance is of hyperkeratotic plaques on sole or palm (i.e. acral, hence the name) that may ulcerate. Patients are middle aged with equal sex distribution.

They can be pigmented and thus resemble a melanoma. Actual malignant change (to a malignant eccrine acrospiroma) is rare but has been reported with propensity for local recurrence and distant metastasis (approximately half).

- Excision is the commonest treatment.

Poroma

This is a benign tumour of skin adnexae (the malignant counterpart is porocarcinoma). They are often referred to as 'eccrine poroma' but recent reports show that they can be either eccrine or apocrine, with the latter possibly being more common.

They present usually as solitary skin-coloured (rarely pigmented), well-circumscribed lesions and affect males and females of any ethnicity equally. Lesions are mostly slow-growing and asymptomatic though pain may be a feature in some.

Poromas are related to acrospiromas, with similar cytological features, but are more superficial being confined to the epidermis and upper dermis whilst acrospiromas are found in the deep dermis or upper hypodermis. They are satisfactorily treated by simple excision/ablation.

Dermal cylindroma (turban tumour, Spiegler's tumour)

These uncommon tumours are derived from the coiled part of sweat glands (part secretory, part duct) and are most commonly found in the scalp and forehead. They appear in early adult life, though solitary forms typically affect an older age group. They were previously thought to be apocrine in nature, thus distinguishing it from 'eccrine' spiradenomas, but there is probably a fair overlap between the two. It is a dermal tumour with no attachment to epidermis; histologically, there are columns of cells interspersed with hyaline material.

Typically, they present as a slow-growing rubbery lesion with pinkish, fleshy appearance on the scalp – multiple lesions tend to coalesce together like a 'turban' hence the name. Multiple lesions may be inherited (autosomal dominant) whilst solitary lesions are not. Most are small but they can grow up to several cm wide and may be painful in some. Malignant change is very rare but has been reported; the tumour is then locally aggressive with significant risk of metastasis. Treatment is typically by surgical excision although ablative lasers have been used with some success, and there are trials with topical sodium salicylate and prostaglandin A1.

- **Brooke–Spiegler syndrome** is an autosomal dominant disease with variable expression, with a predisposition to develop **multiple appendigeal tumours**, e.g. trichoepitheliomas, spiradenomas and cylindromas, others being less common. The gene CYLD has been localized to the 16q chromosome and encodes a deubiquinating enzyme whose exact biological function is yet to be elucidated.

Sweat gland carcinoma

Malignant epithelial tumours of the sweat glands (i.e. adenocarcinoma within the dermis) form a rare heterogeneous group and categorization can often be difficult. Most benign sweat gland tumours have a malignant counterpart and the diagnosis depends on identification of a residual benign portion. There are eccrine or apocrine varieties, though the former is more common and frequently metastasizes.

- Porocarcinoma.
- Syringomatous carcinoma.
- Ductal carcinoma.
- Mucinous carcinoma.
- Syringocystoadenocarcinoma papilliferum is very rare.

In general, sweat gland carcinoma affects patients in their middle age onwards (no sex difference). The most common presentation is of a painful, firm/hard, reddish nodule within the dermis with an irregular border. They can occur anywhere, but mainly affect the scalp and face. Growth is typically slow but may metastasize; excision should be wide, whilst the nodes should be assessed and monitored.

Adenoid cystic carcinoma of the scalp

This malignant tumour usually arises in the salivary glands and less commonly in the lacrimal glands and mucous glands of the upper respiratory tract. It rarely arises in the skin, with most cases affecting the eccrine sweat glands of the scalp – though this remains disputed with some shown to arise from apocrine glands.

Clinically, this is a slow-growing, skin-coloured tumour in the middle aged, which invades fascial planes, nerves and bone. It has a characteristic lattice-type appearance microscopically. It tends to run an indolent course with an average 10 years before diagnosis. It is treated by excision with histological control of margins (requires wide excision) but tends not to spread distantly. It is not radiosensitive.

B. Malignant melanoma

I. Epidemiology and overview

Malignant melanoma is a malignant tumour of epidermal melanocytes that accounts for < 5% of all skin cancers but > 75% of deaths from skin cancer. It was first described by John Hunter in 1799 as a 'cancerous fungous excrescence' behind the jaw in a 35-year-old man.

Incidence

- 6 per 100 000 per year in the UK.
- 33 per 100 000 per year in Australia.

It is the commonest cancer in young adults (20–39 years, rare before puberty) and the incidence is increasing rapidly, especially in men. The lifetime risk in the USA is 1.4%; it is estimated that people born in 2000 will have a 1:75 risk of developing melanoma sometime during their lifetime.

- It is more common in Celtic races and uncommon in black populations; the risk is related to the Fitzpatrick skin type (highest in types I and II).
  - The risk in redheads and blondes is 3× and 2.5× that compared with patients with dark hair.
- Female:male ratio is 2:1.
- There is a family history in 10% and the familial type tends to present younger.

Other risk factors

- Sunlight – it is more related to **non-occupational ultraviolet light** (UVB) exposure i.e. short, intense episodes of sun exposure particularly resulting in sunburn, rather than total or occupational (i.e. daily) exposure.
  - The current British Association of Dermatologists (BAD) guidelines (Marsden JR. *Br J Derm* published online 2010; DOI 10.1111/j.1365–2133.2010.09883.x) reinforce this and recommend limiting recreational exposure through life (level I evidence) and those most at risk are those with freckles, red/blond hair, those who burn, those with increased numbers of naevi and those with a family history of melanoma. It is also recognized that insufficiency of vitamin D in the UK is becoming more common and thus those not in the risk categories above should still be careful about sun exposure but not greatly limit it (vitamin D supplementation may be needed).
  - Higher socioeconomic group – possibly related to travel. Case–control studies have not shown a reduction with sunscreen use, though in Australia the incidence of melanoma among young Australian adults declined from 1983 to 1996.
  - The incidence of melanoma is higher in those who tend to burn rather than tan.
  - Note however that up to 75% of melanoma occurs on relatively unexposed areas and are difficult to produce experimentally with ultraviolet light.
- Immunosuppression.

Predisposing conditions

- **Significance of a pre-existing naevus**. The vast majority of melanocytic naevi are benign – each adult has 30 naevi on average. Only ~10% of melanomas actually arise in a pre-existing naevus i.e. most tumours arise *de novo*. The lifetime risk of malignant change in an individual naevus is difficult to quantify, with the highest risk in congenital and dysplastic naevi. Prophylactic excision of naevi or small congenital naevi (< 5 cm) in the absence of suspicious features is not recommended (BAD 2010, level III, grade B).
  - Atypical mode syndrome: > 100 naevi > 6 mm in diameter that are present in birth and increase at puberty. Larger numbers (> 10) of larger (> 8 mm) naevi.
  - Dysplastic naevus: 6–10% risk.
  - Giant congenital naevus 4% (2–42%). These patients are deemed to be at greatly increased risk and current BAD guidelines recommend that these patients be monitored by an 'expert' for their lifetime (BAD 2010, level III, grade B).
- Lentigo maligna (LM).
- Xeroderma pigmentosum (1000× incidence), albinism.

Clinical features

There are commonly described characteristic features which should alert suspicion: ABCD.

- **Asymmetry**.
- Irregular **border** – this feature is most commonly found in superficial spreading melanoma (SSM) and lentigo maligna melanoma (LMM) whilst nodular melanoma are often symmetrical with a well-defined border.
- **Colour** irregularity, i.e. variegated pigmentation and irregular surface.
  - Typically a melanoma has a haphazard array of brown–black though nodular lesions are often blue-black.

  ○ Red lesions indicate a host inflammatory
    response.
  ○ Depigmentation indicates either an amelanotic
    area or a focus of regression; an asymmetric
    halo around an asymmetrical lesion is strongly
    indicative of a melanoma. Amelanotic lesions
    will still stain positively for tyrosinase.
- **Diameter** > 6 mm.
- E could be included to stand for '**evolving**' –
  particularly significant is a recent history of
  changing size or pigmentation ('major signs' with
  good positive predictive value). Absolute size or
  the presence of bleeding or itching, are less
  predictive ('minor signs'). Ulceration is suggestive
  of malignancy.
  ○ Note that 'E' is not part of the original criteria,
    neither is 'F' for something that looks 'funny'.

Growth phases

The growth of a melanoma is described as having two
phases.

- **Radial growth phase**: this is the proliferation of
  neoplastic melanocytes within the epidermis with
  only focal/single cell invasion of papillary dermis.
  This is typical of SSM, LMM, acral lentiginous
  MM.
- **Vertical growth phase**: this is the invasion of
  malignant melanocytes into papillary and reticular
  dermis and is typical of nodular MM and late
  LMM. Invasive melanocytes are spindle-shaped
  and infiltrate along neurovascular structures.

II. Melanoma subtypes

Superficial spreading melanoma (pagetoid melanoma)

This is the most common type of melanoma (50–70%
of all) in Whites and may occur in pre-existing naevi.
It is usually found on the backs and legs in women
whilst in men it is more common on the trunk. The
radial growth phase may be as short as 6 months or as
long as 6 years. The lesions are often flat with irregular
border, pigmentation and surface; invasion is usually
heralded by ulceration. Dense lymphocytic and fibroblast aggregations indicate regression. It can be difficult to distinguish histologically from Paget's disease
when located at the nipple.

Nodular melanoma

These comprise 0–20% of all melanoma and are characterized by concurrent radial and vertical growth – the

relatively early vertical growth phase means that these
lesions tend to be better demarcated. It is twice as
common in women, whilst 5% are amelanotic.

Lentigo maligna melanoma (5–10% of all melanoma)

These are most commonly found on sun-exposed skin,
especially the face, of older patients (more in women).
Lesions have a prolonged radial phase and may take up
to 30 years before the vertical growth phase begins.

Lentigo maligna melanoma is said to be the invasive counterpart of lentigo maligna (LM, which is
in situ melanoma, also known as Hutchinson's mela-
notic freckle); 3–5% of LM will become invasive (lifetime risk), appearing as darkened nodules/foci within
areas of pre-existing LM. Standard excision of LM with
5 mm margins will be insufficient in 50% and Mohs
micrographic surgery is recommended (McKenna JK.
Dermatol Surg 2006;**32**:493–504).

- Johnathan Hutchinson (1828–1913) was a
  Yorkshire-born surgeon who trained at St
  Bartholomew's and was mentored by James Paget.

Acral lentiginous melanoma

Acral lentiginous melanoma (ALM) comprise 2–8% of
melanoma in Whites but up to 60% in dark-skinned
races. In the former group, it usually affects the elderly
(> 60 years) with lesions most commonly found on
palms, soles, mucocutaneous junctions and in subungual locations (black streaks in nails – melanonychia).
Radial growth is followed by vertical growth after ~2
years. It is histologically similar to LMM but is more
locally aggressive and more likely to metastasize.

- **Subungual melanoma** (1–3%) affects the great toe
  in ~50% of cases with the thumb the next most
  common. It is typically a pigmented lesion of the
  nail bed, often with splitting of the nail, paronychia
  and nail dystrophy – it can be difficult to
  distinguish from pigmented naevus of the nail
  matrix. It is treated by amputation of the affected
  digit; the level of amputation does not seem to
  affect local recurrence or survival. There is a high
  incidence of amelanotic lesions in subungual
  melanoma (~30%; 7% of all cutaneous melanoma
  are amelanotic). Isolated limb perfusion (ILP)
  reduces local recurrence but does not affect
  survival (Lingam LK. *Br J Surg* 1995;**82**:1343–
  1345). Hutchinson's sign – broad streaks of
  variegated pigmentation within the nail plate are
  associated with subungual melanoma.

Subungual melanoma of the hand
Quinn MJ. *J Hand Surg Am* 1996;**21**:506–511.

This is a series of 38 patients with mean tumour thickness 3 mm and age at presentation 58 years (later than other melanoma). The mean duration of symptoms before diagnosis was ~12 months, often having been treated for a 'fungal' infection and often associated with a history of trauma. Male patients were more common whilst upper limb melanoma overall is more common in females. Survival rates were lower than for melanoma overall.

The authors recommend distal (or functional) amputation: either through the neck of the proximal phalanx of the thumb or through the PIP joint of the fingers. (The term 'distal' is used as previous surgeons had proposed amputation through the tarsometatarsal or carpometacarpal joints.)

- This recommendation is supported by Finley RK. *Surgery* 1994;**116**:96–100. The study with 22 patients showed that more distal amputations preserved hand function without compromising survival or local control.

Functional surgery in subungual melanoma
Moehrle M. *Dermatol Surg* 2003;**29**:366–374.

The authors described their results with 64 patients with stage I and II melanoma. They recommend 'functional surgery' with partial resection of the distal phalanx only and 3-dimensional histology to ensure clearance, and their figures suggest that it does not negatively affect the prognosis whilst improving function and cosmesis. Patients with amputation at or proximal to the DIP joint did not fare better. However, there is selection bias as the decision for conservative excision was based on the pathological results of the initial excision.

Subungual melanoma: management considerations
Cohen T. *Am J Surg* 2008;**195**:244–248.

This series describes the Memorial Sloan Kettering experience with 49 patients with subungual melanoma treated after they began to use sentinel node mapping (30 patients).

- Female patients were more common (63%) in contrast to the Quinn study.
- Toe lesions were thicker with an overall Breslow depth of 2.1 mm.
- Sentinel node positive rate was 17% and all underwent complete node dissection.
- For the majority of invasive lesions, they performed amputation at MTP for the toe and PIPJ/middle phalanx for digit lesions as their **standard operation**. In their experience, wide local excision (WLE) was associated with local recurrence and eventual formal amputation.

Desmoplastic melanoma
This rare subtype (1%) occurs most commonly in the head and neck and may be non-pigmented. Histologically there is desmoplastic spindling stroma with melanocytic dysplasia; special stains may be needed for diagnosis. There is a tendency for local recurrence due to perineural infiltration and lymphatic spread.

Secondary melanoma (no identifiable primary)
In these cases it is assumed that the primary lesion has regressed. This accounts for ~5% of melanomas, usually presenting as lymph node disease though non-lymph node metastatic sites include skin, brain, lung, bone, spinal cord and adrenals. Abdominal presentation of MM is most commonly obstruction or intussusception, usually from a metastatic deposit that is usually amelanotic. Radiotherapy may offer effective palliation of brain metastases whilst surgery may be indicated for a solitary brain metastasis.

Tumour markers
At present, there is no true 'tumour marker' that is of value in the early detection of melanoma, but other tests may be helpful in other ways.

- Polymerase chain reaction assay of **tyrosinase activity** is often used to assess occult (micrometastasis) tumour burden e.g. in sentinel nodes.
- **S-100 and TA-90** has been used on tissue samples to aid the histopathological diagnosis of melanoma whilst serum S-100 may be helpful in detecting progression (increased volume of disease), and serum TA-90 has been used to assess the risk of metastasis (a positive test is associated with a 5-year survival of 44% vs. 89% if negative; Chung MH. *Ann Surg Oncol* 2002;**9**:120–126).
- **HLA-DQB1*0301** is a genomic marker that independently identifies melanoma patients in whom recurrence is more likely, and is potentially useful in selecting those most likely to benefit from adjuvant therapy (Lee JE. *Int J Cancer* 1994;**59**:510–513). However there has been sparse research published on this since.

III. Excision margins

The initial excision biopsy should be excised with 2 mm normal skin and a cuff of fat, with the axis orientated along the axis of limbs if possible. Shave or incisional biopsies are not recommended; the latter may be acceptable in lentigo maligna or ALM, but should only be performed by those within the melanoma multidisciplinary team.

Excision margins in high risk malignant melanoma
Thomas JM. *New Engl J Med* 2004;**350**:757–766.

This study presented outcome data from the UK Melanoma Study Group trial (*n*= 900, > 2 mm thick) assessing 1 cm vs. 3 cm margins, and found that 1 cm margin was associated with a significantly increased risk of local recurrence, but overall survival was similar in the two groups. This is commonly referred to as the BAPS/MSG study.

Surgical excision markings for primary cutaneous melanoma
Sladden MJ. *Cochrane Database Syst Rev* 2009.

Included trials are:

- BAPS/MSG Thomas JM. *New Engl J Med* 2004;**350**:757–766.
- French study: Khayat D. *Cancer* 2003;**97**:1941–1946.
- Intergroup Study Balch CM. *Ann Surg Oncol* 2001;**8**:101–108.
- Swedish study: Cohn-Cedermark G. *Cancer* 2000;**89**:1495–1501.
- WHO study: Cascinelli N. *Sem Surg Oncol* 1998;**14**:272–275.

This systematic review summarizes the evidence regarding width of excision margins for primary cutaneous melanoma. None of the five published trials, or the meta-analysis, showed a statistically significant difference in overall survival between narrow or wide excision.

The summary estimate for overall survival **favoured wide excision by a small degree** [Hazard Ratio 1.04; 95% confidence interval 0.95–1.15; P = 0.40], but the result was not significantly different. This result is compatible with both a 5% relative reduction in overall mortality favouring narrower excision and a 15% relative reduction in overall mortality favouring wider excision. Therefore, a small (but potentially important) difference in overall survival between wide and narrow excision margins cannot be confidently ruled out.

The summary estimate for recurrence-free survival favoured wide excision margins [Hazard Ratio 1.13;

Table 8.1 Summary of recommendations for wider excision margins for melanoma.

Breslow thickness	UK (2010)	Australia (2008)	US (2009)
In situ	2–5 mm	5 mm	5 mm
≤ 1 mm	1 cm	1 cm	1 cm
1.01–2.00 mm	1–2 cm	1–2 cm	1–2 cm
2.01–4.00 mm	2–3 cm	1–2 cm	2 cm
> 4 mm	3 cm	2 cm	2 cm

95% confidence interval 0.99–1.28; P = 0.06] but again the result did not reach statistical significance (P < 0.05 level).

The conclusion was that current randomized evidence is insufficient to address optimal excision margins for primary cutaneous melanoma.

In the main, a 2 cm wider excision margin is often the upper limit for most lesions with 3 cm used in certain circumstances (particularly in UK practice). Current national guidelines are given in Table 8.1.

Head and neck malignant melanoma: margin status and immediate reconstruction
Sullivan SR. *Ann Plast Surg* 2009;**62**:144–148.

Immediate reconstruction is safe except for patients with locally recurrent, ulcerated or thick (T4) tumours as the risk of a positive margin after WLE is increased in these cases. The tendency to be more conservative with resections in the head and neck leads to higher rates of incomplete excision and subsequent recurrence (9 and 13% respectively) compared with the extremities (1 and 6%). Immediate frozen sections are generally regarded as not being that reliable, thus in these cases temporary coverage was needed until paraffin sections confirm clearance of tumour. Some have suggested (delayed) skin grafting to facilitate monitoring but tissue transfer has not been found to hinder follow-up for recurrences.

IV. Prognosis and prognostic indicators

Clinical variables

Better prognosis in:

- Thinner tumours.
- Node negative. The 2-year survival of patients undergoing positive radical neck dissection approaches zero.

Table 8.2 Summary of the important tumour trials relevant to excision margins.

Trial	Design	Number of patients	Follow-up	Local control	Overall survival
Veronesi (WHO) *New Engl J Med* 1988	1 vs. 3 cm WLE for MM < 2 mm	612	5 years	No difference	No difference
Cohn-Cedermark (Swedish Melanoma Study Group) *Cancer* 2000	2 vs. 5 cm WLE for primary MM 0.8–2.0 mm trunk or extremities	989	11 years	No difference	No difference
Balch (Intergroup Melanoma Surgical Trial) *Ann Surg Oncol* 2001	2 vs. 4 cm WLE for primary MM 1–4 mm trunk/upper limb	468	10 years	No difference	No difference
Khayat (French Co-operative Study) *Cancer* 2003	2 vs. 5 cm WLE for primary MM < 2.1 mm	337	16 years	No difference	No difference
Thomas (MSG study) *New Engl J Med* 2004	1 vs. 3 cm WLE for MM >2 mm	900	5 years	Increased local recurrence in 1 cm group	No difference

WLE, wide local excision; MM, malignant melanoma.

- Women.
- < 50 years old (but the elderly tend to have thicker lesions and more acral lentiginous melanoma).
- From pre-existing naevus (20% of cases).
- The significance of upper back, posterior arm, posterior neck, and posterior scalp (BANS) lesions is disputed.

Pathological variables

- Tumour thickness (**Breslow** – Breslow A. *Ann Surg* 1970;**172**:902–908): measured from the stratum granulosum to the deepest part of the tumour.
- Level of invasion (**Clark** – Clark WH. *Cancer Res* 1969;**29**:705–726).
  - I – confined to the epidermis.
  - II – invasion of papillary dermis.
  - III – filling of papillary dermis.
  - IV – invasion of reticular dermis.
  - V – invasion of subcutaneous fat.
- Ulceration.
- Neurovascular invasion.
- Microscopic satellites.
- Mitotic activity.

Final version of the AJCC staging system for cutaneous melanoma

Balch JM. *J Clin Oncol* 2001;**19**:3635–3648.

Drawing on a database of 30 450 patients with full data on 17 600 available for production of survival data, this paper produced updated staging information for the 2002 staging system. The main differences between this and the previous edition can be outlined.

- Level.
  - Was – used as alternative to thickness.
  - Now – not used except for T1 lesions.
- Ulceration.
  - Was – not used.
  - Now – a secondary determinant of T and N staging, it upstages tumour.
- Nodes.
  - Was – size.
  - Now – number.
- Metastatic volume in nodes.
  - Was – not used.
  - Now – included as secondary determinant of N staging. Micrometastases are detected by sentinel lymph node biopsies (SLNBs) whilst macrometastases are palpable nodes confirmed pathologically or nodes with gross extracapsular spread.
- Lactate dehydrogenase (LDH).
  - Was – not used.
  - Now – used in M category.
- Satellite lesions.
  - Was – considered separately from in-transit.
  - Now – merged with in-transit lesions in N category and consider stage III disease.
  - **In-transit metastases** can be defined as non-nodal cutaneous or subcutaneous deposits

between the primary site and draining nodal basin i.e. in transit to the node. Rapid development of in-transit metastases often coincides with development of distant disease.

- **Satellite lesions** by definition are those that occur within 5 cm of the site of the primary lesion (i.e. satellite of the primary) but are probably biologically the same entity as in-transit disease, and in the 2002 and 2010 staging manuals are grouped together.
- Pathological staging.
  - Was – not used.
  - Now – SLNB results incorporated into definition of pathological staging. There is large variability between clinical and pathological staging; the latter is recommended before entry of patients into melanoma trials.

Pathological staging is based upon further information about the regional nodes following SLNB and completion of lymph node dissection (LND) and thus subdivides stage III disease by N stage. Positive SLNB upstages the patient to stage III, irrespective of tumour thickness but survival in a patient with a *non-ulcerated* melanoma and micrometastases in the sentinel node only (stage IIIa) is likely to exceed survival in a patient with stage IIc disease, i.e. a thick, *ulcerated* primary (69% and 45% survival at 5 years, respectively).

AJCC Staging manual 7th edition
Final version of the 2009 Melanoma staging and classification
Balch JM. *J Clin Oncol* 2009;**27**:6199–6206.

The staging system was updated again and was effective from 1 January 2010. The main differences between this and previous edition are:

- Histological level of invasion.
  - Was – used only for defining T1 lesions.
  - Now – is used only in the unusual circumstances of the mitotic rate being indeterminate.
- Ulceration.
  - Was – a secondary determinant of T and N staging.
  - Now – same. It implies locally advanced disease.
- Mitotic rate per mm^2.
  - Was – not used.
  - Now – used for T1 lesions; a rate of greater than or equal to 1/mm^2 defines T1b. From the data,

its predictive value is almost as strong as thickness and better than ulceration.
- Immunochemistry for nodal metastasis.
  - Was – not used.
  - Now – used; at least one marker e.g. HMB-45, Melan-A, MART-1 with cellular features of malignant morphology.
- Threshold of defined N+.
  - Was – implied to be 0.2 mm and required formal H&E staining.
  - Now – deposits < 0.1 mm with histological or immunohistochemical criteria, i.e. there is no lower limit.
- Elevated serum LDH.
  - Was – a secondary determinant of M staging.
  - Now – same; a repeat confirmatory test is recommended if elevated.
- Clinical vs. pathological staging.
  - Was – sentinel node results incorporated into latter.
  - Now – sentinel node biopsy/staging encouraged as standard care, and is required before entry into clinical trials.

Other comments included:

- The staging committee also recommends that the **microsatellite** – any discontinuous nest of metastatic cells > 0.05 mm in diameter clearly separated by normal dermis from the main invasive component by at least 0.3 mm – be retained in N2c.
- For metastatic disease from an **unknown primary** arising in nodes, skin or subcutaneous tissues is stage III rather than stage IV.
- **Stage III disease is very heterogeneous** and depending on the number of nodes, presence of ulceration and nodal tumour burn (micro- vs. macrometastases), 5-year survival may range from 81.5% (single micrometastasis in node, non-ulcerated tumour) to 29% (four or more macroscopically involved nodes with an ulcerated primary tumour).

The removal of a lower limit for the definition of nodal and the acceptance of immunohistochemistry for the diagnosis, means that even one metastatic cell is enough and many more patients will be diagnosed as stage III. This is likely to be the point that is most debated – some feel that micrometastases smaller than 0.1 mm carry a prognosis almost as good as no micrometastasis at all.

Table 8.3 TNM (tumor-node-metastasis) staging for melanoma.

Tumour	Thickness	Ulceration/ Mitosis
Tis	NA	NA
T1	≤ 1.00 mm	a: Without ulceration and $1/mm^2$ b: With ulceration or $\geq 1/mm^2$
T2	1.01–2.00 mm	a: Without ulceration b: With ulceration
T3	2.01–4.00 mm	a: Without ulceration b: With ulceration
T4	>4.00 mm	a: Without ulceration b: With ulceration

Nodes	Number involved regional nodes	Nodal metastatic mass
N0	0	NA
N1	1	a: Micrometastases b: Macrometastases
N2	2–3	a: Micrometastases b: Macrometastases c: In-transit/satellite *without* nodal disease
N3	4 +, or matted nodes, or in-transit/satellite *plus* nodal disease (micro- or macroscopic)	

Metastasis	Site	Serum lactate dehydrogenase
M0	No distant metastasis	NA
M1a	Distant skin, subcutaneous or nodal involvement	Normal
M1b	Lung	Normal
M1c	All other visceral	Normal
	Any	Elevated

V. Management of lymph nodes in melanoma

Sentinel lymph node biopsy (SLNB) and staging of malignant melanoma

The argument for elective lymph node dissection (ELND) assumes that it identifies nodal metastases and prevents subsequent recurrences in the same (dissected) basin, that metastases may exist in the regional lymph nodes in the absence of distant disease, and that removal of nodal metastases prevents subsequent spread to distant sites.

Early non-randomized retrospective studies did demonstrate an advantage over delayed therapeutic lymph node dissection (TLND) but subsequent randomized prospective trials did not confirm this – suggesting the opposite, that lymph node metastases may be markers of systemic disease and distant metastasis may occur without involvement of regional nodes. Neither ELND nor delayed TLND became universally accepted, and as a result of this controversy Morton DL (*Arch Surg* 1992;**127**:392–399) devised a selective lymph node biopsy based on intra-operative lymphatic mapping i.e. SLNB.

- The sentinel node is the first lymph node to which lymph drainage from the area of the lesion is received.
- National Institute for Health and Clinical Excellence (NICE) guideline (2006): SLNB should be undertaken in centres with experience of procedure and normally only in context of ethically approved clinical trials.

According to McMasters KM (*J Clin Oncol* 2001;**19**:2851–2855) the main benefits of SLNB in melanoma are:

- **Accurate staging** (for prognostic assessment). The hazard ratio for survival for those with a positive SLN was 6.53 compared with 1.23 for tumour thickness and 1.62 for tumour ulceration. The 3-year survival rates for patients with negative and positive SLNB are 96.8 and 69.9% respectively. There is currently no other way to reliably stage lymph nodes – positron emission tomography (PET) has limits of 3 mm in the best studies.
- Identification of early micrometastasis in lymph nodes to **direct therapeutic lymph node dissection**. Truncal melanoma exhibits unpredictable drainage patterns in up to 32%. Morton DL (*New Engl J Med* 2006;**355**:1307–1317) conclude that SLNB may identify patients with nodal metastases whose survival may be prolonged potentially by immediate nodal surgery.
- Identification of those who may benefit from adjuvant IFN-2-α.
- Delineation of populations for trials.

Table 8.4 Clinicopathological staging for melanoma.

Clinical staging				Pathological staging			
Stage	**T**	**N**	**M**	**Stage**	**T**	**N**	**M**
0	Tis	0	0	0	Tis	0	0
IA	1a	0	0	IA	0	0	0
IB	1b or 2a	0	0	IB	0	0	0
IIA	2b or 3a	0	0	IIA	0	0	0
IIB	3b or 4a	0	0	IIB	0	0	0
IIC	4b	0	0	IIC	0	0	0
III	Any	>0	0	IIIA	Any (no ulceration)	1a or 2a	0
				IIIB	Any (ulcerated)	1a or 1b	0
					Any (no ulceration)	1b or 2b or 2c	0
				IIIC	Any (ulcerated)	1b or 2b or 2c	0
					Any	3	0
IV	Any	Any	M	IV	Any	Any	M1 (a,b,c)

Clinical staging (and 5-year survival)

Stage I: Localized disease, T2a or less.
Localized disease, T2a or less.
- 5-year survival Ia – 95%, Ib 90%.

Stage II: Localized disease, T2b or more.
  o IIa – 80%, IIb – 65%, IIc – 45%.

Stage III: Nodal disease.
  o IIIa – 65%, IIIb – 50%, IIIc – 25%.

Stage IV: Metastatic disease.
  o 8%.

Clinical staging includes microstaging of the primary melanoma and clinical/radiological evaluation for metastases. By convention, it should be used after complete excision of the primary melanoma with clinical assessment for regional and distant metastases.

Pathological staging includes microstaging of the primary melanoma and pathological information about the regional lymph nodes after partial (i.e. sentinel node biopsy) or complete lymphadenectomy. Pathological stage 0 or stage IA patients are the exception; they do not require pathologic evaluation of their lymph nodes.

Surgical management of regional lymph nodes in primary cutaneous malignant melanoma
Stone CA. *Br J Surg* 1995;**82**:1015–1022.

This is a literature review with a good historical overview.

- Collaborative study of 1786 patients in Alabama and Sydney (Balch and Milton respectively, in 1982) demonstrated that results of elective LND acts as an independent prognostic variable for lesions 0.76–3.99 mm thick.
- Series of ELND indicates that 40% of node metastases are subclinical, and frequency of occult disease increases with depth (38% > 1.5 mm) and level of invasion (58% > level V). ELND offers a survival advantage over TLND only if < 10% of the node basin harbours occult disease.
- The overall discordancy between predicted and actual drainage patterns averages 40%, especially for head and neck lesions – 10% drain to contralateral nodes.
- The argument against ELND was mainly based on the Veronesi (WHO) study in 1977, however this had a gender bias (women > men) and lesion bias (mostly lower limb – better prognosis in women).

Long term results of a multi-institutional randomized trial comparing prognostic factors and surgical results for intermediate thickness melanoma (1.0 to 4.0 mm). Intergroup Melanoma Surgical Trial
Balch CM. *Ann Surg Oncol* 2000;**7**:87–97.

The Intergroup Melanoma Surgical Trial (1983–1989) aimed to determine the role of ELND for patients with intermediate thickness melanoma and included 740 patients prospectively randomized to ELND or observation groups.

Ten-year survival rates favoured those with node dissection with approximately 30% survival benefit for non-ulcerated melanomas, tumours 1–2 mm and tumours of the limbs. The risk of distant metastatic disease in patients with ulcerated melanomas and tumours > 4 mm offsets potential benefits of ELND. The authors suggested that **ulceration and tumour thickness** are dominant predictive factors for staging of stage I and II tumours and made a case for including them in the T classification.

This study did not analyse the survival difference between positive ELND patients versus those in the observation arm that subsequently needed TLND patients.

Immediate or delayed dissection of regional nodes in patients with melanoma of the trunk: a randomised trial
Cascinelli N. *Lancet* 1998;**14**:793–796.

This is a multicentre trial on behalf of the WHO with 240 patients under 65 years of age with truncal melanoma > 1.5 mm randomized to either ELND or observation and TLND (median tumour thickness was comparable in both groups). The 5-year survival in *positive* ELND patients was 48.2% compared to 26% in patients undergoing TLND when nodes became clinically obvious. Their interpretation was that node dissection may increase survival in patients with nodal metastasis only and suggested that **SLNB may be a tool** to identify those with occult metastasis.

Efficacy of selective lymphadenectomy as a therapeutic procedure for early stage melanoma
Essner R. *Ann Surg Oncol* 1999;**6**:442–449.

This study compared the outcome in 267 matched pairs of patients undergoing either SLNB/completion or ELND, matched for gender and age, and site and thickness of the primary tumour. There was no overall significant difference in survival or number of tumour-positive dissections but there was a significant increase in number of tumour-positive dissections in the SLN group for **intermediate thickness** primaries (related to immunohistochemical diagnosis of occult microscopic disease). There was a similar incidence of same-basin recurrence (4.8% in SLNB group) and in-transit disease (3%) after tumour-negative dissection.

Elective, therapeutic and delayed lymph node dissection for malignant melanoma of the head and neck: analysis of 1444 patients from 1970 to 1998

Fisher SR. *Laryngoscope* 2002;**112**:99–100.

This was a retrospective analysis of 1444 patients with head and neck melanoma with **positive neck dissections** grouped by:

- ELND at time of diagnosis (within 2 months) – 24% 5-year survival.
- Delayed LND for regional recurrence > 3 months from diagnosis, 56% 5-year survival.
- TLND for palpable nodes within 30 days of diagnosis (99/112 positive), 36% 5-year survival.

Eleven per cent of ELND were positive i.e. had occult disease whilst those who did not have any initial LND had a 12% nodal 'recurrence' rate which was deemed comparable. The authors tried to explain the poor prognosis with ELND by postulating that micrometastatic disease may stimulate T-cell activation and that removal by ELND **may adversely** affect survival. However, it is important to note that the number in the ELND group was small (27).

Lymphatic mapping and sentinel lymphadenectomy for early stage melanoma
Morton DL. *Ann Surg* 2003;**238**:538–550.

This study came from the John Wayne Cancer Institute with 1599 stage I/II patients who underwent SLNB. They had a median tumour thickness of 1.43 mm and positive sentinel nodes in 322 (20%).

- The **risk of metastasis to nodes is directly proportional to the thickness** of the primary tumour. Tumours less than 1 mm have a low incidence of sentinel metastasis, whilst intermediate thickness lesions (1–2 mm) may have sentinel-only metastasis (non-sentinel nodes not involved), whereas thicker lesions may have additional nodes and distant sites involved.
- **Afferent lymphatics drain in a compartmentalized fashion into the node**: specific areas of skin map to specific compartments within the node. RT-PCR facilitates detection of micrometastases that are missed by serial sectioning (with 12–20 sections this represents about 1% of total node volume).
- In some patients, the SLN harbours cells that, after a latent period of growth, are responsible for later haematogenous spread (**incubator hypothesis**). A critical mass of cells must be achieved in order to allow passage of cells along the lymphatic chain (postulated generation of immunosuppressive factors). The incubator hypothesis of spread supported by

observation of 15-year survival in up to 32% of patients undergoing therapeutic LND, i.e. node removal before progression to distant metastases. It implies that there is a therapeutic window.

- In other patients, SLN positivity is simply a marker for metastatic disease that has bypassed the node (**marker hypothesis**).

Analysis of overall survival in 287 pairs of patients matched for clinical/pathological stage showed improved survival in the SLNB/completion lymph node dissection group compared with delayed LND (73% and 51% survival at 5 years, respectively).

Five years experience of sentinel node biopsy for melanoma: the St George's Melanoma Unit experience
Topping A. *Br J Plast Surg* 2004;**57**:97–104.

This was the largest UK series at the time of publication with prospective data on 347 patients undergoing SLNB (1996–2001). The indications were Breslow thickness > 1 mm or < 1 mm if > Clark III. Pre-operative lymphoscintigraphy (Nanocoll) was performed for surface marking of the node and then intra-operative patent V dye was injected around the biopsy scar for visual localization of the SLN and hand-held gamma probe for the 'hot' node. Wide lesion excision was then performed with 1-cm margin (if primary < 1 mm) or 2 cm (primary >1 mm). Positive SLNB was followed by completion LND within 3 weeks in all patients; the false-negative rate was 2%.

- The rate of positive SLNB was 17.6% and 87% had no further disease in the same node basin. Eleven patients subsequently died of disseminated disease; two of these had further disease in the nodal basin at completion lymphadenectomy.
- The ratio of negative:positive SLNB was related to the tumour thickness from 19:1 for < 1 mm to 2:1 for > 2 mm.
- Patients with a positive SLNB were 6× **more likely to die** from their disease than patients with a negative SLNB during the follow-up period; it is an independent prognostic indicator for survival but was not as significant as tumour thickness.

Sentinel-node biopsy or nodal observation in melanoma
Morton DL. *New Engl J Med* 2006;**355**:1307–1317.

This study presented the results of the MSLT group with 1269 patients with intermediate (1.2–3.5 mm) thickness melanoma randomized to:

- Wide excision and observation, with lymphadenectomy for nodal relapse (15.6%).
- Wide excision, SLNB with immediate completion lymphadenoctomy if positive (16%).

There was no difference in the 5-year survival rates, contradicting Morton (2003) which suggested an advantage to early lymphadenectomy. In the SLNB group, the 5-year survival was 72.3% in those with positive SLNB compared with 90.2% in negative SLNB. Finally, in those with nodal disease, either positive SLNB or nodal relapse during observation, the former group had better survival at 72.3% vs. 52.4%. The authors thus conclude that SLNB may identify patients with nodal metastases whose survival may be prolonged potentially by immediate nodal surgery.

Postoperative morbidity of lymph node excision for cutaneous melanoma-sentinel lymphonodectomy versus complete regional lymph node dissection
Kretschmer L. *Melanoma Res* 2008;**18**:16–21.

This was a clinical study of 315 patients with axillary or groin dissections – 275 sentinel lymphonodectomies (SLNE) and 90 complete regional lymph node dissections (CLNDs). The overall incidence of at least one complication after SLNE was 13.8% (all were mild – wound problems especially seroma (6.9%) and infection (3.6%) as well as pain (0.7%), haematoma (2.5%)) vs. 65.5% after CLND (50% incidence of both short- and long-term complications, including swelling (37.1%) and functional deficit (16.8%)).

The microanatomic location of metastatic melanoma in sentinel lymph node predicts nonsentinel lymph node involvement
Dewar DJ. *J Clin Oncol* 2004;**22**:3345–3349.

Positive SLNs from 146 nodal basins were examined for intra-nodal location of metastases. The extent, anatomical site of metastases and depth of involvement of the SLN correlated with non-sentinel node involvement at completion lymphadenectomy e.g. subcapsular vs. deeper parenchymal (0% vs. 19%) and multifocal/extensive disease (37–42%). They suggest that in those with only subscapular deposits (26% of cases in this series) in the sentinel node, completion node dissection may be safely avoided.

Patterns of recurrence after SLNB
- The frequency of SLNB positivity tends to depend on the stage of the primary.
- SLNB-negative patients have fewer nodal recurrences and better disease-free survival.

● False-negative sentinel node biopsy has been described – some ascribe this due to obstruction of lymphatics by metastatic melanoma (Lam TK. *Melanoma Res* 2009;**19**:94–99) and suggest that ultrasound of the nodal basin may reduce this occurrence.

There have been many published articles in this area; the following are a selection of 'classic' papers.

Sentinel lymph node biopsy in cutaneous melanoma: the WHO melanoma program experience

Cascinelli N. *Ann Surg Oncol* 2000;**7**:469–474.

Eighteen per cent of 829 patients participating in this WHO SLNB (used blue dye only) programme had positive SLNB. Of the SLNB-negative patients, 6% developed regional nodal recurrence, 7% developed distant metastases and 3% developed in-transit disease. **SLN positivity, tumour thickness and ulceration** were independent prognostic variables by multivariate analysis.

Multi-institutional lymphatic mapping experience: the prognostic value of sentinel node status in 612 stage I and II melanoma patients

Gershenwald J. *J Clin Oncol* 1998;**3**:976–983.

This was a follow-up study of 243 patients of 612 who had negative SLNB. One per cent and 4.1% of all patients developed recurrent or in-transit disease respectively; 5.8% developed nodal disease in the biopsied node basin whilst 7.4% developed distant disease.

Sentinel lymph node biopsy in the management of patients with primary cutaneous melanoma: review of a large single-institutional experience with an emphasis on recurrence

Clary BM. *Ann Surg* 2001;**233**:250–258.

This was a review of 332 sentinel node biopsy procedures (positive 17%) over a 7-year period; lesions had a mean Breslow thickness 2.7 mm with ulceration in 29%. SLNB-negative patients had better disease-free survival at 3 years (75% vs. 58%) and fewer recurrences (14% vs. 40%) compared with SLNB-positive patients.

Re-evaluation of selected negative SLNB samples by PCR in patients developing recurrent disease showed that most (7/11) actually had metastatic disease that was undetected at the time.

Patterns of early recurrence after sentinel lymph node biopsy for melanoma

Chao C. *Am J Surg* 2002;**184**:520–524.

This presented data from the Sunbelt Melanoma Trial group with 1183 patients that had 233 (19.7%)

positive SLNB then followed by completion lymphadenectomy with or without adjuvant interferon alpha-2b. Predictors of tumour recurrence included **Breslow thickness/Clark level, ulceration and positive SLNB and number of positive nodes at SLNB**. After positive SLNB, patients had a lower rate of recurrence in the nodal basin (after completion), but higher rate of in-transit and distant recurrences, compared with patients with negative SLNB.

Is sentinel node biopsy beneficial in melanoma patients? A report on 200 patients with cutaneous melanoma

Doting MH. *Eur J Surg Oncol* 2002;**28**:673–678.

In this study 200 patients underwent SLNB for stage I/II melanoma and 24% had positive nodes. The results of completion lymphadenectomy showed that risk of positive nodes increased with **tumour thickness**. They postulated reasons for cases of recurrence in the biopsied nodal basin: biological failure (in-transit cells yet to reach nodal basin and advocate introducing time delay between diagnosis and SLNB), technical failure (SLN not correctly identified, wrong node harvested) or pathological failure (metastatic cells not identified within the SLN). The authors conclude that SLNB provides accurate staging and important prognostic information.

Clinical outcome of stage I/II melanoma patients after selective lymph node dissection: long-term follow up results

Vuylsteke RJ. *J Clin Oncol* 2003;**21**:1057–1065.

This is a 5-year follow-up study of 209 patients following SLNB with or without completion lymphadenectomy. Forty had a positive sentinel node (19%) and of these, none had regional node recurrence but 32% developed in-transit recurrence and 22.5% developed systemic disease. Compared with those with negative SLNB, there was a higher rate of nodal recurrence but lower incidence of in-transit and distant disease. The overall survival at 5 years was 92% in SLN-negative compared with 67% in SLN-positive.

Patterns of initial recurrence and prognosis after sentinel node biopsy and selective lymphadenectomy for melanoma

Wagner JD. *Plast Reconstr Surg* 2003;**112**:486–497.

This study from Indianapolis included 408 patients with melanomas > 1 mm that were staged by SLNB (mean thickness 2.8 mm); 20.8% of SLNB were positive, of these 21.4% had positive completion

Table 8.5 Summary of recurrence rates after negative SLNB.

Negative SLNB	Biopsied nodal basin	In-transit	Distant
Gershenwald, 1998	4.1%	5.8%	7.4%
Essner, 1999	4.8%	2.6%	4.0%
Clary, 2001	4.4%	2.8%	5.6%
Chao, 2002	0.4%	1%	2.7%
Wagner, 2003	2%	5%	5.9%
Doting, 2002		4%	
Estourgie, 2003	6%	7%	12%
Vuylsteke, 2003	2.4%	6.5%	4.8%
Topping, 2004	2%	0.7%	2.8%

lymphadenectomy. They reported a false-negative rate of 4.5%. Compared with SLN-negative patients, SLN-positive patients are **more likely to experience distant recurrence**.

Review and evaluation of sentinel node procedures in 250 melanoma patients with a median follow-up of 6 years
Estourgie SH. *Ann Surg Oncol* 2003;**10**:681–688.

This is a single institution review from the Netherlands. Their patients had a mean Breslow thickness of 2.7 mm and 24% had a positive SLNB – they were at high risk of in-transit metastases (23%) or distant disease (42%) within the follow-up period. Sentinel node positivity confirmed as a poor prognostic indicator: disease-free survival was better for SLNB-negative than for SLNB-positive (80% at 5 years vs. 53%). Minor local wound complications and mild limb oedema occurred in about 9%.

VI. Axillary dissection

The guidelines are that radical nodal dissections should only be performed by those who do a minimum of 15 cases a year of axillary and groin dissections for skin cancer.

- The risk of locoregional recurrence is 16–32% despite radical surgery.

Anatomy

The axilla contains the axillary artery, axillary vein, lymph nodes and brachial plexus.

- Floor: axillary fascia.
- Anterior wall: pectoralis major, pectoralis minor, subclavius and clavipectoral fascia.

- Posterior wall: subscapularis, teres major, tendon of latissimus dorsi.
- Medial wall: serratus anterior.
- Lateral wall: the intertubercular sulcus of the humerus.
- Apex: outlet/inlet bounded by outer edge of first rib medially, clavicle anteriorly and scapula posteriorly.

Axillary artery

There are three parts to the artery relative to the pectoralis minor muscle, with the second part behind the muscle which arises from the third, fourth and fifth ribs to insert into the coracoid process and assists serratus in protraction of the scapula but is of no great functional significance.

- Superior thoracic artery arises from the first part which is superior to the muscle.
- From the second part, are the thoraco-acromial and lateral thoracic arteries (follows inferior border of pectoralis minor lying on the fascia investing serratus anterior). This part of the artery is clasped by the cords of the brachial plexus.
- Third part: subscapular artery (largest branch) which runs down the posterior axillary wall and divides into the circumflex scapular and the thoracodorsal arteries, and the medial and lateral circumflex humeral arteries.

The **axillary vein** lies on the medial side of the axillary artery in the apex of the axilla and is not invested by the fascia projected off the paravertebral fascia – the axillary sheath, and hence is free to expand. It receives the cephalic vein in its first part (above pectoralis minor).

Lymph nodes

There are between 35 and 50 in number that are arbitrarily divided into surgical groups I, II and III, lying lateral, beneath and medial to the pectoralis minor respectively.

Anatomical groups

- **Anterior** (pectoral) – medial wall of axilla, along the lateral thoracic artery at the lower border of pectoralis minor, drain the majority of the breast (level I).
- **Posterior** (subscapular) – medial wall of axilla in its posterior part, along the subscapular artery, drain the posterior trunk and tail of the breast (level I).

- **Lateral** – along the medial side of the axillary vein, drain the upper limb (level II).
- **Central** – within the fat of the axilla, receive lymph from all the above groups (level II).
- **Apical** – at the apex of the axilla, receive lymph from all the above groups (level III).

Brachial plexus; nerves in the axilla

- **Long thoracic nerve C5, 6, 7.** It emerges from the posterior aspect of nerve roots to lie posterior to the mid-axillary line where it lies upon and supplies serratus anterior.
- **Thoracodorsal nerve C6, 7, 8.** From the posterior cord, the nerve runs down the posterior axillary wall closely related to the subscapular artery and enters latissimus dorsi on its deep surface.
- **Intercostobrachial nerve.** This is the lateral cutaneous branch of the second (occasionally third) intercostal nerve that supplies an area on the medial aspect of the upper arm.
- **Lateral pectoral nerve C6, 7, 8.** Arising from the lateral cord, it crosses the axillary vein to enter the deep surface of the pectoralis minor, and then through to the pectoralis major – positioned more medial to the medial pectoral nerve.

Technique

- A skin flap is raised with an inverted U-shaped incision with the arm in abduction and the fat is **swept off the pectoralis major**, continuing on its deep surface whilst taking care to preserve the lateral pectoral nerve.
- The arm is then flexed to relax the pectoralis major and allow access to the apex of the axilla and the **pectoralis minor** (**dividing** its insertion).
- The fat is **dissected off the axillary vein**, following it from medial to lateral, tying off tributaries. The specimen is swept downwards and off the medial wall of the axilla, preserving the long thoracic nerve anteriorly and the thoracodorsal nerve and subscapular artery posteriorly.

Nodes in level I–III should be included in the dissection specimen.

VII. Groin dissection

Anatomy

Femoral triangle

The boundaries of the femoral triangle include the inguinal ligament superiorly, the medial border of sartorius laterally and the medial border of adductor longus medially i.e. a small triangle. The gutter-shaped floor is formed by pectineus, psoas and iliacus (from medial to lateral). The femoral sheath containing the femoral vessels (artery in lateral compartment, vein in intermediate) lies in this gutter but the nerve is lateral to and outside the sheath. In the medial compartment of the femoral sheath is the femoral canal, which allows dilatation of the medially placed vein as well as transmitting lymphatics from the deep inguinal nodes to the iliac nodes. Cloquet's node lies in the femoral canal and drains lymph of the clitoris/glans penis.

Femoral artery, vein and nerve

The **femoral artery** has four branches in the thigh, arising just below the level of the inguinal ligament:

- Superficial circumflex iliac.
- Superficial epigastric.
- Superficial external pudendal.
- Deep external pudendal.

The profunda femoris artery comes off the femoral artery just beneath the distal edge of the femoral sheath, passing medially deep to adductor longus. The (superficial) femoral artery passes into subsartorial canal (adductor/Hunter's, along with the vein and the saphenous nerve) to emerge as the popliteal artery in the popliteal fossa.

The **femoral vein** receives four tributaries corresponding to the arterial branches as above plus the long saphenous vein.

The **femoral nerve** gives off:

- Muscular branches to the extensor compartment of the thigh.
- Sensory branches: intermediate and medial cutaneous nerves of the thigh.
- Saphenous nerve.

Other nerves that are nearby include:

- Lateral cutaneous nerve of the thigh, which passes deep to the inguinal ligament at the origin of sartorius at the lateral upper corner of the femoral triangle.
- Femoral branch of the genitofemoral nerve (L1), which pierces the femoral sheath to supply the skin overlying the femoral triangle.

Lymphatics and lymph nodes

Lymphatics accompany the long saphenous vein. The superficial inguinal nodes include:

- Vertical group along the termination of the long saphenous vein drains the leg.
- Lateral group below the lateral inguinal ligament drains the buttocks, flank, etc.
- Medial group below the medial part of the inguinal ligament drains the anterior abdominal wall below the umbilicus and the perineum.
- Deep inguinal nodes lie medial to the femoral vein and communicate with superficial nodes via the cribriform fascia at the saphenous opening.

Technique

The patient is positioned with the hip extended, slightly abducted and externally rotated. There are various types of skin incision described, each with their pros and cons. In general, vertically orientated incisions allow wider access particularly if a deeper/higher dissection is needed but skin flap necrosis may be a problem; whilst horizontal incisions parallel to the inguinal ligament have better vascularity, access is more limited.

For vertical incisions, begin 5 cm above the inguinal ligament, two-thirds along its length from the pubic tubercle and curve down to the inferior apex of the femoral triangle. Flaps are raised to include the fascia to reduce wound necrosis/breakdown. Fat is cleared to the margins of the femoral triangle working from above infero-laterally; some recommended tying off of the lower portions of the dissection rather than using diathermy to reduce lymph leak. 'Sartorius switch' procedure to cover the femoral vessels is recommended by many surgeons and two large drains are commonly used.

Whilst other superficial vessels are usually sacrificed during a groin dissection, the superficial circumflex iliac and deep external pudendal arteries are usually preserved as they lie deeper along the floor of the femoral triangle, and this may help reduce skin necrosis.

Complications of lymphadenectomy

- Intra-operative – accidental damage to vessels and nerves.
- Early post-operative – skin necrosis, dehiscence, infection, seroma, DVT/PE.
- Late post-operative – numbness and dysaesthesia, lymphoedema, hernia.

Superficial vs. radical inguinal node dissection

- **Inguinal node clearance** includes the femoral triangle up to inguinal ligament, also called superficial inguinal node dissection.
- **Iliac node clearance** includes the iliac and obturator nodes up to bifurcation of common iliac artery (or further up to aortic bifurcation if nodes clinically enlarged), and is also called deep or extended dissections.

Patients with deep inguinal (iliac) nodes have a poor prognosis with a high likelihood of distant disease, and iliac node dissection may significantly increase morbidity particularly of lymphoedema. The data are conflicting on the survival benefit following radical clearance of deep nodes.

The risk of pelvic nodes is about 36–40% if there is gross inguinal disease, whilst it is 14–19% if there is microscopic inguinal disease. Some others prefer to predict the likelihood of pelvic nodes using either Cloquet node histology (79% risk of pelvic node if positive) or the number of inguinal nodes (12% for 1–3 nodes compared with 44% for more than three positive superficial nodes).

There is more debate over groin dissections than for the axilla and current guidelines recommend a pelvic dissection in those with:

- More than one clinically palpable inguinal node.
- CT or ultrasound evidence of more than one inguinal node or of pelvic node involvement.
- More than one microscopically involved node at SLNB.
- A conglomerate of inguinal or femoral triangle lymph nodes.
- Microscopic or macroscopic involvement of Cloquet's node (level III, grade B).

Superficial inguinal and radical ilioinguinal lymph node dissection in patients with palpable melanoma metastases to the groin
Kretschmer L. *Acta Oncol* 2001;**40**:72–78.

Thirty-five per cent of 69 patients undergoing extended clearance had positive iliac nodes which correlated with a significant increase in mortality compared with iliac node negative patients (5-year survival 6% vs. 37%). As there was **no difference in overall survival** between extended and superficial dissection groups, on this basis the authors recommend that unless there is evidence for pelvic nodal disease, a superficial node clearance is preferred.

Prognosis and surgical management of patients with palpable inguinal lymph node metastases from melanoma
Hughes TM. *Br J Surg* 2000;**87**:892–901.

Table 8.6 Summary of recurrence rates after positive SLNB.

		Recurrence		
	Positive SLNB rate	Biopsied nodal basin	In-transit	Distant
Essner, 1999	15.7%	12%	10%	16.7%
Clary, 2001	17%	5.4%	12.5%	17.9%
Chao, 2002	20%	0.4%	2%	10.3%
Doting, 2002	24%		8%	
Estourgie, 2003	24%	8%	23%	42%
Vuylsteke, 2003	19%	0%	32%	22.5%
Wagner, 2003	20.8%	4.7%	9.4%	16.5%
Leiter U. *Ann Surg Oncol* 2010;**17**:129–137.	11.2%	7.3%	8.3%	5.5%

Retrospective analysis of 132 patients showed that the presence of pelvic node metastases reduced 5-year survival from 47% (iliac node negative) to 19% (iliac node positive). Other prognostic factors were extracapsular spread and number of positive superficial nodes. There was **no significant increase in morbidity** following extended dissections in comparison with superficial lymphadenectomy, whilst providing additional prognostic information and optimal regional control.

Pelvic lymph node dissection is beneficial in subsets of patients with node-positive melanoma
Badgwell B. *Ann Surg Oncol* 2007;**14**:2867–2875.

The benefit of deep pelvic LND (DLND) continues to be debated. This study from the M. D. Anderson Cancer Center reviewed the records of 332 patients (235 underwent SLND, 97 underwent combined SLND and DLND). They found that age ≥ 50 years, number of positive superficial nodes and positive imaging, were predictors of deep nodes. The 5-year survival was 51% for those with negative deep nodes vs. 42% for positive deep nodes. The overall survival of those with three or fewer deep nodes (treated) was comparable to those with no deep nodes and the authors suggest that deep pelvic disease should be classed as stage III and not stage IV (distant) disease. Those with risks factors for deep node involvement may benefit selectively from a combined node dissection.

VIII. Distant metastasis

Imaging and investigations of stage III/IV melanoma

Current British Association of Dermatologist guidelines are:

- Stage III – CT head, chest, abdomen and pelvis will adequately exclude metastases in most cases and is most useful in stage III disease before planning a regional node dissection or regional chemotherapy.
- Stage IV – CT of the head and whole body when stage IV disease is suspected; PET/CT potentially increases yield but is unlikely to be clinically relevant (level III, grade D) – except where metastectomy is planned and a PET/CT may exclude other disease that may make such surgery inappropriate.

There is no indication for bone scans in the absence of bone symptoms.

Management of metastatic disease

- Surgery can be considered for metastatic disease in sites such as skin, bowel or brain, or to prevent pain or ulceration.
- Dacarbazine is the chemotherapy agent of choice but is largely palliative (level II, grade B).
- Radiotherapy may palliate symptomatic metastases.

Regional non-nodal metastases of cutaneous melanoma
Cascinelli N. *Eur J Surg Oncol* 1986;**12**:175–180.

This is a review of 1503 patients with approximately equal distribution into groups who underwent ELND at the same time as excision of the primary lesion, patients who underwent delayed ELND or TLND and patients who did not have nodal surgery. The overall incidence of non-nodal metastasis after excision of a primary melanoma was as high as 19%.

In-transit recurrences occurred in 8.9% of patients who had no nodal surgery compared with 12.5% in patients who had positive nodal disease. There was no significant difference in incidence of post-lymphadenectomy in-transit disease in patients subjected to in-continuity vs. discontinuity dissection. Median survival following the diagnosis of in-transit disease was 30 months; distant disease was diagnosed in 22% of patients at the time of appearance of in-transit disease. The authors conclude from their data that local recurrences, satellites and in-transit metastases are similar and are similar in prognosis to distant skin metastasis.

Metastatic pathways and time courses in the orderly progression of melanoma
Meier F. *Br J Dermatol* 2002;**147**:62–70.

At total of 3001 patients with stage I/II disease were followed for 20 years; 466 patients developed metastases – the first recurrence were satellite or in-transit (21%), regional node (50.2%) and distant metastases (28.1%).

Patients with lower limb primaries were most at risk of developing in-transit disease (31.8%, median interval 17 months) whilst upper limb and trunk primaries were most at risk of developing distant disease as first recurrence (35%, about 25 months). The median time to the development of regional node metastases was 14 months.

- 51.5% of patients with in-transit disease were subsequently diagnosed with systemic disease.
- 20.8% of patients with in-transit disease subsequently developed nodal disease.
- 59% of patients with nodal disease subsequently developed distant disease.

Locoregional cutaneous metastasis in patients with therapeutic lymph node dissection for malignant melanoma: risk factors and prognostic impact
Kretschmer L. *Melanoma Res* 2002;**12**:499–504.

This is a review of 224 patients subjected to axillary or inguinal lymphadenectomy. Sixty-five (29%) developed in-transit metastases during the course of their disease; thicker primaries and lower limb primaries were predictive of the development of in-transit disease.

In patients who developed in-transit disease after nodal or distant recurrence following TLND, the 5-year survival was 0%. Those who developed it before palpable nodes or as first recurrence after TLND had a 5-year survival rate 27–28%.

Management of in-transit metastases from cutaneous malignant melanoma
Hayes AJ. *Br J Surg* 2004;**91**:673–682.

Patients with in-transit metastases are staged with either IIIB or IIIC disease and have a 5-year survival of 18–60%. Treatment of in-transit disease is generally palliative.

- Complete excision (narrow margins acceptable) or carbon dioxide laser therapy.
  - Kandamany N (*Lasers Med Sci* 2009;**24**: 411–414) suggest laser therapy as a first-line therapy and described a subgroup that did not show systemic progression for unknown reasons.
- Isolated limb perfusion with melphalan or dacarbazine with good response rates reported.
- Radiotherapy with 52% response rate reported by Fenig E (*Am J Clin Oncol* 1999;**22**:184–186).
- Chemotherapy for widespread truncal or head and neck in-transit disease, that is not amenable to surgery.
- Amputation is only considered for palliation of fungating disease or exsanguinating haemorrhage.

In general, regional/local techniques are preferable, having better control and reduced operative morbidity, whilst systemic therapy has considerable toxicity and marginal response (Gimbel MI. *Cancer Control* 2008;**15**:225–232).

FDG–PET scanning for staging of melanoma

18F-Fluorodeoxyglucose–positron emission tomography (FDG–PET) is being used increasingly in melanoma. **The threshold for sensitivity seems to be 80 mm^3 of tumour** (Wagner JD. *J Surg Oncol* 2001;**77**:237–242); it detects all nodal metastases ≥ 10 mm in diameter, 83% 6–10 mm in diameter and 23% of those less than 5 mm in diameter (Crippa F. *J Nucl Med* 2000;**41**:1491–1494).

It is neither as sensitive nor as specific as SLNB for nodal metastasis but as it provides a wider area of imaging than CT and MRI, it can detect distant metastasis that may alter patient management. The AJCC recognizes the useful of FDG–PET as a staging tool in selected patients with recurrent or metastatic disease (stage III/IV) but the bulk of literature does not support its role for stage I/II.

Fluorodeoxyglucose-positron emission tomography and sentinel lymph node biopsy in staging primary cutaneous melanoma
Havenga K. *Eur J Surg Oncol* 2003;**29**:662–664.

FDG-PET was compared with SLNB in staging 55 patients with primary cutaneous melanoma > 1.0 mm thickness and no palpable regional lymph nodes. FDG–PET scan was performed before SLNB.

SLNs were retrieved in 53 patients and metastases were found in 13 patients; FDG–PET detected the metastases in two of these 13 and the explanation was that SLN biopsy reveals regional metastases that are too small to be detected by FDG–PET.

However, in some patients FDG accumulation was recorded in a regional lymph node basin where the SLNB was negative (five) and increased activity at a site of possible distant metastasis (eight) with metastatic disease confirmed in only one patient. No explanation for the positive FDG–PET result could be found in five cases.

They conclude that FDG-PET should **not** be considered in patients with primary cutaneous melanoma ≥ 1.0 mm Breslow thickness, and no palpable regional lymph nodes. They suggest that it may be of value in stage III, IV or for patients with recurrent melanoma.

The role of fluorine-18 deoxyglucose positron emission tomography in the management of patients with metastatic melanoma: impact on surgical decision making
Gulec SA. *Nucl Med* 2003;**28**:961–965.

Forty-nine patients with known or suspected **metastatic** melanoma underwent extent-of-disease evaluation using CT of the chest, abdomen and pelvis, and MRI of the brain. After formulation of an initial treatment plan, patients underwent FDG–PET imaging and more metastatic sites were identified in 27 of 49 patients (55%). In six of these, PET detected disease outside the fields of CT and MRI. Forty-four of the 51 lesions that were resected were confirmed to be melanoma. All lesions larger than 1 cm were positive on PET whilst 2 of 15 lesions smaller than 1 cm were detected. **The results of PET led to treatment changes in 24 patients (49%).**

The authors suggest that FDG-PET provides a more accurate assessment than conventional imaging in patients with **metastatic carcinoma**.

Clinical applications of fluorodeoxyglucose-positron emission tomography in the management of malignant melanoma
Kumar R. *Curr Opin Oncol* 2005;**17**:154–159.

False-negatives may arise due to micrometastases or lesions smaller than 10 mm whilst false-positives may be due to inflammation related to surgery, other inflammatory conditions or benign tumours. The authors

conclude that although it is non-invasive and more sensitive than CT for detecting metastases, particularly in unusual sites, it is of limited use in early stage (I/II) disease and those with small metastases in lung/brain. It **cannot replace SNLB** for detecting node disease.

F-18 fluorodeoxy-D-glucose positron emission tomography scans in the initial evaluation of patients with a primary melanoma thicker than 4 mm
Maubec E. *Melanoma Res* 2007;**17**:147–154.

This is a prospective study in 25 patients newly diagnosed with T4 melanomas who had FDG-PET as well as SLNB in those without palpable nodes. After correlation of results, they found that the scan detected 1 of 6 primary melanomas, 0 of 6 nodal micrometastases, 4 of 4 nodal macrometastases (palpable) and no distant metastases. FDG-PET also led to an unnecessary node dissection i.e. false-positive and three other sites of false-positive distant metastasis. They conclude that **PET is not useful for the initial work-up** of patients with melanoma, even for thick lesions.

Adjuvant therapy

Radiotherapy

Radiotherapy is not part of the traditional treatment approach to melanoma. Survival gains from adjuvant radiotherapy may be limited because patients with involved nodes usually die from distant metastasis. A review of the literature by Ballo MT (*Surg Clin North Am* 2003;**83**:323–342) suggests that there is a possible role for radiotherapy in certain situations including as primary treatment for large facial lentigo maligna melanoma in the elderly, and as adjuvant therapy in certain groups at high risk of recurrence e.g. desmoplastic tumours, thick tumours and after therapeutic neck dissection. It may also be indicated for palliation of metastatic disease.

Is adjuvant radiotherapy necessary after positive neck dissection in head and neck melanomas?
Shen P. *Ann Surg Oncol* 2000;**7**:554–559.

This is a retrospective review of 217 patients undergoing positive neck dissection (80% therapeutic and 20% positive elective); the majority of patients in this study did not receive radiotherapy. Fourteen per cent developed recurrence in the dissected nodal basin with extracapsular spread being the strongest predictor. A similar proportion of recurrence was found in those who received post-operative radiotherapy but the numbers were insufficient for statistical analysis. The authors suggest, with caveats, that there is **no role** for **routine** adjuvant radiotherapy unless there is widespread extracapsular spread.

Survival and prognostic factors in patients with brain metastases from malignant melanoma
Meier S. *Onkologie* 2004;**27**:145–149.

This is a retrospective review of the factors influencing survival in 100 patients with brain melanoma treated between 1966 and 2002. The overall median survival time was 4.8 months. Multivariate analysis demonstrated that aside from tumour thickness, radiotherapy (partial and whole brain), chemotherapy and especially surgery and stereotactic radiosurgery significantly prolong survival.

A multi-institutional retrospective analysis of external radiotherapy for mucosal melanoma of the head and neck in Northern Japan
Wada H. *Int J Radiat Oncol Biol Phys* 2004; **59**:495–500.

This is a multi-institutional retrospective study of the efficacy of external radiotherapy as the **definitive treatment** modality for localized mucosal melanoma of the head and neck in 31 patients. Radiotherapy alone was performed in 21 patients whilst 10 received adjuvant radiotherapy for gross post-resectional disease – the total dosages were 32–64 Gy (median 50 Gy) with a fraction size 1.5–13.8 Gy.

- Complete response in 9/31 patients and partial response in 18/31 patients. Most incidences of local recurrence and distant metastasis developed within 2 years. Age the only significant prognostic factor by multivariate analysis.
- Radiotherapy provided no significant locoregional control or survival benefit in patients with gross post-resectional disease.

The authors concluded that **local control** is achievable using radiotherapy at a dose of 3 Gy or more per fraction in patients with localized mucosal melanoma of the head and neck. This was most beneficial in younger patients and the authors could not explain this.

Immunotherapy

Immunotherapy is using the patient's own immune system, directly or indirectly, to act against the melanoma; the major use is to reduce recurrence after surgery (including metastasectomy) in those who are at risk. Many have been promising and have subsequently fallen from favour e.g. Canvaxin (produced from whole tumour cells) and antibody to GM2.

- **Interferon α (IFN α) and interleukin-2 (IL-2)** (aldesleukin) are the most studied. (Riker AI. *Expert Opin Bio Ther* 2007;**7**:345–358).
  - Meta-analysis of phase III trials has concluded that IFN α reduces recurrence by 26% and improves survival by 15% (NS, P = 0.06) (Wheatley K. *Cancer Treat Rev* 2003;**29**: 241–252). The small benefit needs to be weighed against the significant side-effects and cost. IFN α-2b was given **FDA approval** in 1995 as immunotherapy for IIB/III melanoma.
  - IL-2 is **FDA-approved** (1998) as immunotherapy for metastatic melanoma, and has a low but consistent response rate of 13–17%; optimal dosage regimes have not been determined and there is no way to predict which patients will or will not respond.
- Vaccines are largely experimental.
  - Antibody to CTLA-4 (cytotoxic T-lymphocyte associated antigen 4; the antibody blocks this to potentiate antitumour T-cell response) – **Ipilimumab**. Recent phase III trial with 676 patients with inoperable metastatic disease demonstrates that it increases 2-year survival from 14% to 24% (Hodi FS. *New Eng J Med* 10.1056/ NEJMoa1003466, published online 5 June 2010).

Interferon α-2b adjuvant therapy of high-risk resected cutaneous melanoma: the Eastern Cooperative Oncology Group Trial EST 1684
Kirkwood JM. *J Clin Oncol* 1996;**14**:7–17.

This reported on the results of a trial of maximum-dose interferon α-2b in patients with T4 primary melanoma or regional nodal disease (N1 – 1 node either microscopically or macroscopically involved) and compared with observation only in a total patient group of 287. The median follow-up was 6.9 years.

The conclusion was that high-dose IFN α-2b prolongs the relapse-free interval and overall survival in high-risk resected melanoma patients.

High- and low-dose interferon α-2b in high-risk melanoma: first analysis of intergroup trial E1690/ S9111/C9190
Kirkwood JM. *J Clin Oncol* 2000;**18**:2444–2458.

A total of 642 patients were enrolled in to three treatment arms following resection of high-risk (IIB/ III) melanoma (608 eligible).

- High-dose IFN α-2b for 1 year (HDI).
- Low-dose IFN α-2b for 2 years (LDI).
- Observation.

The 5-year relapse-free survival with IFN α-2b (44% high dose, 40% low dose) was better than no treatment (35%) but there was no overall survival benefit.

Adjuvant interferon in high-risk melanoma: the AIM HIGH Study
Hancock BW. *J Clin Oncol* 2004;**22**:53–61.

This was a randomized controlled trial involving 674 patients evaluating low-dose extended-duration interferon α-2a as adjuvant therapy in patients with thick (> or = 4 mm) primary cutaneous melanoma and/or locoregional metastases and those with radically resected stage IIB and stage III disease. The interferon was given at 3 megaunits 3 times per week for 2 years or until recurrence.

The overall survival and recurrence-free survival were 44% and 32%, respectively and **not** significantly different from control. Interferon-related toxicities were modest including fatigue or mood disturbance in 7% and 4%, respectively; there were 50 withdrawals (15%) due to toxicity. The authors concluded that extended-duration low-dose interferon is **no better** than observation alone in the initial treatment of completely resected high-risk malignant melanoma.

Adjuvant therapy with pegylated interferon alfa-2b versus observation in resected stage III melanoma
Bottomley A. *J Clin Oncol* 2009;**27**:2916–2923.

This trial recruited 1256 patients with stage III melanoma post-lymphadenectomy, randomized to either observation or pegylated (PEG) IFN α-2b, and a standardized quality-of-life questionnaire was used. After a median follow-up period of 3.8 years, for the primary end point of recurrence-free survival (RFS), risk was reduced by 18% in the treatment arm (a significant improvement) but there was a negative effect on health-related quality of life (HRQOL; key factors were social functioning, appetite loss and fatigue).

Some authors (Janku F. *J Clin Oncol* 2010;**28**: e15–16) feel that that the price in terms of side-effects and reduced quality of life is too high. Adjuvant interferon does not reduce the overall risk of recurrence or death, but **may delay disease recurrence in a small subset** (many for less than a year). Thus if a patient is destined to die of melanoma, interferon may delay it for only a short while but with significant side-effects.

Current BAD 2010 guidelines do not recommend interferon as standard of care for adjuvant treatment of primary or stage III melanoma (level Ia, grade A) as the effect on disease-free survival is small and of uncertain clinical significance and it has significant toxicity.

Sentinel-node technique will change design of clinical trials in malignant melanoma
Kretschmer L. *J Clin Oncol* 2002;**20**:2208.

Microscopic nodal staging is necessary in order to compare treatment outcomes in adjuvant therapy trials. In analysing a heterogeneous group of high-risk patients with clinically negative nodes (T4N0M0) **without node surgery**, some patients may have micrometastases (N1a or N2a disease) while others may have true N0 disease but the former group will have a worse prognosis compared with the latter group of patients. Thus unequal distribution of these patients into cohorts comparing treatment vs. observation will affect results. This criticism was levelled at the E1684 trial.

Systemic chemotherapy

Chemotherapy can be given as single agent or in combination; however there is little evidence for any survival benefit in patients with disseminated disease.

Dacarbazine

This is the most commonly used drug for advanced disease and is the **only FDA-approved** chemotherapy treatment for melanoma. It causes tumour shrinkage in 15–20% for 6 months before tumours resume growth; to date it has **not** been shown to significantly prolong survival (indeed some authors have commented that it also has not been shown not to shorten survival).

Combination regimes (e.g. Dartmouth or CVD) have not been shown to be significantly more effective than dacarbazine alone but have more side-effects.

Temozolomide

This is a well-tolerated oral alkylating agent with activity in the CNS (Agarwala SS. *J Clin Oncol* 2004;**22**: 2101–2107). Overall, the early promise has not been borne out by more recent trials.

Randomized phase III study of temozolomide versus dacarbazine in the treatment of patients with advanced metastatic malignant melanoma
Middleton MR. *J Clin Oncol* 2000;**18**:158–166.

This study included 305 patients with advanced metastatic melanoma. Temozolomide was as effective as dacarbazine (7.7 months median survival vs. 6.4 for dacarbazine), was easy to administer and was associated with greater improvements in some QOL domains.

Extended schedule, escalated dose temozolomide versus dacarbazine in stage IV malignant melanoma
Patel P. 33rd ESMO Congress 2008 Abstract LBA8.

The EORTC 18032 trial included 859 patients with stage IV melanoma. Temozolomide showed better overall response compared with dacarbazine (14.4% vs. 9.8%) but progression-free survival was very similar as was median overall survival. The recommendation seems to be to **consider temozolomide** in patients with poor venous access, liver failure or asymptomatic brain metastases, if cost is not an issue.

Isolated limb perfusion

Isolated limb perfusion (ILP) is a regional administration of high-dose chemotherapeutics and can be used for locally advanced disease. The main agent used is **melphalan**, but alternatives include cisplatin and recombinant TNF-α. It requires general anaesthesia and mild hyperthermia (38–43 °C); a pump oxygenator is used to perfuse Ringer's lactate and 95% O_2 and 5% CO_2 with drugs added at ~200–400 ml/min. Catheters are placed via direct arteriotomy and venotomy; at the end of the procedure, the toxic levels of treatment solution is flushed out with 1 unit of blood and the vessels are repaired. Complications include: death, amputation and life-threatening leukopenia, all < 1%; it is conventional to avoid synchronous lymphadenectomy.

- A treatment regime of TNF + melphalan + IF-γ yields a complete response rate of 90%.
- Elective ILP for melanomas of 1.5–3.0 mm demonstrates a locoregional control advantage but no survival benefit.
- Reduces local recurrence rate of subungual melanoma but does not influence survival.
- Prophylactic ILP with melphalan offers no benefits (Koops HS. *J Clin Oncol* 1998;**16**:2906–2912).

Management of in-transit melanoma of the extremity with isolated limb perfusion
Fraker DL. *Curr Treat Options Oncol* 2004;**5**:173–184.

A limited number of in-transit metastases (1–3 nodules) can be managed by simple surgical excision with minimal negative margins (no role for wide excision) plus staging of distant disease. Indications for isolated limb perfusion (ILP) include:

- Rapidly recurrent in-transit disease.
- Disease out of local surgical control.

Isolated limb perfusion was continued for 60–90 minutes within an extremity using an extracorporeal circuit whilst the limb was heated to mild hyperthermia (38.5–40 °C); at the end of treatment, the limb was flushed from the extremity and normal perfusion was re-established. Typical treatment regimens use melphalan at 10 mg/l limb volume for lower extremities (13 mg/l limb volume for upper extremities).

The authors report response rates between 80% and 90% though complete response rates are lower, between 55% and 65%. Between 20% and 25% of the total patient population have sustained complete responses, typically 9 to 12 months. Side-effects include skin erythema, myopathy and peripheral neuropathy.

Regional isolated limb perfusion of extremities for melanoma: a 20-year experience with drugs other than L-phenylalanine mustard
Ariyan S. *Plast Reconstr Surg* 1997;**99**:1023–1029.

In this study, the authors reported on 43 patients treated with therapeutic ILP for in-transit/local recurrences (a few patients had several perfusions, lower limb 4× more than upper) whilst 17 were treated prophylactically for high-risk melanoma. Isolated limb perfusion was performed with a pump oxygenator for 1 hour using non-melphalan drugs including DTIC, cisplatin and carboplatin. The overall complication rate was 21% including oedema (permanent in 11), seroma, dehiscence, infection and pulmonary embolism (non-fatal). There were no reports of systemic toxicity.

- 11 patients alive and disease free at ~5 years (median figure).
- 12 of the 17 patients treated prophylactically were alive and disease free at ~6.5 years.

Their conclusion was that non-toxic drug alternatives to melphalan enable safe palliation and achieve good locoregional control.

Isolated limb infusion

Isolated limb infusion (ILI) is essentially a low-flow ILP performed without oxygenation via percutaneous catheters. Under LA and sedation, contralateral limb vessels are cannulated under radiological guidance and with the tips sited in the affected limb, the therapeutic agents are infused manually for > 15–20 min. It is considered to have the same efficacy as ILP but with reduced side-effects and may be the preferred option in the future.

Prognostic factors after isolated limb infusion with cytotoxic agents for melanoma
Lindner P. *Ann Surg Oncol* 2002;**9**:127–136.

In 135 patients treated by ILI, the overall response rate in the treated limb was 85% (complete and partial response rates 41% and 44%) with the median response duration 16 months and median patient survival 34 months. In those with a complete response, this was 24 and 42 months respectively. Overall, patients aged > 70 years had a better response than younger patients. Other factors associated with an improved outcome were:

- Earlier stage of disease.
- Final limb temperature > 37.8 °C.
- Tourniquet time > 40 minutes.

The conclusion was that the frequency and duration of responses after ILI were comparable to those achieved by conventional ILP. The ILI technique is particularly useful for older patients who might not be considered suitable for conventional ILP.

Isolated limb infusion for melanoma: a simple alternative to isolated limb perfusion
Mian R. *Can J Surg* 2001;**44**:189–192.

Nine patients were treated with ILI for extensive in-transit limb melanoma. There were no peri-operative deaths but one patient had deep venous thrombosis and pulmonary embolism. Control of in-transit metastases was achieved to some degree in all patients and the response was complete in four patients. The conclusion was that ILI provides effective palliation in patients suffering from multiple, advanced in-transit melanoma metastases with limited morbidity and a safe, quick, inexpensive alternative to isolated limb perfusion with comparable results.

Melanoma and pregnancy

Current management of patients with melanoma who are pregnant, want to get pregnant or do not want to get pregnant
Schwartz JL. *Cancer* 2003;**97**:2130–2133.

The prognostic factors for pregnant patients are the same as for non-pregnant patients (sentinel node status, tumour thickness and ulceration). SLNB may be performed as radiation doses involved (5 milli-Grays (mGy) exposure to the fetus) are far below levels known to induce fetal malformation (100 mGy), but **the risk of anaphylaxis to isosulfan blue** may preclude its use. Transplacental metastases are extremely rare (19 cases reported) so termination is not indicated although histological evaluation of the placenta is recommended.

Patients with melanoma who want to get pregnant are advised that it is important to avoid the development of metastatic disease during pregnancy and advice is therefore related to the prognostic indicators of the primary tumour. Patients with low-risk lesions may be advised to wait longer than patients with high-risk lesions (e.g. 5 years from diagnosis). Patients with a poor prognosis tumour are also advised to consider the effect of losing a mother in early childhood.

There is no evidence to show that either the oral contraceptive pill or hormone replacement therapy adversely affects outcome in melanoma patients.

Pregnancy and early stage melanoma
Daryanani D. *Cancer* 2003;**97**:2248–2253.

Age- and stage-matched pregnant and non-pregnant controls showed similar 10-year disease-free survival and overall survival. Contrary to popular belief, growth or change in **pre-existing naevi** during pregnancy is uncommon and should be treated as suspicious by expedient biopsy.

Malignant melanoma and hormone replacement therapy
Jeffrey SLA. *Br J Plast Surg* 2000;**53**:539–542.

This short review of studies from Sweden and Denmark confirmed the conclusions of a previous review (Franceschi S. *Tumori* 1990;**76**:439–449) i.e. no identifiable increased risk with HRT, thus female melanoma patients should continue with HRT where indicated.

Melanoma in children

Classification of pre-pubertal melanoma:

- Congenital melanoma acquired through transplacental spread.
- Melanoma arising *de novo*.
- Melanoma arising in **giant congenital naevi**.

Cutaneous malignant melanoma in children and adolescents in Scotland, 1979–1991
Naasan A. *Plast Reconstr Surg* 1996;**98**:442–446.

Only 1% (50) of the 4700 cases of melanoma in Scotland in the study period have occurred in patients under 18 years (male:female = 2.5:1), with 15 in the pre-pubertal age range (< 14 years) with equal sex distribution. Nine developed metastatic disease (all lesions were > 1.5 mm thick), and eight died with maximum survival of 4 years. Half had a reliable history and one-third of these (eight) described a pre-existing naevus. The disease behaves similarly in children as in adults and the treatment should be the same; errors in diagnosis may occur due to histological similarity with Spitz naevi.

Cutaneous malignant melanoma in the young
Zhu N. *Br J Plast Surg* 1997;**50**:10–14.

Forty-seven of 3246 (1.4%) melanoma patients (1967–1993 at Frenchay Hospital) were < 21 years with female:male = 2:1. Ten were pre-adolescent (< 14 years). The vast majority (83%) were SSM; 4% nodular, 2% acral lentiginous and the remainder unclassified. Sixteen arose in pre-existing naevi (but none in giant congenital melanocytic naevus). The authors concluded that SSM is much more common than other subtypes in the young.

Non-cutaneous melanoma

These are uncommon (2%); they usually present late and have a poor prognosis. More common subtypes include mucosal and ocular melanoma.

Anorectal melanoma

Anorectal melanoma is an uncommon aggressive tumour with poor prognosis (less than 20% 5-year survival) and early metastatic spread. Melanoma accounts for < 1% of all anorectal malignant tumours and patients usually present in the fifth–sixth decade with rectal bleeding that may be mistaken for haemorrhoidal bleed, pain and a palpable mass. 20% of lesions are amelanotic.

Abdominoperineal resection (APR) may improve local control but not overall survival, it is only indicated for bulky disease where local excision transgresses tumour.

Sphincter-sparing local excision and adjuvant radiotherapy for anal–rectal melanoma
Ballo MT. *J Clin Oncol* 2002;**20**:4555–4558.

In this study, 23 patients with anorectal melanoma (median primary tumour thickness 5 mm) were managed by local excision and radiotherapy (hypofractionated regimen of 30 Gy, 5 fractions over 2.5 weeks). Fifteen died from melanoma within a median follow-up period of 32 months. The actuarial 5-year local control was 74% (nodal control 84%) – no patient had locoregional failure as the only site of failure. The actuarial 5-year disease-specific survival was 31%. The authors conclude that sphincter-sparing local excision with adjuvant radiotherapy is well tolerated and reduces the morbidity of APR whilst effectively providing local control.

Surgical management of primary anorectal melanoma
Pessaux P. *Br J Surg* 2004;**91**:1183–1187.

This review of 40 patients demonstrated no difference in overall survival between patients treated by wide local excision or by APR, hence the former is recommended. The median overall survival was 17 months.

Management of anorectal melanomas: a 10-year review
David AW. *Trop Gastroenterol* 2007;**28**:76–78.

This study reviewed the results of 17 patients. One had inoperable disease at presentation whilst four had metastatic disease. Ten had APR whilst two had wide local excision; the stage-specific disease-free survival and overall survival were 8 vs. 10 months and 13 vs. 27 months respectively. The authors confirm that wide local excision is preferred when complete excision with negative margins can be achieved.

Outpatient follow-up
Recurrence of thin melanoma: how effective is follow-up?
Moloney D. *Br J Plast Surg* 1996;**49**:409–413.

A total of 602 patients were followed for a minimum of 5 years following excision of thin primary lesions < 0.76 mm. There was recurrence in 14 within 5 years with mean time to recurrence of ~4.5 years. **Only 5/14 were treatable** (1% of all patients) including a need for TLND.

- In four of the five treatable cases, treatment resulted in survival beyond 5 years and all of them presented within 2 years of primary excision.
- The other nine patients with recurrence returned with disseminated disease.

After 5 years there were a further 10 recurrences (4 treatable and 6 non-treatable), but none survived > 10 years. Hence, total number of recurrences was 24/602 (4%). Their conclusion was that as the **treatable** recurrences were all detected **within 2 years of primary excision**, the need for continued follow-up beyond this point can be debated.

There is currently no consensus for follow-up, and little in the way of evidence to support one practice over another. The BAPS/BADS guidelines are:

- *In situ* disease – discharge.
- <1 mm – 3 years at 3/12.
- >1 mm – 3 years at 3/12, 2 years at 6/12 and then discharge after 5 years.

Multiple primary melanomas: data and significance
Ariyan S. *Plast Reconstr Surg* 1995;**96**:1384–1389.

It is demonstrated that 5% will develop a second primary i.e. histologically confirmed not to be in-transit metastases or satellite lesions. This was a 10-year review of the Yale Melanoma Unit with 423 patients. It found that 22 developed a second primary whilst five developed three (several were those with multiple dysplastic naevi). In 30% this occurred within 1 month and was considered to be synchronous. First primaries were between 0.2 and 6.0 mm thick but all subsequent primaries were *in situ* or < 1 mm (which the authors suggested may be due to earlier diagnosis or some altered host immune response). The patient's **prognosis is related to the thickness of the thickest lesion** and thus developing more than one melanoma does not necessarily change the prognosis.

C. Non-melanoma skin cancer

I. Risk factors and premalignant conditions

The causes tend to be multifactorial, with an interaction between host-related and environmental factors.

Immunological factors

Cell-mediated immunity is a major host defence mechanism against subdermal invasion of cutaneous malignancies.

- Ageing reduces the effectiveness of immunity and DNA repair.
- Immunosuppression increases risks of malignancies, possibly by depressing immune surveillance against newly transformed cells.

Ultraviolet light

Ultraviolet light causes formation of pyrimidine dimers that are usually dealt with by nucleotide excision repair (NER) – excision of the damaged sequence by endonucleases, then repaired by DNA polymerase

and sealed by a ligase. The **ozone layer** absorbs radiation about 290 nm, i.e. 95% of UVA and 5% of UVB reaches the Earth.

- UVA 400–315 nm – initially regarded as relatively harmless but now regarded as a potentiator of the effects of UVB (co-carcinogen).
- UVB 315–290 nm – most carcinogenic through direct photochemical damage to DNA and DNA repair mechanism.
- UVC 290–200 nm – a potent carcinogen but most is filtered by the ozone layer.

Other environmental factors may also act as co-carcinogens, increasing the sensitivity to UV radiation.

- Ionizing radiation – accumulated dosage also important.
- Chemicals e.g. polycyclic aromatic hydrocarbons, psoralens and UVA (PUVA therapy for psoriasis), arsenic. These may also be direct carcinogens.

It is common to divide sun exposure into:

- Occupational: e.g. farming, construction.
- Non-occupational/recreational: e.g. sunbathing, sports, fishing. Skiers should be aware that UVB increases 10% for every 1000 feet of elevation.

Sunscreens

- A cotton T-shirt provides the equivalent of less than SPF 10.
- Chemical sunscreens absorb UV radiation. SPF > 15 is needed before a reduction is seen in actinic keratoses and malignancies.
- Physical or reflective sunscreens reflect radiation and are usually opaque e.g. zinc oxide; they provide the best protection.

Sunscreen should be applied generously and frequently; it needs to be reapplied after swimming or sweating. However, outcome data on cancer reduction through sunscreen shows only limited success; programmes designed to increase awareness have little measurable effect on behaviour including that of medical students.

Conditions associated with skin cancer

Xeroderma pigmentosum

Kaposi first described the condition in 1874 though the term was not coined by him until 1882. Xeroderma pigmentosum is a group of rare familial disorders (2 in a million, autosomal recessive) in which there are deficiencies in the DNA repair processes (NER defects are most common) and DNA damage becomes cumulative and irreversible. This leads to photosensitivity and a predisposition to cutaneous malignancy – BCC and SCC (median age 8 years compared with 58 in the normal population) and a 2000× risk of melanoma. Eighty per cent have eye problems whilst 20% have neurological problems. It is usually detected at age 1–2 after having apparently healthy skin at birth.

There are eight subtypes based on their repair defect (A is the 'classical' form but C and D are most common, whilst V is a 'variant').

- First stage – at 6 months, erythema, actinic changes and freckles/lentigines on exposed areas initially, followed by other areas – the skin is dry and pigmented, hence the name. There is sensitivity to **sunburn e.g. first sun exposure** of baby. The changes diminish in winter until the disease progresses.
- Second stage – poikiloderma – skin atrophy, telangectasia and dyspigmentation.
- Third stage – malignancies as early as 4–5 years and then relentless thereafter. Most die in their 30s from SCC and melanoma (Kraemer KH. *Arch Dermatol* 1987;**123**:241–250). 90% survive to 13 years, 70% to 40 years; overall life expectancy is reduced by 28 years.

Management

- Patients need to adhere to strict sun avoidance – sunscreens, clothing and eye-care and caution even with fluorescent and quartz halogen lights.
- Frequent skin, eye and neurological examinations.
- Treat lesions early: actinic keratosis may be treated with 5-FU or cryotherapy; isotretinoin may be considered in those with multiple tumours but side-effects include irreversible calcification of tendons and ligaments.

Some studies have been conducted with DNA repair enzymes delivered via liposomes but these are a little way from clinical use; gene therapy is still pretty much experimental/theoretical.

Gorlin's syndrome (Gorlin–Goltz syndrome, naevoid basal cell carcinoma syndrome, basal cell naevus syndrome)

This affects 1 in 100 000 and demonstrates autosomal dominant inheritance (40% are new mutations). There are multiple BCCs (> 2), odontogenic keratocysts or in

bone of the jaw, and pits of the palm and soles (3 or more), calcification of the falx cerebri and a first-degree family history of the syndrome – these are **major criteria** (Kimonis VE. *Am J Med Genet* 1997; **69**:299–308). The diagnosis is made with two major criteria or one major with one minor. Other features include sebaceous cysts, medulloblastoma, lymphomesenteric cysts, hypertelorism, widened nose, frontal bossing, and abnormalities of ribs (e.g. bifid) and vertebrae (scoliosis). There is an abnormality of the PTCH gene on chromosome 9q.

- Patients usually present in their 20s for removal of jaw cysts; BCCs do not appear until 30–40s. These are treated in the usual manner including photodynamic therapy (PDT), 5-FU and imiquimod but radiotherapy should be avoided as patients seem to be very sensitive to radiation (imaging with ionizing radiation should also be minimized). Isotretinoin may be used as chemoprevention to reduce the risk of future tumours. The so-called basal cell naevi are true BCCs.
- Robert J. Gorlin (1923–2006) described it in 1960 along with R. Goltz.

Albinism (*albus*, Latin for white)

This is an autosomal-recessive inherited lack of melanin that greatly increases the risk of SCC in particular. There is no sex or race predisposition. The most common forms are oculocutaneous albinism (Types 1–4 with differing levels of pigment) and ocular albinism (five forms). Eye disorders are common in albinism, particularly nystagmus and strabismus. It may be part of a syndrome e.g. Chediak–Higashi.

Porokeratosis

Porokeratosis is an uncommon autosomal-dominant inherited condition characterized by abnormal skin keratinization that leads to malignant degeneration – risks being 7.5–11%. Typical lesions are annular plaques with horny borders and flattened centres. There are various forms with disseminated superficial actinic porokeratosis (DSAP) being most common. Experience with 5-FU, imiquimod, oral retinoids and PDT have been described but none are entirely satisfactory.

Premalignant skin conditions

Actinic (solar) keratosis

Actinic (solar) keratosis is the commonest premalignant skin lesion, seen in almost half of the Whites over

40 living in Australia. These are patches of keratosis (thickened, rough, dry, scaly skin) in sun-damaged skin that also features telangiectasia and sometimes keratin/cutaneous horns. It is most commonly found on the face and dorsum of hands. Histopathologically, the cardinal feature is **epithelial dysplasia** (variable thickness), with hyperplasia, hyperkeratosis (thickening of the keratin layer which is otherwise normal) and acanthosis. There are basaloid cells adjacent to basement membrane and elastotic degeneration in the dermis may be pronounced.

These are the earliest identifiable lesions that can eventually develop into invasive SCC. Clinical conversion into SCC occurs after 10 years (increased risk in those with multiple lesions – 10% progress in a 5-year study; Marks R. *Lancet* 1988;**1**:795–797). These tumours tend to be slow growing and unlikely to metastasize. Sunlight is the strongest aetiological factor – UVB-specific p53 mutations have been found; they are increased in the immunosuppressed and the association with HPV is unclear.

Treatment

Generally treatment is conservative; treatment if required includes cryotherapy or non-surgical topical therapies. There is FDA approval for 5-FU, imiquimod, topical diclofenac and PDT D-ALA, that are preferred to excision/curettage but the latter is needed when SCC is suspected or lesions fail to respond. Parentheses in the following list show 2006 BAD guidelines with strength recommendation and quality of evidence scores.

- **Skin care** (sun avoidance and sunblocks, with or without emollients). Some evidence that up to 25% will regress within one year (A, II–ii). Applying block twice daily may help prevent further lesions after treatment.
- **5-fluorouracil** (5%) twice daily for 6 weeks is effective for up to a year (A, I). It inhibits thymidylate synthetase and causes death in proliferating cells. It may cause irritation which makes it a less popular choice; some use salicylate pretreatment.
- **Imiquimod** may be used for 4 months or more (B, I) but the longevity of its effects are unclear and there may be irritation similar to 5-FU. It up-regulates cytokine response and there may be a memory effect from up-regulating T cells, thus reducing risk of recurrence. It costs almost 20× the

price of 5-FU and is thus used mostly on a named patient basis.
- **Topical diclofenac** gels (3%) twice daily for 3 months have moderate efficacy and low morbidity (B, I). The duration of benefit is unclear. The mechanism is unknown.
- **Topical salicylic acid ointment** (A, III) is sometimes used before 5-FU to remove superficial keratin. In a 2% concentration it acts as an emollient as well as a mild keratolytic; also a component of facial peels.
- **Tretinoin cream** (B, I). Some evidence of benefit but probably needs to be used for about a year. Overall, the effects are not much better than sunblock, emollient and 2% salicylic acid.
- **Facial peels** or other resurfacing techniques may be helpful but are not really treatments solely for actinic keratosis (C, III).
- **Cryotherapy** (A, I) for thicker lesions that would be less responsive to topical creams, but leaves scars that are often hypopigmented (melanocytes most sensitive).
- **Photodynamic therapy** (B, I) has good results with superficial and confluent actinic keratoses, with a similar efficacy to 5-FU though optimal protocols have not been definitively established. It is expensive, but good healing/less scarring make it preferable for sites known for poor healing e.g. lower leg.
- **Systemic retinoids** (B, I) for high-risk e.g. immunosuppressed or organ-transplant patients. There is a rebound effect if discontinued.

Bowen's disease

This is intra-epidermal carcinoma (and thus strictly not a premalignant lesion) that appears usually as red hyperkeratotic plaques that are well demarcated. The potential for transformation into an invasive SCC (which tends to be fairly aggressive) is approximately 3–5%; appearance of ulceration is often an indication of invasion. The intact basement membrane defines its intra-epidermal or *in situ* nature. There is squamous proliferation, acanthosis and atypia (nuclear and cellular pleomorphism, hyperchromatism and frequent mitoses); there may be loss of intercellular connections. It may be difficult to distinguish from full thickness solar keratosis. Most patients are elderly (women twice as often, but many say equal distribution). The limbs are particularly affected but it can occur anywhere on skin or mucosal surfaces including non-sun-exposed regions.

- Erythroplasia of Queyrat is Bowen's disease of the glans penis, with 20% risk of SCC.

The main aetiological factor seems to be sun damage; others include exposure to arsenicals (medical solutions including Fowler solution previously used to treat psoriasis, contamination), immunosuppression, viral infection (HPV). There is a reported association with internal malignancy which may be an association with arsenic, but currently the prevailing opinion is that Bowen's disease is not paraneoplastic.

Suspicious lesions should be biopsied and a full skin examination performed. Confirmed lesions should be excised (A, II-iii) with **margins of 5 mm or more**, Mohs surgery and also for selected lesions, curettage (A, II-ii) and ablative lasers. Alternatives include 5-FU applied 1–2 times a day for 6–16 weeks with a margin around the lesion (B, II-i), PDT (A, I), imiquimod (B, I) and cryotherapy (B, II–i) with caution in the pretibial area of the elderly. Radiotherapy is not a common therapy currently but it is reported to be radiosensitive (B, ii–iii). BAD 2006 guidelines are in parentheses – strength of recommendation and quality of evidence.

- Fernández-Vozmediano J. Infiltrative squamous cell carcinoma on the scalp after treatment with 5% imiquimod cream. *J Am Acad Dermatol* 2005;**52**:716–717.
- JT Bowen described the disease in 1912.

Bowen's disease and internal malignancy: a meta-analysis

Lycka BAS. *Int J Dermatol* 1989;**28**:531–533.

The authors pooled the data from 12 studies and found no association between Bowen's disease and internal malignancies, thus extensive investigation in patients is not needed.

II. Basal cell carcinoma

This is a malignant tumour composed of cells derived from the pluripotential cells of the epidermis or outer root sheath of the hair follicle. It is the commonest malignant skin tumour in Whites and 75% of patients are over 40 years old. Men are affected more frequently except for lower extremity lesions (where the female: male ratio is 3:1). The estimated lifetime risk in the USA for Whites is 23–39% (men are at the higher end of the range, women at the lower).

There is an increased prevalence in locations of high sunlight exposure particularly non-occupational exposure (i.e. intermittent exposure including sunburn). The face is at much greater risk than other sun-exposed areas (this may be related to density of pilosebaceous follicles). It is less common in non-Whites but the tendency for pigmented variants (up to three-quarters in Chinese) is increased.

Aetiology

The most important factor is UV (B > A) (see Fitzpatrick skin types). Other factors include:

- Ionizing irradiation.
- Immunosuppression e.g. transplant patients.
- Malignant change in sebaceous naevi and other adnexal hamartomas.
- Burn and vaccination scars.
- Arsenicals.
- Occasionally has a familial inheritance or is syndromic, e.g. Gorlin's, Xeroderma pigmentosum, albinism and Bazek's (multiple BCC with follicular atrophoderma and local anhidrosis).

Classically the tumour cells with varying degrees of atypia are arranged in **palisades** with a well-organized surrounding stroma. Mucin accumulation and central necrosis are characteristic of cystic lesions. Clinically, the typical lesion is a pinkish, pearly nodule (often pigmented in Asian patients) with telangiectasia; it may be ulcerated or encrusted. BCCs are usually slow growing and very rarely metastasize. Long-standing tumours may invade deep into subcutaneous tissues, and in combination with central ulceration gives rise to the appearance of a **rodent ulcer**.

Subtypes (there are 26 different types identified in the literature and a third may have a mixed pattern) include:

- Nodular – most common (50–60%) and appearance as above. Some may also be:
  - Cystic.
  - Pigmented – and may resemble melanoma.
- Superficial – (10–15%) often multiple and found on upper trunk/shoulders as red scaly patches.
- Morpheaform/sclerosing -uncommon (2–3%). The scar-like appearance seems to come from fibroblast proliferation.
- Infiltrative (7%).
- Basisquamous – potentially more aggressive. Elevated levels of collagenase enzymes have been

isolated from BCCs including basosquamous and may account for more aggressive behaviours.

Treatment

- **Excisional biopsy**: 2–5 mm margins depending on the location of the tumour and on how well-demarcated the border is. Some recommend antibiotic cover if the tumour is ulcerated.
  - For well-defined lesions up to 2 cm in size, a 3-mm margin will clear the tumour in 85% whilst 4–5 mm will increase this to 95% (Telfer NR. *B J Derm* 1999;**141**:415–423). Morpheic lesions require 15 mm to achieve > 95% clearance.
  - Thomas DJ. *Plast Reconstr Surg* 2003;**112**: 57–63. For well-marcated lesions 3 mm is adequate, whilst for others 4 mm will give a 96% complete rate.
  - Bisson MA. *Br J Plast Surg* 2002;**55**:293–297. 3 mm gives a 96% complete excision rate.
- **Mohs micrographic surgery** – excision with horizontal topographical map, 99% cure rate. This may be most useful in recurrent cases, non-nodular, size > 2 cm in high-risk sites such as ear, eyes, lips, nose and nasolabial folds.
- Curettage and electrodesiccation – overall cure rate 75% but for selected small tumours it approaches 95%.
- Cryotherapy – cooling to −40°C, with repetitive freeze–thaw cycles. This will leave hypopigmentation and prolonged swelling.
- 5-FU, imiquimod (6 weeks) or photodynamic therapy (Metvix) for superficial lesions.
- Radiotherapy (one 18 Gy dose, or 35 Gy in five doses) in the older age group with a cure rate of 92% but late results can be poor due to contraction.

Follow-up

There is a 35% risk of developing another non-melanoma skin cancer in 3 years, 50% in 5 years.

Recurrence may take up to 5 years, and up to 18% may present after this. In one large review (Rowe DE. *J Dermat Surg Oncol* 1989;**15**:315–328):

- 1 year – less than 1/3 recurrences present.
- 2 years – 50%.
- 3 years – 66%.

The evidence points to follow-up for at least 3 years to detect recurrences/new lesions but studies looking at UK practices for follow-up show that there is a wide range of 'protocols' with more than half offering one or no follow-up for primary BCCs. Patient attendance is also low, particularly after the first visit.

- Regular follow-up is probably most useful in those with high-risk lesions or multiple/recurrent BCCs.

Incompletely excised BCCs

Depending on the series, this occurs in about 4.5–7%; the best published result is 0.7% (Emmett AJJ. *Aust NZ J Surg* 1981;**51**:576–590) with two experienced surgeons operating on 1411 private patients. Bread-loafing at 4 mm intervals of an elliptical excision with 2 mm margins is about 44% sensitive at detecting residual tumour at the surgical margin.

About 30–41% of incompletely excised tumours recur and re-excision of incompletely excised tumours shows residual tumour in only 45–54% of cases. When offered a choice, older patients are more likely to opt for observation over re-operation.

Audit of histologically incompletely excised basal cell carcinomas: recommendations for management by re-excision

Griffiths RW. *Br J Plast Surg* 1999;**52**:24–28.

This was a retrospective review of 99 incompletely excised BCCs (approximately 7% of one surgeon's cases over 10 years). Incomplete excision was more common for periorbital and nasal lesions (13% and 12% respectively). The lateral margin was involved most frequently (55%), whilst the deep margin was involved in 36% and both lateral and deep margins involved in 9%.

Seventy-four of 99 were re-excised and residual tumour found in only 40 specimens (54%). For the subset of periorbital lesions that were re-excised, only 25% contained residual tumour and none of five patients with incompletely excised tumours developed recurrence without further treatment after a mean follow-up period of 2 years.

Incomplete excision of basal cell carcinoma

Kumar P. *Br J Plast Surg* 2002;**55**:616–622.

The overall incidence of incomplete excision in this study is 4.5%. The authors note that the incidence of incomplete excision is inversely proportional to the excision margin (lowest rates with margins 5 mm or more).

- Trunk and extremity BCCs less frequently incompletely excised than facial BCCs.
- Recurrent and multifocal lesions most prone to incomplete excision, whilst superficial BCCs are least prone.

Recurrence in the face may be related to tumours along areas of embryonic lines of fusion and the difficulty of reconstruction. The authors did not elaborate on their management of incompletely excised lesions except to say that approximately half were observed whilst the others had further excision (one had radiotherapy).

Incomplete excision of basal cell carcinoma: a prospective trial
Yu SY. *Plast Reconstr Surg* 2007;**120**:1240–1248.

During the 2-year period of study, 1214 BCCs were excised; 11.2% were incompletely excised. Risk factors identified by the authors included: location on the head, non-nodular subtypes (morpheic, superficial, infiltrative), lesions larger than 2 cm, multiple lesions and recurrent/incompletely excised lesions. They suggest that these criteria can be used to identify those most at risk.

Incompletely excised basal cell carcinomas: our guidelines
Longhi P. *Onco Targets Ther* 2008;**1**:1–4.

This is a retrospective review of 982 patients treated for BCC: 116 had margin involvement according to the pathological report; 36 were re-excised whilst the others were followed up (only 39 of 80 could be located for follow-up).

- They found 72% of re-excision margins had residual margins.
- 16 of the 39 observation-only cases had recurrences, with several after 5 years.

They concluded that their policy was to recommend immediate re-excision in cases of margin involvement. They also found that those with clear but close margins (< 1 mm) were safe for follow-up only with only 1 in 40 recurring after 6 years of follow-up.

III. Squamous cell carcinoma

Squamous cell carcinoma is a malignant epidermal tumour whose cells show maturation towards keratin formation. It is strongly associated with UV irradiation particularly total and occupational exposure; it is uncommon in dark-skinned races. The rate of SCC doubles for each 8–10° of latitude decline. SCCs appear from late middle age onwards; males are affected twice as often as females.

Other causes include:

- Burn scar (Marjolin) or other chronic scar wounds (1–2% with latency of about 30 years) including osteomyelitis sinuses, granulomatous infections, hidradenitis suppurativa and venous ulcers. These tend to be more aggressive and 30% have lymph node metastasis at the time of presentation.
- Immunosuppression (> 200× risk in renal transplant patients).
- Industrial carcinogens and oils.
- Premalignant conditions such as actinic keratoses, Bowen's disease and leukoplakia.
- Xeroderma pigmentosum and dermatoses such as poikiloderma.
- Viruses e.g. HPV; their exact role is unclear.

Histopathologically, there are variable degrees of cellular atypia and differentiation; well-differentiated tumours exhibit parakeratosis and keratin pearls.

The clinical appearance varies depending on the level of differentiation – the most common mode of presentation is a firm skin tumour on the dorsum of hands, scalp and face; it may have everted edges with a keratotic crust. Well-differentiated tumours have a keratin horn whilst less well-differentiated lesions are flat and ulcerated. Lymph node metastases may be present; the risk of occult nodes is 2–3%. The presence of nodal disease reduces the 5-year survival from over 90% for early tumours to 30%.

- Keracanthoma may be regarded as a well-differentiated SCC.

Classification
There are several different methods:

- Broder's based on level of differentiation.
- Tumour thickness – 2 mm or less (low risk of recurrence and metastasis), 4–10 mm (high risk), more than 10 mm (very high risk).
- Histological subtype e.g. verrucous.
- Growth pattern.

Treatment

- Excision with histology confirmed is the standard care (antibiotic cover if ulcerated). Margins according to Broadland DG and Zitelli AJ (*J Am Acad Dermatol* 1992;**27**:241–248) are 4 mm for low-risk tumours and 6 mm for high-risk tumours; this provides an overall 95% cure. In practice, it is common to use 5 mm for lesions on the face and 1 cm elsewhere.
  - Mohs is used less than it is for BCCs.

○ Curettage or cryotherapy may be indicated for small early lesions.

- Radiotherapy is not a primary treatment modality but there is a response rate of up to 90% in T1 lesions (and some choose it for incomplete excision); the long-term cosmetic outcome can be poor. It may be more useful for sites such as the lip, nasal vestibule and ear.
  ○ Radiotherapy may be palliative in large inoperable or recurrent SCC.
  ○ Chemotherapy has little role in SCC.

Therapeutic lymph-node dissection may be needed for clinical node disease. Elective prophylactic node dissection has been proposed for skin SCC thicker than 8 mm (or lip thicker than 8 mm) but the evidence is rather weak (strength of recommendation is C). The risk of metastases seems to be related to the location:

- Trunk and metastases 2–5%.
- Face and dorsum of hand 10–20%.
- Scars 38%.

Some predictive risk factors include degree of differentiation, depth of invasion and presence of perineural spread.

Multiprofessional guidelines for the management of the patient with primary cutaneous squamous cell carcinoma
Motley R. *Br J Plast Surg* 2003;**56**:85–91.
This is a review of the overall management of SCC including surgical and adjuvant treatment modalities that was also published in the *British Journal of Dermatology*. The metastatic potential of SCC is determined by:

- Location of tumour – highest in sun-exposed areas including lip.
- Diameter of tumour – **tumours > 2 cm** are twice as likely to recur locally and 3× more likely to metastasize than smaller tumours.
- Depth of invasion – **tumours > 4 mm thick** most likely to metastasize (> 45% incidence).
- Histological differentiation – **poor differentiation and perineural involvement** correlate with local and distant recurrence.
- Host immunosuppression.

These are often described as 'high risk SCC'.

Audit of clinical and histological prognostic factors in primary invasive squamous carcinoma of the skin
Griffiths RW. *Br J Plastic Surg* 2002;**55**:287–292.

This is a retrospective review of one surgeon's experience. Eight of 93 patients available for follow-up died of their disease within 5 years. In these patients tumour thickness and tumour diameter were greater compared with surviving patients. The lateral excision margins were similar in surviving and non-surviving patients (7 and 6 mm, respectively).

The eight patients who died from the disease developed nodal disease as their first presentation of metastatic disease and none developed local recurrence. The mean interval from primary surgery to first metastasis was 9 months (range 1–34 months).

Follow-up

Early detection and treatment of recurrent disease improves patient survival. In contrast to BCCs, 95% of SCCs are detected within 5 years but the British Association of Dermatologists guidelines 2002 (still the most current) does not offer more guidance than this.

D. Soft tissue sarcomas

I. General

Soft tissue sarcomas (STS) are relatively rare, comprising 1% of all cancers. They are ranked as the 21st most common cancers in the UK with 2.5 cases per 100 000 population per year. Non-specialists may see only one or two in their career and it is well established that soft tissue sarcomas are more effectively treated in specialist centres, particularly true for large (> 10 cm), high-grade and trunk/retroperitoneal tumours (Gutierrez JC. *Ann Surg* 2007;**245**:952–958).

- 60% are found in the limbs, the remainder are trunk/retroperitoneal/intra-abdominal.
- 20% are found in the head and neck, with more in adults compared with children.

Sarcoma means a **tumour of connective tissue** (or mesenchymal tissue) from Greek *sarkos* for flesh, *sarcoma* for fleshy substance. There are various histopathological subtypes that have their own characteristics and it is difficult to make sweeping statements that apply to all. Overall it is a heterogeneous group (WHO-STT 1994 classified 15 subtypes) and only the commonest types will be discussed; the commonest adult STS are malignant fibrous histiocytoma (MFH) (elderly), liposarcoma (middle aged) and leiomyosarcoma (young) whilst the commonest in children is the rhabdomyosarcoma (RMS).

- It is important to note that soft tissue sarcomas (80% of sarcomas) demand a very different approach from primary bone sarcomas.

Aetiology

In most cases, there is no clearly defined aetiology, however in some cases, soft tissue sarcomas are related to **genetic conditions**:

- **Neurofibromatosis** – NF1 (schwannoma, benign and malignant) and NF2 (meningiomas and schwannomas) and neurofibrosarcomas.
- **Retinoblastoma** – the original eye cancer can often be cured but survivors are at high risk of developing another cancer decades after, particularly osteosarcoma or other sarcomas. This is probably due to the RB-1 gene mutation as well as the radiation treatment given (though tumours may occur outside the radiation field e.g. leiomyosarcoma).
- **Li–Fraumeni syndrome** – this is a rare autosomal dominant condition that increases cancer susceptibility due to germline mutations of the p53 tumour suppressor gene. There is an increased risk to a wide variety of cancers including sarcomas (STS and bone) or breast, brain, leukaemias, often at a **young age** (below 45) and at multiple times.
- Familial polyposis coli.
- Gorlin's syndrome (gene PTC (Chr 9q22.3)) with increase in mediastinal sarcomas – fibrosarcoma and rhabdomyosarcoma particularly.
- **Gardner's syndrome** (Eldon Gardner, 1909–1989, was a geneticist who described the condition in 1951) – mutation of APC gene on chromosome 5q21 (autosomal dominant inheritance) is associated with epidermoid cysts, desmoid tumours (15%), osteomas and colonic polyps, that are numerous and have malignant potential (100% risk unless the colon is removed). It is distinct from the more common familial adenomatous polyposis but shares the same gene that is mutated.

Genetic alterations (due to unknown causes) are relatively common in sarcomas including:

- Alterations in cell regulatory genes, e.g. Rb-1 and p53 detected in substantial proportion of sarcomas.
- Translocation in Ewing's sarcoma.

- Presence of TLS-CHOP fusion protein; which is now a definitive diagnostic tool for myxoid liposarcoma.

Acquired conditions

- **Radiation exposure** particularly in treatment of carcinomas of breast and cervix, as well as lymphoma, typically appearing 7–10 years after. Such tumours tend to have a poor prognosis.
- **Lymphoedema** (lymphangiosarcoma), e.g. filarial and 'surgical' especially after breast surgery (mastectomy and irradiation). Such sarcomas are not regarded as radiation-induced as they are usually found outside the irradiated zone.
  - **Stewart–Treves syndrome** – aggressive lymphangiosarcoma (often multifocal) in those with post-mastectomy lymphoedema (1948). The incidence ranges from 0.07% to 0.45% of 5-year survivors. The most common cause of death (8–16 months after diagnosis) is metastasis to lungs and chest wall; metastasis and local recurrence is common even after radical excision.
- Some chemicals e.g. vinyl chloride and liver angiosarcoma. In some, chemical agents are important, such as phenoxyacetic acids (herbicides), vinyl chloride, arsenic, chlorophenols (wood preservatives) and thorotrast (radioactive contrast agent).
- Virus e.g. HPV8 in Kaposi's sarcoma.

Age and sex

Sarcomas are slightly more common in males than females and in general the incidence increases with age. Some subtypes are more common in certain age groups:

- Malignant fibrous histiocytoma – elderly.
- Liposarcoma – middle age.
- Leiomyosarcoma – young.
- Rhabdomyosarcoma – children.

Anatomical site

The most common sites involved are the extremities particularly for liposarcoma, MFH, fibrosarcoma and tendosynovial sarcoma.

- Retroperitoneal – liposarcoma, leiomyosarcoma.
- Trunk – desmoid tumour, liposarcoma.

The most important prognostic variables are **grade, size and location of tumour**. To a certain extent, these determine the mode of presentation e.g. superficial tumours as a mass, deep tumours due to compression/distortion will cause pain.

Cutaneous metastatic malignant tumours

This is relatively uncommon but may arise from, in order of frequency: breast, stomach, lung, uterus, large bowel, kidney, prostate, ovary, liver and bone. The trunk and scalp are the most commonly affected areas of skin whilst para-umbilical metastases may occur secondary to intra-abdominal malignancy (Sister Joseph's nodule).

- Histologically, these tumours are usually poorly differentiated and may resemble a primary lesion; a foreign-body type inflammatory reaction may be present.
- Tumour deposits can be treated by excision or laser to prevent fungation.

II. Assessment, biopsy and staging

Clinical assessment

- Size of tumour and skin involvement (and likely defect).
- Pulses and sensation (for vascular and nerve reconstruction).
- Involved muscle groups (for tendon/vascularized muscle transfer).
- Age and fitness for surgery.
- Lifestyle (for limb preservation).

Radiological assessment

- Ultrasound may exclude benign soft tissue swellings such as lipomata or Baker's cysts.
- MRI provides most information particularly size of tumour and its relationship to surrounding structures, e.g. nerves and vessels. Fatty tumours can be identified by suppression on T2 images.
- CT is required for assessment of bone involvement whilst it is also useful for staging (chest and abdomen/pelvis).
- PET can also be used for staging.

Referral to a soft tissue sarcoma service

The Department of Health UK advises urgent referral (within 2 weeks) if a patient presents with a palpable lump that is:

- Mass > 5 cm.
- Deep to fascia, fixed or immobile.
- Enlarging.
- Painful.
- Recurrent.

Ten per cent will have regional metastasis at the time of presentation particularly if high grade. Delays in referral to specialist centres may lead to a poorer prognosis; several papers have found that medical professionals are the source of greatest delay (Brouns F. *Eur J Surg Oncol* 2003;**29**:440–445; Hussein R. *Ann R Coll Surg Engl* 2005;**87**:171–173).

In general, the advice is that suspected sarcomas **should not be biopsied** prior to referral to a specialist sarcoma centre. Inadequate excision by non-specialists results in a difficult situation with regards to further excision as well as its magnitude.

- About half will turn out to have no residual tumour on re-excision. At present there is no way to detect microscopic spread pre-operatively; MRI is the most useful method to define the limits of detectable residual disease but can be falsely negative in up to one-quarter.
- The role of adjuvant therapy after further WLE is unclear but chemotherapy is of no benefit in most deep, high-grade lesions whilst radiotherapy is routinely used in most centres for lesions greater than 5 cm or with close margins.

Biopsy of STS

- Clinical evaluation of soft tissue sarcoma is often inaccurate due to a variety of factors including vague history (often with misleading history of trauma) and inaccurate palpation.
- Imaging is often non-specific – the majority of soft tissue masses/tumours are post-traumatic, inflammatory or benign.

Large masses below the level of the fascia should be considered malignant until proven otherwise – there is thus often a need to biopsy soft tissue masses. Biopsy in itself is simple, but the following points should be borne in mind:

- Biopsies should be large enough to obtain adequate tissue (open or large core) without interfering with definitive surgery. Avoid breaching the **deep** border. The biopsy tract will need to be excised at the time of definitive excision.

- Open (incisional/excisional) or closed (FNA/trephine/core).
  - Trephine/core preserve the architecture and have an overall accuracy of 80%. Caution is advised with cystic/myxomatous tumours. Directed core biopsies e.g. by high PET activity may be useful in heterogeneous lesions.
  - FNA is less accurate diagnostically but should still be able to differentiate malignant from benign in 90%, and grade in 75%. Positive reports are more useful than negative.
  - Closed techniques are popular due to low risk of complications such as haematoma and infection and little need for anaesthesia/hospitalization. However, they do make interpretation more difficult and thus should not be used in centres that see these tumours only occasionally.
  - Open biopsy is usually reserved for failed core biopsy and it is important to avoid crushing (use sharp dissection). It may potentially upstage tumours by transgressing compartments and the biopsy scar will need wide excision. However, it is the most reliable by providing ample tissue for diagnosis which is particularly useful for low-grade and rarer tumours.
  - Although FNA can be used prior to imaging and may successfully diagnose high-grade tumours, core biopsy, on the other hand, should **only** be undertaken **after imaging** to avoid disruption of images by haematoma.
- The person doing the biopsy is often not the person/team who will ultimately treat the patient and where possible there should be consultation with the responsible surgeon.

Ideally, biopsy should be **the final step** in the evaluation of the patient with all local imaging done – this will provide the maximum information for the person doing the biopsy of the mass, for the pathologist examining the specimen and will reduce artefacts affecting imaging. In some situations, biopsy may be CT-guided to target the most suspicious or most representative areas.

Principles of biopsy

- Aseptic technique.
- Choose a site in the tumour that can be excised en bloc with the tumour; thus the doctor performing the biopsy should be aware of potential flaps to avoid compromising them by tumour contamination.
- The most frequent site is usually at the vertex of the tumour away from vital structures e.g. away from medial neurovascular bundle in the arm, away from sciatic and femoral areas in the lower limb. The **deep surface should not be violated**.
- Longitudinal incisions in the limbs are preferable.
- Good haemostasis is vital to avoid contaminating haematomas.
- Drains should be closed and in line with the incision.
- Light compression and elevation.

Potential hazards.

- Bad planning.
- Complications e.g. haematoma, infection, contamination.
- Studies have shown that there are more problems if biopsy is performed outside of specialist centres. Open biopsies are more likely to cause problems that significantly alter management.

AJCC Staging 2002 – tumour, node, metastasis, grade (TNMG)

- Based on tumour grade, size and location.
- Lymph-node metastasis is uncommon but is associated with a poor prognosis.
- **Grade is one of the most important prognostic factors** – a pathologist with expertise is vital but this may be difficult because of the low incidence – pathologists may only see one case per year.

Primary:

- TX cannot be assessed.
- T0 no evidence of primary tumour.
- T1 tumour 5 cm or less in greatest dimension (a superficial, b deep).
- T2 tumour more than 5 cm in greatest dimension (a superficial, b deep).

Regional nodes:

- NX cannot be assessed.
- N0 none.
- N1 regional nodes.

Distant metastases:

- MX, M0, M1

  Histological grade G (G1/2 would be low grade):

- GX cannot be assessed.
- G1 well differentiated.

Table 8.7 Staging of sarcoma.

Stage		
T1	< 5 cm	Stage Ia G1/2 T1
T1a	Superficial to fascia	
T1b	Deep to fascia	
T2	> 5 cm	
T2a	Superficial to fascia	Stage Ib G1/2 T2a
T2b	Deep to fascia	Stage IIa G1/2 T2b
N1	Regional node involvement	Stage IV N1
M1	Distant metastases	Stage IV M1
G1	Well differentiated	
G2	Moderately differentiated	
G3	Poorly differentiated	Stage IIb G3/4 T1
		Stage IIc G3/4 T2a
G4	Undifferentiated	Stage III G3/4 T2b

- G2 moderately differentiated.
- G3 poorly differentiated.
- G4 undifferentiated; many institutions use a 3-tiered system.

Enneking stage 1980 TMG

- T1 intracompartmental.
- T2 extracompartmental.
- G1 low grade.
- G2 high grade.
- M0 no metastasis.
- M1 metastasis (regional or distant).
- Stage Ia – G1, T1, M0.
- Stage Ib – G1, T2, M0.
- Stage IIa – G2, T1, M0.
- Stage IIb – G2, T2, M0.
- Stage III – M1.

Memorial Sloan-Kettering staging 1992

Stage is related to the number of favourable features:

- 0 – 3 favourable
- I – 2 favourable.
- II – 1 unfavourable, or 1 favourable and 2 unfavourable.
- III – 3 unfavourable.
- IV – metastasis.

Table 8.8 Favourable versus unfavourable features for sarcomas.

	Favourable	Unfavourable
Size	< 5cm	> 5cm
Depth	Superficial	Deep
Grade	Low	High

Treatment

Planning of treatment should happen within a multi-disciplinary team environment.

- **Surgery** is the mainstay of treatment: consider anatomical margins of excision and requirements for flap reconstruction e.g. skin, nerve and functional muscle. Frozen section can be used for histological control of the margins – the best area to sample is around the pseudocapsule–tumour interface where the tumour is most viable.
  - Small/low-grade lesions can often be treated with wide excision only; larger/higher-grade lesions may benefit from adjuvant treatments.
  - **Compartectomy** means to excise a whole musculofascial compartment (corresponds to 'radical'). Muscles are excised from origin to insertion where possible. Main arteries are dissected free unless encased by tumour as they are rarely invaded by tumour in comparison to veins which are usually sacrificed unless it is a major vein e.g. femoral, common iliac or subclavian. Tumour is dissected off nerves taking along the perineurium.
    - Intralesional – partial removal of tumour.
    - Marginal – through reactive zone and may leave residual microscopic disease.
    - Wide – entire tumour with cuff of normal tissue.
    - Radical – entire compartment containing tumour.
  - Amputation is reserved for otherwise unresectable tumours (sometimes for recurrent tumours). Studies have shown no survival advantage over limb-sparing surgeries (Willard WC. *Surgery* 1992;**175**:389–396).
- Consider **neoadjuvant therapy** for high-grade tumours; isolated limb perfusion with TNF-α may be considered for locally advanced and inoperable extremity tumours with poor prognosis as an alternative to limb amputation.

- Plan **adjuvant therapy**:
  - Post-operative radiotherapy for marginal excisions and high-grade tumours >5 cm; consider brachytherapy if radiosensitive tissues are nearby. The general effect is to reduce local recurrence with little improvement in overall survival. There is no consensus on pre-operative (to reduce tumour size for limb-sparing surgery) or post-operative irradiation, and the choice depends largely on the preference of individual centres. Pre-operatively, tumour cells are better oxygenated and thus more responsive but neoadjuvant therapy may delay surgery, complicate histological evaluation and increase wound complications.
  - Post-operative chemotherapy for high-grade tumours and chemosensitive tumours; possible role also in palliation. There are many different regimes, including combinations – these may be preferred in rapidly progressive disease, but at the cost of increased toxicity. There is an improvement in disease survival at 10 years in dermatofibrosarcoma with anthracycline from 45% to 55% but no significant increase in overall survival. The most commonly used agents include:
    - Doxirubicin – cardiotoxicity may be reduced by continuous infusion or liposomal formulations.
    - Ifosfamide – prodrug activated by liver metabolism, urothelial toxicity.
    - Paclitaxel – good response rate in angiosarcoma.
    - Gemcitabine, methotrexate, cisplatin, mitomycin C.
  - Isolated limb perfusion with melphalan, TNF-α and interferons has been effective (albeit transiently) and may be useful to reduce tumour size for limb-sparing surgery.

Metastatic spread

Local recurrence after incomplete excision does not necessarily correlate with earlier development of distant disease. The vast majority (90%) of metastatic disease is pulmonary; other sites are rare – lymph nodes (10%), bone (8%) and liver (1%).

- Consider also the risk of nodal metastases: SLNB reported for rhabdomyosarcoma, epithelioid and synovial sarcoma.

- Metastatic disease is usually incurable, but benefit is still possible from chemotherapy or local control methods; higher-grade lesions respond better to chemotherapy.

Follow-up

- Clinical assessment: 3-monthly for 2 years then 6-monthly for 3 more, and then annually if appropriate until year 10.
- Radiological follow-up.
  - Local tumour site (MRI).
    - Superficial tumours: only if clinical suspicion of recurrent disease.
    - Deep tumours: baseline post-operative imaging at 6–12 months with further imaging annually for up to 5 years.
  - Distant site imaging.
    - For high-grade tumours, a plain chest X-ray at each clinical review with CT chest if any change from previous film, or annual CT chest.
    - Low-grade tumours rarely metastasize and an annual chest X-ray is sufficient.

III. Tumours of fibrous tissue

Nodular fasciitis is a benign subcutaneous tumour due to reactive proliferation of fibroblasts. Lesions consist of spindle-shaped fibroblasts in a myxoid stroma that can infiltrate fat or muscle bundles. It presents as a rapidly growing (< 2 weeks), often tender mass (1–3 cm diameter) beneath the skin, most commonly in the forearm. It can occur at any age but is commonest in middle age. Treatment of choice is excision; resolution may still follow incomplete excision.

Histiocytoma

Histiocytes are monocytes derived from the bone marrow that populate areas of acute or chronic inflammation of the skin. **Histiocytomas** are closely related to foreign body giant cells and epithelioid cells. Histologically, they are proliferations of histiocytes, fibroblasts and vascular endothelial cells with iron inclusion bodies and foam cells.

Histiocytomas show a predilection for females and often occur on the lower extremities, presenting as a firm brownish nodule with smooth or warty surface up to 3 cm diameter. Around 20% may be preceded by trauma or insect bite. A dermatofibroma is a histiocytoma with maturation of cells towards fibroblasts.

Tumours of fibrous tissues:

- Benign – fibrous histiocytoma, dermatofibroma.
- Intermediate – atypical fibroxanthoma, dermatofibrosarcoma protuberans.
- Malignant – storiform pleomorphic tumour, myxoid tumour.

Treatment of choice is excision; resolution may follow incomplete excision but 5–10% may recur.

Malignant fibrous histiocytoma

Malignant fibrous histiocytoma (MFH) may represent malignant change in a benign histiocytoma or may arise *de novo*. More than 80% demonstrate cytogenetic abnormalities including 7q32 which seems to predict a worse outcome. It is one of the commonest soft tissue sarcomas overall comprising about 20% of all diagnoses and mostly affecting patients in **late adult life** with a slight male predominance.

Typically there is a subcutaneous nodule that is composed of histiocytes and fibroblast-derived cells in different proportions with storiform-pleomorphic, myxoid, giant cell and inflammatory subtypes. More recent evidence has shown no true histiocytic differentiation and that MFH may be a final common pathway in tumours that undergo undifferentiation (the WHO declassified it as a diagnostic entity, renaming it **undifferentiated pleomorphic sarcoma NOS**) but the MFH name continues to be widely used.

WHO 2002 classification for undifferentiated pleomorphic sarcoma (MFH):

- Pleomorphic high grade (most common 70%) also known as storiform-pleomorphic.
- Myxofibrosarcoma also known as myxoid (20%).
- Pleomorphic with giant cells.
- Pleomorphic with prominent inflammation.

It is most common in the abdomen and extremities especially the **thigh** (only 1–3% in the head and neck). It has been reported to arise in burn scars; many report preceding trauma, but trauma does not cause MFH – it draws attention to the lesion. MRI is the best investigation before biopsy.

Treatment of choice is wide excision (compartment or 3 cm) with post-operative radiotherapy for close/positive margins; chemotherapy (doxorubicin) for distant metastasis (or at high risk of), in the context of a trial. However local recurrence (20–40%) and

metastases (20% especially if high grade and > 5 cm) are common. Overall mortality is 40% but it is age related (70% for over 70s, 30% for under 40s).

Advances in the surgical management of sarcomas in children

Andrassy RJ. *Am J Surg* 2002;**184**:484–491.

Malignant fibrous histiocytoma is the second most common non-rhabdomyosarcoma soft tissue sarcoma (NRSTS) in children and surgical excision is the mainstay of treatment. Poor prognostic indicators included size >5 cm and involved surgical margins.

Atypical fibroxanthoma

This is a locally aggressive cutaneous tumour of the head and neck that may represent a superficial variant of pleomorphic malignant fibrous histiocytoma. It occurs most commonly on the ears and cheeks of elderly people, with a predilection for sun-damaged skin and areas of previous radiotherapy. A typical lesion is a red, fleshy mass with granuloma-type appearance consisting of fibroblasts, histiocytes and multinucleate giant cells and may become ulcerated. Histologically it is a **diagnosis of exclusion** after immunohistochemistry, looking very similar to melanomas, spindle cell SCC and leiomyosarcomas. It has invasive potential; lesions may recur locally after excision, though metastasis is rare. Lesions should be excised with margins > 1 cm.

Desmoid tumour (aggressive fibromatosis)

The name comes from *desmos* (Greek for band-like or tendon-like); the tumour was first described in 1832 by McFarlane and named in 1834 by Müller. The estimated incidence is 2–4 per 1 000 000. These are firm, irregular tumours arising typically from the muscular aponeurosis of the abdominal wall, especially below the umbilicus, though extra-abdominal lesions have been described. It can be regarded as an aggressive fibromatosis with fibroblast proliferation with variable collagen deposition and mucoid degeneration that is prone to **aggressive local invasion and local recurrence** if inadequately excised but is unlikely to metastasize (however, death may still result from the aggressive local invasion). Desmoid tumours have a predilection for parous women in their 30s–50s and have an association with Gardner syndrome. The aetiology is unknown but possible aetiological factors include:

- **Trauma** – reports of desmoid tumours arising in scars e.g. Caesarean section and desmoid reported in the capsule surrounding a breast implant. Some say that surgical trauma may stimulate tumour growth particularly in familial adenomatous polyposis (FAP).

- **Hormonal factors:** extra-abdominal desmoids may express **oestrogen receptors** and increased growth is observed during pregnancy, with a peak incidence in post-pubertal and pre-menopausal women. Tumours may regress during menopause, after tamoxifen or combined oral contraceptive (COC) treatment.
- **Genetic factors:** Gardner syndrome (FAP with *APC* gene mutation on chromosome 5) –desmoid tumours are 1000× more common (incidence of 10–15%). Familial multicentric fibromatosis – desmoid tumours usually occur singly in non-FAP patients but can occur multifocally without evidence of Gardner syndrome in some patients.

Beta-catenin gene (*CTNNBI*) mutations have been implicated in pathogenesis and agents blocking this pathway are under study.

Treatment

- **Surgery** – wide local excision is recommended; positive histological margins increase risk of local recurrence but it is not inevitable. Musculoaponeurotic lesions are more likely to be multifocal. Recurrence after surgery alone is relatively high (25–40%) being more common in younger patients.
  - Intralesional injections e.g. acetic acid, radiofrequency ablation reported.
- **Radiotherapy** is useful in those who cannot have surgery or as an adjunct, except for intra-abdominal tumours. Radiographic evidence after radiotherapy (typically 6–8 weeks) may take many months to be evident.
- **Medical** – NSAIDs (especially sulindac) and anti-oestrogens (e.g. tamoxifen at breast cancer doses – there is no evidence for higher dosages). These two types of drugs are often used in combination –they will improve symptoms in approximately half but chances of major shrinkage are low.
- **Chemotherapy** – generally low-toxicity regimes e.g. of methotrexate and vinblastine; most reserve high-dose regimes for tumours unresponsive to other therapies.

Extra-abdominal desmoid tumours peak in incidence between 25 and 35 years of age. They may arise primarily in musculoaponeurotic tissue or elsewhere (e.g. breast) and are sometimes multifocal. They are histologically identical to abdominal desmoids with spindle cells, abundant collagen and few mitoses.

Dermatofibrosarcoma protruberans

Dermatofibrosarcoma protruberans (DFSP) is an uncommon tumour of dermal fibroblasts (6% of all soft tissue sarcomas) that may occasionally be preceded by trauma. There is no overall sex preference though it is reported to be **hormone sensitive** with accelerated growth during pregnancy. More than 90% have a reciprocal chromosomal translocation t(17:22), a rearrangement that leads to constitutive activation of **PDGF receptor** (fusion with *COL1A1* collagen gene) thus providing a rationale for therapy in those with advanced unresectable disease, i.e. **imatinib**, a selective inhibitor of PDGFR tyrosine kinases.

Histologically it is a locally malignant tumour of dermal fibroblasts with a distinct storiform (cartwheel) pattern extending from the dermo-epidermal junction into subcutaneous tissues. It spreads in an infiltrating manner laterally but metastasis is rare (5%, usually to lungs). Malignant fibrous histiocytoma in DFSP has been described (Gorgu M. *Eur J Plast Surg* published online 30 April 2010 DOI 10.1007/s00238–010–0439-z).

Typically DFSP appears in early adult life and though rarely diagnosed during childhood, congenital DFSP has been reported (Weinstein JM. *Arch Dermatol* 2003;**139**:207–211). **Anti-CD34** immuno-histochemistry may be useful but not 100%. Typical lesions are red dermal nodules with a firm/rubbery touch and are intimately fixed to the overlying skin. Most commonly they appear on the front of the trunk, extremities and the head as a painless (15% or less have pain) mass that tends to grow slowly but may enter a more rapid growth phase which usually prompts the patient to seek attention.

Local recurrence is common if inadequately excised; generally wide local excision with a wide margin is advised.

- Historically, margins as high as 5 cm were used, recent guidelines suggest **2–4 cm** (NCCN, National Comprehensive Cancer Network 2007) along with complete circumferential peripheral and deep margin assessment (CCPDMA, of which Mohs surgery is an example) – taking the deep and lateral faces for complete frozen section examination to avoid the false negative error inherent in 'bread loafing'.

- Parker TL. *J Am Acad Dermatol* 1995;**32**:233–236. Margins of 2.5 cm clear all lesions, whilst 1.5 cm is sufficient for lesions less than 2 cm wide. 3 cm margins have been associated with 11% recurrence.
- Some propose Mohs surgery.

The evidence to support a role for radiotherapy is limited.

Fibrosarcoma

This is a relatively uncommon malignant tumour consisting of cells resembling fibroblasts that mostly affects patients in their 30s–60s (slightly more common in males). It may be more common in irradiated skin (10-year delay), burns scars (30-year delay) and xeroderma pigmentosum patients (these patients more commonly develop SCCs, BCCs or sebaceous carcinomas).

Histologically, lesions show atypical fibroblasts with generous blood supply; there may be large amounts of mucin (low-grade fibromyxoid sarcoma). Less well-differentiated tumours may be best described as anaplastic sarcomas. Better techniques have shown that many lesions previously labelled as fibrosarcoma were actually MFH, synovial sarcoma etc.; this means that earlier literature should be interpreted cautiously.

Fibrosarcomas usually present as painless slow-growing masses of the deep tissues of the **thigh or the trunk**; if close to the skin, then it is usually a red–purple nodule with a smooth surface. There may be some fluctuance due to intralesional haemorrhage whilst anaplastic lesions tend to ulcerate. The tumour has a tendency to metastasize via blood or lymphatics.

The treatment of choice is wide excision though local recurrence may occur even after apparent complete excision with negative margins. Radiotherapy has also been used primarily for close or positive margins. Poor prognostic factors include high grade, > 5 cm, positive margins (with invasion to vessels, nerves, bone or skin). The variant that occurs in infants (< 5 years old) has a much better prognosis.

Epithelioid cell sarcoma

This is a malignant connective tissue tumour comprised of epithelioid cells; tumours are often multifocal. It is found most commonly in adolescents and young adults, mainly in the subcutaneous and deep tissues of the extremities, especially palm/flexor surface of fingers. Deeper nodules may be associated with fascia, periosteum, tendon and nerve sheaths. They ulcerate sometimes and then are commonly mistaken for ulcerated SCCs. Prognosis is poor with local recurrence common and metastases frequent.

IV. Tumours of vessels

Glomus tumour

Glomus is Latin for 'ball'. A glomus body is a highly convoluted arteriovenous shunt (i.e. no intervening capillary bed) with rich sympathetic innervation. It is involved with thermoregulatory activity. The central coiled canal is lined by endothelial cells and is surrounded by smooth muscle fibres containing rounded specialized pericytes called **glomus cells**; there are numerous unmyelinated nerve fibres. A glomus tumour is an encapsulated dermal tumour (strictly a hamartoma) of sheets of proliferating glomus cells surrounding small vascular channels. They arise from the arterial portion of the glomus body. These were originally described as 'painful subcutaneous tubercles' by William Wood in 1812.

Glomus tumours arise from late childhood onwards, most common in the 30–40s, with a female preponderance (2–3×) for subungual lesions whilst extradigital lesions tend to have equal distribution. They are relatively rare (1% of all hand tumours); the malignant counterpart, glomangiosarcoma, is exceptionally rare.

- They are usually **solitary** (75%) small lesions about 10 mm in size and occur spontaneously (some report a history of prior trauma) as pink-purple painful nodules on the extremities (75%), especially subungual (most common, 'haemangioma like lesion' with nail deformity), deep palm.
- There is an autosomal-dominant familial inheritance in some cases with multiple tumours – these are often painless and may be associated with limb malformations.
- Rarely, larger tumours may be situated elsewhere e.g. stomach, sinuses where glomus bodies do not normally exist and may not be painful.

The **classic triad** is of pinpoint tenderness, severe paroxysmal pain and extreme cold sensitivity (place finger in ice water for a minute, 100% accurate) in decreasing order of frequency; the diagnosis is primarily clinical.

- **Love's test** is the provocation of pain isolated to the area of a pin head/paper clip/wire on skin/nail over tumour, with relief when released. It is supposed to be 100% sensitive (Bhaskaranand K. *J Hand Surg Br* 2002;**27**:229–231).
- **Hildreth's test** is also reliable (92% sensitive, 91% specific) – exsanguinate arm by elevation then apply a tourniquet inflated to 250 mmHg (pain and tenderness should be reduced) – the test is 'confirmed' if release of the tourniquet causes sudden increase in pain. Giele H. *J Hand Surg Br* 2002;**27**:157–158.

Imaging has variable success: X-ray may show erosion of bone with a thin reactive sclerotic margin (14–60%). Ultrasound is inconsistent, CT is useful whilst high-resolution MRI is regarded as gold standard with a high signal on T2 images and enhance brightly with gadolinium.

Treatment

Excision (with capsule to reduce local recurrence) provides relief in all cases. Use Love's test to localize the tumour and then excise under direct vision. Subungual lesions may need nail removal with meticulous nail-bed repair afterwards but a lateral paronychial approach may be better for deeper or more lateral lesions. Incisions through hyponychium may cause nail deformity.

Glomus tumours of the hand

van Geertruyden J. *J Hand Surg Br* 1996;**21**:257–260.

This series had 51 patients and 80% had spontaneous pain, with sensitivity to touch in 100% and to cold in 63%. One-third of patients have radiological evidence of indenting of distal phalanx. Patients may have multiple tumours on one finger; tumours may also arise on metacarpals, wrist, neck, thigh, knee and leg.

The average duration of symptoms before treatment was 10 years. Excision, if incomplete, leads to recurrence usually within a few weeks (recurrence after years is usually due to a new solitary tumour).

Kaposi's sarcoma

Kaposi's sarcoma is a malignant, multifocal tumour of proliferating capillary endothelial cells and perivascular connective tissue cells, with lymphocytic inflammatory response. The original description was of a very aggressive tumour that killed within 2–3 years, but then came to describe a less common, more indolent tumour found in older people of Mediterranean

origin that often involutes spontaneously but may be associated with leukaemia/lymphoma.

The tumour is now more common due to AIDS/HIV (non-classic or 'epidemic') – it develops in up to 50% of these patients, presenting as multifocal blue–purple macular plaques on skin and sometimes mucosa which grow and coalesce. They usually appear on the extremities (legs more commonly in non-HIV patients) which become lymphoedematous; tumours may develop in internal organs without skin manifestation. Lymphadenopathy may be a feature.

- **Type 1:** chronic, originally restricted to eastern European Ashkenazi Jews and Mediterranean races i.e. 'classic KS'. Patients usually die of other causes.
- **Type 2:** lymphadenopathic.
- **Type 3:** transplantation associated, affects less than 1% of transplant patients. Similar to HIV type.
- **Type 4:** related to HIV infection. At its peak, it was the presenting symptom for undiagnosed AIDS in 14%, affecting up to 40% overall. Antiretroviral therapy has reduced the overall prevalence to 15%. It is more aggressive than classic KS with a significant mortality rate due to disseminated disease or opportunistic infection.

Treatment

The disease runs a variable course; lesions may involute or ulcerate and fungate. Excision is a common treatment but other options include:

- Localized lesions – local injection with cytotoxic agents or cryotherapy. Laser may palliate mucosal lesions.
- Extensive localized disease – radiotherapy.
- Systemic or aggressive disease – liposomal anthracycline or liposomal doxorubicin. In AIDS, neutropaenia is a limiting factor for this type of treatment. Interferons and beta HCG have been used with some success.

Angiosarcoma

Angiosarcoma is one of the least frequent soft tissue sarcomas (< 1%) with very poor prognosis generally. It is more frequent in men (3×). The tumour is derived from endothelial (vascular – haemangiosarcoma or lymphatic – lymphangiosarcoma) cells. Histologically, endothelial cell markers such as factor VIII will be positive and there will be Weibel–Palade bodies (storage granules of endothelial cells with VWF and Pselectin, microtubular-like bundles) on electron microscopy (if well differentiated). There are four clinicopathological types:

- **Cutaneous angiosarcoma** – uncommon type that affects scalp/face in elderly patients especially post-irradiation. Lesions are often well differentiated.
- **Angiosarcoma of the breast** – that may follow radiotherapy for breast cancer and is associated with lymphoedema in the breast. These tumours are often high grade.
- Angiosarcoma of the deep soft tissue.
- Angiosarcoma of the parenchymal organs, e.g. liver lesions that may be related to vinyl chloride exposure (not associated with angiosarcomas of other regions).

Other risk factors include extremity lymphoedema > 10 years. High-grade lesions tend to present with pain and bleeding from multiple ulcerated lesions, whilst low-grade lesions tend to be asymptomatic painless red nodules. Adjacent satellite lesions are common that suggests multifocality which partly explains the high recurrence rate.

The usual treatment is excisional surgery (> 3 cm) and radiotherapy. Some recommend regional **node dissection** for scalp lesions or those with palpable lymphadenopathy. The role of adjuvant chemotherapy is unclear though there have been recent reports of paclitaxel use. Overall there is a recurrence rate of over 50%.

V. Tumours of nerves

Neurofibroma (Molluscum fibrosa)

Neurofibromas are benign tumours derived from peripheral nerves and supporting stromal cells including neurilemmal cells i.e. a mixed cell population – Schwann cells and fibroblasts. Tumours usually appear at an early age, e.g. before age 10, and are usually soft and fleshy; they can be sessile or pedunculated.

- Visceral – appendix, gastrointestinal tract, larynx.
- Peripheral – from peripheral nerve, usually solitary and not associated with neurofibromatosis (and its other features).
- Plexiform, usually in association with the fifth cranial nerve – diffuse type of neurofibroma arising from a superficial/cutaneous nerve and characterized by myxoid degeneration. These can be very disfiguring and their vascularity can make surgery difficult.

Some lesions can lead to functional abnormalities such as paraesthesia, some may be associated with gigantism. There is a risk of sarcomatous change (3–10%, especially if >10 years) which is usually manifested by an increase in size and pain; this is commoner in non-cutaneous lesions (<15%) than cutaneous (1%). The prognosis of malignant nerve sheath tumours/neurofibrosarcomas is poor (20% 5-year survival) even after radical surgery.

Neurilemmoma (schwannoma)

These benign nerve sheath tumours are most common in the middle aged (equal sex distribution), presenting as an asymptomatic eccentric slow-growing nodule **extrinsic to a nerve**; it can be excised/separable **except for the one involved fascicle**. The aetiology is unknown but many show genetic aberrations e.g. ring chromosome 5 (this chromosome includes the NF2 gene on band 22q12).

They are the commonest nerve tumour and are usually solitary (multiple in neurilemmatosis which is a variant of neurofibromatosis NF2); the head and neck, and flexor surfaces of limbs are the commonest sites. Occasionally there may be paraesthesia, numbness (sensory nerves are more commonly affected) or weakness. It resembles neurofibromas but with no neurites within the tumour; there are Antoni A and B areas.

Imaging with MRI or ultrasound is usually diagnostic. Indications for excision include enlargement causing concern or disfigurement, symptomatic e.g. pressure effects or neurological. They can be removed without sacrifice of the main nerve. Recurrence is rare and malignant transformation is practically zero.

- Neurofibromas occur in the substance of a nerve whilst neurilemmomas occur on the surface, and thus the latter can usually be 'shelled out' whilst the former need excision. They can be distinguished by MRI and NCS.

Malignant peripheral nerve sheath tumour (malignant schwannoma)

Malignant peripheral nerve sheath tumours form 2–3% of malignant tumours and affect adults between 20 and 50 years of age. They may arise *de novo* or in pre-existing neurofibromas. There are three groups:

- Neurofibromatosis related (neurofibrosarcoma).
- Post irradiation.
- Solitary.

Most are associated with the major nerves of the extremities or trunk. They are typically clinically aggressive with *high metastatic potential*, with up to 90% mortality. Solitary lesions tend to have a better prognosis. They are treated with wide excision/amputation, as sensitivity to radiotherapy or chemotherapy is poor.

Neurofibromatosis is the occurrence of multiple neurofibromas.

Neurofibromatosis type 1 (NF1) – 1 in 3000, autosomal-dominant inheritance with half due to a new mutation affecting the *NF1* gene at chromosome 17q11.2. Diagnosis is made from two or more of the following criteria:

- Six or more café au lait spots – > 5 mm pre-puberty, > 15 mm post-puberty.
- Two or more neurofibroma or one plexiform neurofibroma.
- Axillary or inguinal freckling.
- Two or more Lisch nodules (pigmented iris harmatoma).
- An osseus lesion e.g. sphenoid dysplasia or long bone cortical thinning.
- Optic glioma.
- First-degree relative with NF1.

Other associated features include:

- Neural: meningioma, phaeochromocytoma, mental disability.
- Cardiovascular: obstructive cardiomyopathy, renal artery stenosis, orbital haemangioma, pulmonary fibrosis.
- Bony: scoliosis, fibrous dysplasia.

Generally patients present with skin lesions for excision, with large facial mass/asymmetry (plexiform neurofibromas) or rarely, sarcomatous change. Most individuals with NF1 lead healthy and productive lives. Neurofibromas can be excised with primary nerve repair if possible.

Neurofibromatosis type 2 (NF2) or 'central NF' due to involvement of intracranial tumours is less common (1 in 50 000) and is also autosomal dominant (95% penetrance) but is due to a gene defect on chromosome 22q12 (encoded protein is called merlin). It is more commonly associated with acoustic neuroma (actually more accurately a vestibular schwannoma), the excision of which may lead to facial palsy and the need for reanimation surgery.

- Bilateral VIII nerve masses confirmed on MRI/CT.
- First-degree relative with NF2 and either unilateral VIII mass or two of the following:
  - Neurofibroma, meningioma, glioma, schwannoma.
  - Juvenile posterior subscapular lenticular opacity.

The condition usually presents in adolescence with hearing loss or tinnitus. Neurofibromas and café au lait spots may also be present but in fewer numbers than NF1.

Cutaneous meningioma

These are typically soft dermal or subcutaneous masses (2–10 cm) found in the scalp and paraspinous regions in children and young adults. The histological features are similar to the intracranial type of meningioma (i.e. psammoma bodies).

Merkel cell tumours

The Merkel disc is the expanded cutaneous nerve ending responsible for mechanoreception. Merkel cell tumours (or trabecular cell carcinoma, small cell carcinoma of the skin) are aggressive malignant tumours arising from dermal Merkel cells; tumours are masses of small dark cells with positive immunostaining for **neuro-endocrine** differentiation.

They are typically found in elderly females (4× males), presenting as a reddish-blue nodule most often on the head and extremities. It is usually an aggressive tumour with early lymphatic spread though spontaneous regression has been reported.

- Friedrich Sigmund Merkel (1845–1919) was a German anatomist. He described the large clear oval cells intimately associated with nerve endings in vertebrate skin in 1875 and named them 'Tastzellen' (touch cells).

Merkel cell carcinoma of the skin
Al-Ghazal SK. *Br J Plast Surg* 1996;**49**:491–496.

The authors suggest the combination of radiotherapy after wide resection due to a high recurrence rate after surgical excision alone. Combination chemotherapy followed by radiation therapy may be suited for advanced locoregional disease and metastatic disease.

The authors suggest that the condition is amenable to sentinel lymph node biopsy.

Predictors of survival and recurrence in the surgical treatment of Merkel cell carcinoma of the extremities

Senchenkov A. *J Surg Oncol* 2007;**95**:229–234.

This is a retrospective study of 38 patients with Merkel cell tumours of the limbs treated by wide local excision or Mohs technique. They found no difference in local recurrence rates between these two groups. Positive nodes were treated whilst negative nodes were either observed or staged with SLNB. Node dissection did not offer any survival benefit but helped predict the risk of regional recurrence. Radiotherapy did not improve survival but reduced the local recurrence rate.

VI. Tumours of muscle

Leiomyosarcoma

Leiomyosarcoma is a malignant tumour of smooth muscle composed of spindle-shaped cells containing myofibrils with cytological atypia. Typical patients are > 60 years of age. The most frequently affected site is the uterine wall, but it may also be found in the retroperitoneum where typically it presents as a metastatic deposit. The tumour invades muscle and spreads along fascial planes and blood vessels. Distant spread occurs by both haematogenous (20% at presentation) and lymphatic routes (less common). The average length of survival is 2 years. Treatment of choice is wide local excision with adjuvant therapy where indicated.

- **Leiomyoma** is the benign counterpart of leiomyosarcoma. It is a smooth muscle tumour arising from erector pili muscle (leiomyoma cutis) most commonly on the extremities. It may also arise from tunica media of blood vessels (angiomyoma) or panniculus carnosus of the genitalia or nipple (dartotic myoma). Lesions present as painful/tender pinkish dermal nodules and adjacent nodules may coalesce to form plaques. Excision is curative. Familial lesions are often multiple.
- **Cutaneous leiomyosarcoma** is a distinct biological entity presenting as a smooth reddish dermal nodule. They tend to run a more indolent course than subcutaneous or deep lesions. These account for 1–2% of all soft tissue sarcomas and may be associated with premalignant leiomyomas, physical trauma and radiation. They arise from dermal smooth muscle, arrector pili and the smooth muscle surrounding eccrine glands. There is a relatively high risk of local recurrence but metastases have never been reported.

Cutaneous leiomyosarcoma

Porter CJ. *Plast Reconstr Surg* 2002;**109**:964–967.

This is a retrospective review of eight patients over 12 years with mean patient age 62.2 years. Four lesions were located on head and neck, whilst the remainder were found on the extremities. The authors reported that there were no local or distant recurrences despite narrow margins in some patients.

Rhabdomyosarcoma

Rhabdo is Greek for rod.

Soft tissue sarcomas account for approximately 7% of all childhood cancers and rhabdomyosarcoma (RMS) alone accounts for over half of these. It is the **most common soft tissue sarcoma in children** (still only 2–3% of total childhood tumours and uncommon in adults) with 40% arising in those under 5 years of age. The incidence in Asians is lower than in Whites. It has been associated with specific chromosomal abnormalities but the aetiology is otherwise unknown.

Most cases are sporadic but after a thorough assessment, some (10–20%) are associated with identifiable genetic risk factors:

- **Li–Fraumeni** cancer susceptibility syndrome (germline p53 mutations) 20–30× risk of sarcomas.
- Beckwith–Wiedemann syndrome.
- NFS type I (4–5%).
- Costello syndrome (germline HRAS mutations), characterized by postnatal growth retardation, typical coarse facies, loose skin and developmental delay.
- Gorlin syndrome.

There is said to be an increased risk in children whose parents use marijuana or cocaine (Grufferman S. *Cancer Causes Control* 1993;**4**:217–224).

Tumours generally present as painless enlarging masses with or without localized symptoms and signs such as overlying erythema. The commonest sites are orbit, nasopharynx, temporal bone and sinonasal. Parameningeal tumours may cause indirect symptoms such as facial nerve or other palsies, ear/nasal discharge etc.

- One-third in the head and neck region particularly orbital (10% of all RMS), parameningeal (middle ear, nasal cavity, paranasal sinuses, nasopharynx or infratemporal fossa). Non-parameningeal tumours affect the scalp, parotid, oral cavity or larynx.

- Genitourinary tumours (1/4) bladder, vagina, testes. More common in males (3×).
- Extremity tumours (1/5) with inguinal node involvement in up to 50%. These tend to be the most aggressive types growing to a large size within weeks.

Tumours arising from the orbit, non-parameningeal head and neck and the genital tracts are often considered to be 'favourable'.

Pathology

The tumours arise from skeletal muscle precursors; some tumours may exhibit skeletal muscle and nerve differentiation (Triton tumours). There are various pathological subtypes with different behaviours e.g. alveolar has a much poorer prognosis with high risk of metastasis; botryoid (shaped like a bunch of grapes) has the best prognosis.

- **Embryonal** (60%) – primitive spindled rhabdomyoblasts.
- **Alveolar** (cancer cells form hollow spaces or 'alveoli'; 20%) – increasing in proportion with age i.e. adolescents and are common in larger muscles of extremities.
- Botryoid embryonal – genitourinary tumours and other mucosal cavities (5%).
- Anaplastic, previously known as **pleomorphic** – the rarest at 1% (higher proportion of adult RMS at 20%).
- Spindle cell embryonal.

Investigations

- CXR, CT, MRI especially head and neck.
- Biopsy – with cytogenetics/FISH, RT-PCR if available.

Staging sytems

Older **group** staging system is the IRS (intergroup RMS staging) on post-surgical margins (complete resection, gross resection with positive margins, gross residual disease or metastases). Staging is related to survival (group I 90%, II 80% and III 70%).

Surgicopathological clinical group with Roman numeral:

- Group I – localized disease, completely resected.
  - Limited to muscle of origin.
  - Beyond muscle of origin.
- Group II – gross total resection.

  - Microscopic residual disease in tumour bed.
  - Microscopic disease in regional nodes.
- Group III – incomplete resection, gross residual disease.
  - Essentially a biopsy.
  - More than 50%.
  - Resected.
- Group IV – distant metastatic.

The Union Internationale Centre le Cancer (**UICC**) **TNMG** does not take extent of surgery into account:

- T stage is determined by site, size and degree of confinement to anatomic site. T1 and T2 are differentiated by confinement to site of origin or otherwise.
- Nodal and distant metastasis, 1 to denote presence.
- Grades 0–4.

Combined for staging:

- Stage I – T1, NX or N0, M0.
- Stage II – T2, NX or N0, M0.
- Stage III – Any T, N1, M0.
- Stage IV – Any T, any N, M1.

RMS staging with Arabic numerals:

- Stage 1 – localized disease in favourable regions e.g. orbit, head and neck (not parameningeal), genitourinary (not bladder or prostate),
- Stage 2 – other locations, N0/X, tumour less than 5 cm.
- Stage 3 – nodal involvement or tumour larger than 5 cm.
- Stage 4 – metastasis.

Treatment

There have been recent advances in the treatment of rhabdomyosarcoma. **Multimodality** management with surgery, chemotherapy and radiotherapy can lead to a 5-year survival in up to 70% (and is better than any single modality); late relapse is uncommon but risk increases in those with gross residual disease in unfavourable sites, or with metastatic disease at diagnosis. The very young (under 1 year of age) who cannot withstand the full course of therapy have poorer results. **Mutilating surgery is avoided**.

Local surgical therapy in the form of **complete resection with 2-cm clear margins** provides the best chance of cure, but there is the potential problem in the head and neck where narrower margins may have to be accepted, or the extremities where compartmentectomy is preferred to amputation, and in such situations radiotherapy as well as chemotherapy plays a major role in control of patients with microscopic or gross residual disease. Durable remissions are possible even in metastasis, with chemotherapy and radiotherapy to the primary site and metastatic sites.

- With only surgery and local RT, there is a recurrence rate involving other sites of up to 80%, hence there has been a shift towards chemotherapy, particularly earlier rather than later.
    - ○ Induction (neoadjuvant) chemotherapy. There has been a shift towards giving combination chemotherapy first, followed by surgery and radiotherapy. In particular, orbital, vaginal and bladder rhabdomyosarcomas show good response and this facilitates more limited surgery.
- Definitive radiotherapy, though may be complicated by growth disturbance and induction of secondary tumours.
- Adjuvant chemotherapy: mainstay is VAC (vincristine, actinomycin D, cyclophosphamide). The Intergroup Rhabdomyosarcoma Study–IV compared cyclophosphamide (VAC) with ifosfamide (VAI) but showed no difference. Stem cell reconstitution seems to have no survival benefit.

Elective or therapeutic **dissection of regional nodes**; node sampling/SLNB staging rather than radical dissection is preferred.

The 5-year disease-free survival rate can be as high as 90% orbit, 69% parameningeal and 80% in other head and neck sites. Many with local recurrence are curable with salvage surgery particularly if primary therapies were complete. Chemotherapy for metastatic disease usually only has temporary effects (slows progression) and 5-year survival is 30% or so. Solitary lung metastases are very rare and confirmation of diagnosis by biopsy is required.

VII. Miscellaneous sarcomas

Liposarcoma

Liposarcomas are relatively common (20% of all STS) and are found in patients in their middle age onwards, affecting males more frequently (in comparison,

Table 8.9 Summary of the different tumour subtypes.

Subtype	5-year survival (%)	Recurrence rate (%)
Well differentiated	85–100	29–62
Myxoid	77–95	33–57
Pleomorphic	21–45	43–73
Round cell	13–55	63–86

benign lipomas tend to be more common in females). The aetiology of these lesions is unknown, but a variety of cytogenetic abnormalities have been described. Liposarcoma arising in pre-existing lipomas has been described but most believe that the majority are distinct lesions with separate origins.

It appears as a diffuse nodular swelling of subcutaneous fat, most commonly the lower limb or buttock, but may appear in retroperitoneal and mesenteric fat. Lesions demonstrate haematogenous spread but well-differentiated lesions are unlikely to metastasize. The histological grade has predictive value and is the single most important criterion.

It is a **malignant tumour of mesenchymal cells resembling fat cells**. Histologically there are uniglobular and multiglobular fat cells and undifferentiated sarcoma cells. There have been reports of well-differentiated liposarcoma de-differentiating to high-grade MFH.

Treatment of choice is excision with a wide margin (3–5 cm; despite an apparent capsule lesions are infiltrative); radiotherapy may have a role as an adjunct for well-differentiated or myxoid subtypes. Local recurrence and survival is related to the pathological subtype.

Synovial sarcoma

This is relatively rare (6–10% of all STS) but most common in adolescents and young adults (males 2× more frequent) (second to rhabdomyosarcoma), arising from soft tissues in the vicinity of large joints of the extremities (it has no relation to synovium per se, and is called synovial because of its histological appearance). Lesions are generally high grade with poor prognosis with local and distant (including lymphatic) recurrence being common.

Pathological subtypes – a reciprocal translocation t(X;18)(p11.2;q11.2) has been identified:

- Biphasic with epithelial and sarcomatous cells.
- Monophasic fibrous.
- Monophasic epithelial.

All synovial sarcoma are classified as high grade by the AJCC. Lymph node metastases are rare (5%) but distant metastases (usually lungs) are fairly common (50%).

Excision with post-operative radiotherapy is the commonest treatment (radiotherapy reduces recurrence rates from 60–90% to 28–49%). Chemotherapy (ifosfamide) may be beneficial for distant metastasis.

Advances in the surgical management of sarcomas in children
Andrassy RJ. *Am J Surg* 2002;**184**:484–491.

Synovial sarcoma is the most common non-rhabdomyosarcoma soft tissue sarcoma (NRSTS) in children; 30% of all patients with synovial sarcoma are under 20 years of age.

- Most are found on lower extremity.
- Lymph node metastases occur in up to 15% of cases and SLNB is used to assess nodal status.
- Distant metastatic disease mostly to the lungs.

All tumours should be regarded as high grade and the best treatment is adequate negative surgical margins plus adjuvant radiotherapy; chemotherapy is generally ineffective. Late relapse is possible therefore long-term follow-up is advocated.

Clear cell sarcoma

This mainly occurs in young adults and typically presents as a subcutaneous mass around the knee. Histologically, lesions are S-100 and HMB45 positive and some regard it as a variant of malignant melanoma. The prognosis is poor with local and distant (including lymphatic) recurrence being common.

Gastrointestinal stromal tumours

Gastrointestinal stromal tumours (GiST) mostly affect patients aged 40–60. Approximately half affect the stomach and another quarter the small intestine. It has been related to KIT mutation.

Treatment
- Surgery is usually the primary treatment but there is a high recurrence rate.
- Standard chemotherapy is rarely effective but good responses to imatinib mesylate have been described (possibly needed indefinitely).

VIII. Resection margins

Positive resection margins, local recurrence and survival
If positive margins are resected, then there is residual tumour in about 55% (Zagars 2003 vide infra) and margin status is an important predictor. Local recurrence does not always have to be strongly related to a positive resection margin (particularly if planned and if low grade; Gerrand 2001 vide infra) due to adjuvant therapies (Eilber 2003 vide infra).

Local recurrence is often taken to be a marker of an aggressive tumour that is more likely to metastasize but the exact relationship between local tumour recurrence and survival is yet to be fully defined.

Classification of positive margins following resection of soft tissue sarcoma of the limb predicts the risk of local recurrence
Gerrand CH. *J Bone Joint Surg Br* 2001;**83**:1149–1155.

The authors suggest that positive surgical margins may occur after limb-sparing excision of soft tissue sarcoma for the following reasons:

- **Group 1 – Planned positive margins** with **low-grade liposarcomas** that often present as large tumours. Planned marginal excision will help to preserve vital structures such as blood vessels and nerves with the rationale that the lesion seldom recurs locally and rarely metastasizes, behaving quite differently from soft tissue sarcomas of other histological types.
- **Group 2** – Planned positive margins due to deliberate marginal resection of tumours other than low-grade liposarcoma to preserve vital structures **after decision to accept positive margins** agreed at MDT planning meeting.
- **Group 3 – Unplanned positive margin at re-excision** of an incompletely excised and previously unrecognized sarcoma (first attempt at excision usually by a non-sarcoma surgeon).
- **Group 4 – Unplanned positive margin due to primary surgery** performed by the sarcoma team but surgical margins found to be histologically positive – further excision always considered in such cases.

Their retrospective review of a database of 566 soft tissue sarcoma patients at Mount Sinai Hospital showed 87 patients with positive margins after limb-sparing surgery for extremity soft tissue sarcoma. All had had neoadjuvant radiotherapy and a post-operative radiotherapy boost. The local recurrence rate (at mean follow-up of 5.4 years) was 3.6–4.2% vs. 31.6–37.5% in groups 1 and 2 (planned) and groups 3 and 4 (unplanned), i.e. there was a **low rate of recurrence following excisional surgery with planned positive margins**.

High grade extremity soft tissue sarcoma: factors predictive of local recurrence and its effect on morbidity and mortality
Eilber FC. *Ann Surg* 2003;**237**:218–226.

This was a retrospective review of 753 patients treated for intermediate to high-grade extremity sarcoma at UCLA.

- 607 patients were treated for primary tumours – 10% developed locally recurrent disease.
- 146 patients were treated for locally recurrent tumours – 20% developed locally recurrent disease. Reduced overall survival at 5 years 67% vs. 71% in primary tumours.

Microscopically positive margins (2%) were treated by additional local re-excision, additional radiotherapy, amputation or no further treatment. Of the 92 patients who developed locally recurrent disease, only five had positive resection margins – i.e. **positive resection margin was not a significant risk factor for the development of local recurrence**. Instead significant risk factors for development of local recurrence in order of hazard ratio were:

- Malignant peripheral nerve sheath tumour.
- High histological grade.
- Age > 50 years.
- Failure to receive neoadjuvant treatment was the only risk factor in patients treated for already locally recurrent disease.

Significant risk factors for **decreased survival** in order of hazard ratio:

- Local recurrence.
- High histological grade.
- Leiomyosarcoma.
- Size.
- Age > 50 years.
- Lower extremity location.
- Male gender was a risk factor in patients treated for already locally recurrent disease.

Surgical margins and reresection in the management of patients with soft tissue sarcoma using conservative surgery and radiation therapy

Zagars GK. *Cancer* 2003;**97**:2544–2553.

This paper reviewed the MD Anderson Cancer Centre experience of 666 patients in whom **macroscopic** tumour clearance had been achieved *prior to* tertiary referral.

Histological margins were defined as:

- **Negative** if tumour was not actually present at the inked margin. The actual distance was not regarded as significant (n = 129).
- **Positive** with presence of microscopic disease at the surgical margin (n = 63).
- **Uncertain** if there was no comment upon margin of clearance on the pathology report from the referring centre (n = 220).

Re-resection was undertaken only when the primary surgery was judged as inadequate and when it could be undertaken without significant functional morbidity. **Residual tumour was identified in 46% overall**, about half of those with uncertain or positive margins and surprisingly one-third of patients with negative margins (but a small group). Local control at 5, 10 and 15 years was better in those who had re-resection at each time point. The most significant predictors of local recurrence were:

- Age > 64 years.
- Positive or uncertain resection margins (primary or re-excision).
- Recurrent tumour at presentation to the specialist unit.
- Tumour size > 10 cm.

The most important predictor of **lymph node recurrence** was histopathological tumour type – epitheloid sarcoma, rhabdomyosarcoma and clear cell sarcoma.

Predictors of distant metastases

- Tumour size > 5 cm, tumour grade and margin status.
- Negative margins achieved by re-resection still qualified as negative and patients in whom negative margins were not achieved by re-resection had shorter disease-free and overall survival. This effect was most significant for tumour of the extremities or superficial trunk and least significant for head and neck tumours.

Major amputation for soft tissue sarcoma
Clark MA. *Br J Surg* 2003;**90**:102–107.

This was a retrospective review of 40 major amputations (forequarter/hindquarter) undertaken at the Royal Marsden Hospital for soft tissue sarcoma over a 10-year period. 31/40 were performed for recurrent disease following limb-sparing surgery and 37/40 were performed with curative intent.

The median hospital stay was 10.5 days. 50% were disease-free at 12 months and 23% were alive and disease-free beyond 2 years. Phantom pain or sensation occurred in 75% (severe in one-quarter).

Soft tissue sarcoma of the upper extremity: a five year experience at two institutions emphasizing the role of soft tissue flap reconstruction
Lohman RF. *Cancer* 2002;**94**:2256–2264.

This was a review of 100 patients requiring resection of an upper extremity soft tissue sarcoma. 29% underwent intralesional (positive histological margins) or marginal (within the tumour pseudocapsule) resection whilst 70% of patients underwent wide excision (cuff of normal tissue) or compartmental resection. The size of the resection margin was often dictated by the proximity of vital structures when undertaking limb-sparing surgery.

29% of patients required soft tissue reconstruction (two free fillet flaps); in the others, the defect was closed primarily. **Wound complications were common in both groups of patients (about one-third) and recurrence rates were also similar**.

- The indications for flaps included: insufficient soft tissue for primary closure, coverage of neurovascular structures or implant material and to fill dead space. Flaps were most commonly needed around the elbow.

Soft tissue sarcomas of the upper extremity
Popov P. *Plast Reconstr Surg* 2004;**113**:222–230.

This is a retrospective review of 95 upper extremity soft tissue sarcomas treated at the Helsinki University Hospital over a 12-year period. Their definitions of surgical margins were:

- **Compartmental** (entire compartment resected en bloc with tumour) included 'myectomy' for intramuscular tumours.
- **Wide** (nearest margin > 2.5 cm or < 2.5 cm but intact anatomical barrier, e.g. fascia).
- **Marginal** (< 2.5 cm but negative histological margins).
- **Intralesional** (macroscopic or microscopic disease at margin).

The aim of surgery was preservation of function whilst excising widely. If wide excision was impossible then they performed a planned marginal excision (clear but < 2.5 cm) supplemented by adjuvant radiotherapy. Reoperation for positive margins was performed where possible.

- The arm was amputated only when a major nerve, bone or joint was infiltrated by tumour (n = 10).

At 5 years, there was 79% overall local control rate and 68% overall metastases-free survival.

- **There was no difference in recurrence rates between wide excision or marginal excision plus radiotherapy**.
- Metastases were more common with extracompartmental primaries and large tumour size.

E. Vascular lesions

I. Haemangiomas

Mulliken and Glowacki demonstrated that there are only two major types of vascular birthmarks based on differences in clinical, histological, haematological and radiological/skeletal features. The histological features are the most important differentiating factors – haemangiomas have plump endothelia, increased mast cells, and multilaminated basement membranes whilst vascular malformations have flat endothelia, normal mast cell numbers, and a thin basement membrane.

- **Haemangiomas**: increased turnover of endothelial cells, proliferate and involute (e.g. strawberry naevus); they may be superficial, deep or combined.
- **Vascular malformations**: these arise due to inborn errors of vascular morphogenesis, and are thus permanent and may be progressive. They are classified according to their flow characteristics and their composition – capillary, lymphatic, venous, arterial, combined.

Haemangiomas are **benign neoplasms** (with increased endothelial cell turnover, multilaminated basement membranes) of vascular tissue with a well-defined life cycle of rapid proliferation and slower involution. They are the most common tumours of infancy and the most common birthmark (20× more common than port wine stain) and are seen in up to 10% of White children. Haemangiomas are more common in

White females (3×) born to older mothers particularly if premature or in multiple births. 90% appear within the first month of life though up to one-third may be seen at birth. Precursor lesions are those that appear prior to the actual proliferation of the haemangioma and include pale patches, telangiectasia, macular erythema or bluish discolouration that may be confused with port wine stains.

These lesions grow rapidly in the first year of life and then intravascular thrombosis and fibrosis results in regression with a colour change from bright to dull red, then with central greying. Involution also corresponds with **mast cell infiltration** and as a general rule, 50% involute aged 5 years, 60% aged 6 and 90% aged 9. Whilst most resolve without major complications, often there is a pale pink or wrinkled scar and the regression of bulkier lesions tends to be incomplete, leaving an atrophic or dented (anetoderma) scar in many cases. Early onset of resolution leads to a better cosmetic outcome whilst the rate of resolution is generally unaffected by ulceration, size or depth of lesion. Spontaneous resolution is said to be more common in premature infants.

Although these can be subdivided by their depth their clinical behaviour is similar.

- **Superficial** also known as capillary haemangioma, haemangioma simplex, capillary naevus, strawberry haemangioma or naevus due to its colour.
- **Deep** also known as cavernous haemangioma; bluish colour and may be confused with a venous vascular malformation.

Most haemangiomas are localized but larger ones may occupy a dermatomal type distribution and are called segmental haemangiomas that tend to occur earlier and grow bigger and become unsightly. These may be associated with other anomalies (**PHACE syndrome** – posterior fossa abnormalities e.g. Dandy Walker malformation, haemangiomas of head and neck, arterial cerebrovascular anomalies, cardiac defects and eye anomalies – some add an 'S' for sternal clefts; **PELVIS syndrome** – perineural haemangioma, external genitalia abnormalities, lipomyelomeningocoele, vesicorenal abnormalities, imperforate anus and skin tags). Some family history e.g. autosomal-dominant inheritance pattern in some patients and may be associated with other congenital abnormalities. Associated syndromes are less common than with vascular malformations.

The exact cause is unknown but hypoxia seems to be an important factor.

- VEGF expression decreases with resolution but bFGF levels remain high.
- Mast cell population dramatically increases in involuting lesions.
- Levels of matrix metalloproteinases and bFGF seem to be correlated with proliferating lesions.

Most occur in the region of the head and neck (60%) with about 30% on the face or scalp; **visceral lesions** can occur without cutaneous lesions. 80% are single, whilst multiple haemangiomas are more common in multiple births and may be associated with internal haemangiomas of CNS and viscera. Those with more than four skin haemangiomas should have a CT (liver) to rule out visceral involvement. The most common parotid tumour of childhood is a haemangioma; there is a risk of ear canal obstruction with conductive hearing loss.

- In **diffuse neonatal haemangiomatosis** there are multiple, small uniform cutaneous lesions that may be associated with visceral lesions in the liver, gut and central nervous system. These may be asymptomatic but there may also be high-output cardiac failure, obstructive jaundice or haemorrhage/coagulopathy. Lesions (both cutaneous and visceral lesions) tend to involute by age 2 years.
  - Symptomatic patients should be treated; ultrasound or MRI studies are indicated – lower midline back lesions may be associated with spinal dysraphism.

Non-operative treatments

- **Observation** only with dressings for minor bleeding etc. Reassurance after explanation of the condition is sufficient in most cases; photography may be useful. The child is reviewed in regular follow-up visits.
- **Corticosteroids**.
  - **Oral steroids** – there are many different regimes, some suggest a short course of high-dose steroids (4 mg/kg/day for 2 weeks) followed by a gradual tailing off whilst others say 2–3 mg/kg/day for 4–6 weeks). There is close to 100% response in proliferating lesions that some may rebound on withdrawal and some may require an additional course.

Steroids are used for the treatment of **rapidly growing** haemangiomas but must be used under close supervision e.g. by a paediatrician. Immunizations should be withheld until the patient has stopped steroids for 1 month. Side-effects include increased appetite, change in sleep patterns, increased risk of infection and adrenal suppression.

○ The use of **intralesional steroid** injections (triamcinolone, 3–5 mg/kg/dose) has been reported for periorbital haemangiomas but complications include local (globe perforation, blindness, eyelid necrosis, retinal artery embolization, soft tissue/fat atrophy, bleeding) and steroid-related – systemic absorption is significant.

○ **Topical** high potency corticosteroids may be effective in small very superficial haemangiomas but are not commonly used.

● Propranolol has been recently reported.

● **Pulsed-dye lasers** may be used for superficial lesions and may improve outcome especially for ulcerated lesions. The use of intralesional argon lasers for deeper tissues has been described but is not a standard procedure.

● **Interferon** (anti-angiogenic) can be used for lesions not responsive to corticosteriods including non-proliferating lesions. Due to the side-effects, it is generally reserved for use in life-threatening lesions only, e.g. systemic haemangiomatosis. There is a 10–25% incidence of potentially severe side-effects including fever, neutropenia, spastic diplegia (5%, potentially permanent but may be reversible with early discontinuation) and motor delay.

● Others include compression e.g. for limb lesions, cryotherapy, imiquimod, radiation and vincristine.

Propranolol for severe hemangiomas of infancy

Leaute-Labreze C. *New Engl J Med* 2008;**358**:2649–2651.

In this letter, the authors report on their experience with the use of oral propranolol in 11 children with haemangiomas. They report discernible changes within 24 hours of starting treatment. They speculate on the mechanism of action.

Since then, multiple reports have appeared in the literature – many have described successful use of the drug though the optimal dosage is not yet known, whilst others are concerned about the potential side-effects.

In a review by Storch CH (*Br J Dermatol* 2010;**163**:269–274) the early effects seem to be related to vasoconstriction due to reduced nitric oxide release, intermediate effects due to inhibition of angiogenic signals (VEGF, bFGF and matrix metalloproteinases (MMPs)) and long-term effects may be due to induction of apoptosis.

Life-threatening infantile haemangioma: a dramatic response to propranolol

Theletsane T. *J Eur Acad Dermatol Venereol* 2009: **23**:1465–1466.

A dosage of 2 mg/kg/day was effective within 24 hours in reducing stridor in an infant not responding to oral steroids.

Propranolol for infantile hemangiomas: early experience at a Tertiary Vascular anomalies center

Buckmiller LM. *Laryngoscope* 2010;**120**:676–681.

This paper reports on 32 children treated with oral propranolol (2 mg/kg/day in three divided doses). 97% showed improvement (50% excellent responders). Therapy continued until 1 year of age, or until observable benefit ceased – weaning was required – halving the dose for 1–2 weeks and then stopping. Side-effects were reported in 10 patients including somnolence, gastroesophageal reflux and a rash. Patients had baseline investigations including ECG. A history of asthma, cardiovascular illness or hypoglycaemia was specifically elicited by questioning of parents.

Lawley LP (*J Eur Acad Dermatol Venereol* 2010;**27**:320–321) suggests that older children may have outpatient treatment (baseline ECG and blood glucose) but recommend those under 3 months of age should have inpatient treatment in a hospital setting with continuous monitoring. Yamada K. (*J Eur Acad Dermatol Venereol* 2010;**27**:319–310) suggests starting at 0.5 mg/kg/day in 3 divided doses for a week, then 1 mg/kg/day for another week before going to 2 mg/kg/day. Hypoglycaemia seems to be the most commonly reported complication (Bonifazi E. *Ped Dermatol* 2010;**27**:195–196).

The rapid action makes it suited for more urgent situations such as airway or orbital haemangiomas (Li YC. *Clin Exp Ophthalmol*, published on line 2010 doi: 10.1111/j.1442–9071.2010.02327.x).

Complications

● Ulceration (more common in rapidly growing lesions and in the diaper area); recurrent problematic bleeding is rare as these are low flow lesions.

- Large/diffuse complex lesions may be associated with skeletal distortion or high-output cardiac failure.
- Late complications include scarring, residual colour/mass, redundant skin, telangiectasia and hypopigmentation.

Indications for surgery

Uncomplicated haemangiomas should, in general, be left alone until complete involution and late scar revision are performed. However, selected lesions may be excised e.g. very small lesions, with psychological morbidity (including anxious parents), can be easily excised and directly closed. In addition, nasal tip and vermilion lesions are notoriously slow to involute whilst congenital haemangiomas tend not to involute.

- Obstruction e.g. oral cavity, airways; neonates are obligate nasal breathers.
- Impingement on visual axis (mechanical ptosis) causing amblyopia whilst deformation of the growing cornea may cause astigmatism.
- Severe bleeding or ulceration unresponsive to conservative treatments.

Kasabach–Merritt syndrome is a sequestration of platelets leading to thrombocytopaenia, localized consumption coagulopathy (low platelets and fibrinogen decreased, but PT/PTT minimal change) and DIC with a mortality rate of 30–40%. It is associated with haemangioendothelioma or tufted angioma and not the common types of haemangioma. Treatment options include excision, interferons or systemic corticosteroids.

Management of haemangioma of infancy
Achauer BM. *Plast Reconstr Surg* 1997;**99**:1301–1308.

This is a retrospective review of treatment outcomes in 245 patients. Complications seen included obstruction, ulceration, bleeding, infection and pain. Their data showed that laser therapy was most efficacious in terms of volume reduction, colour and texture compared with observation, steroids, surgery or combined modalities. The authors recommend that its early use be considered in complicated haemangiomas and to avoid psychological morbidity.

Vascular lip enlargement: Part I. hemangiomas – tenets of therapy
Zide BM. *Plast Reconstr Surg* 1997;**100**:1664–1673.

Lip lesions may cause difficulty in eating and drinking along with psychosocial morbidity. Steroids can control endothelial cell proliferation with a 30–90% response rate if used during the proliferative phase but may cause growth retardation. Waiting for involution and subsequent scar revision is psychologically debilitating. In such cases, early intervention is advocated to avoid teasing and childhood depression (2–3 years of age). Debulking procedures described include horizontal and vertical elliptical/wedge excisions. Reduction of haemangioma bulk should be conservative; avoid lip denervation by central or paracentral reduction. Mucosal advancement may be needed to reconstruct vermilion.

Intralesional photocoagulation of peri-orbital haemangioma
Achauer BM. *Plast Reconstr Surg* 1999;**103**:11–16.

Twenty-three patients were treated with bare tip KTP or Nd:YAG laser introduced **into** the haemangioma. The aim in treating periorbital haemangiomas was to avoid amblyopia secondary to a mechanical ptosis. Two-thirds had a > 50% reduction in bulk at 3 months without affecting the overlying skin though there was ulceration in four patients.

A NICE review in 2004 concluded that intralesional photocoagulation is of uncertain efficacy; **facial nerve damage** is an important potential complication (Burstein FD. *Ann Plast Surg* 2000;**44**:188–194; two cases in 100 patients, with small burns in two and superficial ulceration in 20).

Pyogenic granuloma

Pyogenic granuloma are vascular nodules comprised of proliferating capillaries in a loose stroma, although histologically they are 'haemangiomas' – they are reactive rather than neoplastic. They often follow trauma with rapid growth and the tendency to bleed easily. The proliferating vessels extend deep into dermis, thus recurrence is likely after simple cautery e.g. with silver nitrate sticks, and excision is preferred.

II. Vascular malformations

Mulliken and Glowacki classification 1982

- Low flow: capillary (PWS), venous and lymphatic.
- High flow: arterial and arteriovenous.

Port wine stain

Port wine stains (PWS) are capillary vascular malformations related to developmental weakness of vessel walls leading to progressive ectatic dilatation of mature superficial dermal vessels. The frequent distribution along with the branches of the fifth cranial nerve suggest a neurogenic pathogenesis. Most lesions occur in the head and neck; 50% of facial PWS are restricted to one trigeminal sensory region, the remainder involve more than one, cross midline, or are bilateral.

Port wine stains occur with an incidence of about 0.3% of neonates with equal sex and racial predilection. They are almost always present at birth with growth in proportion to the child. They start off as a flat patch with a deep red–purple colour but may progress to become nodular (cobblestoning) and hypertrophic over time (supposedly related to density of sympathetic innervation – relative deficiency causes slow growth whilst an absolute deficiency causes an aggressive, rapidly growing lesion).

- **Sturge–Weber syndrome.** A facial PWS (particularly V1) may be associated with congenital glaucoma or ipsilateral leptomeningeal angiomatosis causing neurological symptoms such as seizures (may be intractable) and mental disability. Imaging may demonstrate railroad track calcifications. PWS of the V2 and V3 regions only have a low risk of brain involvement. Proper assessment and follow-up is needed in those with V1 lesions. Fundoscopic examination and tonometry are required to monitor for retinal detachment, glaucoma or blindness.
- **Klippel–Trenaunay syndrome** – there is soft tissue hypertrophy and bony overgrowth of an extremity, in association with a capillary malformation. The overgrowth is not present at birth but may eventually lead to significant limb length discrepancy. There are no associated CNS or visceral anomalies. Treatment is usually limited to premature epiphyseal closure as surgical debulking is usually not feasible because of the **lateral** varicose veins that may represent the only venous outflow for the limb, though this is being challenged. A similar clinical picture occurs in **Parkes–Weber syndrome** with arteriovenous malformations (AVM).

Differential diagnoses

- Flat haemangioma.
- **Naevus flammeus neonatorum** – fading macular stain that affects 50% of neonates, in the supratrochlear or supraorbital nerve territories; one-half resolve spontaneously whilst the remainder persist but never progress.

- **Salmon patch.** These are pink patches found most frequently on the nape of the neck; they occur in up to 50% of infants but usually disappear within a year. Transient flushing may be seen during crying and exertion. The lesion is composed of ectatic superficial dermal capillaries, and is thought to reflect persistence of fetal-type dermal circulation.

Treatment

Pulsed-dye lasers (PDLs) were a major breakthrough and are the treatment of choice for PWS. Although multiple treatments are required (average 6.4), there are few side-effects; however only 10% of lesions will be completely ablated, 60–70% will have improved but 20% will have no benefit.

- No anaesthesia is needed for treatment of smaller lesions in adults; whilst topical anaesthesia is sufficient for pain control, a general anaesthetic is usually needed in infants and children, particularly with large lesions. There seems to be evidence that aggressive treatment of infants and young children at earlier ages improves PWS clearance; early treatment takes advantages of 'optical' advantages to allow deeper penetration into tissues.
  - Less cumulative ultraviolet light exposure results in less epidermal melanin which competes for the absorption of laser light.
  - Less collagen in the skin results in less scatter.
  - Due to the heterogeneous size/calibre of vessels in a PWS, many suggest combining several different lasers – shorter wavelengths first to target smaller vessels, then longer wavelengths and pulses for residual, deeper and larger vessels.
- Improvements include selective epidermal cooling permitting the use of higher light dosages and better clearing.
- The response does seem to vary according to anatomical area: the central face responds less well compared with the lateral face.
- Some reports suggested that up to 50% may 'recur' or redarken (Huikeshoven M. *New Engl J Med* 2007;**356**:1235–1240) after 4 years but this is probably due to deeper vessels working their way up to the surface, rather than the previously treated vessels 'reforming' i.e. not a true 'recurrence'. Criticisms made against the Huikeshoven study include the fact that the patients were treated with older machines without cooling and that the average age of the patients was 13.

Skin grafting and cosmetic camouflage were the only options prior to PDL and can still be considered for the non-responders; there are trials with 1064 nm long pulse and IPL 590 nm filter.

Comparison of intense pulsed light (IPL) and pulsed dye laser (PDL) in port-wine stain treatment

Drosner M. *Med Laser Appl* 2008;**23**:133–140.

This study from Munich included 100 patients with PWS who were divided into left–right sides for treatment with IPL and PDL, repeated 6–8 weekly until one side showed improvement or had side-effects at which point patients were given a choice. Superior clearing by IPL was found in 57.5% vs. 13.8% for PDL; patients elected to continue with IPL in 59% vs. 19% preferring PDL.

Vascular lip enlargement: Part II. Port-wine macrochelia

Zide BM. *Plast Reconstr Surg* 1997;**100**:1674–1681.

Lasers are effective in treating surface colour but do little to reduce bulk. As PWSs do not involute, there is no rationale for delayed surgery – generally lip reduction surgery to debulk (with slight over-reduction) with post-operative laser. It is a low-flow lesion so bleeding is not excessive but oozing should be expected.

Venous malformations

These are soft blue skin/subcutaneous swellings composed of superficial or deep venous lakes that empty with compression and elevation, and demonstrate no pulsation. They are often multiple; 85% occur in the head and neck; the lips are commonly involved, usually laterally, as well as the tongue.

They are non-proliferative and thus generally non-progressive but may enlarge with episodes of trauma or infection (thrombophlebitis), or crying, straining in an infant/Valsalva manoeuvre; lesions are also sensitive to the hormonal environment. They show no tendency for involution and may form phleboliths which is said to be pathognomonic.

They can be hereditary.

Large facial lesions may show deep involvement of masseter and parotid but bony involvement is rare (mandible is commonest). It is generally a cosmetic deformity in the main, though functional sequelae are possible e.g. orbital venous malformation can cause enophthalmos or exorbitism (depending upon filling) or may communicate with the infratemporal fossa via the inferior orbital fissure. Some patients, particularly those with large/multiple lesions, may have a coagulopathy due to decreased fibrinogen.

Treatment

- Conservative. Compression garments can help.
- Intralesional sclerotherapy – 95% ethanol or sodium tetradecyl sulphate 3% (maximum 30 ml a time), staged injections every 3 months. Complications include skin necrosis, blistering or nerve injury.
- Discrete lesions can be considered for excision – a prior course of sclerotherapy 4 weeks before surgery may be considered. The extent of involvement of the soft tissues should be carefully defined e.g. with MRI (T1-weighted image – isointense with muscle, T2-weighted image – hyperintense, phleboliths appear as dark holes). Fluid–fluid levels may be present.

Evaluation and treatment of head and neck venous vascular malformations

Pappas DC. *Ear, Nose Throat J* 1998;**77**:914–922.

Digital subtraction angiography with percutaneous puncture and injection of contrast allows the lesion to be defined. Sclerotherapy with 95% ethanol is effective in reducing the size of the lesion with immediate coagulation, followed by an intense inflammatory response that causes late fibrosis. Sclerotherapy is contraindicated if malformations communicate with the ophthalmic veins to avoid cavernous sinus thrombosis. Extravasation may cause soft tissue necrosis. Surgery was reserved for residual disease when assessed at least 4 months following sclerotherapy.

Evaluation of vascular birthmarks

Birthmarks that still present at the 4-week check-up should be examined by a vascular birthmark specialist.

- In the **V1 dermatome**, Sturge–Weber syndrome should be ruled out. A paediatric eye specialist should also rule out glaucoma; MRI to rule out meningeal involvement.
- In the **V3 dermatome**, paediatric ENT surgeon should rule out airway, palate and gum involvement. Stridor suggests airway involvement.
- At the base of skull/base of spine and rapidly proliferating – a neurologist should rule out nerve involvement, especially for large, rapidly growing lesions.
- In the periorbital area, a paediatric eye specialist should rule out vision impairment.
- Lesions of the nasal tip, particularly if rapidly proliferating – an ENT surgeon should assess early to reduce the risk of cartilage erosion.

- Lesions involving a wide area and very rapidly proliferating – Kasabach–Merritt syndrome should be ruled out; a paediatric haematologist should also be consulted.
- On the extremities and/or trunk area – consider referral to a paediatric orthopaedic specialist to assess for Klippel–Trenaunay syndrome.

Infants with cutaneous lesions with symptoms suggesting **internal lesions** always require imaging.

- Distended abdomen and enlarged liver – possibly haemangiomas of the liver.
- Stridor.
- Seizures.
- Blood in the stool.

Arteriovenous malformations

Schobinger classification

International Workshop for the Study of Vascular Anomalies 1990.

- Stage 1 – AV shunting – quiescence.
- Stage 2 – thrill, pulsation, bruit – expansion.
- Stage 3 – ulceration, bleeding, pain – destruction.
- Stage 4 – high output cardiac failure – decompensation.

Arteriovenous malformations (AVMs) are due to errors of angiogenesis during weeks 4–6. Although present at birth, at least at a microscopic level, they may not be immediately obvious – most patients have a cutaneous blush during infancy or at birth, resembling a PWS. They may be localized or diffuse with the middle upper lip a common site; intracranial lesions are more common than limbs, trunk or viscera.

They may be first noticed following puberty; they are often undiagnosed until adulthood when discolouration or a pulsatile mass is noted. AVMs are generally high-flow, warm, pulsatile with thrills/bruits. They may ulcerate causing bleeding (in one-third, either spontaneously or after trauma such as after dental extraction – a loose tooth in a bleeding socket should be treated with caution) and pain. Puberty or pregnancy may provoke progression from stages 1 to 2 or 3.

Treatment

Treatment is directed predominantly at stage 3/4 lesions.

- **Embolization** alone causes recruitment of other feeding vessels and so is inadequate as a standalone treatment.

- Commonly pre-operative angiography and embolization is followed by surgery within 24–48 hours. High-grade lesions may involve skin, making skin excision mandatory, as it can be the source of recurrence. Some recommend excision early in life (Kohout 1998).

Arteriovenous malformations of the head and neck
Kohout MP. *Plast Reconstr Surg* 1998;**102**:643–654.

In a retrospective review of 81 patients, there was bony involvement in 22 patients – cranium, maxilla or mandible. Most patients were treated by embolization combined with resection. Bony resection and reconstruction was secondary to soft tissue procedures and most soft tissue defects were closed with local tissues or skin grafts, with free flaps in 11 patients. The outcome was adversely affected by increasing Schobinger stage and intervention at stage 1 to prevent progression may be indicated in children with discrete scalp and lip lesions. Treatment with laser and steroids was not effective.

Large arteriovenous malformations of the face: aesthetic results with recurrence control
Bradley JP. *Plast Reconstr Surg* 1999;**103**:351–361.

The authors used highly selective embolization and resection to treat 300 facial AVMs. 'Cure is elusive and recurrence can be rapid' – in particular, resection of scalp AVMs must include the periosteum to avoid recurrence. They noted that hypovascularity develops in neighbouring tissues making them of dubious reliability for expansion.

Lymphatic malformations

Classification

- **Microcystic** (previously known as lymphangioma, tend to be firm) tend to be diffuse lesions that violate tissue planes. Commonly facial or cervicofacial.
- **Macrocystic** (previously known as cystic hygroma, tend to be soft) are localized and respect tissue planes, thus tend to shell out easily.

Lymphatic malformations are a focus of abnormal development of lymphatics that grow in proportion with growth of the child. Most lymphatic malformations will present at birth though they may only manifest themselves during late childhood or adolescence. The head and neck is most commonly affected, particularly the posterior triangle; in this region, lymphatic malformations are often a combination of macro- and microcystic disease.

- Lymphatic malformations do not involute – they fill and empty, and any sudden enlargement may be due to intralesional bleeding or in response to infection e.g. **upper respiratory tract infection** (URTI) or cellulitis secondary to minor trauma. Overall 17% have an episode of infection; 6–8 weeks of antibiotics is recommended.
- Some may have a significant venous component i.e. lymphovenous malformation though intralesional bleeding may cause confusion. Phleboliths seen in some patients may be secondary to intralesional bleeding.
- Local mass effects may cause compression – **airway obstruction**, difficulty feeding.
- It is a known cause of **macroglossia**. Infiltration of soft tissues of the oral cavity, especially tongue, may also lead to dental caries secondary to difficulty in access for cleaning and speech problems.
- Secondary bony **hypertrophy** especially mandible; may lead to abnormal bite/occlusion.
- Thoracic lymphatic malformations involving the mediastinum may cause pleural and pericardial effusions whilst lesions in the groin can cause lymphoedema and limb hypertrophy.

Investigations

- **Transillumination test**.
- Fluid levels on **MRI** scan are diagnostic: 'rim enhancement' (gadolinium) and hyperintense (T2).

Management

- Antibiotics and NSAIDs if inflamed.
- Support garments if needed.
- Sclerotherapy with 95% ethanol or sodium tetradecyl sulphate 3% is often used before surgery. Alternatives include OK-432 (denatured group A *Streptococcus pyogenes*) or doxycycline.
- Surgical excision should be carefully planned after imaging has defined the full extent as recurrence is almost inevitable following incomplete excision (more than 40%), as the lymphatics regenerate. Complete macroscopic excision may still have a 20% recurrence rate.
- Laser (Nd:YAG) has been used for cutaneous lesions.

The surgical management of giant cervicofacial lymphatic malformations

Lille ST. *J Paediatr Surg* 1996;**31**:1648–1650.

Although inadequate excision led to a high recurrence rate, surgical excision remains the definitive management. Infiltration along tissue planes sometimes meant extensive involvement of intra-oral structures and nerves and skin involvement, in which skin had to be excised and reconstructed. Mandibular osteotomy improves intra-oral access.

Cervicofacial lymphatic malformations

Padwa BL. *Plast Reconstr Surg* 1995;**95**:951–960.

Massive cervicofacial lesions account for ~3% of lymphatic malformations. Priorities are airway problems, for which a tracheostomy is frequently required (two-thirds in this series), and to establish a feeding line.

The authors described their protocol of staged debulking, where resection was limited to a defined anatomical region at each stage e.g. tongue reduction. Mandibular surgery, particularly the correction of class III malocclusion and anterior open bite, was performed after completion of skeletal growth, usually with a segmental mandibulectomy, inferior border resection or Le Fort I osteotomy. Lymphatic malformation could be present within medullary bone.

Surgery was complicated by injury to facial and hypoglossal nerves in some cases.

Cystic hygroma of the chest wall

Ardenghy M. *Ann Plast Surg* 1996;**37**:211–213.

Seventy-five per cent of macrocystic lymphatic malformations (cystic hygromas) occur in the neck with predilection for the left side, mainly in the posterior triangle. Ultrasound scan demonstrates multiloculated cysts, and CT or MRI were used to define the relationship of the lymphatic malformation with surrounding tissues. The authors recommend treatment by conservative excision.

Syndromes associated with vascular malformations:

- Klippel–Trenaunay – venous and lymphatic malformations, capillary malformation.
- Parkes–Weber (CM-AVM) high-flow AVM or fistula, with capillary malformation of skin, limb hypertrophy. May have *RASA1* mutation in familial cases.
- Maffucci's syndrome – venous malformations, multiple enchondromas (1/4 malignant change).
- Blue rubber bleb nevus syndrome (BRBNS) – venous malformations of skin and gut which may be painful. Gastrointestinal haemorrhage is common cause of death.

- Proteus syndrome – PWS, partial gigantism, macrocephaly, epidermal naevi.
- Wyburn–Mason syndrome – retinal and CNS AVM, facial PWS.
- Riley-Smith syndrome – cutaneous venous malformation, macrocephaly.
- Cobb syndrome – venous malformations of spinal cord, truncal PWS.
- Bannayan–Zonana syndrome – subcutaneous/visceral venous malformation, lipomas.
- Gorham's syndrome -venous and lymphatic malformations involving skin and skeleton – osteolytic bone disease.

Acquired vascular malformations

- Campbell de Morgan spots are AV fistula at the dermal capillary level found mostly in sun-exposed skin in older patients.
- Spider naevus is an angioma appearing at puberty and disappearing spontaneously; it also affects two-thirds of pregnant women and disappears in the puerperium.

F. Miscellaneous

I. Hyperhidrosis

Hyperhidrosis is excessive sweating, mostly from the eccrine sweat glands affecting axillae, palms and soles of feet. Patients complain about social embarrassment and staining of clothing.

- Primary hyperhidrosis affects up to 1% of the population, predominantly young adults.
- Secondary hyperhidrosis may be due to:
  - Endocrine disorders, e.g. hyperthyroidism, menopause.
  - Neurological disorders, e.g. syringomyelia.
  - Drugs, e.g. antidepressants.
  - Neoplastic disease, e.g. Hodgkin's lymphoma, carcinoid, phaeochromocytoma.

Eccrine sweat glands:

- Found on almost entire body surface and secrete a salty, watery solution under control of cholinergic sympathetic nerves.

Apocrine sweat glands:

- Are more localized: axillae, periareolar area, perianal area, eyebrows.

- Secrete a mixture of fat, cholesterol and salt onto hair shafts under adrenergic sympathetic nerve control.
- They are ten times larger than eccrine glands.
- They are present in equal numbers as eccrine glands in the axilla.

Hyperhidrosis: a review of current management
Atkins JL. *Plast Reconstr Surg* 2002;**110**:222–228.

Conservative treatment

- Topical agents such as aluminium chloride hexahydrate in alcohol (Driclor).
- Systemic agents such as anxiolytic drugs, e.g. benzodiazepines to reduce anxiety-provoked symptoms and glycopyronium bromide (anticholinergic side-effects).
- Iontophoresis is useful for palmar and plantar disease although the exact mechanism of action is not fully understood. On average, 15 treatments are required.
- Botulinum toxin provides effective but temporary relief of symptoms. After a starch iodine test, multiple intradermal injections given in a grid pattern (approximately 50 units of botulinum toxin A per treated area). General anaesthesia may be required for palmar and plantar injections due to the pain involved.

Surgery

- Excision of skin and/or subcutaneous tissue (direct closure, Z-plasty or S-shaped closure) effective but risks of wound infection, dehiscence, haematoma, delayed healing common.
- Alternatives include:
  - Axillary liposuction, particularly superficial (subdermal) liposuction.
  - Thoracoscopic sympathectomy is more suited to palmar than axillary hyperhidrosis; response rates are good but Horner's syndrome, thoracic duct injury and phrenic nerve injury reported, and the skin tends to be vasodilated, dry and fissured. Furthermore, compensatory sweating on trunk, limbs or face in up to 50% of patients, especially if sympathectomy bilateral (treat dominant hand only).

II. Bromidrosis

Bromidrosis is an offensive odour due to the bacterial degradation of apocrine sweat gland secretions. Alternative terms include 'bromhidrosis' or 'osmidrosis'.

Some say that osmidrosis is the problem of odour and bromidrosis is the combination of osmidrosis and hyperhidrosis.

Sweat itself is relatively odourless but alterations may make it pungent:

- Propionic acid from amino acid breakdown by propionibacteria ('vinegary').
- Isovaleric acid from *Staphylococcus epidermis* ('cheesy').

Surgical management of axillary bromidrosis – a modified Skoog procedure by an axillary bipedicled flap approach
Wang HJ. *Plast Reconstr Surg* 1996;**98**:524–529.

In this technique, parallel incisions are made in the axilla to allow a bipedicled strip of skin to be raised, and turned over for careful thinning with scissors which divides sweat gland ducts and generates fibrosis. Further parallel incisions can be added as needed to extend the treated area. The authors report good resolution of hyperhidrosis and bromidrosis in their series of 110 patients, with reduction in sweating in 92% of operated axillae at 30 months. Complications include haematomas in four patients and mild dehiscence in six.

- Technique is similar to that originally described by Skoog 1963 – raised four flaps (staggered + shape).

Effectiveness and complications of subdermal excision of apocrine glands in 206 cases with axillary osmidrosis
Qian JG. *J Plast Reconstr Aesthet Surg* 2010;**63**:1003–1007.

The authors used a single 3-cm incision in the axilla to elevate the skin flaps that were thinned/defatted. In this series, up to 97% had reduction of odour after surgery; all reported reduction in sweating. A side-effect was reduced hair growth in 95% that seemed particularly welcomed by the female patients. Complications include haematoma, seroma and wound infection in 1% each roughly but superficial epidermal necrosis of 37% (the surgeons seemed to thin out the skin significantly).

Ultrasound-assisted lipoplasty treatment for axillary bromidrosis: clinical experience of 375 cases
Hong JP. *Plast Reconstr Surg* 2004;**113**:1264–1269.

The authors used very superficial UAL in patients under sedation, with cold irrigation externally to reduce thermal injury; the end point was bloody aspirates and erythema of the skin. A drain was used along with bulky dressings.

In this review with an average follow-up period of 18.8 months, 91.7% had satisfactory reduction of odour. Complications included mild skin sloughing (3.2%), haematoma (1.3%) and temporary sensory alteration of the hand (0.3%).

Treatment of axillary hyperhidrosis/bromidrosis using VASER ultrasound
Commons GW. *Aesthetic Plast Surg* 2009;**33**:312–323.

This is a small series with 13 patients treated with VASER liposuction to the axilla under local anaesthetic. Eleven had significant reduction of symptoms with no significant recurrence at 6 months. They reported a lack of complications.

III. Hidradenitis suppurativa

This is an inflammatory disease of apocrine sweat glands causing recurrent deep abscess-like swelling in axillae and groins. It affects mostly young females (3×) with peak incidence in second and third decades. It is still poorly understood.

- It may be familial in some patients (autosomal dominant inheritance).
- Disease seems to be associated with obesity (exacerbating rather than causative, weight loss may help), acne and hirsutism (i.e. androgen related).
- Strongly linked with smoking.

Clinical appearance

- Early lesions are tender subcutaneous nodules that are deep and round without pointing. They may resolve or progress to discharge to the skin.
- Isolated lesions may resolve spontaneously or continue uncontrolled to sinus formation.

Traditionally, surgery consists of excision to fascia under antibiotic cover, with reconstruction as indicated by the defect; delayed wound healing after surgery is common.

Hidradenitis suppurativa: pathogenesis and management
Slade DE. *Br J Plast Surg* 2003;**56**:451–461.
  Non-surgical management

- Oral clindamycin 300 mg twice daily (including peri-operative infection prophylaxis).

- Cyproterone acetate (antiandrogen) improves symptoms in females.
- Acitretin 25 mg twice daily (retinoids reduce sebaceous gland activity).
- Laser treatment with CO_2 laser with healing by secondary intention.

Surgical management includes incision and drainage of acute abscesses, or excision of hair/gland-bearing skin with reconstruction by:

- Healing by secondary intention.
- Primary closure of small defects.
- Reconstruction of larger defects e.g. split skin graft +/− VAC, pedicled flaps especially from scapular region.

Chronic axillary hidradenitis–the efficacy of wide excision and flap coverage
Soldin MG. *Br J Plast Surg* 2000;**53**:434–436.

A review of 59 patients (94 axillae) treated surgically for hidradenitis suppurativa by either

- Limited i.e. only diseased skin.
- Wide i.e. excision of all hair-bearing skin including a 2 cm margin.

The defects were reconstruction with closure, split skin graft or flap reconstruction (Limberg, fasciocutaneous and parascapular flaps) as required by the defect. There seems to be less disease recurrence observed with more radical excision (3/39 versus 7/26) although no significant advantage seen otherwise. Wound breakdown was observed in all modalities of closure; most importantly, scar contracture observed in one-third of axillae reconstructed with split skin grafts.

Pyoderma gangrenosum
Pyoderma gangrenosum is an uncommon condition characterized by cutaneous ulceration with a purple undermined border; in some, there are multiple skin abscesses with necrosis that continues to enlarge. It can occur in any part of the skin but most often in the lower leg/pretibial area. Histologically, there are intense dermal inflammatory infiltrates composed of neutrophils with little evidence of a primary vasculitis. Gram-negative streptococci are frequently cultured from wounds but their role is unclear.

Classic pyoderma gangrenosum may be associated with symptoms of pain, fever, malaise, myalgia and arthralgia and has also been described in early childhood (4%).

The aetiology is unclear but seems to be related to altered immunological reactivity. ~50% of cases are associated with a specific systemic disorder: inflammatory bowel disease, rheumatoid arthritis, non-Hodgkin's lymphoma, Wegener's granulomatosis (especially head and neck lesions) and myeloproliferative disorders. The other 50% have no identifiable risk factors.

- The diagnosis is based on clinical and histopathological findings (characteristically a neutrophilic infiltration). There is no specific test; biopsy is used mainly to rule out other causes.

Pyoderma gangrenosum has also been reported in:

- Fasciocutaneous flaps and complicating breast reduction (Gudi VS. *Br J Plastic Surg* 2000;**53**: 440–441).
- DIEP flap breast reconstruction (Caterson SA. *J Reconstr Microsurg* 2010;**26**:475–479)

Management

- Surgery may exacerbate the disease and is usually avoided.

The commonest reported treatments include steroids, azathioprine and cyclosporine.

Genitourinary and trunk

A. Principles of surgical management of hypospadias

I. Relevant anatomy and embryology

Embryological development of the penis and urethra (Sadler TW. *Langman's Medical Embryology*, 11th Edn.)

During the 3rd week of development, primitive streak mesenchymal cells migrate around the **cloacal membrane** to form the cloacal folds which fuse cranial to the membrane to form the **genital tubercle**.

- The fetus is sexually indeterminate until the 6th week of gestation when the cloacal membrane divides into urogenital and anal membranes whilst the cloacal folds also divide into **urethral folds** anteriorly and anal folds posteriorly with **genital swellings** lateral to them (these form the scrotal swellings in the male and labia majora in the female).
- During the 6th to 11th weeks, the genital tubercle elongates to form the **phallus** under the influence of androgens. As the phallus develops, it pulls the urethral folds forwards to form the lateral walls of the **urethral groove** which extends only up to the

distal part of the phallus – here the epithelial lining is of endodermal origin and is known as the **urethral plate** (glandular urethra).

- During the 12th week, the urethral folds come together and close over to form the penile urethra (the glandular part of the urethra is not canalized at this stage).
- During the 13th week, the glandular urethra becomes canalized by the inward migration of ectodermal cells to form the **external urethral meatus** and the genital swellings enlarge to form each half of the scrotum.

Anatomy of the penis

The root of the penis consists of the **bulb** of the penis (posterior part of the corpus spongiosum) and the **lateral crurae** (posterior ends of the corpora cavernosa).

- The **ischiocavernosus** muscles are attached to the perineal membrane and the ramus of the ischium, passing forwards to insert into the upper part of the corpus cavernosum; they act to move the erect penis.
- **Bulbospongiosus muscles** are attached to the perineal body and pass forwards to attach to the

corpus spongiosum, with some fibres passing around to the corpus cavernosum; when they contract, they empty the urethra of semen/urine.

The body of the penis is the portion that lies between the root and the glans. The urethra runs through the ventral **corpus spongiosum**, which is related on its dorsolateral surface to the **corpora cavernosa**. The corpora are bound by a fibrous sheath called the **tunica albuginea**; a reflection of the tunica forms the **suspensory ligament** that suspends the penis to the undersurface of the symphysis pubi.

The deep fascia of the penis is called **Buck's fascia**; it is a continuation of the Colles' fascia, and envelopes the tunica albuginea. The dorsal arteries, deep dorsal veins and dorsal nerves lies beneath this, whilst a loose areolar tissue (Dartos fascia), containing the superficial dorsal vein, covers Buck's fascia which is then enveloped by skin.

Blood supply

There are three pairs of arteries which are all branches of the internal pudendal artery (internal iliac artery).

- **Artery to the bulb**: supplies the posterior part of the corpus spongiosum.
- **Dorsal artery** of the penis: supplies the corpus spongiosum, skin, fascia and glans (hence an anastomosis exists between the artery to the bulb and the dorsal artery). The arteries run either side of the deep dorsal vein in the groove between the corpora cavernosa.
- **Deep artery**: supplies corpus cavernosum and its sole function is erectile.

Although some venous drainage from the penis follows the venae comitantes draining into internal pudendal veins, most of it flows along the deep dorsal vein, draining into the prostatic venous plexus.

- The superficial dorsal vein drains skin only and joins with the superficial external pudendal and great saphenous veins.
- Lymphatic channels accompanying the superficial dorsal vein, drain into the superficial inguinal nodes whilst the glans and corpora drain to the deep inguinal nodes/internal iliac nodes.

Nerve supply

The skin of the penis is supplied by the posterior scrotal and dorsal branches of the pudendal nerves (sacral plexus, S2, 3, 4).

- **Erection** is mediated by parasympathetic pelvic splanchnic nerves (nervi erigentes) from the sacral plexus (S2, 3, 4) via the superior and inferior hypogastric plexuses. This causes dilatation of blood vessels and closure of arteriovenous anastomoses (AVAs) that normally allow bypass of the corpora, along with some contraction of the ischiocavernosus muscles, that compress veins with decreased venous outflow.
- **Emission** is mediated by sympathetic nerves (L1 root from the sacral ganglia) via the superior and inferior hypogastric plexuses. It is the process of the movement of sperm from the epididymis, mixed with secretions from accessory sex glands to the prostastic urethra – this is caused by smooth muscle contraction in epididymis, vas, seminal vesicles as well as closure of sphincter of bladder.
- **Ejaculation** is mediated by contraction of skeletal muscles of ischiocavernosus and bulbospongiosus muscles supplied by perineal branch of the pudendal nerves. The force moves semen toward the glans.

Anatomy of the male urethra

- The urethra is lined by transitional epithelium except for the part just proximal to the external urethral meatus, the navicular fossa, which is lined by stratified squamous epithelium and has blind-ending lacunae. The empty urethra is horizontal in cross section whilst the external meatus forms a vertical slit, hence the urine stream spirals. The urethral glands of Littré open into the urethra on its anterior and lateral aspect, 'against' the stream.

There are three points of constriction along the urethra: internal meatus (bladder neck), proximal end of navicular fossa and the external meatus. The three dilatations are prostatic urethra, bulb and navicular fossa.

II. Assessment of hypospadias

Hypospadias results from incomplete closure of the urethral folds during the 12th week of development and may represent abnormal fusion between endodermal and ectodermal processes. It occurs in 1 in every 300 live male births and seems to be increasing; it is characterized by:

- Ventral meatal dystopia i.e. ventral position of the meatus.
- Dorsal hooded foreskin.

- Ventral curvature on erection (chordee).
  ○ This is a fibrous remnant of the corpus spongiosum causing ventral penile curvature. Dissection of the urethral plate alone will not correct the curvature. In > 90% of cases chordee is due simply to ventral skin shortage.
- Deficiency of ventral skin.
- Clefting of the glans, and in the most severe cases scrotal bipartition.

Seventeen per cent of cases have associated urogenital abnormalities including undescended testes and inguinal hernia. Patients with *proximal* hypospadias should be screened for abnormalities of the urinary tract (renal ultrasound, isotope renogram).

Aims of correction of hypospadias:

- Allow micturition while standing with a non-turbulent stream.
- Achieve a natural appearance with slit-like meatus located at the distal extent of the glans.
- Allow normal sexual function.

Aetiology

Aetiological factors include environmental oestrogens, intersex states and genetic influence (familial hypospadias).

- Environmental (oestrogenic chemicals).
- Androgen hyposensitivity (especially if associated with micropenis, severe hypospadias, hypogonadism, undescended testes and inguinal hernia).
- Genetic: with an affected male, his sons will have a 8% risk whilst his brothers have a 14% (Bauer SB. *Urol Clin N Am* 1981;**8**:559–564); however, identical twins do not necessarily both have hypospadias, hence the aetiology is multifactorial.
- Factors such as increased maternal age and drug exposure have not stood up to follow-up studies. There is no association with the use of oral contraceptives during pregnancy.

There is a link with cleft palate and hypertelorism i.e. Schilbach–Rott syndrome, which is very rare (Joss SK. *Am J Med Genet* 2002;**113**:105–107).

Classification

Classification is based on the position of the abnormally proximal opening of the urethral meatus, from distal to proximal. There are many different variations on the theme:

- Glanular/coronal/subcoronal.
- Distal shaft/mid-shaft/proximal shaft.
- Penoscrotal/scrotal or perineal.

History

- Family history of hypospadias.
- Maternal drugs, occupation of the father, etc.
- Any urinary tract infections (which may be manifested as failure to thrive) or known abnormalities of the upper genitourinary tract.
- Any curvature during witnessed erections.

Role of maternal smoking and maternal reproductive history in the etiology of hypospadias in the offspring
Kallen K. *Teratology* 2002;**66**:185–191.

This study of data from the Swedish health registry showed that, of 1 413 811 infants born between 1983 and 1996, 3262 had hypospadias. There was a negative association between hypospadias and maternal smoking but a positive association with primiparity.

Examination

- Penis – size, degree of meatal dystopia i.e. position of meatus, depth of urethral groove, chordee, dorsal hooding.
- Preputial involvement (circumcision or preputial reconstruction).
- Assessment of associated anomalies:
  ○ Position of testes – descended/undescended, size – cryptorchidism in up to 10%.
  ○ Inguinal hernia/open processus vaginalis 9–15%.

Investigations

Investigations should include general examination and exclusion of an intersex state in severe anomalies with ambiguous genitalia (genetic and endocrine work-up).

- Urinary stream.
- Urea and electrolytes (U&Es), renal ultrasound or isotope renogram if concerned about upper genitourinary tract (not affected except in very severe forms of hypospadias).

III. Surgical principles

Timing of surgery

This is quite variable and opinion is divided. Traditionally (up to the 1970s) surgery was deferred until after 3 years of age (before children went to school, and so could urinate standing up at school) but it is now generally accepted that earlier repair (6–18 months) will reduce psychological impact of the condition as young children will have little memory of their hospital stay. However, there is no true consensus internationally.

- Single stage –12 months.
- Two stage: stage 1 at 12 months and stage 2 at 18 months.

Waiting makes little difference to the size as the penis grows less than 1 cm during the first 3–4 years.

Administering pre-operative testosterone, DHT or β-chorionic gonadotrophin may be useful for those with a small penis, or for repeat surgery.

There have been different techniques described in the literature:

- 1932 Mathieu (flip–flap one stage).
- 1949 Browne (modified Duplay).
- 1952 Cecil–Culp (modified Duplay).
- 1962 Cloutier (two-stage preputial FTSG).
- 1963 Devine and Horton (modified Mathieu).
- 1965 Mustarde (modified Mathieu).
- 1977 Van der Meulen (modified Duplay).
- 1980 Duckett (transverse preputial island flap).
- 1981 Duckett (meatoplasty and glanuloplasty – MAGPI).
- 1984 Harris (split preputial flap technique).
- 1987 Elder and Duckett (onlay island flap).
- 1994 **Snodgrass** (tubularized incised plate).
- 1995 **Bracka** (modified Cloutier).
- 1997 Turner-Warwick (bulbar elongation and anastomotic meatoplasty – BEAM).

Surgical techniques

Use of loupes is common. Techniques to repair hypospadias can be divided in to one-stage or two-stage repairs. The early techniques were two-staged, but technical developments allowed a single-stage procedure to be performed safely and applied to the vast majority of cases of hypospadias. There is renewed interest in two-staged repair, particularly in that it can improve results in most severe forms of hypospadias.

One-stage repairs can be classified as:

- Urethral advancement techniques.
- **Onlay** techniques in which vascularized tissue is transposed onto the urethral defect to close the tube.

- **Inlay** techniques in which a tubed flap of vascularized tissue is transposed into the defect to reconstruct the whole circumference of the tube.

Older one-stage techniques were based on the Mathieu flip–flap procedure; newer alternatives include transverse preputial island flap (Duckett) or split preputial flap (Harris) techniques (preputial flap techniques cannot be used if the child has been circumcised). The Snodgrass technique is quite popular currently.

Older **two-stage techniques** were based on the Duplay procedure (preputial skin flaps supplementing ventral skin then tubularized (or buried – Dennis Browne) to form a neo-urethra). The Bracka two-stage repair is probably the most popular two-stage technique currently used.

One-stage surgery involves fewer operations for the patient, is less expensive overall and is said to cause less psychological trauma. However, there are some advantages to a two-stage repair (particularly the Bracka):

- Greater versatility for dealing with a wider spectrum of hypospadias and thus less need to master a greater number of techniques.
- Surgery is technically easier and produces more reliable results, with a low fistula rate of ~ 3%.
- It avoids a circumferential anastomosis, a potential site of stricture and achieves a more natural-looking and distal slit-like meatus.
- Some argue that psychosexual adjustment is more related to appearance than number of operations.

Anaesthesia

General anaesthesia may be supplemented with:

- Dorsal penile block – fails to fully anaesthetize ventral skin/glans.
- Penile ring block.
- Caudal block – also anaesthetizes mucosa and there is less bladder neck spasm; it allows a lighter general anaesthetic to be administered with lower opiate requirements but causes semi-erection.

Release of chordee

- Deglove penis (skin chordee).
- Excision of genuine chordee (fibrous tissue on ventral penis); the urethral plate does not cause curvature in most cases.

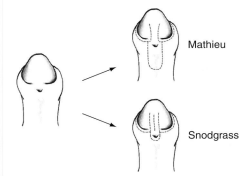

Figure 9.1 Common techniques for more distal types of hypospadias.

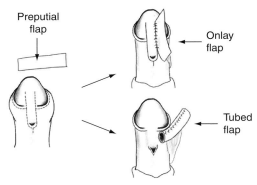

Figure 9.2 Other techniques for hypospadias using preputial flaps.

- Residual chordee is usually due to disproportion of the corpora and requires straightening by dorsal orthoplasty (modified Nesbit).

Preserving the urethral plate

The mainstay of surgery is to preserve the well-vascularized plate and to utilize it for urethral reconstruction.

- If the plate is wide, it can be tubularized as per Thiersch–Duplay.
- If the plate is too narrow for tubularizing, then a midline relaxing incision can be used as per the Snodgrass technique. This is primarily used for distal hypospadias – the complication rate with proximal defects is higher.
- If the plate is too narrow or too unhealthy:
  ○ Proximal defect, use onlay technique.
  ○ Distal defects, many choices e.g. Mathieu, urethral advancement etc.
- If the continuity of the plate cannot be preserved then either a tube onlay or inlay–onlay flap is used to prevent urethral strictures, usually using islanded flaps. A two-stage technique may be useful.
  ○ If preputial/penile skin is not available (including balanitis xerotica obliterans (BXO)) then buccal mucosa can be used if onlay or two-stage.

Suture materials

- Subcuticular 6/0 to glans, 7/0 to skin.
- 7/0 vicryl is often described as being the suture of choice whilst vicryl rapide is also useful, lasts ~2 weeks.

- Polydioxanone (PDS) is avoided as it dissolves quickly when exposed to the urinary tract.

Post-operative management

- Urinary diversion for 2–6 days, fix catheter carefully.
  ○ Size 8–10F silicone catheter, 15 mm diameter in children and use paediatric drainage system – adult bags can give rise to air locks and obstruction.
  ○ 25 mm/size 12 catheter in adults – fix catheter carefully.
  ○ Urine can be drained with a transurethral dripping stent or suprapubic catheter but some do not drain after distal repairs.
- Circular dressings with slight compression, antibiotics.
  ○ There is a wide range of practice for dressings and drainage and there is not strong evidence to make any specific recommendations.
- Ketoconazole 400 mg tds – rapid control of erections.
- Treat bladder neck spasm with oxybutynin 1 mg 8 hourly.
- 0.75% plain marcaine continuous dorsal penile block, 1 ml 4 hourly.

Follow-up

The main aim of follow-up is primarily to monitor for stenosis (also fistula and aesthetics) – the onset of spraying is usually indicative of a stenotic process. Patients are seen regularly for ~3 years and then intermittently until after puberty.

Complications

- Early – haematoma, infection, dehiscence (all of which may lead to fistulae).

- Late – fistula (turbulent flow – salvage surgery 10%; primary surgery 3%), stenosis (early 2%; overall 7%; late strictures mainly due to BXO developing in preputial FTSGs), poor aesthetics.

Revision

- Revision of the first stage: 3.7% (further chordee release, meatoplasty, etc.).
- Revision of the second stage: 5.5% (aesthetic adjustments).

Is prophylactic antimicrobial treatment necessary after hypospadias repair?

Meir DB. *J Urol* 2004;**171**:2621–2622.

This is a prospectively randomized clinical trial evaluating the role of oral cephalexin in hypospadias repair by tubularized incised plate urethroplasty, with a urethral catheter *in situ* for a mean of 8 days postoperatively. The incidence of bacteriuria was halved in the cephalexin group and there was higher proportion of urinary tract infection, fistulae and meatal stenosis. There was also difference in pathogens – *Pseudomonas aeruginosa* was commonest in the prophylaxis group, whilst in the control group it was *Klebsiella pneumoniae*. The author recommends broad-spectrum prophylaxis.

The efficacy of dihydrotestosterone transdermal gel before primary hypospadias surgery

Kaya C. *J Urol* 2008;**179**;684–688.

This is a prospective randomized controlled trial including 75 consecutive children with primary hypospadias undergoing tubularized incised plate urethroplasty. One group had 2.5% transdermal gel applied daily; the control group did not. They found a significant reduction in post-operative complications and improvement of the cosmetic results; the authors attributed this to increased blood flow.

Fistulae

The suture lines in a hypospadias repair may be under adverse conditions, being continually bathed in urine under pressure, and the skin may be under tension due to oedema, erections and post-operative haematomas. In addition, multiple operations may have left tissues friable or scarred. There is also an element of infection.

All of the above means that there is a significant risk of fistula formation; 90% are detectable within 1 week of operation.

- Early fistulae due to post-operative obstruction, extravasation, haematoma, infection.

- Late fistulae are usually said to be due to turbulent flow.

Repair of fistula. It is important to ensure that there is no distal obstruction prior to reoperation; it is generally advisable to wait for the tissues to soften and for inflammation to settle.

The defect in the urethra should be closed carefully, avoiding overlapping suture lines. Some propose using an interpositional fascial flap (including elevation of glans and placement of fascial flap for coronal fistula).

- Test integrity of repair at end of procedure and do not use catheters.

IV. Specific techniques

One-stage repairs

Flip–flap one stage [original article in French]

Mathieu D. *J Chir* 1932;**39**:481.

This is a turnover of a ventral penile skin flap, distally based at the meatus and with parallel incisions, into the glanular groove to form the neo-urethra. However, as it uses abnormal urethral plate in the repair (which tends to be scar-like tissue), it is prone to problems with wound healing. It is suited for midshaft to coronal hypospadias.

The technique has withstood the test of time, though its main drawback is the meatus that tends not to be very natural/aesthetic.

The following two are regarded as being modifications of Mathieu's technique.

One stage hypospadias repair

Devine PC. *J Urol* 1961;**85**:166–172.

Subcoronal incision is extended onto the ventral surface of the penis, encircling native urethra. Chordee is released and triple glans flaps are raised:

- Central 'V'-shaped flap with its apex at the native urethra.
- Distally based 'V'-shaped ventral penile skin flap raised and tubularized to the 'V'-shaped central glans flap.
- Lateral glans flaps cover the neo-urethra, shaft skin defect is closed by preputial flaps.

If the native meatus is more proximal, FTSG is used to reconstruct the anterior urethra beyond the limits of the flip–flap.

One-stage correction of distal hypospadias: and other people's fistulae
Mustarde JC. *Br J Plast Surg* 1965;**18**:413–422.

Diverting perineal urethrostomy was used in this series. After release of chordee, a distally based ventral skin flap, with its base at the ectopic meatus, is elevated.

- One or two catgut sutures are used to minimally tubularize the flap and this tubed flap is fed through a tunnel created in the glans. Dog-ears are excised.
- Prepuce is opened out and button-holed (Ombrédanne, 1932), the glans is fed through the button-hole to allow reconstruction of the ventral skin defect.

Transverse preputial island flap technique for repair of severe hypospadias
Duckett JW. *Urol Clin N Am* 1980;**7**:423–430.

This technique is described as being suitable for anterior urethral defects of 2–6 cm. The authors used suprapubic catheters for diversion.

- Subcoronal incision, release of chordee and erection test.
- Transverse preputial rectangle is marked out on inner preputial skin, as long as the anterior urethral defect and 12–15 mm in width. This island flap is tubularized around a catheter and raised with Dartos fascia; it is anastomosed to the native urethra and then channelled through glans.
- Ventral skin closure is achieved by splitting the prepuce vertically in the midline and rotating two preputial skin flaps ventrally around either side of the penis (i.e. Duplay).

Island flap techniques are needed when resection of chordee results in discontinuity of the urethral plate.

MAGPI (meatoplasty and glanuloplasty): a procedure for subcoronal hypospadias
Duckett JW. *Urol Clin N Am* 1981;**8**:513–519.

The authors recommend their technique for subcoronal hypospadias, especially where the glans is broad and flat. The aim is to give the appearance of a more terminally located meatus. An incision is made in the cutaneomucosal junction of the prepuce. A deep vertical incision in the glans groove is made and then closed transversely with advancement of the meatus. The ventral lip of meatus is lifted up with a stay suture and glans flaps closed beneath the elevated meatus.

Splitting the prepuce to provide two independently vascularised flaps: a one stage repair of hypospadias and congenital short urethra
Harris DL. *Br J Plast Surg* 1984;**37**:108–116.

This is similar to Duckett's transverse preputial island flap technique; the fistula rate is quoted at 6%. A penile block is used; perineal urethrostomy for drainage and silicone foam dressing to reduce swelling and haematomas.

- Subcoronal incision is made and the plane between Dartos fascia and tunica albuginea is developed to enable release of chordee.
- One central (inverted 'V') and two lateral glans flaps are elevated; the preputial skin is back-cut to allow it to rotate ventrally to the right of the shaft of the penis.
- Incise the free edge of the prepuce and separate the internal skin from the external skin based on a vascularized flap of Dartos fascia.
- **Tubularize the inner preputial** flap around a catheter and anastomose proximally to the native urethra and distally to the central glans flap.
- The external preputial skin is draped over the neo-urethra to reconstruct ventral skin shortage.

Onlay island flap in the repair of mid and distal penile hypospadias without chordee
Elder JS. *J Urol* 1987;**138**:376–379.

The senior author of this paper is Duckett JW. The urethral plate is preserved by 'U'-shaped incision around the meatus and along glandular groove lines. The penile skin is mobilized, fibrous chordee removed – if curvature persists, then dorsal tunica albuginea plication.

- The thin/hypoplastic proximal urethra is excised.
- A transverse preputial island flap is raised but instead of tubularizing, inset into the 'U'-shaped incision as an onlay island flap.
- Close lateral glans flaps and ventral penile skin using preputial skin flaps.

Tubularized incised plate urethroplasty for distal hypospadias
Snodgrass W. *J Urol* 1994;**151**:464.

This technique is suitable for distal hypospadia, or in conjunction with other modern techniques when urethral closure might otherwise be too tight.

- Subcoronal degloving incision and chordee correction by tunica albuginea plication (TAP) (Nesbit).

- Parallel longitudinal incisions at edges of urethral plate are made to create glans wings and a midline incision is made in the urethral plate. The epithelial strips are closed ventrally leaving the dorsal defect to re-epithelialize.
- Waterproofing layer is closed followed by closure of glans wings.

Currently tubularized incised plate (TIP) urethroplasty is one of the most popular techniques for distal (and midshaft) hypospadias.

Bulbar elongation and anastomotic meatoplasty (BEAM) for subterminal and hypospadiac urethroplasty
Turner-Warwick R. *J Urol* 1997;**158**:1160–1167.

This technique relies upon mobilization of the bulbar urethra to gain sufficient length to allow advancement of the distal urethra to the glans tip. Ventral penile curvature may result from over-ambitious stretching; 2–2.5 cm in children and 4–5 cm in urethral length in adults may be gained.

- The bulbar urethra is first mobilized via a perineal approach and then mobilized anteriorly via a subcoronal incision. After mobilizing, the urethra should project, tension free, beyond the glans tip. Where there is a significant glans cleft, the urethra is formally inset after raising glans flaps but where the glans has little clefting, the urethra is tunnelled to a new terminal position.
- Slit-like meatus may be achieved by a Parkhouse procedure (double spatulate the urethra at 6 and 12 o'clock positions and partially resuture, face to face).

Two-stage repair
Duplay described the technique of tubularization of the urethral plate (in French) in 1874, the general principle being that it can be tubularized as far as the tip of the glans. (The Snodgrass technique aimed to overcome difficulties in tubularizing a narrow plate by incising it longitudinally.) In two-stage repair, preputial skin flaps are brought ventrally with second-stage tubularization.

- **Stage one**: Subcoronal incision, release of chordee and glans split. The dorsal prepuce is split in the midline and brought ventrally around either side of the penis with skin closure in the midline.
- **Stage two:** Two vertical incisions from the native meatus to the neomeatus at glans tip and free edges

sutured together to tubularize a neo-urethra. Direct ventral skin closure over this tube is possible due to previously imported preputial skin; close in a double-breasted fashion – one side is de-epithelialized.

Variants
- **Browne modification buried skin strip**. Allow a buried skin strip to tubularize itself without suturing the free edges of the neo-urethra. Popular in the 1950/60s, but most reported a 10–30% fistula rate.
- **Cecil–Culp modification scrotal skin**. Used for proximal hypospadias. At the second stage, a vertical incision is made from the native urethra on to the scrotum and the penis is turned down and inset into the scrotum. At a third stage, the penis is released with ventral closure using scrotal skin.
- **Van der Meulen modification one-stage correction**. In the patient without chordee the anterior urethra can be reconstructed in one operation by using Duplay's second stage only, and incorporating Browne's modification (buried skin strip).

Two-stage preputial FTSG
A method for hypospadias repair
Cloutier A. *Plast Reconstr Surg* 1962;**30**:368–373.

First-stage at age > 18 months: Circumcision and glans split. Transverse coronal incision and correction of chordee. A ventral full thickness preputial skin graft is inset; use of FTSG overcomes the problem of skin shrinkage.

Second stage > 3 months later. Vertical incisions to form free edges of neo-urethra continuous beneath the native meatus and up to the neomeatus at glans tip and excision of mucosa on glans flaps. Lateral skin is undermined and edges are sutured over the skin strip. Dorsal relaxing incision and SSG.

Modified Cloutier technique
Hypospadias repair: the two-stage alternative
Bracka A. *Br J Urol* 1995;**76**:31.

Stage 1 at 3 years of age: tourniquet, 8F urinary catheter, erection test (Horton).

- Subcoronal incision and dissection down to distal ends of corpora cavernosa to release chordee. Verify adequacy of release with repeat erection test.
- The glans is split and inner preputial FTSG placed with Jelonet tie-over dressing (buccal mucosal

graft is preferred in the presence of BXO). **FTSG restores thin skin layer firmly adherent on to glans tissue that flap techniques cannot achieve**. The catheter is left in for 2 days with **trimethoprim** antibiotic prophylaxis. Patient is kept in hospital until dressing change at 5 days under GA or sedation + EMLA cream.

Stage 2 – after 6 months:

- The grafted skin is tubularized around an 8F catheter, starting with a 'U'-shaped incision beneath the native meatus and allowing a width of 14–15 mm of skin for tubularizing.
- Close in two layers and cover with a waterproofing pedicled flap of Dartos fascia/subcutaneous tissue from the prepuce.

In very proximal repairs, insufficient tissue may be available for the waterproofing layer; in this situation use an anteriorly based fascial flap from the scrotum. In most cases the penis is circumcised rather than attempting to reconstruct the foreskin which can often become tight and uncomfortable.

The catheter is left for 6 days and **augmentin antibiotic prophylaxis** is given. In adults or older children, cyproterone acetate is given to reduce erections (started 10 days before); alternatively, 'a sharp icy blast of freeze spray' can be 'kept on the bedside locker for emergency use'!

Typical choice of repair

Distal meatal dystopia

- MAGPI (Duckett).
- BEAM (Turner-Warwick).
- Tubularized incised plate (Snodgrass).
- Two-stage repair (Bracka).

Mid-shaft to coronal meatal dystopia

- Ventral skin flip–flap (Mathieu).
- Transverse preputial island flap (Duckett).
- Two-stage repair (Bracka).

Penoscrotal meatal dystopia

- Transverse preputial island flap (Duckett).
- Two-stage repair (Bracka).
- Two-stage repair (Cecil–Culp).

Overviews

One-stage repairs using dorsal preputial flaps can be separated into two groups: those that transpose the whole prepuce as a double-faced flap (onlay island flap, Elder and Duckett 1987) and those that use two independently vascularized flaps (transverse preputial island flap, Duckett 1980 and split preputial flap technique, Harris 1984).

- Internal preputial skin is vascularized from the Dartos fascia while external preputial skin is vascularized from the subdermal plexus (larger vessels) and a plane that is readily dissectable exists between these two layers. Hence, the internal preputial skin may be islanded as a flap and tubularized to form neo-urethra while external skin may be raised as a cutaneous flap to resurface a ventral defect.
- When the chordee is laterally placed, the urethral plate may be retained and the urethra reconstructed with an onlay flap or ventral flap whilst for a midline chordee, the urethral plate is excised and replaced by a tubed flap.

However, from an embryological perspective, the urethral plate is always abnormal and should be **excised** as is performed in Bracka's technique.

- There are two possible situations. One, where the corpus spongiosum extends to the apex of the corpora cavernosa and chordee is due to ventral skin shortage and condensed fascia lateral to the untubed urethra, thus treatment involves excision of this lateral tissue and reconstructing ventral skin.
- In the other, the corpus spongiosum does not extend the full length of the corpora cavernosa and chordee is due to **midline** failure of differentiation, and needs to be excised along with urethral mucosa and a neo-urethral tube needs to be reconstructed.

The urinary stream should be diverted away from the suture lines of the neo-urethral tube using a suprapubic catheter (oxybutynin to prevent bladder spasm; extravasation of urine may cause fibrosis and stricture formation). A good calibre match between native and neo-urethra must be achieved as turbulence of the urinary stream causes fistulae and ballooning.

The selective use of a single-stage and a two-stage technique for hypospadias correction in 157 consecutive cases with the aim of normal appearance and function
Johnson D. *Br J Plast Surg* 1998;**51**:195–201.

This is a retrospective analysis of 157 repairs (both one- and two-stage; also see below) with particular emphasis upon aesthetics.

Single-stage GRAP (glanular reconstruction and prepucioplasty, Gilpin 1993) repair for distal hypospadias if tourniquet erection test excludes chordee with a well-formed glans sulcus; this applied in up to 40% of cases of hypospadias.

Glans flaps are used to re-create the distal urethra around an 8F silicone catheter unless there is a dense bar of tissue between meatus and glans sulcus. The repair is closed with a waterproofing fascial layer and a foreskin reconstruction (prepucioplasty). The procedure leaves natural-looking meati, no suture marks and no stenosis.

Bracka two-stage repair in > 60% of cases of hypospadias and is particularly suitable for a more proximally situated meatus with no appreciable glans sulcus. Foreskin reconstruction where done happens at the second stage. There is a significant learning curve to reduce fistulae: the rate is halved after first 40 repairs (5% for all primary repairs but > 20% for salvage procedures). It leaves a natural-looking meati, no suture marks and no stenosis.

Treatment modalities for hypospadias cripples
van der Werff JF. *Plast Reconstr Surg* 2000;**105**:600–608.

Hypospadias cripples can be defined as patients with remaining functional complications after previous hypospadias repair such as major meatal dystopia (87%), residual curvature of the penile body (46%), meatal stenosis (20%) and one or more fistulae (5%).

- A mean of two further operations is needed to solve these problems such as circumferential advancement of penile skin, dorsal transposition flap of preputial skin, distally based transposition flap of penile skin and full-thickness skin graft.
- Complications included fistulae, meatal stenosis and residual curvature and functional complaints included spraying at micturition, dribbling and deviation of urinary stream.

The author recommends meticulous technique, delicate tissue handling, and advanced post-operative care.

Outcomes

Long-term review of hypospadias repaired by split preputial flap technique (Harris)
Kumar MVK. *Br J Plast Surg* 1994;**47**:236–240.

This is a 10-year follow-up of 35 patients treated with split preputial flap technique (senior author is Harris).

- The post-operative appearance was objectively assessed as looking normal in 80%; 80% felt confident in peer company, 20% felt penis was too small or abnormally shaped.
- 40% of patients had intermittent spraying, all had a forceful stream.
- All patients 'masturbated to their satisfaction', 83% had straight erections though only a small number had any sexual experience due to young age at follow-up.

Analysis of meatal location in 500 men
Fichtner J. *J Urol* 1995;**154**:833–834.

Analysis of meatal location in 500 men showed that 13% had hypospadias (glandular:coronal ratio = 3:1) and two-thirds of these were unaware of a penile anomaly, all but one (homosexual) had fathered children and all were able to micturate from standing. Only one case of subcoronal hypospadias was associated with penile curvature. Given these observations, the need for meatal advancement for distal hypospadias, potentially complicated by meatal stenosis and fistula formation, is questioned.

Satisfaction with penile appearance after hypospadias surgery
Mureau MA. *J Urol* 1996;**155**:703–706.

There was no correlation between patient and surgeon satisfaction. Patients were less satisfied in general; patients with a glanular meatus were more satisfied than those with a retracted meatus. Satisfaction did not correlate with penile length.

Urodynamic evaluation of hypospadias repair
Van der Meulen JC. *J Urol* 1997;**157**:1344–1346.

There was no difference in flow between different operative techniques (including one- and two-stage).

Sexual behaviours and sexual function of adults after hypospadias surgery
Bubanj TB. *J Urol* 2004;**171**:1876–1879.

This is a questionnaire-based study of 37 adult hypospadias patients and 39 controls.

The self-reported libido was similar in both groups with no difference in achieving erection but hypospadias patients were less completely satisfied with their sex life and had fewer partners. There was downward curvature noted in 40% of hypospadias (2 × controls) and ejaculation difficulties in one-third of patients (spraying/dribbling).

Buccal mucosal grafts in hypospadias surgery: long-term results

Hensle TW. *J Urol* 2002;**168**:1734–1736.

This is a 10-year review of 47 patients in whom buccal mucosal grafts were used for secondary hypospadias surgery. The overall complication rate was 32% and all occurred within 6 months of surgery. There were three patients with BXO in the series and all developed complications, thus buccal grafts may not be indicated in these patients. Apart from this subset, most patients benefited from a durable reconstruction. Onlay grafts were preferred to tubularized grafts.

Long term follow up of buccal, mucosa onlay grafts for hypospadias repair

Fichtner J. *J Urol* 1995;**172**:1970–1972.

This is a retrospective review of 132 patients with buccal mucosal onlay graft for hypospadias repair with an average 6.2 years of follow-up. The overall complication rate was 24%, almost all occurring in the first year thereafter the results were stable and long term.

Most surgeons will agree that buccal mucosa has its advantages and contrary to Hensle TW (*J Urol* 2002;**168**:1734–1737), is a good choice in BXO patients. It is relatively thick, mechanically stiff and elastic; the lamina propria allows rapid graft take.

B. Perineal reconstruction

I. Epispadias and exstrophy of the bladder

Epispadias

Epispadias is embryologically different from hypospadias. It is a developmental abnormality of the abdominal wall that reflects abnormal development of the cloacal membrane due to failure of rupture and mesenchymal in-growth. Epispadias proximal to the bladder neck leads to incontinence. Other features include: diastasis of recti, low-set umbilicus and widening of the pubic symphysis.

- In males: short penis, dorsal chordee, epispadic meatal dystopia, divergent corpora.
- In females: short vagina, wide separation of the labia, bifid clitoris.

Exstrophy of the bladder

Features of bladder exstrophy include abdominal wall defect, separation of the symphysis pubis and absent anterior bladder wall and eversion of the bladder. There is an increased risk of carcinoma if left untreated.

- Exstrophy plus epispadias (commonest combination) – 1 in 30 000.

Staged functional reconstruction:

- Bladder closed as a neonate – 1 week.
- Epispadias repair at 1–2 years of age. Surgery for epispadias is virtually the same as for hypospadias but conducted on the dorsal surface and most common options are flip–flap types of procedure (Devine–Horton) or preputial island flap (Duckett).
- Bladder neck reconstruction at 3–4 years of age.

Iliac osteotomies to allow closure of the symphyseal defect and abdominal wall closure may need rectus muscle flap.

II. Peyronie's disease and balanitis xerotica obliterans

Peyronie's disease

The majority of patients with this condition have upward curvature with thickening on the dorsal surface of the tunica albuginea, with fibrosis extending into septum between corpora; it is a similar phenomenon to Dupuytren's disease. It is rare before 40 years of age and may be related to repetitive trauma, especially to the semi-erect penis. Some suggest a role for TGF-β over-expression.

Medical treatment

- Para-aminobenzoic acid, vitamin E, colchicine, tamoxifen, verapamil.
- Ultrasound.
- Steroid injections.

Surgical treatment

Fifty per cent spontaneous resolution may occur – thus do not operate within 1 year of presentation. Surgery is indicated if the patient is unable to have intercourse, whilst a penile prosthesis is a choice, if the patient is bordering upon impotence.

- Nesbit procedure to plicate the ventral tunica; however, this shortens the penis.
- Excision of plaque and grafting with dermis (the use of dura, fascia lata, AlloDerm, vein and Gore-Tex patch have also been reported); however, these

materials can resorb or produce ballooning of the corpora and compromise erection.

Balanitis xerotica obliterans

Balanitis xerotica obliterans (BXO) is a male genital form of lichen sclerosis of unknown aetiology, though some viral and HLA associations have been reported. It typically occurs in obese patients; a warm, moist uriniferous environment increases the risk. BXO accounts for many hypospadias cripples; chronic BXO may lead on to SSC.

- Early – dyskeratosis and inflammatory changes progressing to
- Late – fibrosis and skin atrophy, prepuce becomes adherent to glans.

There is a white stenosing band at the end of the foreskin whilst a haemorrhagic response to minor trauma leads to phimosis and distal urethral stenosis.

Treatment

- Circumcision (allows glans to dry out) and/or meatoplasty – meatotomy will restricture.
- Trial of steroid creams for early disease in children.
- Surgical excision of advanced disease and thick SSG. Substitution urethroplasty may use buccal mucosal grafts; bladder mucosal grafts fail to keratinize and retain an ugly fleshy appearance.

Recurrence in:

- Genital FTSG: 18 months–2 years.
- Postauricular FTG: > 5 years.
- Buccal mucosa: none yet recorded.

Penile enhancement

- Liposuction of pubic fat pad, fat injection into shaft.
- Partial/complete division of suspensory ligament (drops angle of erection).
- V–Y skin advancement from pubic area.
- Dermofat onlay grafts around tunica to increase girth.
- Stretching with weights for preputial advancement after circumcision.

III. Vaginal reconstruction

Pathology

- Congenital absence (Rokitansky syndrome) or segmental (imperforate hymen, long segment atresia).

- Congenital malformation – female hypospadias.
- Surgical ablation – e.g. mid-section excision for prolapse.
- Radionecrosis – hostile tissues.

Surgical options

- Local tissue e.g. vagina, vulva, skin. Vulval tissue expansion provides appropriate tissue with minimal donor defect and high success rate. However, treatment requires two stages and hospitalization for 6–7 weeks during expansion.
- Split skin grafts (e.g. McIndoe technique for vaginal agenesis; however, skin graft take may be poor and leaves a visible donor site).
- Distant flaps: bilateral groin flaps, TRAM (pedicled through the pelvis on IEA) or pedicled ALT or gracilis.
- Bowel (jejunum) but tend to get stenosis at mucocutaneous anastomosis.

With post-radiotherapy defects, well-vascularized tissue on its own blood supply needs to be imported e.g. TRAM, omentum or gracilis whilst fistulae generally require flap closure.

Vaginal reconstruction for hypoplasia

Vaginoplasty in childhood usually has poor results; procedures are best deferred until after puberty.

- Dilation – should be first line.
- Vaginoplasty.

Pressure dilation techniques

Vaginal oestrogen creams or pessaries are useful for those using dilators; its use results in a 'plumping' up and cushioning of the vaginal tissues and makes it more comfortable to use dilators. Systemic HRT does not always produce an improvement in vaginal symptoms (dryness and atrophy) and vaginal oestrogen may also be needed to improve the condition of the vaginal epithelium.

Intermittent pressure (Frank method, 1938). Self-dilation is carried out with rounded rod-shaped appliances and gentle pressure (enough to cause mild discomfort) is applied, typically once or twice per day for 20 to 30 minutes. The time to completion of treatment can vary from less than a month to over a year. An adequate dosage of oral oestrogen, plus local application of vaginal oestrogen cream may be helpful; a motivated patient is needed.

- Ingram (1981) developed a set of Lucite appliances, and a specialized stool (the 'bicycle seat') which allows dilation to be carried out while the patient is clothed and in a sitting position. Modern dilators are also designed to be used in a seated position, but on an ordinary chair, thus removing the need for the cumbersome stool. They have a design that allows adjustment of their length in very small increments, which helps make the process less uncomfortable.

Continuous pressure (Vecchietti procedure).
The Vecchietti operation (1965) is well accepted in Europe. Pressure is applied in the vaginal area by a dilation 'olive', a plastic bead through which traction sutures or threads are threaded, and run up through the abdominal cavity to a traction device placed on the outside of the abdomen (this can be done with laparoscopic assistance). It is a true dilation-type neovagina. However, in contrast to the intermittent pressure technique using dilators by hand which requires considerable patient effort and time, the Vecchietti method applies constant round-the-clock traction to create a functional vagina (10–12 cm length) in 7–9 days. Intercourse is said to be possible after 3–5 weeks. The Vecchietti procedure is useful when manual dilation is excessively uncomfortable, or when progress in dilation is poor. Its relative advantages over manual dilation are greater when the vagina is initially represented by only a very shallow dimple. It does require flexible/elastic skin and thus is not suitable for those with scarring from previous operations.

Vaginoplasty

The McIndoe method is the most common surgical technique used and is variably attributed to McIndoe, Reed and Abbe. The neovaginal cavity is lined with split skin graft that is held in place with a stent for 7 days. The main problem is the strong tendency for the graft to contract; prevention requires conscientious use of dilators (or intercourse) daily. The graft donor site also seems to be of concern for patients. Variants include lining with FTSGs, or with amnion (Sharma D. *J Gynecol Surg* 2008;**24**: 61–66) which become gradually replaced by vaginal epithelium.

- **Davydov technique** uses peritoneum freed from the pelvic side wall to line a newly excavated vagina; it can be performed laparascopically.

- **Intestinal transposition** and variants: A vagina is formed from a transplanted length of pedicled colon (colovaginoplasty). This is possibly the most invasive of the techniques used and is not recommended as first-line treatment. It has a lower contracture rate compared with the McIndoe procedure but there may be a problem with prolonged mucous discharge (may respond to irrigation with short chain fatty acids/steroids). In rare cases, adenocarcinoma in the segment of bowel has been reported.

Comparison of two methods of vagina construction in transsexuals
Van Noort DE. *Plast Reconstr Surg* 1993;**91**:1308–1315.

Male to female surgery is 3× commoner than female to male. An epithelium-lined cavity must be created between prostate/urethra/seminal vesicles and rectum. Inversion of penile or penile and scrotal skin flaps is the most commonly used technique; scrotal skin is incorporated into neovagina or used to fashion labia. Others include SSG, pedicled flaps or intestinal segments. Regular dilation post-operatively is achieved by stent or vibrator and then intercourse.

Twenty-seven male to female patients were evaluated comparing penile skin inversion with penile and scrotal skin inversion. The combined technique offers a more capacious neovagina but hair growth and skin prolapse are more of a problem.

IV. Sexual differentiation

The sex of an individual will be determined by a series of mechanisms:

- Chromosomal or genetic through the presence or absence of the Y chromosome.
- Gonadal – primary sex determination which is controlled by the testes determining factor TDF, which is the *SRY* gene (Koopman P. *Reprod Fertil Dev* 1995;**7**:713–722).
- Phenotypic – secondary sex determination which is controlled by gonadal hormones.

Disorders of sexual differentiation
Warne GL. *Endocr Metab Clin N Am* 1998;**27**:945–967.

SRY **gene** – the sex-determining region of the Y chromosome is the testis-determining factor and absence of the *SRY* gene means no testis formation and thus leads to formation of the female phenotype.

The mechanism of action of *SRY* is not known; there is the proposal that it acts as a negative regulator of a hypothetical *Z* gene whose role is to repress the testis-forming pathway i.e. a double negative system. Recent work suggests that the fate of the primordial gonad lies in the balance of male-promoting signals e.g. Sox9 and Ffg9 that push towards testis differentiation and Wnt4, female-promoting signals that push towards ovarian differentiation.

Karyotype problems

- **Mixed gonadal dysgenesis** is a condition of atypical gonadal development leading to unassigned sex differentiation. There have been a variety of karotype problems reported but most commonly a mosaic 45,X/46,XY with both male and female gonads (one of which is 'streak') and ambiguous genitalia. Such patients have an increased risk of gonadal malignancy.
- **Hermaphroditism** (46,XY/XX) with both testes and ovaries, male genitalia or ambiguous. This may be familial (there is a high incidence in the Bantu population of South Africa, for example). Most, but not all, such patients are infertile.
- **Turner's syndrome** (45,XO) with streak gonads, female genitalia, short stature and webbed neck, primary (congenital) lymphoedema.
- **Klinefelter's syndrome** (47,XXY) small testes, hypogonadism, gynaecomastia.

Gonadal problems

- **Gonadal dysgenesis**. The loss of primordial germ cells in the gonad leads to **streak gonads** – hypoplastic and hypofunctional gonads consisting mostly of fibrous tissue. Causes include Turner's syndrome, mixed gonadal dysgenesis etc.
- **Androgen-insensitivity syndrome (AIS)** – a set of conditions where the testosterone receptors are insensitive to androgens. Most have a variable degree of undervirilization/infertility in a XY person; those with complete insensitivity (previously known as 'testicular feminization') has male karyotype 46,XY but female genitalia and external appearance.
- Enzyme deficiencies.
  - ○ **Congenital adrenal hyperplasia (CAH)**: several autosomal recessive diseases due to enzyme mutations; 95% are due to 21-hydroxylase deficiency. There is altered development of sex characteristics and only a

small proportion develop a true intersex condition. Classically, those with female karyotype may have ambiguous genitalia due to adrenal androgen excess. 21-hydroxylase deficiency causes precursors involved in the aldosterone pathway to be diverted into androgen synthesis. Salt-losing type may cause hyponatraemia, hyperkalaemia and dehydration in the first week postnatally.
  - ○ **17-α-hydroxylase deficiency CAH** (very rare): enzyme required for synthesis of androgens and oestrogens.
    - – 46,XX females are born with normal female anatomy but at the time of puberty, breast and pubic hair development is impaired due to the adrenals and ovaries being unable to produce sex hormones; milder forms may have relatively normal breasts with irregular menstruation.
    - – 46,XY males have reduced testosterone production and are undervirilized. There is impairment of glucocorticoid synthesis and adrenal hyperplasia.

Hormones

- Leydig cells in the testis secrete testosterone that confers male phenotype through action on Wolffian ducts (epididymis, vas deferens, seminal vesicles).
- Sertoli cells secrete Müllerian-inhibiting substance that cause regression of Müllerian ducts (upper third vagina, uterus, oviducts).
- Virilization of the external genitalia requires conversion of testosterone to dihydrotestosterone via 5-α-reductase.

Intersex disorders

XY females occur due to mutation in the *SRY* gene that leads to deficiencies of 5-α-reductase and 17-α-hydroxylase.

XX males resemble Klinefelter's and the male phenotype due to *SRY* gene translocation from Y to X chromosome. However, the genitalia are ambiguous with a phallus intermediate in size between a penis and clitoris. The most likely diagnoses are:

- CAH.
- 5-α-reductase deficiency.
- Mixed gonadal dysgenesis.
- XY male with persistent Müllerian duct structures due to mutations in the *MIS* gene or its receptor.

- XX female with absent Müllerian duct structures, also known as Müllerian agenesis or Meyer–Rokitansky–Kuster–Hauser syndrome (MRKH), cause unknown but some suggest activating mutation in the *MIS* gene or its receptor.

Management

- Counsel the parents – defer registering or naming the child.
- Surgery:
  - Streak gonads have risk of malignant change therefore must be removed.
  - Androgen-insensitivity syndrome patients have a 9% risk of developing seminoma and should have their testes removed before 20 years (phenotypically female).
- Feminizing genitoplasty e.g. CAH are almost always reared as female and are fertile therefore feminizing genitoplasty reinforces sexual identity.

C. Defects of the chest wall, abdominal wall and trunk

I. Chest wall and sternum

Reconstruction may be required following:

- Clearance of cancer including breast or other chest wall malignancies – palliative surgery may be acceptable for advanced lesions.
- Radiation-induced ulceration. Of note, irradiated tissues tend to be stiffer and show fewer tendencies for paradoxical chest movements post-resection. It may be difficult to distinguish between radiation ulcers and tumour on biopsy – the whole area should be resected, which would also remove tissues of poor vascularity/healing. Vascular tissue in the form of pedicled or free muscle flaps is preferred, allowing at least 6–12 weeks following cessation of all radiotherapy before considering reconstruction.
- Congenital defects e.g. pectus and Poland's syndrome.
- Trauma or post-operative e.g. sternotomy wound dehiscence, bronchopleural fistula, empyema (Clagett's procedure useful: allow cavity to granulate then fill with antibiotic solution).

Flaps for chest wall reconstruction

Most are local flaps.

- Pectoralis major – advancement based on the thoracoacromial axis or turnover flaps based on parasternal perforators (type V). Both sides may be used.
- Pedicled latissimus dorsi (type V) – the use of this myocutaneous flap was originally described by Tansini in 1906 for closure of a chest wall defect. Central back defects can be closed using bilateral latissimus dorsi advancement flaps.
- Pedicled TRAM/VRAM for sternal wounds in particular. The superior rectus can still be raised after use of the internal mammary artery (IMA) for coronary artery bypass graft (CABG), being supplied by the 8th intercostal but the inferior portion below the umbilicus is less reliable.
- Breast sharing (vide infra).
- Omentum (based on right gastro-epiploic artery).
- Serratus anterior for intrathoracic transposition (type III).

Paradoxical chest movement (with reduced mechanical efficiency) may follow if three or more ribs removed (athletes) or two or more ribs removed (elderly) – similarly, those with underlying lung disease will be less tolerant of a chest wall defect whilst those with prior irradiation will be more tolerant due to tissue stiffness. In addition, posterior defects (especially superior ones shielded by the scapulae) may be better tolerated.

Others suggest an absolute size e.g. > 5 cm as a threshold for skeletal reconstruction; protection of internal organs is another consideration. Options for skeletal support include:

- Alloplastics.
  - Marlex mesh (polypropylene) forms a fibrous capsule that is semi-rigid; however, it may fragment or become infected.
  - Gore-Tex is more malleable and also forms a capsule. It is more expensive and more prone to seroma formation.
  - Methyl methacrylate sandwich with a cement layer ~0.5 cm thick – the tissues have to be protected from the exothermic chemical reaction when it is being fabricated. The infection and extrusion rates are moderately high.
- Autologous.
  - Bone or fascia grafts.
  - Muscle or fascial flaps.

Thoracoplasty is a last-resort operation if flaps are not suitable/available; staged removal of ribs allows the chest wall to collapse.

Chest wall reconstruction: an account of 500 consecutive patients
Arnold PG. *Plast Reconstr Surg* 1996;**98**:804–810.

The authors used muscle flaps predominantly: pectoralis major (355), latissimus dorsi (141), serratus, external oblique, rectus and trapezius in that order of frequency; the omentum was used for salvage in 50 patients. Skeletal defects were reconstructed in 116 with polypropylene mesh or autologous rib. 83.1% were alive a month after the operation and had healed.

Design of the 'cyclops flap' for chest wall reconstruction
Hughes KC. *Plast Reconstr Surg* 1997;**100**:1146–1151.

This is essentially an axial pattern flap based upon the lateral thoracic artery and breast tissue is advanced across the midline to leave the nipple in a more central position. The aesthetic result is poor but it is worth keeping in mind, being useful in situations where:

- Scarring in the axilla precludes a pedicled latissimus dorsi or microvascular anastomosis.
- Chest wall defect e.g. full-thickness excision of chest wall precludes use of the internal mammary arteries or may be lost due to previous cardiac surgery.
- The patient may be unfit for a major procedure.

External oblique myocutaneous flap coverage of large chest wall defects following resection of breast tumors
Bogossian N. *Plast Reconstr Surg* 1996;**97**:97–103.

The external oblique flap is a large myocutaneous rotation flap from the whole of the ipsilateral upper quadrant of the abdomen. It is a reliable sensate flap that can be raised quickly without turning. The donor site closes directly with no risk of abdominal hernia as the rectus is intact. It can extend ~3 cm beyond the midline.

The flap is raised superficial to the rectus sheath medially then deep to the external oblique muscle laterally where it is based on perforators from intercostal vessels at the posterior axillary line. Moschella F (*Plast Reconstr Surg* 1999;**103**:1378–1385) includes the anterior rectus sheath in the flap and advances the internal oblique by plicating the abdominal wall.

Sternal wound dehiscence
Sternotomy wound infections occurs in 5% of cardiac procedures particularly IMA harvest – 0.3% of unilateral harvest and 2.4% with bilateral harvest.

- Early – this is often minor and due to superficial wound infection. Treatment includes dressings after opening up the cavity though the wires may need to be removed.
- Late – this is often major including dehiscence of the sternum itself. An important point to note is whether the left internal mammary artery (LIMA) was used.

Pairolero classification
- Type 1 – within first 3 days. There is a serosanguinous discharge with negative cultures. These can be treated with exploration, debridement and closure.
- Type 2 – presents within the first 3 weeks, presenting with a purulent mediastinitis with positive cultures; there may be chondritis with or without osteomyelitis.
- Type 3 – presents late, usually months to years afterwards, typically with a draining sinus that connects to a focus of chronic osteomyelitis. These should be treated with flap coverage after debridement.

Starzynski classification (sternal defects)
- Loss of upper sternal body and adjacent ribs – minimal physiological effect.
- Loss of entire sternal body and adjacent ribs – moderate physiological effect.
- Loss of manubrium and entire upper sternal body and ribs – severe effect.

Reconstructive options
- Vertical rectus (use right side if LIMA was used).
- Omentum (but can be very thin).
- Pectoralis major advancement or turnover.
- Bilateral bipedicled pectoralis major-rectus flaps.
- Latissimus dorsi free flap.

Secondary sternal repair following median sternotomy using interosseous absorbable sutures and pectoralis major myocutaneous advancement flaps
Perkins DJ. *Br J Plast Surg* 1996;**49**:214–219.

The sternum is sutured first (unicortical) with no. 1 PDS interosseus sutures; if the sternum cannot be closed directly then VRAM or pectoralis major turn-over flaps or omentum are used. A VRAM may be still be vascularized by the cardiophrenic artery (anastomoses with intercostal arteries) in the absence of the internal mammary but it is unreliable, particularly distally (past the umbilicus).

The pectoralis major (PM) is raised only as far laterally as the site of the internal mammary artery perforators (approximately 6 cm from the midline) which maintains this part of the muscle which is far away from the thoraco-acromial pedicle.

- If the IMA has already been harvested, the muscle is regarded as having been 'delayed' by the surgery.
- If the IMA is present, the turnover flap is a lifeboat.

The mobilized muscles are then approximated to the midline. Bilateral PM advancement flaps can be combined with **breast reduction** and free nipple graft to reduce breast weight and thus tension on wound closure. Preserving the internal mammary perforators maintains perfusion to the mobilized muscle and also to the medial breast dermoglandular flap of the reduction.

The most consistent place to find the IMA is the **3rd intercostal space**; 40% of the left-sided veins and 70% of the right-sided veins are 3 mm or more in diameter.

Sternal wound reconstruction: 252 consecutive cases
Schulman NG. *Plast Reconstr Surg* 2004;**114**:44–48.

This is a retrospective review of 252 sternal wound closures for post-sternotomy problems. Their work-horse flap is the pectoralis major pedicled on the thoraco-acromial axis, with the latissimus dorsi and rectus flap used less frequently. They report a 3% mortality rate and a 5% reinfection rate.

Free flaps in the management of intrathoracic sepsis
Perkins DJ. *Br J Plast Surg* 1995;**48**:546–550.

The author presents their experience with five cases requiring free flaps. The aim is to evacuate, sterilize and obliterate the cavity. The evacuation is performed by chest drain or open drainage; packing/dressing the cavity for it to granulate may take ~2 weeks.

- Use of a pedicled latissimus dorsi may be precluded by lateral thoracotomy incision.
- Free muscle flaps to the thoracodorsal vessels may be needed e.g. contralateral latissimus dorsi or de-epithelialized TRAM.

Single-stage muscle flap reconstruction of the post-pneumonectomy empyema space
Seify H. *Plast Reconstr Surg* 2007;**120**:1886–1891.

The authors describe their experience in 55 patients. Their treatment algorithm is:

- No bronchopleural fistula – acute chest tube drainage until mediastinum is stabilized then attempt modified Clagett's procedure – and if it fails, then muscle flaps are used.
- With fistula, first use chest tube drainage and follow the above if the fistula closes. If the fistula remains open then an Eloesser procedure may be attempted before using muscle flaps.

Commonly used muscle flaps included serratus anterior, latissimus dorsi, pectoralis major, rectus and omentum. 8.7% had persistent empyema.

- Multiple flaps are needed to close the chest cavity completely; an average of 2.1 flaps were used in patients (Micheals BM. *Plast Reconstr Surg* 1997;**99**:437) along with thoracoplasty in some cases.

II. Chest wall deformities

Poland's syndrome
The chest defect was first described in a post-mortem examination by Alfred Poland in 1841 of a convict called Marc DeYoung; the name was coined by Clarkson PW in 1962 who described a case with similar chest features and hand anomalies. It occurs in 1 in 25 000 live births affecting males 3× more, and is on the right side in 75% of cases. There are many theories regarding its aetiology:

- Intrauterine vascular insult (subclavian artery disruption) or hypoxia during the stage of limb bud development (weeks 6 and 7).
- Genetic – familial tendency has been reported, although most cases are sporadic.

Chest wall defects
- Deficiency of pectoralis major (total aplasia or isolated loss of sternocostal head); variable deficiencies of pectoralis minor, serratus, latissimus dorsi (thus would not be a reconstructive option), deltoid, supra- and infraspinatus.

- Breast hypoplasia or aplasia with a smaller nipple–areolar complex or absent nipples.
- Others.
  - Deficiency of subcutaneous tissue.
  - Contraction of the anterior axillary fold.
  - Abnormalities of the anterior portion of the second–fourth ribs.
  - Thoracic scoliosis, pectus excavatum, Sprengel's deformity.

Limb abnormalities.

- Shortening of digits and syndactyly (simple, complete) – **brachysyndactyly** – the middle phalanges are most affected.
- Hypoplasia of the hand and forearm.
- Foot anomalies.

Cardiovascular abnormalities.

- Dextrocardia.
- Hypoplastic or absent vessels (subclavian, thoraco-acromial, thoracodorsal).
  - Consider angiography before reconstructing breast with latissimus dorsi.

Other associated abnormalities.

- Renal hypoplasia.
- Congenital spherocytosis.
- Increased incidence of leukaemia.

Patients usually present for chest wall management at adolescence or early in adult life.

- Women usually complain of breast maldevelopment.
- Male patients often complain of deficient anterior axillary fold.

The anterior axillary fold can be recreated with latissimus dorsi muscle transposition inserting the tendon into the bicipital groove; however, beware of hypoplastic muscle or absent thoracodorsal vessel – may consider angiography first. In these cases, other options include silicone implants or more uncommonly, de-epithelialized pedicled TRAM or free flaps. CT scans may be useful to define the skeletal anomalies, and the status of the latissimus dorsi.

Management of the chest deformity in male patients with Poland's syndrome
Marks MW. *Plast Reconstr Surg* 1991;**87**:674–678.

The authors suggest an axillary approach to the latissimus dorsi: the muscle is raised and transferred via a subcutaneous tunnel to the chest wall, and the tendon of LD is sutured beneath the clavicular head of pectoralis major.

The authors compared their results using customized silicone implants alone with latissimus dorsi in addition to the implant and found superior long-term results with the combination. There is some over-correction initially with optimum result after atrophy of the muscle (which occurs despite maintaining the thoracodorsal nerve).

Pectus excavatum (funnel chest)
Pectus excavatum tends to present in early childhood with a progressive worsening of the deformity, affecting males $3\times$ more often. This is the most common chest wall abnormality, occurring in about 8 in 1000 live births (some say $10\times$ more common than pigeon chest) – most patients are asymptomatic but some may have cardiopulmonary compromise.

There is a family history in one-third of patients; in one-fifth, there is an association with Marfan's syndrome or scoliosis. A much smaller number may have congenital cardiac abnormalities.

Treatment options include:

- Midline sternal incision or bilateral inframammary incisions, then osteotomies, partial costal cartilage resection/overlapping, sternal elevation.
- Sternal turnover.
- **Ravitch technique** (1949) – sternal osteotomy and retrosternal strut for support. It is a well-documented procedure with good long-term results.
  - Leonard modification (2003) – removal of 4–5 cartilages whilst the perichondrium is left in place; a wedge osteotomy of the sternum is performed and a sheathed wire (instead of a bar) placed behind the sternum and brought up through to the chest wall to be secured to an external brace.
- **Nuss procedure** (1998) – a 'minimally invasive technique'. A curved stainless steel bar is placed thoracoscopically behind the sternum and then 'flipped' to push the anterior chest out, fixation/stabilization is usually needed. The bar is removed after 2–4 years and long-term follow-up has shown less than 5% recurrence. It is less likely to work well in adults. There is a significant learning curve.
- Silicone implant for less severe deformity – 3D reconstructive CT used to guide manufacture of custom-made implants.

Early repair is advocated, with better results during the ages of 2 and 5.

Comparision of the Nuss and the Ravitch procedure for pectus excavatum repair: a meta-analysis
Nasr A. *J Ped Surg* 2010;**45**:880–886.

In this study, data were extracted by three authors from nine studies (there were no randomized trials). There was no difference in patient satisfaction; there were also no differences in overall complications, time to ambulation and length of hospital stay.

The rate of reoperation and haemo/pneumothorax was higher in the Nuss procedure.

There was a trend towards a higher analgesic requirement in the Nuss procedure.

Pectus carinatum (barrel or pigeon chest)

Pectus carinatum is more common in males, with a family history in one-third; there is an association with scoliosis and heart disease in 15%. The problem presents later on than funnel chest, with one study reporting that half are found after about 10 years of age – it is mostly a cosmetic problem with only a minority with pulmonary problems. The mechanism seems to be related to overgrowth of the costal cartilages with displacement and buckling of the sternum.

- Chondrogladiolar protrusion – anterior displacement of sternum, with concavity of the ribs – most common 90%.
- Lateral depression of ribs on the other side, which tends to be more common in those with Poland's syndrome (mixed carinatum and excavatum)
- Chondromanubrial (pouter pigeon chest) – upper prominence with inferior depression (a distal anterior displacement gives it a characteristic Z on lateral X-ray). This is the least common (3%) form and is often noted at birth.

    Orthotic bracing may work in younger patients.

- Correction by Lester's method (1953) is rather radical and is associated with significant blood loss: partial costal cartilage resection/overlapping and wedge osteotomy of the sternum to achieve sternal depression.
- Shamberger and Welch (*J Pediatr Surg* 1988;**23**:319–322) with double or single wedge osteotomies.

Surgery of chest wall deformities
de Matos AC. *Eur J Cardiothoracic Surg* 1997;**12**:345–350.

The author presents experience with 77 patients. Pectus excavatum is more than twice as common as pectus carinatum (53 vs. 24 in this series). Most patients < 15 years of age and are generally asymptomatic. However, there is a possibility of:

- Secondary back problems in later life due to poor posture and spinal scoliosis.
- Psychological morbidity.
- A small number have dyspnoea and abnormal respiratory function tests.
- A minority of patients have associated congenital cardiovascular anomalies (atrial septal defect (ASD), ventricular septal defect (VSD), pulmonary stenosis, etc.).

The position of the sternum is the result of abnormal growth of the costal cartilages. Surgical options include subperichondrial resection of abnormal costal cartilages and sternal osteotomies; the segment is then turned over and fixed with steel rods (Steinmann pin) that can be removed after 6–12 months.

There have been reported problems of avascular necrosis (large bone graft) with sternal turnover procedures.

III. Abdominal wall and perineum

The aim of reconstruction is the restoration of functional integrity of the abdominal wall; it is important to determine which components are missing: skin, muscle, fascia. In addition, whilst immediate closure is usually desirable, it is also important to consider the implications of relocating abdominal viscera that may be swollen into an enclosed space – thus consider pre-operative pulmonary function tests and assess the effect on respiration of closing the abdominal wall (e.g. for large incisional hernias).

Reconstructive options can be 'definitive' closure or as a temporizing stage i.e. debridement and SSG with or without intervening stage of allowing granulate/vacuum closure. The latter option may be more suitable to allow local tissue inflammation (due to bowel fistulae, trauma, surgery or infection) to subside before attempting definitive reconstruction.

- Vacuum-assisted closure (VAC) will assist in increasing granulation tissue, reducing the defect while stabilizing the wound.

413

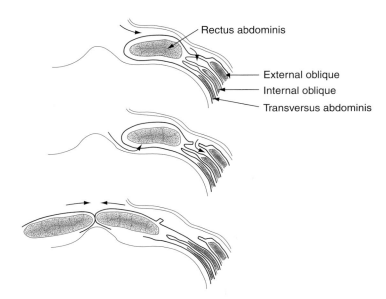

Figure 9.3 The components separation technique involves dissecting the plane between the external and internal oblique muscles, and then incising the rectus sheath to allow advancement of the rectus as a unit with the two inner muscle layers. This was described by Ramirez OM (*Plast Reconstr Surg* 1990;**86**:519–526). Bilateral dissection allows advancement of 10, 20 and 6 cm at the epigastric, umbilical and suprapubic areas respectively.

Indications for abdominal wall reconstruction

Congenital (exomphalos) vs. acquired:

- Fungating tumours.
- Traumatic including burns or iatrogenic e.g. wound dehiscence, incisional hernia.
- Necrotizing fasciitis.
- Post-radiation ulcers, etc.

For the perineum and groin

In simple terms, muscle flaps will bring the best blood supply but fasciocutaneous flaps are thin and potentially sensate. There are a number of pedicled flaps that are usually available.

- Rectus abdominis – muscle, TRAM (high skin paddle including peri-umbilical perforators) or VRAM flaps. This is useful for reconstructing large perineal defects and can be transferred through the pelvis or subcutaneously, and dis-insertion from the pubis allows greater mobility.
- The rectus femoris myocutaneous flap can be applied to most situations of perineal reconstruction but leaves a relatively poor donor site scar.
- Tensor fascia lata (TFL).
- Gracilis muscle or myocutaneous flap.
- Posterior thigh fasciocutaneous flap.

Free flaps – there are a wide choice including latissimus dorsi and TRAM – can be anastomosed to inferior gluteal vessels.

- Full-thickness abdominal wall reconstruction using an innervated latissimus dorsi flap (Ninkovic M. *Plast Reconstr Surg* 1998;**101**:971–978) or autologous fascial grafts (Disa JJ. *Plast Reconstr Surg* 1998;**101**:979–986).

An algorithm for abdominal wall reconstruction
Rohrich RJ. *Plast Reconstr Surg* 2000;**105**:202–216.

Assess size of defect

- Small defects are often closed directly by undermining and local advancement, small random pattern fasciocutaneous flaps or skin grafts.
- Larger defects may be reduced by NPWT then managed as above.
- Defects > 15 cm may require axial flaps, tissue expansion or distant pedicled or free flaps. Distant flap from the thigh region e.g.
  - TFL, rectus femoris, sartorius, gracilis.
  - Often limited by size and arc of rotation, only suitable for lower defects. Large anterior thigh flaps based on either anterolateral or anteromedial perforators have been used to cover large defects of the anterior abdomen up to the level of the xiphisternum (Lin SJ. *Plast Reconstr Surg* 2010;**125**:1146–1156).

Fascial reconstruction

- Prosthetic materials e.g. nylon mesh, Marlex.
- Free or vascularized fascia lata (TFL flap or thigh flaps). If mesh is contraindicated by the presence of

potentially contaminated tissue, autologous fascia lata grafts can be used instead, but take care to leave the tendon of the iliotibial tract to maintain lateral knee stability.

- Collagen substitues (e.g. Permacol™ – acellular porcine collagen).

Wound closure in large defects

Midline defects: **component separation** or lateral releasing incisions to advance fasciocutaneous flaps medially.

Lateral defects:

- Upper third
  - Superiorly based rectus abdominis from the other side.
  - External oblique.
  - Extended latissimus dorsi flap.
  - Extended TFL, subtotal thigh.
- Middle third.
  - Rectus abdominis (including extended deep inferior epigastric flap).
  - External oblique.
  - TFL, rectus femoris, subtotal thigh.
- Lower third.
  - Inferiorly based rectus abdominis (including extended deep inferior epigastric flap).
  - Internal oblique.
  - TFL, rectus femoris, vastus lateralis, gracilis, groin flap, subtotal thigh.

Free tissue transfer

The freedom of movement with free flaps means that they may be applied to upper, middle and lower third defects.

- Free latissimus dorsi myocutaneous flap which can be anastomosed to the superior epigastric pedicle and re-innervated by coaptation of the thoracodorsal nerve to intercostal nerves supplying rectus abdominis which in theory provides muscle contraction to the abdominal wall and can avoid a mesh.
- Alternatively TFL with innervated muscle transfer as described by Ninkovic.
- Subtotal thigh flap.
- Other recipient vessels include:
  - Deep inferior epigastric vessels.
  - Deep circumflex iliac vessels.
  - Internal mammary vessels.

Abdominal wall expansion in congenital defects
Byrd HS. *Plast Reconstr Surg* 1989;**84**:347–352.

Tissue expansion was used to reconstruct the lower abdominal wall defect of two children with cloacal exstrophy. Tissue expanders were placed in the space between transversus abdominis and internal oblique via incisions in the lateral part of the rectus sheath and expanded over ~10 weeks (requiring GA each time). One patient suffered from colonic dysmotility and constipation during the course of the expansion.

The authors subsequently applied the same technique to an adult patient with an abdominal defect following necrotizing pancreatitis with initial closure by skin grafts. He placed them in the same plane; Livingston D (*J Trauma* 1992;**32**:82–86) placed expanders under the subcutaneous fascia superficial to the external oblique.

IV. Posterior trunk

Apart from tumours and infections, defects of the posterior trunk may result from:

- Spina bifida.
- Spinal surgery wound dehiscence.

Upper third: trapezius myocutaneous flap based on transverse cervical artery.

Middle third: latissimus dorsi based on thoracodorsal pedicle.

Lower third:
  - Latissimus dorsi turnover flap.
  - Lumbar artery perforator flaps.
  - Gluteus maximus or S-GAP flap.
  - Bipedicled fasciocutaneous flaps, keystone flaps.

Other options include:

- Tissue expansion.
- Vacuum closure and SSG.

Management of massive thoracolumbar wounds and vertebral osteomyelitis following scoliosis surgery
Mitra A. *Plast Reconstr Surg* 2004;**113**:206–213.

This is a review of a series of 33 patients (11–65 years) with large thoracolumbar wounds following scoliosis surgery with exposed metalwork, dead bone/osteomyelitis and large dead space. Patients may present with pain, tenderness, erythema, pyrexia. The metalwork was able to be retained in all patients.

Principles of management:

- Expedient return to theatre.
- Wound irrigation and primary closure if possible.

- Thorough excisional debridement of non-viable bone and soft tissue.
- Specimens for culture.
- Closed suction drainage.

Superior wounds:

- Myocutaneous extended **latissimus dorsi flap** – the fasciocutaneous extension of the flap, beyond the inferior muscle edge, is de-epithelialized and turned in to the defect to help obliterate dead space. The secondary defect is skin grafted.

Inferior wounds:

- Whole **gluteus maximus muscle** islanded on the superior gluteal vessels and rotated in to the defect after insertions on the iliac bone, sacrum and gluteal fascia are divided, and also released laterally from iliotibial tract and the femur.
  - All patients reconstructed with this flap were non-ambulatory.
  - Some wounds may also require inferiorly based fasciocutaneous skin flaps to supplement closure.

Chapter 1

Aesthetic

I. Lasers: principles and safety

- 1916 – Einstein's theory of stimulated emission of radiation.
- 1957 – Townes, Schawlow and Gould – laid down the principles for light amplification by stimulated emission of radiation (LASER, which followed on from MASER related to microwaves which had been developed recently). As always, at the time there was a side story with patents, law suits etc. between the protagonists.
- 1960 – Maiman built the first laser using a synthetic ruby crystal placed inside a coiled flash lamp inside a Fabry-Pérot etalon (two parallel flat semi-transparent mirrors in a tube – light that enters is reflected multiple times and the resulting interference modulates the beams).

Soon after this, developments came thick and fast; the helium neon, neodymium:yttrium aluminium garnet (Nd:YAG), CO_2 and argon lasers were all developed in the early 1960s.

Components of a laser:

- Energy source
  - Electricity (argon laser).
  - Flashlamp (pulsed-dye laser).
  - Another laser (CO_2 laser).
- Laser medium – solid or gas.
- Laser cavity (resonator).

The laser medium is energized to excite electrons into a higher energy state (singlet state in an unstable orbit around the nucleus). As electrons move back into a stable orbit, a photon of light of a particular wavelength is emitted. Photons hitting excited atoms generate more photons, i.e. **stimulated emission**.

Photons move randomly in the resonator but through the action of a pair of mirrors, they become a parallel or collimated laser beam all with the same wavelength.

Energy (J) is proportional to the number of photons.
Power = energy/s, i.e. rate of delivery of energy (W).

- $1\ W = 1\ J/s$.
- Rate of **input** of energy to create the laser beam.

Irradiance = power per unit area (W/cm^2).
Fluence = energy/cm^2 (J/cm^2).

Continuous wave lasers may be broken intermittently by a mechanical shutter to form a pulsed wave (pulsed-dye laser) with higher energy and peak temperature.

- Q-switching: electromagnetic switch produces ultra-short pulse duration.

When the laser beam contacts the target, the light can be:

- Reflected.
- Transmitted – passes through unchanged.
- Refracted – passes through with a directional change.
- Scattered – by dermis (collagen).
- **Absorbed** – clinical effects occur when laser light is absorbed by 'chromophores' such as haemoglobin, melanin, tattoo pigments and water. Different

chromophores maximally absorb light at different wavelengths.

The shorter the wavelength, the more scatter and reflectance, or the corollary is that longer wavelengths allow better penetration. **Absorption coefficient** of tissues also determines penetration. The depth of penetration is proportional to:

- Degree of scatter.
- Absorption by chromophores.
- Energy delivered.
- Wavelength of the laser beam.

Gaussian distribution of heat within the laser spot means that 10% overlap is usually not harmful. **Multiple passes** do not produce additive effects – the first pass causes coagulation and changes the optical properties of the tissue, thus a second pass achieves only 50% coagulation compared with the first.

Selective photothermolysis: precise microsurgery by selective absorption of pulse radiation
Anderson RR. *Science* 1983;**29**:524–527.

The principle of selective photothermolyis (Anderson and Parrish) aims to **target** with:

- **Wavelength** of laser light specific to chromophores of that tissue.
- **Pulse width** to maximize destruction of chromophores without collateral damage:
  - A pulse width less than the thermal relaxation time of the tissue (T_r = time to cool to 50% of initial temperature achieved) limits thermal diffusion and thus minimizes unwanted collateral damage.
  - Diameter of a vessel determines its thermal relaxation time.
- **Fluence** above threshold for destruction of that chromophore.
  - Pulsed delivery of laser light delivers higher energy.

For example, the argon laser (457–514 nanometres (nm)) aims to target haemoglobin (and cause coagulation) but the chromophore absorption peaks and T_r are:

- Melanin (500–600 nm) – 1 μs.
- Haemoglobin (577–585 nm).

Thus, if an argon laser is used to treat vascular malformations, it will cause depigmentation because melanin also absorbs this wavelength. The darker a patient's skin colour, the more likely that there will be pigmentation changes after laser treatment.

Laser safety

- Laser plume can contain viable bacteria and viruses including human papillomavirus (HPV), HIV and hepatitis B (HBV), although the actual infection risk is difficult to quantify. Good smoke evacuation systems and protection in the form of masks and gloves are needed.
  - Tissue splatter with Q-switching.
- Goggles are needed for eye protection (patient and doctor) and are not interchangeable between lasers.
- Fire and electrical shock hazard.

Individual lasers

Argon laser

- 457–514 nm blue–green light, continuous wave and mechanical shutter.
- Usual chromophores are haemoglobin and melanin. It is effective in treating PWS but
  - Shallow penetration depth ~1 mm and increased energy required which increases risk of scarring.

Pulsed-dye laser

- Fluorescent dye absorbed in water or alcohol; flashlamp stimulates emission of light that is tuned between 400 and 1000 nm depending upon the dye used, but usually 577–585 nm (yellow) for most clinical applications.
  - The pulse duration is very short.
  - Penetration 1.2 mm at 585 nm.
- It is good for vascular malformations with a high concentration of oxyhaemoglobin; there will be transient purple discoloration when used in the treatment of PWS.

Nd:YAG laser

- Laser media are the yttrium aluminium garnet (YAG) crystals in which neodymium is an impurity (YAG crystals can also be grown in erbium – Erb:YAG 2940 nm). It emits light at 1064 nm; it is poorly absorbed by haemoglobin, melanin, and water allowing greater penetration. Machines are usually Q-switched.
  - 1064 nm (infrared) useful for pigmented lesions and hair removal, particularly in darker-skinned patients.

○ Haemangiomas and vascular malformations at 532 nm (green yellow, frequency doubled); used in ophthalmology for retinal photocoagulation.

Ruby laser

- Flash lamp stimulation produces 694 nm (red) light.
- May be used for tattoos or hair removal (only safe for those with very pale skin).

Alexandrite laser

- Emits light at 755 nm (red).
- It can be used for hair removal but is not safe for darker skins.

CO_2 laser

- Gas mixture includes helium and nitrogen – helium provides targeting beam as for laser pointers. The 10 600 nm wavelength is in the infrared spectrum and is absorbed by water in the tissues and leads to vaporization of the superficial layers of skin.
- It is often used as a surgical scalpel in neurosurgery and ENT surgery or for superficial ablation/rejuvenation. Leukoplakia, warts with no pigmentation, and other superficial cutaneous or mucosal lesions can also be ablated with CO_2 laser.

II. Lasers in plastic surgery

Laser treatment of vascular lesions

The pulsed-dye laser (PDL, 585 nm) is often used for vascular malformations including PWS and superficial haemangioma; it is also used in treatment of hypertrophic scarring.

- Small vessels 30–40 μm, e.g. PWS can be treated with argon (488 nm), pulsed-dye laser.
- Medium sized 100–400 μm, e.g. haemangioma with a KTP laser.
- Large vessels > 400 μm, e.g. venous malformation with a Nd:YAG laser (> 100 ms).

Note that lesions such as PWS may have variable appearances in terms of colour, texture and distribution, probably representing different vessel configurations; these will respond differently to specific lasers, e.g. light pink-red lesions respond much better to PDL than darker lesions.

The most commonly treated vascular lesions are PWS (see also Vascular lesions) which seems well established; use of lasers for haemangiomas is more controversial. There may be a role in superficial involuting or ulcerating lesions but probably not in those with deeper components. Local or topical anaesthesia may be needed for larger lesions.

Surface cooling has been useful to reduce superficial damage whilst also allowing higher energies to be delivered to the vessels targeted. Candela's VBeam is a PDL (595 nm for deeper penetration) with a Dynamic Cooling Device (DCD) which delivers a pulse of cryogen spray just before the laser pulse. Other methods of tissue cooling include gels, contact and air-cooling; the timing may be pre-, parallel or post-cooling.

- Excessive cooling can cause epidermal damage and hyperpigmentation (Handley JM. *J Am Acad Dermatol* 2006;**55**:482–489).

Randomized controlled study of early pulsed dye laser treatment of uncomplicated childhood haemangiomas Batta K. *Lancet* 2002;**9354**:521–527.

In this study 121 infants (< 14 weeks) were randomized to pulsed-dye laser treatment (topical local anaesthesia) or observation only. Large, deep or complicated (obstructing vital structures) lesions were excluded.

Follow-up at 1 year showed no difference between observational and laser-treated groups in terms of clearance of haemangioma but skin atrophy and hypopigmentation rates were higher in the treatment group. The authors concluded that PDL is not better than 'wait-and-see' in simple lesions.

Pulsed-dye laser penetrates skin to approximately 1.2 mm and so can only treat superficial early haemangiomas in the preproliferative or early proliferative growth phase; 93% were apparently < 1 mm in height in this study.

Kolde G (*Lancet* 2003;**9354**:348–349) criticized the study for including infants that were too young. In his opinion, early haemangiomas have solid cell nests that are not yet perfused and thus less susceptible to PDL. Results from others studies suggest that matured lesions (at least 11 weeks old) and slightly nodular lesions responded better than initial macular lesions. On the other hand, some suggest that early treatment when lesions are still flat would be better; emphasizing the need for more controlled studies on the subject.

Outcomes of childhood hemangiomas treated with pulsed-dye laser with dynamic cooling
Rizzo C. *Dermatol Surg* 2009;**35**:1947–1954.

This is a retrospective study of 105 haemangiomas in 90 patients (median age 3 months) treated with 595 nm long pulse PDL with DCD at 2–8 weeks intervals. Those with previous treatment (laser, surgery or steroids) were excluded. They reported near-complete/complete clearance of colour in 81% and thickness in 64%. There were pigmentation problems in 18%. The author concludes that PDL is a safe treatment but the study suffers from the lack of controls for comparison.

Treatment of pulsed dye laser-resistant port wine stain birthmarks
Jasim ZF. *J Am Acad Derm* 2007;**57**:677–682.

This paper reviewed the options for PWS that do not respond to 577/585 nm PDL – most studies suggest that less than 20% can be lightened almost completely, 70% will lighten by half or more whilst 20–30% respond poorly, particularly the central face and the limbs. The reasons for variable response are unclear but may be related to the vessel configurations and depth (PDL penetrates about 1 mm). Strategies to improve PDL treatment include use of 595 nm with cooling, longer pulse duration/larger spot sizes for deeper lesions and pulse stacking. Other options discussed include intense pulsed light (IPL) with cooling, alexandrite (755 nm), nm diode (810 nm) and Nd:YAG (1064 nm).

Laser treatment of tattoos

Different lasers with different wavelengths are needed for different pigments thus multicoloured professional tattoos will need repeated treatments with different machines. Other types of tattoos include amateur (usually blue/black and superficial but inconsistent placement) and traumatic (usually following inadequate cleaning of abrasions). The majority of lasers used for tattoo removal are Q-switched lasers.

- Initial tattoo causes an inflammatory response with subsequent fibrosis and trapping.
- Laser fragments tattoo pigment and facilitates phagocytosis.

Red and black are easiest to remove, green and purple more difficult and yellow/orange tattoos tend to respond most poorly. Amateur tattoos are generally easier to remove – less ink and more black pigment, but at less consistent levels therefore not as predictable.

Hypopigmentation (10%) and scarring are potential complications.

- Blue/green – Q-switched ruby laser (red light, 694 nm but high risk of complications) or alexandrite (755 nm).
- Red – QS frequency doubled Nd:YAG (532 nm).
- Black – Nd:YAG (1064 nm), all lasers are effective for black pigment.

Tattoos may undergo colour shifts following laser treatment (Peach AH. *Br J Plast Surg* 1999;**52**:482–487) e.g. conversion of ferric oxide (Fe_2O_3) to ferrous oxide (FeO) in red pigments may darken tattoo; thus it is usually wise to try a test area first.

Laser treatment of tattoos
Bernstein EF. *Clin Dermatol* 2006;**24**:43–55.

In this paper, the author reviewed the use of lasers for tattoo removal and also commented on the pitfalls:

- Using the wrong device – only QS lasers should be used.
- Using too high an energy resulting in complications – often trying to remove residual pigment that is probably deeper in the skin. A better strategy would be to switch to another laser or accept partial removal.
- Failing to consider endogenous melanin – darker-skinned patients are prone to dyspigmentation after laser treatment.
- Allergic reactions to pigment – most often red – these areas are usually nodular and scaly to begin with; check with the patient for skin reactions when the tattoo was first applied.
- Tattoo darkening.

Laser hair removal

The target cells are the pluripotential cells responsible for hair growth in the bulge/bulb region, that are 4 mm or so below the skin surface; they are destroyed indirectly by heat conducted from the melanin in the follicle. Anagen follicles are most sensitive to laser energy, thus repeated treatments are needed to catch hairs in this state.

There are many laser systems available, and most current options focus on long-pulsed lasers.

- Ruby (694 nm): success of 50% reduction at best, less commonly used.
- Alexandrite (755 nm): only safe for lighter-skinned patients.

- Diode (810 nm), Nd:YAG (1064 nm) and IPL are more commonly used at present.

Although there can be good results in well-selected patients e.g. dark hair (easier to remove than light hair) in lighter skins, individual responses cannot be predicted/guaranteed. Painless treatment (without any anaesthesia, including topical) is not likely to be effective.

- Individual follicles targeted therefore must not use other forms of hair removal e.g. plucking or waxing (shaving is alright) for 6 weeks pretreatment.

Laser scar treatment

Just as not all lasers are the same, not all scars are the same.

- Ablative lasers may be suited for acne scarring.
- PDL lasers may treat hypertrophic scars with some success.

Fractional lasers

Fractional lasers are a relatively new development in lasers. An array of tiny areas of laser energy delivery produce microthermal zones (MTZ). Leaving intact tissue in between the minute cores of coagulative necrosis results in faster, better healing.

Efficacy and safety of a carbon-dioxide ablative fractional resurfacing device for treatment of atrophic acne scars in Asians
Manuskiatti W. *J Am Acad Dermatol* 2010;**63**:274–283.

In this study, 13 patients with skin phototype IV and atrophic acne scars were treated with three sessions. After 6 months, 85% of patients rated at least 25–50% improvement of their scars, whilst objective measures of scar volume and surface smoothness also improved. There was temporary hyperpigmenation in 92%.

Fractional nonablative 1540 nm laser resurfacing of atrophic acne scars. A randomized controlled trial with blind response evaluation
Hedelund L. *Lasers Med Sci* Published online 17 June 2010. DOI 10.1007/s10103–010–0801–1

This study used a fractional erbium YAG laser which produces minute zones of thermal damage, making it strictly ablative, but due to the low level of epidermal disruption it is classified as non-ablative fractional resurfacing.

They treated 10 patients with acne scarring; improvements in scars were noted on blinded clinical evaluations. Half of the patients noted moderate improvement in their scars.

Pulsed-dye laser treatment of hypertrophic burn scars
Alster TS. *Plast Reconstr Surg* 1998;**102**:2190–2195.

In this study, 40 hypertrophic scars (half due to burns and half following CO_2 laser resurfacing) were treated with 585 nm PDL and had symptomatic improvement after only one treatment. After 2.5 treatments, there was decreased redness, and scars were softer and more pliable.

- Kono T. (*Ann Plast Surg* 2005;**54**:487–493) noted similar improvement in hypertrophic scars in Japanese patients (22 scars in 15 patients) treated with 585 nm PDL with cryogen cooling, with 40.7% and 65.3% improvement in scar height and redness respectively.
- Parrett BM. (*Burns* 2010;**36**:443–449) discussed the use of PDL in post-burn hypertrophic scarring (See Burns).

Laser treatment of pigmented lesions

For laser treatment to be successful there must be pigment/melanocytes within range of the laser.

- **Dermatoses** e.g. naevus of Ota, naevus of Ito, blue naevus can be treated with Q-switched ruby laser or Q-switched Nd:YAG.
- **Naevi**: Two-thirds of benign naevi respond to laser but dysplastic naevi should not be treated by laser. Congenital naevi may be treated by laser but the malignant potential still exists and complete clearance is very unlikely.

Some lesions are known to respond well to laser, e.g. café au lait. Response in others can be first observed in a test patch.

Predicting the outcome of laser treatment for pigmented lesions
Grover R. *Br J Plast Surg* 1998;**51**:51–56.

This study used 2 mm punch biopsy and immunohistochemistry in 32 patients to predict outcome following laser treatment. They found that unfavourable indicators were depth of melanocytes > 0.3 mm and significant amelanocytosis (> 20%) – amelanotic melanocytes are refractory to treatment but following treatment may form melanin and be a cause of hyperpigmentation.

Congenital naevi and lasers

- Incidence of naevi > 10 cm diameter ~1/20 000 with lifetime malignant potential ~4%.
- The larger the naevus the more likely that deeper structures will be involved.
- Complete eradication of risk may require disfiguring surgery.
- There are no reports of melanoma at sites of successfully curetted naevi but curettage is not always successful and may be difficult in the perineum, etc. It also leads to blood loss and scarring.

Successful treatment of a giant congenital naevus with the high energy pulsed carbon dioxide laser
Kay AR. *Br J Plast Surg* 1998;**51**:22–24.

Pulsed CO_2 laser was used to treat a giant congenital hairy naevus in a 44-day-old infant who had been unsuccessfully treated by curettage. This laser relies upon vaporization of superficial cells rather than selective photothermolysis directed at melanin.

Laser treatment caused immediate reduction in superficial pigmentation with 4–6 passes with the pattern generator head and residual pigmentation was treated by a single pass using a 3 mm collimated hand piece. Post-operative colloid resuscitation was given as plasma loss was observed during treatment. Near-full healing was achieved by 2 weeks.

The authors' conclusions were:

- Laser ablation is a good alternative to curettage.
- The size of the area that can be treated may be limited by plasma loss.
- Close follow-up is mandatory.

Arons MS (*Br J Plast Reconstr* 1998;**51**:570–571) responded to the article above to highlight the point that it was premature to say that the lesion had been 'successfully' treated after only 4-month follow-up.

Combined use of normal and Q switched ruby laser in the management of congenital melanocytic naevi
Kono T. *Br J Plast Surg* 2001;**54**:640–643.

Normal mode ruby light (NMRL) was used first to remove the epidermis and facilitate greater penetration of the high energy of the Q switched ruby laser (QSRL) that effectively destroys naevus nests. QSRL was used in short pulse duration to reduce thermal injury to neighbouring dermis.

A similar strategy was used in giant congenital melanocytic naevi by Michel JL (*Eur J Dermatol*

2003;**13**:57–64). Kishi K (*Br J Dermatol* 2009;**161**:345–352) used **early QSRL** alone, and it took an average 9.6 treatments to reduce the colour of lesions in their nine patients to within 0–20% of baseline.

III. Facial resurfacing

Causes of facial ageing

It is conventional to divide up ageing into chronological and actinic ageing but there is overlap and the relative contributions can be difficult to define.

- Chronological ageing – histologically there is thinning of dermis, reduced elastic fibres, blood vessels, fibroblasts and mast cells. Gravitational forces cause soft tissue descent and deep furrows whilst the contractile forces of the underlying muscles cause wrinkles.
- Actinic damage – characterized by fine rhytids, skin laxity and dyschromia; elastin accumulates in abnormal arrangements whilst collagen content is both reduced and more disorganized.

Choosing between surgery (vide infra) and non-surgical methods of facial rejuvenation (this section) or others such as tissue fillers, botulinum toxin and radiofrequency, comes after discussion; the patient decides on the most unsatisfactory parts of their face and to accept realistic goals including:

- Non-operative methods are generally not as effective as nor have the longevity of surgery.
- Resurfacing will be especially useful for actinic damage and aims to initiate dermal collagen reorganization and new collagen synthesis, but has a significant downtime that increases with deeper resurfacing.

Laser resurfacing

Fitzpatrick skin types

The Fitzpatrick classification categorizes patients according to their skin response to ultraviolet light; the skin type also impacts on their response to laser treatment and scarring after surgery.

General points

Lasers can be non-ablative or ablative – with the common examples being CO_2 or Er:YAG.

Facial resurfacing with the CO_2 laser is an alternative to dermabrasion or chemical peel (comparable peels being 35% trichloroacetic acid or 50% Baker–

Table 10.1 Fitzpatrick skin types and their characteristics.

Skin type	Skin colour	UV sensitivity	Sunburn history
I	White	Very	Always burns, never tans
II	White	Very	Usually burns, sometimes tans
III	White	Sensitive	Burns sometimes, tans gradually
IV	Light brown	Moderately	Burns minimally, tans well
V	Brown	Minimally	Never burns, tans easily to dark brown
VI	Black	Insensitive	Never burns, deeply tans

Gordon phenol), being more controllable and predictable than chemical peels in particular. Deep phenol peels will remove deep wrinkles but result in permanent lightening of the skin.

Pulsed and scanning CO_2 lasers (10 600 nm) introduced in the 1990s with shorter pulse duration than traditional continuous wave lasers allowed much better results than before.

- Typical energies used in the 300–500 mJ range will remove fine wrinkles but are not suitable for the treatment of loose facial skin and deep nasolabial folds.
- Short pulse duration < 1 ms minimizes conduction of heat to neighbouring dermis cells to reduce dermal scarring.

The light energy targets water as the 'chromophore'. It vaporizes the entire epidermis with the first pass and the whitish eschar needs to be removed with a damp swab otherwise it will act as a heat sink, increasing thermal damage. Dermal collagen shrinkage begins with subsequent passes: eyelid skin needs only 2 passes whilst the rest of the face needs 3–4 passes. The yellow reticular dermis is the usual clinical point.

- Phenomenon of collagen shrinkage (by 10–30%) at 55–60 °C, relative shrinkage decreases with successive passes.
- There may also be some collagen remodelling and laying down of new shorter collagen over several months post-treatment that continues to contribute to the skin tightness. The aim is for the damaged disorganized collagen of the papillary dermis to be replaced by normal compact collagen.
- Re-epithelialization from the adnexal structures occurs in 7–10 days and there is **erythema** that lasts for several months. The most common adverse reaction is **hypopigmentation** particularly in the fair skinned.

Erbium: YAG lasers

The pulsed erbium:YAG laser was introduced in 1996 with infrared wavelength 2940 nm. It is closer to the peak absorption for water than the CO_2 laser and thus is absorbed 12–18 × more efficiently and with less thermal diffusion, hence it is more precise with less collateral tissue damage. The penetration depth of 2–5 μm is less than the 20–30 μm for the CO_2 laser meaning a faster recovery/shorter downtime and fewer side-effects (erythema lasts for 2–4 weeks only, hypopigmentation and transient hyperpigmentation).

- However, as it is less coagulative, there will more intra-operative bleeding – the clinical endpoint is punctate bleeding.
- Less collagen shrinkage and less stimulation of remodelling means less pronounced and shorter-lasting effects.

Thus it is usually reserved for **milder** photodamage, rhytids and dyspigmentation (Alster TS. *Plast Reconstr Surg* 1998;**103**:619–632).

Contraindications to laser therapy

Patients should be encouraged strongly to give up smoking.

- Absolute.
  - **Isotretinoin** (used in the treatment of acne) within the last 2 years.
  - Infection (bacterial, HSV).
- Relative.
  - Collagen, vascular or immune disorder.
  - Keloid tendency.
  - Perpetual UV light exposure.

Skin preconditioning

Topical vitamin A (retinoic acid) with glycolic acid preconditioning regimens are often used before laser resurfacing or chemical peels to increase the effectiveness of these therapies. These agents increase the metabolism of the skin, accelerate cellular division, boost collagen synthesis and reduce the thickness of the stratum corneum.

Retinoic acid

Different formulations/products are available.

- Tretinoin 0.05% (Retinova) topical cream for photodamaged skin and mottled pigmentation; excellent treatment for solar-induced lentigines on the dorsum of the hands.
- Tretinoin 0.025% (Retin-A) topical cream for acne treatment.
- Isotretinoin capsules 5 mg (Roaccutane) used for acne treatment; isomer of tretinoin.

Topical tretinoin increases papillary dermal collagen, **glycosaminoglycan** (GAG) synthesis and angiogenesis and exfoliates the stratum corneum. It thus makes the skin more sensitive to peels, for example. Pretreatment with **topical retinoids** may help to reduce post-treatment hyperpigmentation but may contribute to post-operative erythema. It has a rejuvenating effect, partially due to generating dermal oedema, but overall it is **not proven** as a worthwhile pretreatment and is also contraindicated during early pregnancy due to its teratogenicity.

Note that **isotretinoin** is **not** used as a pretreatment. It will cause delayed healing and atypical scarring, and if it is being used it should probably be stopped at least 6 months (many insist on a much longer interval) before laser therapy as it inhibits re-epithelialization from adnexal structures.

Hydroquinolone is a tyrosine inhibitor i.e. it reduces melanin production. It does not alter/lighten pre-existing pigment but can reduce post-treatment/inflammatory hyperpigmentation.

Simultaneous face lifting and skin resurfacing
Fulton JE. *Plast Reconstr Surg* 1998;**102**:2480–2489.

The authors described their results with resurfacing (CO$_2$ laser or superficial TCA peel 20–30%) followed by liposuction and SMAS facelift. Ancillary procedures (brow lift, blepharoplasty, platysmal band surgery, etc.) were also performed under the same anaesthetic.

- They suggest that tumescent low pressure liposuction before raising the skin flaps reduces bleeding and defines the appropriate plane more clearly.
- Preconditioning with glycolic acid and vitamin A is recommended.

'Dramatic' results were reported by the authors with convalescence and complications similar to facelift alone. However, phenol peels should not be combined with facelifts as the risk of flap necrosis would be increased.

- Weinstein C (*Plast Reconstr Surg* 2001;**107**:586–592) combined treatment using the erbium:YAG laser and a range of facelift techniques (most were subcutaneous lifts with SMAS repositioning). Laser fluence was reduced over lateral cheek areas in this group.

A quantitative method for the assessment of facial rejuvenation: a prospective study investigating the carbon dioxide laser
Grover R. *Br J Plast Surg* 1998;**51**:8–13.

This study used pre-operative silicone casts to measure the depth of wrinkles (rhytids) by electron or light microscopy. Patients were treated with Silktouch CO$_2$ laser (200 µm spot scanned > 3 mm diameter area for 0.2 s and power 7–14 W) – **yellow discoloration** indicated penetration into the reticular dermis and was used as the endpoint. Post-operative regime included antibiotics and suncare.

The post-operative moulds demonstrated > 91% reduction in wrinkle depth at 6 weeks. Erythema lasted for ~2 months.

Long-term assessment of CO$_2$ facial laser resurfacing: aesthetic results and complications
Schwartz RJ. *Plast Reconstr Surg* 1999;**103**:592–601.

There was some recurrence at 1 year – predominantly in dynamic areas e.g. periorbital (56% improvement) and circumoral (59%) compared with forehead (61%) and cheeks (77%).

Histological changes in the skin following CO$_2$ laser resurfacing
Stuzin JM. *Plast Reconstr Surg* 1997;**99**:2036–2050.
Collawn SS. *Plast Reconstr Surg* 1998;**102**:509–515.

- **Pretreatment skin**: actinic damage with epidermal atrophy, dermal elastosis (thickened, curled elastin fibres) and increased number and size of melanocytes in the basal layer of the epidermis with uneven distribution of melanin.
- **After one pass**: the epidermis is totally removed. There is elastin degradation and fibroblast necrosis in the remaining papillary and reticular dermis. However, there is little compaction of collagen.
- **After second and third passes**: there is sequential and graded compaction of collagen (it loses its

striations and the fibrils widen); there is also loss of extracellular GAG matrix. Visible skin tightening occurs.

- **Post-operative progress:**
  - 7–10 days: re-epithelialization from adnexal structures.
  - 3 months post-treatment:
    - Epidermal atypia corrected, polarity restored.
    - Melanocyte numbers back to normal with **even distribution of melanin**.
    - **Neocollagen formation**, elimination of elastoses and decreased GAG ground substance.
  - 6 months post-treatment:
    - Resolution of inflammatory changes.
    - Fibroblasts are hypertrophic.

Similar histological changes were observed in pigmented and White skin.

Post-treatment regimens

Resurfacing with two passes of the CO_2 laser at 500 mJ results in healing at 7–10 days. There are many different regimes but a typical post-treatment care regime may include:

- Antibiotics (broad spectrum e.g. cephalexin) post-operatively, some suggest fluconazole to prevent fungal infections but this is less commonly used.
- Sunscreens post-operatively – avoiding sunlight for 3 months.
- Topical steroids (1% hydrocortisone twice daily for 6 weeks) to decrease erythema and swelling, mainly used in the USA.
- Acyclovir treatment for all patients pre- and post-operatively until re-epithelialized (or 1 week) as laser resurfacing can provoke herpes infection in individuals with or without a history of herpes (12% and 6%, respectively, **despite prophylaxis**).
  - Some limit the use to those with a history of herpes infection, others suggest it for all.
  - Weinstein C (*Plast Reconstr Surg* 1997;**100**:1855–1866) advocates 24-hour pretreatment prophylaxis as well as post-treatment.

For fair skin types (I–III) the above regime is adequate, but for darker skins (IV–VI) it may be worthwhile adding:

- Hydroquinone 2.5% twice daily.
- Retinoic acid 0.05% twice daily.

Open vs. closed dressings

- Moist wound healing – petroleum jelly, lipid-based ointments or semipermeable dressings, e.g. Omniderm.
- Closed dressings decrease pain and allow faster re-epithelialization but are now less popular as the incidence of infections does increase.
- Open technique allows patient to shower/wash 3–4 × daily for 4 days then apply moisturizer (after dressings for first 24 h).
  - Anti-milia regime: wash face 2–4× daily, glycolic acid 15%, oil-free moisturizer.

The use of topical Bactroban (mupirocin) may reduce infection rates.

Complications of laser resurfacing

- **Pigment changes** – hypo- (3%) or hyper-pigmentation (7%).
  - Hyperpigmentation is more common in darker-skinned individuals (Fitzpatrick types IV–VI) although initially there may also be hypopigmentation in this group.
  - **Pretreatment** bleaching with **hydroquinone** (toxic to melanocytes/inhibits tyrosinase) may reduce hyperpigmentation although not licensed for this use in the UK. It may also be used post-operatively to **treat** hyperpigmentation.
- **Prolonged** erythema > 10 weeks (6%) may occur. It is important to warn patients of this; it will also get redder when they blush.
- Superficial infection (bacterial 7%, viral 2% overall).
- Flare up of herpes simplex.
- Hypertrophic scarring (1%) which in some cases may lead to ectropion.
- Under-correction of rhytids.
- Acne and milia due to greater production of sebum. Acne/milia may be reduced by avoiding the use of paraffin jelly and treating with retinoic acid, glycolic acid and hydroquinone at night (comedolysis). Some authors suggest using oral tetracyclines.

Good to excellent results in 98% of patients; complications are uncommon (skin slough in smokers; temporary ectropion and lower eyelid synechia reported).

Non-ablative laser and other therapies

The advantage of non-ablative therapy is that recovery is much quicker when there is no epidermal vaporization. The beneficial effects come mainly from heating up the dermal layer which induces an inflammatory response, with collagen reorganization and production leading to skin tightening.

Fractional lasers (vide supra)

Tierney EP (*J Drugs Dermatol* 2009;**8**:723–731) described safe and effective use of fractional CO_2 laser for neck resurfacing in 10 patients.

Neodymium:yttrium aluminium garnet (Nd:YAG)

Ng:YAG is a laser with a wavelength of 1064 nm that has rather non-specific absorption including blood vessels, collagen and melanin with rather non-specific tissue heating, but has relatively good tissue penetration up to 5–6 mm with scattering, meaning that the greatest effects are in the dermal layer – collagen reorganization and production. The epidermis is not ablated and overall the effects are less dramatic when compared with ablative laser treatment.

Radiofrequency

This technique aims to remodel the dermis through RF energy and so bring about skin tightening and is often used for the lower face and neck. The energy is applied by a probe onto skin with simultaneous cryogen cooling to reduce pain (which is often the limiting factor). The surface epithelium remains intact whilst the underlying collagen remodels. As expected, it is not as effective as ablative resurfacing and multiple treatments are needed, but the downtime is minimal (24 hours of mild erythema).

Intense pulsed light

Intense pulsed light (IPL) is not laser light but rather light in a broad range – 500–1300 nm with multiple potential effects:

- 550–580 nm water and haemoglobin.
- 550–570 nm superficial pigment.
- 590–755 nm deeper pigment.

Filters can be used to target components more selectively depending on the effect required. IPL can be useful for a variety of problems, particularly:

- Vascularity – telangectasia, rosacea, flushing.
- Pigmentation – lentigo, melasma, freckles (and hair removal).
- Skin texture, particularly reduction of pore size.

Pretreatments are not required; IPL can be combined with hydroquinones and/or topical retinoids. There is usually erythema for 24 hours or so – possibly with some purpura, oedema or scabbing. Repeated treatments are needed with sun avoidance/block in-between.

Contraindications include unrealistic expectations, tanned skin or Fitzpatrick skin type VI (V is a relative contraindication).

Chemical peels and dermabrasion

A chemical peel is a controlled chemical burn that removes the surface layers and stimulates collagen remodelling in the residual dermis, thus treating dyschromia, rhytids and uneven skin. They are classified according to the chemical composition as well as the depth of peel.

- Superficial – alpha-hydroxy acids (AHAs), Jessner's solution, salicylic acid.
- Medium – trichloroacetic acid (TCA).
- Deep – phenol.

The depth of the peel is related to the level of actinic damage (Glogau classification of photoageing) that requires treatment. Those with Fitzpatrick skin types IV–VI are at greatest risk of post-inflammatory hyperpigmentation and this modifies the type of treatment. They are **cheaper than laser resurfacing** with less dermal thinning but more erythema and early swelling.

Glycolic acid peel

Alpha-hydroxy acids (AHAs) include:

- Glycolic acid from sugar cane, lactic acid from soured milk.
- Citric acid from citrus fruits, tartaric acid from grapes and malic acid from apples.

AHAs are found in many cosmetics in very low concentration; their main use are as an exfoliant by reducing keratinocyte adhesion. In low concentrations they may be used as a primer/preconditioner for chemical peel or laser resurfacing, but at concentrations of 30–70% become a chemical peel. They rejuvenate the stratum corneum in a manner similar to vitamin A.

- The depth of penetration is related to concentration and duration of treatment but usually results in a superficial peel.
- After the initial erythema, there are areas of white eschar (epidermolysis) but full frosting as for TCA peel is not desirable as it indicates dermal destruction. End by diluting with water or neutralizing with $NaHCO_3$.
- Post-treatment management includes avoiding sun exposure and the use of emollients – also consider topical antibiotics and acyclovir.

After epithelialization, alpha-hydroxy acids (weak), retinoic acid and hydroquinone may be reinstated along with make-up.

Jessner's solution

Components include Resorcinol, salicylic acid and lactic acid; it acts mainly as a keratinolytic with the depth related to the number of coats applied (7 coats gives an intermediate depth peel). It is neutralized with water when frosting occurs; it is fairly easy to use and can be repeated every 3 months approximately.

Complications of peels in general

- Hypopigmentation proportional to increasing depth of peel – invariable after phenol peel, may be permanent.
- Hyperpigmentation – inflammatory melanocyte response that usually resolves.
- Erythema.
- Viral and bacterial infection.
- Milia for 2–3 weeks after re-epithelialization due to occluded sebaceous glands.
- Scarring.

Rejuvenation of the skin surface: chemical peel and dermabrasion
Branham GH. *Facial Plast Surg* 1996;**12**:125–133.

Trichloroacetic acid peel

Trichloroacetic acid peel (TCA) causes a coagulative necrosis/protein denaturation and the surface layers slough off subsequently. The depth of TCA peel is proportional to the concentration of the TCA but also depends on the anatomical site (skin thickness) and pretreatment.

- ~10–25% produces a superficial peel (epidermis only).
- ~30–40% produces a medium-depth peel (papillary dermis) though this carries a higher risk of scarring. It is indicated for moderately photo-aged skin and field change early actinic damage. However, it is usually better to repeat treatments than overdo the concentration of TCA.

No systemic toxicity has been reported with the use of TCA.

- Pretreatment with Retin-A or glycolic acid/AHA is recommended.
- Use acetone to remove oily secretions (also helps to remove stratum corneum); stretch the skin to flatten wrinkles and apply with cotton gauze in even strokes in cosmetic units and wait for frosting before removal with dry gauze. Repeat.
- The patient should expect some darkening of the skin and peeling (as for sunburn) afterwards.

TCA-based blue peel: a standardized procedure with depth control
Obagi ZE. *Dermatol Surg* 1999;**25**:773–780.

The rationale for this technique was the observation that the variable results associated with chemical peels were due to lack of control over depth of peel. Shallow rhytids that disappear on light stretching respond to a 'skin tightening' (more superficial) peel whereas those that do not disappear require a 'skin levelling' (deeper) peel.

The TCA **blue peel** facilitates treatment of the papillary and immediate reticular dermis (junction of reticular and papillary dermis). An even blue colour confirms the evenness of application whilst it also allows the endpoint of the peel to be easily recognizable. No systemic side-effects or toxicity have been reported.

- The peel is made by adding TCA at fixed concentration (15% or 20%) and volume with the blue peel base that contains glycerin, saponins and a non-ionic blue colour base.
- The depth of the peel is dependent upon concentration and volume of TCA; one coat of a 15% blue peel solution (30% TCA diluted by an equal volume of blue peel base) exfoliates stratum corneum whilst four coats reaches the papillary dermis. Two coats of 20% blue peel solution reaches the papillary dermis but is more uncomfortable compared with the 15% solution and may require sedation.
- Frosting occurs as a result of protein denaturation; pink frost develops as the papillary dermis is reached, becoming white as the peel acts at a deeper

level, i.e. the immediate reticular dermis which is the maximum recommended depth of peel.

- Period of relative resistance – there is a lag (~2 minutes) before the blue peel solution begins to exert its action due to initial acid neutralization by dermal protein. Wait 2 minutes before repainting.
- Post-treatment re-epithelialization is complete by 7–10 days. Two or three blue peels, spaced 6–8 weeks apart, are recommended for maximum effect.

Complications:

- Scarring and pigment changes are possible with increasing depth of peel.
- Erythema lasting 3–7 days.
- Bacterial or viral infections.

Phenol peel

The Baker–Gordon formula was first described in the 1960s and is the most common one in use; an alternative is the Hetter croton oil peel (Hetter GP. *Plast Reconstr Surg* 2000;**105**:227). The chemicals cause protein coagulation and penetrate into the reticular dermis, i.e. a deep peel. This has been used for field change actinic damage including actinic keratoses, superficial BCCs and solar lentigos, as well as moderate rhytids and acne scarring.

- Acne scarring often needs 3–4 treatments spaced 1 year apart. Ice-pick scars are best excised individually followed by CO_2 laser resurfacing.

The use of phenol peels is contraindicated in patients with a history of **cardiac disease**; patients should be monitored for **cardiotoxicity** especially those undergoing full-face peels. 80% is excreted unchanged in the kidney and thus it is also contraindicated in **renal disease**; patients should be well hydrated before undergoing the peel.

- Ideal patients are skin types I–III as darker skins will be **bleached** and erythema may persist for some months.
- It is more painful than TCA therefore anaesthesia/ analgesia/sedation is needed.
- Apply slowly in cosmetic units after acetone – wait 15 min between cosmetic units to allow for renal excretion. Avoid contact with the eyes.
- Some advocate creating a mask with overlying tape (occlusive technique) that is left on for 24 hours. This increases depth of peel but the removal of the

mask is painful. Pretreatment will also increase the depth of the peel.

Dermabrasion

This is the gradual removal of layers of skin using a diamond burr on a drill, scratch pad or sandpaper i.e. a mechanical peel. The indications are similar to chemical peel and ablative lasers, working well for fine rhytids and providing minor skin tightening, but it is also useful for focal problems such as uneven superficial scars. It is a useful adjunctive treatment of rhinophyma.

The depth of resurfacing is controlled by the coarseness of the abrasive, pressure on the skin and the speed and length of treatment – the usual clinical endpoint is bleeding from the superficial papillary dermis. Some use gentian violet to paint the area and guide treatment for spot/regional dermabrasion; a refrigerant topical anaesthetic is often used (Gold MH. *Am J Clin Dermatol* 2003;**4**:467–471).

- Re-epithelialization 7–10 days.
- Erythema 1–2 weeks with pinkness and some swelling for up to 3 months.
- Collagen remodelling takes up to half a year.

Results thus tend to be quite operator dependent. The side-effects and complications are similar to laser resurfacing – over-dermabrasion will lead to hypertrophic scarring, thus it is important not to extend through the reticular dermis. Scarring will also be worse in patients who have taken Roaccutane (isotretinoin) within 2 months.

- **Microdermabrasion** uses mild suction to pull the skin into the hand piece which removes dirt, dead skin, surface debris and oil by passing a jet of particles (aluminium or zinc oxide) towards the skin causing mild mechanical abrasion or exfoliation of the stratum corneum (other machines use a roughened surface e.g. 'diamond' microdermabrasion). The depth of treatment can be controlled by the flow rate of these particles and the strength of suction. Repeated treatments are needed. It has been reported to exacerbate rosacea and telangectasia and so should be avoided in these conditions, as well as any areas of active infection including herpes, impetigo and warts.

The effect of chemosurgical peels and dermabrasion on dermal elastic tissue
Giese SY. *Plast Reconstr Surg* 1997;**100**:499–500.

Elastin production does not decrease significantly until after age 70 years but elastosis (altered elastin) occurs in photodamaged skin. Whilst the effect of chemical peels and dermabrasion on collagen (homogenization) and melanin granules (depletion) is well defined, the effect on elastin is not.

- This study showed that a single application of 25–50% TCA peel and dermabrasion in pigs did not result in any change in dermal elastin at 6 months.
- A single application of Baker's phenol peel decreased the amount of elastin and there were morphological changes (thinner, immature elastin resulting in a stiffer, weaker skin).

In the discussion, the authors suggest that the effect on the elastin may simply be due to a deeper peel rather than a specific reaction to individual chemicals.

IV. Tissue fillers and botulinum toxin

Tissue fillers

There are many choices for volume replacement of the soft tissues; the 'ideal filler' does not exist. Important considerations include safety and ease of use with predictable results that are potentially reversible if needed.

Autologous

- Autologous fat enhances subcutaneous volume and is not a dermal filler. The survival of the injected fat is somewhat dependent on the technique of harvesting, preparation and injection (small aliquots to increase revascularization) – the Coleman technique is one of the most frequently used. In general, most surgeons quote a 50% survival rate but it does depend on the area in which it is injected – it survives better in static areas and thus has been combined with the use of botulinum toxin.
  - Adipose derived stem cells (ADSC) and platelet rich plasma (PRP) are new strategies that are being reported increasingly frequently, in order to improve fat survival/results of fat grafting.
- Isolagen – is made of cultured autologous fibroblasts prepared from a 3 mm punch biopsy. It takes about half a year for the effects to become apparent and lasts for about a year and a half.
- Autologen – is collagen prepared from a biopsy of the patient's own skin (a larger area is needed than

for Isolagen) and takes about 2 months to be produced.

Non-autologous

Biological

- **Bovine collagen.**
  - Zyderm I and II (double concentration) – for superficial injection to correct fine wrinkles.
  - Zyplast (glutaraldehyde cross linkage for more resistance to degradation and less immunogenicity) – for deeper dermal injections with aim of contour correction e.g. nasolabial folds.
  - There is a 3.5% allergy/sensitivity rate, and two separate **skin tests** are suggested before injecting but even then, there is a significant sensitivity rate of about 1%. The effects last for about 6–9 months.
- **Human collagen.**
  - Cosmoderm I and II – human-derived culture from human dermal fibroblasts for fine lines, whilst Cosmoplast is intended for deeper dermal injections. No skin testing is required.
- **Hyaluronic acid** has been very popular and has largely replaced collagen as the commonest tissue filler. It is a normal component of connective tissue (ground substance) and no skin testing is required. It is very hydrophilic and tends to expand slightly due to water absorption after injection.
  - Hylaform from rooster combs.
  - Restylane from bacterial fermentation (NASHA – non-animal source hyaluronic acid).
  - It is injected at the desired location and can be massaged somewhat to spread the material and prevent lumpiness.

Synthetic

- **Calcium hydroxyapatite** (Radiesse) intended for deep dermal injection and regarded as semi-permanent filler. Lumps occur in about 10%.
- **Poly-L-lactic acid** (PLLA, Sculptra) – the material degrades and is replaced with collagen – it is important not to over-correct. It was approved for correction of facial lipoatrophy in HIV patients but more recently (July 2009) has also been approved for aesthetic indications. It does need to be reconstituted at least 2 hours beforehand (preferably 24 hours or even up to a week) and can be injected deeper (deep dermal, subcutaneous or

periosteal). It is regarded as semi-permanent and usually lasts about 2 years. There are some cases of granuloma formation after injection.

- **Polymethylmethacrylate** (PMMA) ArteFill/ ArteColl is composed of collagen-covered PMMA beads and is regarded as a permanent filler for deeper lines (subdermal injection).

Fat injection

The injection of the patient's own fat is theoretically ideal; it is totally biocompatible with potential for full integration. It remains soft and changes in proportion to patient's weight gain and loss. However, early results were poor and the technique was criticized and largely abandoned (and with advent of other fillers) until better results were demonstrated with changes in technique.

Fat cells are very fragile and each step of the process (harvest, preparation, injection etc.) can potentially increase damage, thus the results are very technique-dependent, with the lower eyelid being one of the most challenging places to treat. It is more successful in younger than older patients. On average, a 50% survival rate is quoted. **The optimal technique is unknown** – there is no consensus but many favour the Coleman technique.

- Scientific proof is lacking but generally favours **blunt** cannula techniques, centrifugation without washing or growth factors and immediate injection of small amounts by multiple passes. The choice of donor does not seem to matter but this is debated.
- Storage: some studies show decreasing yield in stem cells with room temperature and cryopreservation (−80 °C fridge), and more than 24 hours of 4 °C; other studies suggest cryopreservation may be viable. Many keep leftover fat in the fridge for a week until the first follow-up appointment, injecting more if needed, though the viability at this point is largely unknown.
- Complications include damage to structures, intravascular embolization, contamination causing infection etc. Lumpiness can be treated by puncture and massage. Migration of injected fat is unusual unless injecting excessive amounts and if used in very mobile areas. The results of fat injection stabilize after 4–5 months, but the proportion that remains can be quite variable. Thaunat O. (*Plast Reconstr Surg* 2004;**113**:2235–

2236) described a case of cerebral fat embolism after facial fat injection.

Technical points

- **Harvest:** 3–4 mm incisions are made with no. 11 blade and a blunt needle is used to infiltrate adrenaline 1/400 000 (with or without lidocaine e.g. 0.08% depending on use of general anaesthesia), minimal infiltration, approximately 1:1 i.e. not superwet/tumescent – some use Ringer's lactate instead of saline due to the pH differences. The fat is harvested with low suction by hand with a blunt needle, three-way tap and 10 ml syringe, avoiding suction plungers.
- **Processing:** centrifuge at 3000 rpm for 3 minutes (some use lower speeds e.g. 600–1000 rpm) to separate out the layers and then remove blood, fat and water layers and transfer to 1 ml syringes. Some leave the fat to stand and separate by gravity, others pass it through gauze and some promote commercial lipodialysis kits.
- **Placement:** 20G on 1 ml syringe for greatest precision. Inject in at least 2 directions per area and use blunt rather than sharp needles to allow movement in more natural tissue planes, and preferably with side holes injecting on withdrawal in **very small aliquots** (< 0.1 ml). The aim is to deposit fat in such a way as to have maximal contact surface area (and thus nutrition) for better graft survival and fewer irregularities but this requires time and patience. The degree of over-correction suggested is variable but of the order of 10–20%.
- **Post-operative:** some swelling is to be expected with significant tissue oedema that lasts 3–4 days typically but possibly longer in others. Cover wounds with Tegaderm and advise light massage for 'lymph flow'. Firmer massage is counterproductive – indeed some advocate immobilizing the area with dressings for up to a week.

Botulinum toxin

Botulinum toxin is the exotoxin of the spore-forming anaerobe *Clostridium botulinum* which has a similar structure to tetanus toxin. Seven serotypes have been isolated (A–G) of which 'A' is the most potent and commonly used sub-type. It is a potentially lethal toxin with a lethal dose of about 3000 Units (U) for a 70 kg male (extrapolated from LD_{50} in rats).

Mechanism of action

- The toxin binds to presynaptic cholinergic receptors and then becomes internalized, entering lysosomes by endocytosis.
- The toxin undergoes cleavage to release a light chain component into the cytoplasm which catalyses proteolytic cleavage of membrane proteins responsible for exocytosis of acetylcholine.
- The result is presynaptic inhibition of acetylcholine release.

Clinical effects

- Denervation of striated muscle (useful for certain neurological disorders).
- Anhidrosis (useful for hyperhidrosis and Frey's syndrome).
- Onset of dose-dependent activity after 1–7 days, peak 7–14 days and lasting for several months, until the sprouting of motor axons and formation of new motor-end plates.
  - Reassess patients after 2 weeks and touch up if necessary.
- Formation of neutralizing antibodies may gradually reduce efficacy.

Type A is manufactured as Botox° (Allergan, 100 U per vial) or Dysport° (Ipsen, 500 U per vial).

- Manufactured in a small volume of human albumin solution.
- Store as per manufacturer's instructions and reconstitute with normal saline – keep refrigerated and use within around 4 hours of reconstitution according to manufacturer though many report efficacy when stored in the fridge for several weeks.
- Licensed for use in spasmodic torticolis, blepharospasm and hemifacial spasm.
  - FDA approval for glabellar frown lines (all other aesthetic uses are off-label) and hyperhidrosis.
- Avoid in pregnancy/lactation and patients with myaesthenia gravis, areas of active infection, those with known allergy to human albumin solution or taking aminoglycoside antibiotics (may potentiate clinical effect).

Side-effects

- Pain, swelling, bruising and redness at injection sites.

- Unwanted muscle weakening.
  - Intrinsic muscles of the hand (palmar hyperhidrosis).
  - Extraocular musculature (causing diplopia and ptosis) and dry eyes when treating periorbital rhytids (from Greek *rhytis* for 'wrinkle'). Adrenergic eye drops e.g. apraclonidine 0.5%, can be used for unintended ptosis.
- Anaphylaxis has not yet been reported following cosmetic injection in humans (two cases of severe reaction after injection for muscle spasticity).
- The maximum recommended dose in a 70 kg adult is 400 U of Botox; commonly used cosmetic doses are around 25 U Botox or 125 U Dysport per patient – the greater the target muscle mass the higher the dose requirement.

Areas commonly treated in cosmetic practice

- Glabellar lines: procerus and corrugator supercilii.
  - Injection into the glabellar and medial supraorbital areas, 20 U in females/30 U in males per injection site up to 6 in total.
- Forehead creases: frontalis.
  - 10 U females/20 U males in a horizontal line across the middle of the forehead.
- Periorbital rhytids (crow's feet): orbicularis oculi.
  - Inject 10–20 U into the lateral orbicularis oculi (2–5 points per side). Use the lower lid snap test to assess those at high risk of ectropion, in which case lower injections should be avoided.
- Less commonly used to treat perioral rhytids and platysma bands.
  - Targeting the orbicularis oris reduces vertical wrinkles of the upper lip; relaxing the muscle also results in fuller lips. Inject 4–10 U per site (up to 7) symmetrically around the lips within 5 mm of the vermilion border and avoiding the commissures to prevent drooping. Beware of the effects on singers and musicians.

Technique

- Avoid skin alcohol preparation (which is supposed to inactivate toxin).
- Use small-gauge needle and inject into muscle directly using anatomical knowledge of insertion points, demonstration by voluntary contraction and manual palpation.
  - Orientate injection away from the orbit to avoid inadvertent paralysis of extraocular muscles.

V. Lifts

Facelifts

Clinical changes with age

The skin is thinner, more fragile and less elastic.

- Brow and eyelid ptosis.
- Wrinkles (crow's foot, circumoral).
- Jowls.
- Submental skin excess.

Histological skin changes with ageing

- Changes in the collagen composition of the dermis – loss of type III collagen.
- Loss of elastin – elastin production ceases > 70 years.
- Reduction in glycosaminoglycans (GAGs) component of matrix (ground substance).
- Flattening of the dermo-epidermal junction.
- Depletion of Langerhans cells and melanocytes (will lead to immunological changes).

There are also volume changes in the soft tissue and skeletal framework. In simple terms, facelifts address the gravitational effects on the face and are **not** a treatment for fine wrinkling; deep wrinkles may be improved but not eliminated. There is redistribution but not removal of fat (e.g. removal of the buccal fat pad makes the patient look older). It 'sets the clock back but does not stop it ticking'.

Skin creases on the face may arise due to:

- Animation – found perpendicular to direction of muscle pull.
- Loss of skin elasticity – fine and shallow.
- Solar elastosis, epidermal atrophy, soft tissue descent – coarse and deep.

Resurfacing options (chemical peel or laser) are more suited to patients with finer rhytids and solar-damaged skin. Photoageing is different from ageing:

- Thickened elastic fibres in dermis.
- Increased ground substance.
- Decreased collagen but increased proportion of type III.

The best results will most likely involve a combination of approaches including lifts, resurfacing and/or volume restoration, depending on the identifiable problems.

Assessment of the ageing face

Pre-operative photographs are essential. Relevant history includes patient's complaints and expectations; medical history should include smoking, diabetes, hypertension, drugs affecting coagulation and wound healing including herbal remedies. Examination should follow the zones from up to down.

- General.
  - Skin quality, thickness, elasticity and laxity.
  - Asymmetry, distribution of excess tissue, distribution of wrinkles.
  - Facial movement and sensation.
- Forehead.
  - Level of hairline and quality of hair.
  - Ptosis and wrinkles.
  - Glabellar lines and contraction of corrugator supercilii and procerus muscles.
- Mid-face.
  - Circumoral wrinkles.
  - Nasolabial folds, Marionette lines.
  - Ptosis of the malar fat pad and jowls.
- Jaw.
  - Submental fat deposits, 'witch's chin'.
  - Platysma bands, divarication.

Patients in whom lifts are to be avoided are:

- Increased bleeding risk with hypertensives and those on aspirin, steroids, warfarin etc.
- Smokers.
- Poor skin quality/keratoses.
- Thick, glabrous skin with deep creases.
- Collagen/connective tissue diseases.

Ultimately those with unrealistic expectations, particularly those who have had previous facial surgery, should be counselled against having surgery.

Anatomy

The blood supply comes almost completely from the external carotid artery (small contribution from ophthalmic artery).

- Anteriorly, there are musculocutaneous perforators from the facial artery (and labial branches), supratrochlear and supraorbital arteries.
- Laterally, there are fasciocutaneous perforators from the transverse facial, zygomatico-orbital, anterior auricular and submental arteries. These

are divided in a typical facelift operation, thus the face becomes dependent on the first group.

- Forehead and scalp – superficial temporal, posterior auricular and occipital.

Sensation to the mid and lower face is supplied mostly by the maxillary and mandibular divisions of the trigeminal nerve.

- The great auricular nerve (C2, 3) is the most commonly injured nerve during facelifts and may result in earlobe numbness.
- The auriculotemporal nerve (secretomotor to parotid) may also be at risk.

The temporal branch of the facial nerve is the most commonly injured nerve, usually at the zygomatic arch where it lies deep to the superficial musculo-aponeurotic system (SMAS) and immediately superficial to the superficial layer of the deep temporal fascia.

According to classic descriptions, there are five layers to the face (these are condensed over the zygomatic arch):

- Skin.
- Subcutaneous fat.
- SMAS – **the superficial musculo-aponeurotic system** layer in the face is continuous with the temporoparietal fascia in the temple, the platysma in the neck and the galea in the scalp. The SMAS is an extension of the superficial fascia. The muscles are arranged in 4 layers.
  - Depressor anguli oris, zygomatic minor, orbicularis oris.
  - Depressor labii inferioris, risorius, platysma.
  - Zygomaticus major, levator labii superioris alaeque nasi.
  - Mentalis, levator anguli oris, buccinator – the facial nerve is superficial to these (and deep to the three other layers).
- Facial nerve.
  - It innervates the muscles of facial expression on their deep surface, with the main exception being the buccinator that lies **deep** to the buccal branch.
  - 70% of subjects have communicating branches between buccal and zygomatic branches.
  - The marginal mandibular nerve may lie above the inferior border of the mandible at its posterior extent.

- The temporal branch runs beneath a line drawn from the tragus to a point 1.5 cm above the lateral margin of the eyebrow and along with the superficial temporal vessels lies beneath the temporoparietal (superficial temporal) fascia.
- Deep fascial layer (parotid fascia, deep temporal, cervical fascia).

The fascial layers form two layers

- Superficial: galea – temporoparietal fascia – SMAS (below zygomatic arch).
- Deep: pericranium – deep temporal fascia (over temporalis) – splits into two leaves, superficial to the zygoma (innominate fascia) and deep to the zygoma (blends with the parotid fascia).

There is also a system of 'ligaments' or zones of adhesion between the skin and the deeper tissues.

- Osteocutaneous – zygomatic ligament from zygoma to malar fat and dermis, orbitomalar ligament in the upper face.
- Musculocutaneous – parotid ligament, masseteric ligament.

Fat pads

- Malar – superficial to SMAS layer and prone to descent that contributes to deepening of nasolabial fold.
- Buccal – composed of a larger central mass (like an egg yolk in size and colour) with temporal, pterygoid and buccal extensions. It contributes to the cheek contour.

Forehead anatomy

The frontalis muscle elevates the eyebrows causing transverse skin creases and thus opposes actions of corrugator supercilii, procerus and orbicularis oculi. It is supplied by the temporal or 'frontal' branches of the facial nerve (usually 2–5) that enter the muscle on its deep surface after passing deep to SMAS over the zygomatic arch.

- Corrugator arises from the supra-orbital rim and inserts into the medial eyebrow, pulling it downwards and inwards to create a scowling appearance and resulting in **vertical** creases.
- Procerus arises from the nasal bones and inserts into skin in the glabellar area to create **transverse** wrinkles across the bridge of the nose.

Sensation to the forehead is by the supratrochlear and supra-orbital nerves (ophthalmic division of V):

- Supratrochlear nerve is superficial to corrugator.
- Supraorbital nerve is deep to corrugator.

Note that 'typical' brow heights are different:

- Males – level with the supra-orbital rim.
- Females – just above the supra-orbital rim.

Facelift techniques
Incisions
- Temple.
  - In front of hairline – for repeat lifts and those with short sideburns.
  - Behind hairline – often used as continuation of open coronal brow lift.
- Preauricular.
- Postauricular.
  - High for moderate skin redundancy.
  - Low for moderate to excessive skin redundancy.
  - Occipital hairline for excessive skin redundancy.

Vectors
- SMAS fixed.
  - Vertical to improve jawline and perioral creases.
  - Diagonally to improve neck and submental crease.
- Skin fixed.
  - Posterior.
  - Vertical.

Levels of lift

Infiltrate with adrenaline for haemostasis (with or without lidocaine if general anaesthesia is used – note that it is preferable that muscle relaxants/paralysis are avoided). Hypotensive anaesthesia is not desirable as there may be more bleeding post-operatively.

The key points for skin fixation are 1 cm above the ear and at the apex of the postauricular incision. Other points are:

- Excision and/or liposuction of 'witch's chin'.
- Midline platysma plication – in patients with an obtuse cervicomental angle platysma transection may be beneficial.
- Suction drains.

Subcutaneous facelifts
Subcutaneous undermining from the incision line:

- From lateral to within 1 cm of the lateral orbital rim, to the nasolabial folds, within 1 cm of the oral commissure.
- Inferiorly to the level of the thyroid cartilage.

Choices:

- Subcutaneous only – skin only; early recurrence is to be expected.
- Subcutaneous facelift with SMAS plication/imbrication (incise SMAS – advance for suturing with overlap).

SMAS lift (Skoog 1974)
SMAS and skin are elevated as a single unit and advanced posteriorly – elevating the SMAS from the underlying structures distinguishes it from techniques that only plicate the SMAS. Features include:

- Rotated 'L'-shaped incision, horizontally along the inferior border of the zygoma then vertically 0.5 cm anterior to the tragus.
- Rolled SMAS for malar augmentation, or the SMAS is plicated/excised.

There are many variants on the SMAS lift and terms such as deep plane, sub-SMAS or deep SMAS have been applied.

- Low SMAS technique – below the zygomatic arch. This addresses the lower face only with no effect on the mid-face or eyes.
- High SMAS technique (popularized by Barton) – above zygomatic arch, therefore addresses mid-face and periorbital area.
- **Composite facelift** (Hamra) which carries platysma, subcutaneous fat and orbicularis oculi to lower lid as a single unit, suspending the malar and periorbital areas. The skin and subcutaneous tissues are not elevated separately. Some suggest that this makes it a **deep plane** lift (skin and SMAS together in one layer) as opposed to the **extended lift** where separate skin and SMAS flaps are raised.
- **Foundation facelift** (Pitman) formerly known also as a **deep-plane lift** is characterized by elevation of composite musculocutaneous flaps of face and upper neck soft tissue that is rotated to a more lateral and superior position. It is particularly effective in treating the nasolabial fold.

- **Lamellar high SMAS lift** – the skin and SMAS are elevated as two separate layers and advanced to different degrees, along different vectors and suspended under different tension. The high incision allows a more vertical lift vector for the SMAS to be attached to the deep temporal fascia whilst the skin is pulled more obliquely.

Mini-lifts

It was realized that larger operations did not necessarily produce better results; many variants of a more conservative technique exist. The modern facelift has become more a facial sculpturing, combining tension-free skin redraping with suturing and judicious liposculpture with volume addition. These techniques have limited access to the neck and thus less change in the neck contour; in addition the limited access to the mid-face means that those with prominent nasolabial folds would benefit more from traditional lifts.

Short scar facelift with lateral SMASectomy
Baker DC. *Aesthet Surg J* 2001;**21**:14–25.

A strip of SMAS overlying the anterior parotid and parallel to the nasolabial fold is excised. The author also described a classification to determine which patients were suited for short scar/minimal incision lifts.

- Type I – ideal candidate: a female in her early to late 40s with ageing primarily in the face; early jowls with or without submental and submandibular fat.
- Type II – good candidate: late 40s to early 50s, with moderate jowls and moderate skin laxity. Patients have microgenia with submental and submandibular fat but do not have medial platysmal bands.
- Type III – fair candidate: late 50s to early 70s with significant jowling, moderate cervical laxity, and definite existence of submental and submandibular fat. Midline platysmal banding on animation.
- Type IV – poor candidate: 60s to 70s with significant jowls and active lax platysmal banding. There is severe cervical skin laxity and deep skin creases below the cricoid. These patients are not suitable for any type of minimal incision procedure and require extensive dissection and re-draping of the platysma, necessitating a larger incision.

The MACS-lift short scar rhytidectomy
Tonnard P. *Aesthet Surg J* 2007;**27**:188–198.

In the minimal access cranial suspension (MACS) short scar facelift, the skin-subcutaneous tissue is dissected from the SMAS-platysma layer which is suspended vertically to the deep temporal fascia through a temporal hairline incision to prevent sideburn elevation. The skin is directed along different vectors. Poor skin quality may require lengthening of the skin incision behind the ear. The simple MACS uses two purse-string sutures to correct the lower face and neck, whilst the extended MACS uses a third suture to suspend the malar fat pad.

- **Temporal supraperiosteal dissection** – an endoscopic method for the upper face and malar fat pad suspension was advocated by Byrd HS (*Plast Reconstr Surg* 1996;**97**:928).

Subperiosteal face lift:a 200 case, 4-year review
Heinrichs HL. *Plast Reconstr Surg* 1998;**102**:843–855.

This technique aims to rejuvenate the upper and mid face by lifting all of the facial soft tissue in relation to the bone whilst avoiding extensive skin undermining; it only addresses the upper two-thirds of the face. It is more suited to the younger patient who accepts or desires a possible change in eye appearance to an 'almond' eye shape; it is also suitable for patients who have previously undergone facelift. A subperiosteal lift by itself is not suitable for those with significant skin redundancy.

- Gingivobuccal sulcus incision or subciliary incision for elevation of periosteum over the maxilla including peri-orbital areas and the anterior arch of the zygoma.
- The posterior arch is approached via a tunnel at the level of the tragus after elevating a small flap of SMAS – this aims to reduce risk of nerve injury.
- Elevation was achieved/maintained by placing two stitches into fat below orbicularis oculi and anchoring these to the deep temporal fascia overlying temporalis. The mid-face periosteum is thus elevated as a single unit without SMAS or skin dissection as a separate unit, though skin or SMAS procedures can be combined.

The authors reviewed 200 cases, all of whom also underwent synchronous endoscopic brow lift and 13% also underwent upper lid blepharoplasty. Complications (5%) included:

- Transient temporal nerve and infraorbital nerve injury.
- Haematoma.

Avoiding unfavourable results

- Unnatural pulled-up appearance – this is due to excessive skin tension and/or poor choice of vector.
- Visible scars (too anterior or too wide) – either due to poor placement or excess tension.
- Ear.
  - Tragus deformity with blunting of the pretragal depression or anterior displacement, due to excessive tension.
  - Pixie ear deformity – the lobule is pulled inferiorly by tension.
- Hair.
  - Hairline distortion/displacement – the temporal hairline should be 3–4 cm from the lateral orbit.
  - Alopecia – incisions in the hairline should be made parallel to the hairline, dissection should be deep to the level of the follicles and avoid tension in the suture line.

Complications of facelifts

- Intra-operative: facial nerve injury, bleeding.
- Early.
  - **Skin necrosis** (1–4%, for sub-SMAS dissection and subcutaneous dissection respectively) with a 12× higher risk in smokers. Most common in the retroauricular area.
  - **Haematoma** – this is probably the commonest complication and commoner in males (8% vs. 4%, possibly related to greater blood supply to the beard and sebaceous glands) and hypertension (Grover R. *Br J Plast Surg* 2001;**54**:481–486). General strategies for preventing haematoma include control of hypertension and pain, use of drains and dressings.
  - Facial nerve: transient temporal branch injury, platysma pseudoparalysis (complete recovery is expected) causes asymmetry of lower lip and grin due to injury to cervical branch, marginal mandibular branch.
  - Sensory disturbance that can last for several months.
    - Infraorbital nerve numbness.
    - Great auricular nerve that lies just posterior to the external jugular vein, injury may lead to earlobe dysaesthesia and neuroma.
  - Infection.
  - Salivary fistula – the duct is at risk with extensive undermining of the SMAS layer.
- Late.
  - Alopecia 1–3%.
  - Scarring.
  - Hyperpigmentation.

Effect of steroids on swelling after facelift

Rapaport DP. *Plast Reconstr Surg* 1995;**96**:1547–1552.
Owsley JQ. *Plast Reconstr Surg* 1996;**98**:1–6.

Both studies were prospectively randomized double-blind studies assessing the impact of steroids on facial swelling after SMAS facelift in a total of 80 patients. Neither demonstrated any advantage related to steroid medication in terms of a reduction in immediate or early post-operative swelling.

Parotid salivary fistula following rhytidectomy

McKinney P. *Plast Recontr Surg* 1996;**98**:795–797.
Wolf K. *Plast Reconstr Surg* 1996;**97**:641–642.

According to the authors, fistulae (or subcutaneous salivary collections or pseudocysts) can be managed by:

- Aspirate and test fluid for amylase to confirm diagnosis and to exclude haematoma – early aspiration may prevent fistulation.
  - Insert a suction drain.
  - Antibiotics.
  - Compressive dressing.
- Fistulous tract may need to be excised.

Haematomas

Haematoma is the commonest complication of facelift surgery. Small haematomas can be aspirated while major haematomas require formal drainage in theatre.

The risk of developing haematomas seems to be increased by:

- High pre-operative systolic blood pressure > 150 mmHg.
- Male sex.
- Anterior platysmaplasty.
- Non-steroidal medication within 2 weeks of surgery, smoking.

Late haematoma(> 5 days post-operative) is usually due to bleeding from the superficial temporal vessels and is often associated with physical exertion.

The prevention of haematoma following rhytidectomy

Grover R. *Br J Plast Surg* 2001;**54**:481–486.

In this review of an initial group of 1078, the incidence of major haematoma was 4.4% and no significant difference was observed with or without use of:

- Tumescent solution (~one-third and those who did not receive tumescent solution had adrenaline infiltrated along incision lines) 200 ml each side.
- Adrenaline with or without bupivacaine/lidocaine.
- Triamcinolone, hyaluronidase in 500 ml Ringer's lactate.
- Fibrin glue sealant.
- Suction drains (four concertina suction drains used typically).

The subsequent group of 232 patients received tumescent solution as above but without adrenaline and compared:

- There was a significant decrease in haematoma formation amongst patients who did **not** receive adrenaline. Eleven major and 6 minor haematomas in the adrenaline group vs. 0 major and 1 minor haematoma in the non-adrenaline group.

Deep vein thrombosis and pulmonary embolus after facelift
Reinisch JF. *Plast Reconstr Surg* 2001;**107**:1570–1575.

Thromboembolic complications (deep vein thrombosis (DVT)/pulmonary embolism (PE)) were responsible for 5% of operative deaths in hospital. **Abdominoplasty** is probably the most high-risk aesthetic procedure for thromboembolic complications (Grazer FM. *Plast Reconstr Surg* 1977;**59**:513–317).

- DVT 1.2%.
- PE 0.8%.

This was a survey of 273 US plastic surgeons undertaking aesthetic facial surgery; together reporting a total of 9937 facelifts during the 12-month study period. DVT/PE reported by 31 surgeons i.e. 0.35% and 0.14% respectively; one patient died. That is much lower than for abdominoplasty and a plastic surgeon could expect a thromboembolic complication once in every 200 facelift cases.

- General anaesthesia significantly increases risks compared with local anaesthesia.
- **Operative time** longer in patients developing DVT/PE (5.11 hours compared with 4.75 hours).

The surgeons were also surveyed for their thromboembolic prophylaxis protocols:

- 61% of surgeons had no protocols.
- 20% used pressure stockings.
- 20% used intermittent compression devices.
  - **Only these devices** have been shown to significantly decrease the risk of thomboembolic complications. They are supposed to prevent venous stasis, induce fibrinolytic activity in veins and stimulate release of anti-platelet aggregation factor from endothelial cells.

Supplementary procedures

- Nasolabial folds are prominent.
  - Sub-SMAS facelift that goes through the SMAS to become subcutaneous at the belly of the zygomaticus major to stretch and flatten the fold.
  - Release dermal attachments and fill with fat, dermal grafts or soft-tissue fillers.
- Malar retrusion.
  - The cheeks can be enhanced with implants, fillers or SMAS (rolled up, folded).
  - Resuspension of ptotic fat/cheek mass to the lateral orbit or temporal fascia e.g. via transblepharoplasty approach.
- Lips lengthened.
  - Advance vermilion or excise skin at base of nose.
  - Injection of fat/fillers to augment the lips.
- Jawline, jowls and chin ptosis.
  - Platysma surgery.
  - Chin implants (need to release deep attachments particularly in submental area to allow proper redraping).

Neck lift
The **platysma** is a paired superficial flat muscle arising from the pectoralis and deltoid fascia, running up medially and inserting into the mandible and continuing on to the SMAS layer. It lies between the superficial cervical fascia and deep cervical fascia. When the muscle contracts it draws down the lower lip and angle of mouth, wrinkling the neck.

- Nerve supply comes from the cervical branch of the facial nerve.
  - The marginal mandibular nerve is subplatysmal in the region of the parotid tail, running above the inferior border of the mandible posterior to the facial nerve. It innervates the depressor anguli oris, depressor

437

labii inferioris, mentalis and parts of risorius and orbicularis oris.

- Blood supply comes from the submental and suprasternal arteries.

The **submandibular gland** is grooved/pierced by the facial artery along its posterosuperior border and is crossed superficially by the marginal mandibular nerve. It lies under the platysma/deep cervical fascia and body of the mandible.

The **skin** of the neck region has few pilosebaceous units and thus pronounced scarring, prolonged healing times and hyperpigmentation may be associated with surgery/laser treatment/peels to this region.

The anatomy of the platysma muscle
de Castro CC. *Plast Reconstr Surg* 1980;**66**:680–683.

- Type I – 75%, begins interdigitation within 2 cm of the inferior border of the mandible.
- Type II – 15% begins to decussate about the level of the thyroid cartilage.
- Type III – 10% no interdigitation.

Decussation patterns of the platysma in Koreans
Kim HJ. *Br J Plast Surg* 2001;**54**:400–402.

This more recent study in a different ethnic group shows a different distribution: 43%, 43% and 14% for the three groups respectively. In addition, this study changes the definition of II slightly as decussation/interdigitation beyond 2 cm from the inferior border of the mandible.

Management of platysmal bands
Mckinney P. *Plast Reconstr Surg* 1996;**98**:999–1006.

Prominent platysmal bands are due to lateral laxity in the muscle rather than prominent free medial edges. They can be approached via a submental incision, though this may increase the local wound complication rate including haematoma, infection and a 'leather neck' appearance.

A lack of midline stabilization may result in excessive lateral shift of medial borders of muscle during SMAS lift, and the bands then shift from vertical to oblique, thus the author prefers to undertake midline stabilization prior to lateral SMAS lift but it is important to avoid dehiscence of the midline sutures.

Subplatysmal fat is best treated by liposuction.

Assessment of neck lift patients

The youthful neck has a distinct mandible border with a cervicomental angle of 105–120° with a visible subhyoid depression, thyroid cartilage bulge and anterior SCM borders.

- Skin quality and excess, including jawline and jowls.
- Wrinkles at rest and animated.
- Fat – subcutaneous, preplatysmal, subplatysmal (which is more vascular and fibrous making liposuction of this layer less effective).
- Platysma at rest, dynamic banding.
- Chin projection.

Treatment options

- **Liposuction** via submental or posterior earlobe incisions is indicated for young patients with good skin quality and localized deposits of fat.
- Submental neck lift – under direct vision, excise interplatysmal fat, release the mandibular ligament, perform partial resection of the digastric muscle and piecemeal intracapsular resection of the submandibular gland.
  - Endoscopic neck lift.
- **Short-scar facelift with neck lift** (Baker) may be an option in patients with jowling but no excess of neck skin. There is a combined prehairline incision below sideburn and preauricular retro-tragal incision ending at the earlobe. A SMAS/platysma flap is dissected and elevated up.
- **Full-scar face- and neck lift** may be needed in faces with severe ageing and skin excess. The incision may need to be extended into the retroauricular region, then horizontally into the hairline in females to avoid notching the occipital hairline. The skin is pulled in a posterior and oblique vector whilst the platysmal can be dealt with in a number of ways:
  - Imbricated/plicated.
  - Incised (sectional myotomy of medial edge) – dividing the muscle entirely will lead to a visible defect and is not favoured.
  - Suspended (from inferior border of mandible).
  - **Corset platysmaplasty** – the anterior edges are pulled together (from chin to thyroid cartilage) in a multilayer seam to create a waist; it can be combined with lateral plication particularly over the submandibular gland to reduce its bulging. A platysmaplasty is preferable to using a skin-platysma 'lift' per se which anchors the muscle behind the ears – this leaves postauricular scars, tends to leave a strong

pulling sensation, and the risk of the platysma rebounding back. In certain patients, both a neck lift and a platysmaplasty may be needed but it is preferable to perform the latter first.

Complications

- Haematoma – 8% in males and 4% in females, with greater incidence if the blood pressure is over 150 mmHg.
- Facial nerve damage – buccal and marginal mandibular branches with face- and neck lifts respectively.
- Great auricular nerve damage.
- Infection and skin sloughing especially retroauricular.

Brow lift

Brow anatomy

The frontalis muscle forms a continuous layer with the galea. It inserts into the supraorbital dermis and interdigitates with the orbicularis oculi, whilst the posterior part of the galea passes deep to the muscle and inserts into the periosteum at the supraorbital rim. Other brow muscles include:

- **Corrugator supercilii** with its oblique head (supraorbital rim to medial eyebrow dermis and thus acts as a brow depressor forming the oblique glabellar lines) and transverse head (from medial supraorbital rim to middle third eyebrow dermis, thus moving the brow medially and forming vertical glabellar lines).
- **Depressor supercilii** that runs from medial supraorbital rim to medial brow dermis, thus depressing the brow and forming oblique lines.
- **Procerus** runs from medial supraorbital rim to the dermis of the medial brow, thus depressing the brow forming the nasal root lines that are oblique and horizontal.
- **Orbicularis oculi**, orbital part: the medial part causes medial brow depression whilst the lateral portion causes lateral brow depression and 'crow's feet'.

The corrugator, depressor, procerus and orbital part of the orbicularis are all depressors of the medial brow; they are all affected to a certain degree during lift surgery thus leading to medial brow elevation.

The **orbit (retaining) ligaments** (Knize) are upper face/brow retaining ligaments and are to be zones of attachment that must be released to achieve long-standing lift. They are classed as 'true' dermal to periosteal retaining ligaments, approximately 6–8 mm in length and centred over the zygomaticofrontal suture, tethering the lateral orbital rim here to the superficial temporal fascia and dermis. There is a **periosteal zone of adhesion** that is a wing-shaped band about 2 cm wide running above the supraorbital rims, and because it represents an adherence between deep galaea and periosteum it is described as a 'false' retaining ligament.

Sensation is provided by the supratrochlear and supraorbital nerves (superficial branch to the forehead and deep branch to scalp posterior to the hairline – this is transected with subgaleal and coronal incisions and thus leads to paraesthesia).

Brow aesthetics

The normal eyebrow position:

- Male – at the level of the supra-orbital rim, 6 cm from hairline.
- Female – just above the level of the supra-orbital rim, 5 cm from hairline.

The normal eyebrow shape:

- Medial limit forms a line joining the inner canthus with the lateral alar groove.
- Lateral limit forms a line joining the outer canthus with the lateral alar groove.
- The lateral brow end lies on the same horizontal plane or slightly above the medial end. The medial brow is more club shaped whilst the lateral brow tapers out to a sharper end.
- Highest part of the eyebrow lies directly above the outer limbus of the iris (junction of medial 2/3 and lateral 1/3 of brow).
  - More lateral – cross appearance.
  - More medial – sad appearance.

Brow lift surgery

Brow lift surgery is indicated for brow ptosis and transverse furrows, and may be needed before upper lid blepharoplasty/periorbital surgery. Patients with facial palsy may benefit from skin excision above the eyebrow (supraciliary lift or direct brow lift).

Pre-operative evaluation

- Assess brow (may be modified by plucking).
- Assess hairline position (high or low) and quality (thick or sparse, which may make scar concealment difficult).
- Assess wrinkles.

○ Dynamic – on animation, are best treated with botulinum toxin but surgery may improve them by weakening the responsible muscles.

○ Static – present at rest. May be due to sustained muscle activity and may thus be partially improved by surgery to the muscles but also need some form of skin redraping. Superficial wrinkles are amenable to treatment with fillers or resurfacing.

Incisions

- Direct/supraciliary – with excise of a strip of skin above the brow; it is useful particularly in males with thick brows, and for those with facial palsy.
- Transblepharoplasty – can be used to tack the brow to the periosteum as well as excise corrugator and procerus.
- Midbrow – will advance hairline as well as lift brow, useful for males, those with deep wrinkles.

These incisions may be useful in alopecia patients but the coronal incision or endoscopic approaches are the more common techniques in use.

If a **coronal approach** is used, the incision should be made at least 3 cm behind the anterior hairline (use anterior hairline incision if the brow is high, with extreme bevel).

- Bevel the incision parallel to hair follicles and elevate flap in a subgaleal (or subperiosteal) plane.
- Identify supraorbital and supratrochlear nerves deep and superficial to **corrugator** respectively, then resect muscle to reduce vertical creases.
- Pull back the forehead flap and excise any excess before closure; 1.5 mm of flap retrodisplacement translates to 1 mm of brow lift.
- Temporal incision is the oldest technique and is similar to the coronal but spares the midline.

Plane of dissection

- Subcutaneous – allows preservation of sensation of posterior scalp but at expense of reduced vascularity to the flap, a tedious dissection and making muscle surgery more difficult.
- Subgaleal – quick dissection with direct access to muscles; galea can be fixed to the periosteum.
- Subperiosteal – requires release of arcus marginalis for a better lift and supposedly a more sustained

lift; however, some say it is more related to the fixation rather than the dissection.
- Biplanar/dual plane – subcutaneous dissection of flap from muscle in upper part of flap combined with endoscopic/open subperiosteal dissection (and muscle excision). This is said to allow the hairline to stay in its original position whilst improving forehead rhytids.

Muscle surgery

- Direct excision e.g. corrugator, frontalis (2 cm of frontalis should be left above the brow to maintain animation); some suggest fat graft to glabellar to correct depression from excision).
- Scoring.
- Botulinum toxin.

Securing fixation

The elastic band principle states that the further away the suspension point is from the part to be lifted, i.e. brow in this case, the less effective the lift.

- Skin excision – 2:1 ratio of excision to elevation (some suggest 5:1). Obviously this is not applicable to the endoscopic technique.
- Sutures – cortical tunnels.
- Devices – Endotine (absorbable fan-shaped anchor device), Mitek anchor, screws (percutaneous or internal).

Complications

- Haematoma.
- Skin necrosis.
- Alopecia.
- Frontalis paralysis is rare and usually recovers within 12 months.
- Injury to sensory nerves will lead to forehead numbness; numbness posterior to the skin incision is to be expected.
- Chronic pain/supraorbital nerve dysaesthesia particularly if the patient has a history of migraines.
- Poor cosmesis e.g. asymmetry, displacement of lateral brow.

Endoscopic brow lift: a retrospective review of 628 consecutive cases over 5 years
Chiu ES. *Plast Reconstr Surg* 2003;**112**:628–633.

This was a survey of 21 New York plastic surgeons practising endoscopic brow lift: women were 60×

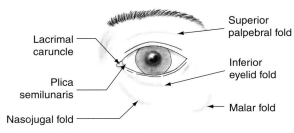

Lacrimal caruncle

Superior palpebral fold

Inferior eyelid fold

Plica semilunaris

Nasojugal fold

Malar fold

Figure 10.1 Features around the eye.

more common than men, and age range was 33–87 years. Observed complications included:

- Alopecia and hairline distortion.
- Asymmetry.
- Prolonged forehead paraesthesia and frontal branch paralysis.
- Implant infection.

The authors noted a progressive decline in the number of endoscopic procedures carried out compared with open brow lift during this period: half use it occasionally, whilst the other half either regularly use the endoscopic lift technique or not at all. They speculate that the decline may possibly be due to:

- More selective use of the technique, recognizing that endoscopic brow lift is ineffective in many patients.
- Increased use of botulinum toxin.

Endoscopic brow lift: a personal review of 538 patients and comparison of fixation techniques
Jones BM. *Plast Reconstr Surg* 2004;**113**:1242–1250.

This was a review of 538 endoscopic brow lifts using a technique based upon that described by Ramirez OM (*Plast Reconstr Surg* 1995;**96**:323). 80% of patients had a simultaneous facelift:

- Lift vector is marked pre-operatively; 2 parasagittal and 2 temporal incisions are made.
- Hydrodissection of the plane beneath the temporoparietal fascia with tumescent solution, followed by surgical dissection with endoscopic elevators to within 2 cm of the supraorbital rim.
- Subgaleal fascial flap is raised from the temporal incisions.
- The fascia at the temporal crease is divided and dissection extended subperiosteally along the zygomatic process of the frontal bone.

- At the supraorbital rim, the supraorbital and supratrochlear nerves are identified and the corrugator supercilii and procerus muscles debulked.
- The brow is then elevated and secured.

Initially fibrin glue was used before the change to sutures passed through drill-hole bone tunnels. The results were longer lasting in the latter group. An alternative method of fixation is the Mitek bone anchor.

VI. Blepharoplasty

Eyelid anatomy
Tarsal plates
The tarsus is composed of fibrous connective tissue with meibomian glands; approximately 2 mm thick.

- Upper tarsus 7–11 mm tall (in Whites) – Müller's and some fibres of the levator are attached. The upper tarsus is narrower in Asians.
- Lower tarsus 4–5 mm tall – capsulopalpebral fascia is attached.

The orbital septum is composed of fibrous tissue and can be viewed as an extension of the orbital periosteum and lies posterior to the orbicularis. It acts as a fascial barrier.

- Upper septum – superior orbital rim to levator aponeurosis.
- Lower septum – inferior orbital rim to capsulopalpebral fascia.

Canthal tendons
These are extensions of the preseptal and pretarsal orbicularis oculi. They act as check ligaments for the lateral and medial recti muscles.

- Lateral canthal tendon attaches to Whitnall's tubercle which is 1.5 cm posterior to the lateral orbital rim.
- Medial canthal tendon is more complex/tripartite (anterior horizontal, posterior horizontal and vertical) and is important for the lacrimal pump.

Fat
Preseptal fat

- Upper lid – ROOF (retroorbicularis fat).
- Lower lid – SOOF (suborbicularis fat).

Orbital fat is physiologically different from other body fat – the cells are smaller, the fat is more saturated, less lipoprotein lipase activity, less metabolically active and is only minimally affected by diet/obesity. The medial fat is usually more vascular, but paler with smaller lobules and more fibrous tissue.

- Upper lid (two pads) medial and central that are separated by the trochlea of the superior oblique.
- Lower lid (three pads) medial, central and lateral. The medial and central fat pads are separated by the inferior oblique (damage e.g. iatrogenic, may cause diplopia that is usually temporary).

Muscles

- Upper lid retractors.
  - **Levator palpebrae** (oculomotor) is the main retractor with 10–15 mm excursion; it arises from the lesser wing of the sphenoid, to Whitnall's ligament and the tarsal plate with some fibres to the dermis (though some dispute this).
  - **Müller's muscle** (sympathetic) provides 2 mm retraction and inserts to the superior tarsal margin.
- Lower lid retractor.
  - **Capsulopalpebral fascia** – 1–2 mm of downward pull from the action of the inferior rectus muscle; it surrounds the inferior oblique.

Lacrimal apparatus

The lacrimal gland has palpebral and orbital portions, separated by the levator aponeurosis. Tears help to lubricate the lid movements over the globe, contribute to nourishment of the corneal epithelium and some components are antibacterial. There are three layers:

- Lipid layer from the meibomian glands and sebaceous glands of Zeiss and Moll.
- Mucoid layer from goblet cells.
- Aqueous layer from the lacrimal gland.

Reflex secretion comes mainly from the lacrimal gland under parasympathetic control whilst passive/baseline tear production comes mainly from the accessory lacrimal glands, mucin goblet cells and meibomian glands.

- The tears flow from lateral to medial, to the puncta of inferior and superior canaliculi that join the lacrimal sac which empties via the nasolacrimal duct to the inferior meatus.

History

- Age, smoking, general health e.g. diabetes, hypertension, coagulopathy.
- Eye disease e.g. dry eyes (sicca syndrome), epiphora, glaucoma.
- Drug history especially anticoagulants.
- Previous scars – quality?

Examination

- Specifically exclude **compensated brow ptosis** – most patients have this to a degree when constant frontalis activity **masks** the ptosis. Following an upper lid blepharoplasty, the frontalis then relaxes and the brow ptosis becomes **apparent** (usually medially first, then laterally). Thus the need for brow lift should always be considered.
  - Ask the patient to look ahead and close their eyes, then immobilize the frontalis and ask them to open their eyes again. A drop in the brow indicates that there was brow compensation. Performing a blepharoplasty in such a patient will cause a drop in the brow post-operatively which is unattractive and unwanted.
  - Brow may have frontalis creases due to contraction to elevate brow.
  - Glabellar lines indicate corrugator (hyper) activity.
- Eye examination.
  - Upper lid.
    - Ptosis and lagophthalmos, skin laxity especially lateral hooding.
    - Position of supratarsal fold (with downward gaze) 8–10 mm from lash line (in Whites).
    - Degree of fat herniation (press gently on the globe).
  - Baseline examination including vision.
  - Bell's phenomenon.
- Facial nerve function.

Counselling

It is important to ascertain the patient's expectations both aesthetically and functionally. They should be advised of:

- Scars and bruising; time off work.
- Possibility of re-operation.
- Gritty/sticky eyes or scleral show.

Upper lid

Aesthetic surgery of the upper eyelid is most frequently directed at dermatochalasis i.e. redundancy of the skin of the lids with or without herniated orbital fat. Soft tissue excess of the upper lid may be due to subcutaneous, preseptal or postseptal fat or lacrimal gland ptosis.

- **Blepharochalasis**, on the other hand, is a rare autosomal dominant condition affecting young adults where there is atrophy of upper lid tissues following recurrent episodes of atopic eyelid oedema. Antihistamines and steroids do not help.
- Steatoblepharon – excess fat protruding through a lax septum.
- Blepharoptosis – drooping of upper lid i.e. 'ptosis'.
- Pseudoblepharoptosis – the eyelid is in a normal position but has the appearance of ptosis due to brow ptosis.

Technique

Basically a caudal incision line is drawn, sparing the supratarsal fold with its connections to the levator mechanism.

- Patients should be marked in an upright position with the upper lid under closing tension. The lower line is marked 9–10 mm above the lash line, the upper line varies – the skin is pinched with a pair of fine (Adson) forceps to determine amount of skin to be removed at various points along the lid. Extend the lower line laterally so that closure occurs within a wrinkle line. This skin is removed.
- Then remove an underlying strip of orbicularis (up to 3 mm) whilst preserving the pretarsal portion – the aim is to allow scarring down to create a crisp supratarsal fold. Muscle excision is conservative to maintain the youthful lid fullness.
  - It is important to not remove too much skin – 30 mm must remain between the lashes and the lower margin of the eyebrow; if too much is removed **and then** brow ptosis is corrected, lagophthalmos will result.
  - Conservative skin/muscle excisions are often best performed in combination with (preferably following) a brow lift and

corrugator excision (bicoronal formal lift, melon-slice lift, direct brow lift or endoscopic lift).
- Incise the orbital septum high up to avoid levator injury; use separate stab incisions. Gentle pressure on the globe accentuates fat herniation from medial and lateral upper lid compartments through the incisions and this is then removed with bipolar cautery.
  - Medial fat is more compact, pale and vascular. Keep resected fat to compare with the other side.
  - Prolapse of 'fat' far laterally is likely to be the lacrimal gland; consider glanduloplasty.
  - Meticulous haemostasis with bipolar diathermy is very important to avoid retrobulbar haematoma.

Complications

- Infection.
- Inadequate correction.
- Muscle injury.
  - Ptosis due to injury to levator.
  - Most commonly damaged extra-ocular muscle is the **inferior oblique** resulting diplopia looking up and out.
- Retrobulbar haematoma and blindness are thankfully rare.

Asian blepharoplasty

The tarsal fixation technique is one technique to create a supratarsal fold for Asians lacking them due to the paucity of fascial connections from the tarsal plate to the overlying eyelid skin, as well as the amount of preaponeurotic fat. The fold ('double eyelid') is created 4–7 mm from the lash line i.e. lower than in eyes of Whites.

There are many different techniques described in the literature; most are variations of either the 'closed' or 'open' techniques.

Closed technique or suture method

The closed technique uses 2–3 sutures to provide static fixation resulting in a static fold i.e. seen when the eye is closed as well as open. 2–3 small stab incisions are made with a no. 11 blade along the chosen line and double-ended sutures are passed from the conjunctival side that is also marked at the same distance (some prefer to re-enter the

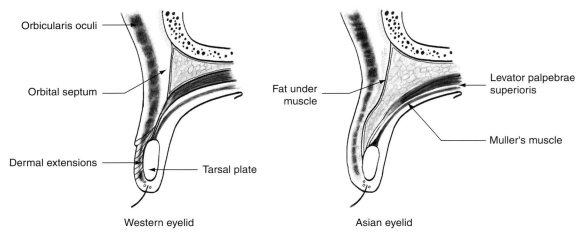

Figure 10.2 Anatomical differences between eyelids of Asians and Whites accounting for the lack of an upper eyelid fold, often referred to as a 'double eyelid'. The tarsal plate in Whites' eyelids is 8–11 mm, whereas it is 6.5–8 mm in Asians.

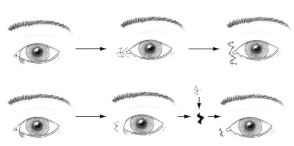

Figure 10.3 Two different methods of dealing with the epicanthal fold. None are entirely satisfactory due to the potential prominent scar; some suggest that the best way of treating epicanthal folds is to augment the nasal dorsum.

same hole, others are less precise at 2–3 mm away, whilst others 'cheese-wire' the conjunctiva) and then tied down.

- This option is said to be more suited to younger patients particularly those with thin lids i.e. no need for fat removal (though some do this through limited incisions). It has a quicker recovery time (a couple of days), but the main disadvantage is that it tends to be temporary, lasting up to several years with a gradual loss of the crease – some studies show 7% loss at 1 year. As there is no rearrangement of internal structures, some describe the technique as being non-physiological.

Full open technique or incisional method

The full open technique is 'definitive' in theory as it changes internal anatomy and provides a dynamic fold i.e. only seen with the eyes open. The incision is similar to a standard blepharoplasty, and thus allows the concomitant correction of any puffiness, ptosis or trichiasis.

- The technique is more suited to older patients with fatter, puffier eyelids that have tissue excess. It is still important to be selective and conservative with any **excisions**. In most of these techniques, the key sutures are those that bring together dermis, tarsal plate and aponeurosis for secure fixation.
  Debulking of pretarsal soft tissue may help reduce bulk and post-operative oedema.

Notable variants include:

- Flowers (1993): 'anchor blepharoplasty' – suture skin to tarsus and levator.
- Sheen (1977): suture pretarsal orbicularis to levator.
- Baker (1977): no sutures are used, instead allow approximately 5 mm of skin to scar down onto the orbital septum overlying the levator.

Lower lid

There is more debate and controversy regarding lower lid blepharoplasty.

Lower lid examination

- Skin – redundancy and crow's feet.
- Examine for **lower lid tone** (it should snap back quickly after being pulled away from the globe). Lax lids are very common and may benefit from canthoplasty or lid shortening (wedge resection). **Scleral show** may be due to tarsal laxity, exophthalmos or middle lamellae contracture.
- There are a variety of lower lid lines/grooves/swellings to note and the inconsistent use of terminology can be confusing. They often coexist.
  - **Palpebral** bags (common eyebags) are the most common and are usually caused by fat protrusion/herniation (Castanares). The fat/swelling lies directly under the eyelid and becomes apparent as the ageing eyelid loses tone (attentuation of orbital septum). This is often bounded inferiorly by the arcus marginalis tethering ('dark circles').
  - **Tear trough** refers to the groove/depression at the boundary of the eyelid and cheek, that is most prominent medially at the nasojugal groove; the name comes from the observation that tears now run obliquely across the face instead of straight down. The medial part is almost level with the infraorbital rim but more laterally, the line runs below the bony rim. More severe forms may be called a tear trough depression whilst a more widespread form, i.e. spreading laterally, is sometimes called 'suborbital volume deficiency'.
  - **Festoons** describe the redundant folds that hang from canthus to canthus; they are soft tissue (usually skin and muscle but may include orbital septum and fat), although they can occur over any part of the upper or lower lids. The term is usually taken to refer to the sagging of the orbital and malar segments of the muscle of the lower lid. A festoon (Latin *festo*, festival garland) is a garland that hangs loosely from two points of attachment. The tear trough bounds the inferior aspect of the festoon.
    - Festoons squinch test – forcible closure of eyes will improve appearance of 'true' **muscle** festoons i.e. ptotic orbicularis oculi (muscle contraction that also pushes any protruding fat back) though the skin redundancy remains.
    - Pinch and traction testing to assess effects of possible surgery e.g. excision, imbricated or tightened laterally as a sling.
  - Palpebral bags should be distinguished from **malar** bags as the latter are rarely corrected by blepharoplasty and probably represent chronic regional oedema of unknown aetiology. Malar bags sit lower and more lateral on the cheek.
  - Palpate the infra-orbital rim to ensure that a prominent bony margin is not mistaken for fat herniation.
- Globe position.
  - Beware of excessive scleral show. Proptosis can be a feature of thyroid disease.
  - Enophthalmos may be post-traumatic e.g. orbital fractures.
  - Perform **lacrimal function tests** in the elderly and those with dry eye symptoms.
    - Schirmer's test 1 – basic and reflex secretion; paper on lateral sclera and more than 10 mm in 5 minutes is normal.
    - Schirmer's test 2 – basic secretion (~40% of above) after topical local anaesthesia.
    - Others are more advanced: tear film break-up, Rose Bengal stain, tear lysozyme electrophoresis.

Blepharoplasty surgical technique

Traditionally lower lid blepharoplasty was an operation to remove skin and fat in the lower eyelid to deal with the wrinkling and bulging from orbital fat hernation. Post-operatively this made the lower eyelid smoother and usually deeper; however, removal of fat leads eventually to collapse of the skin cover and even more wrinkles than before.

- Elevate a **skin–muscle flap** with the skin incision just below the lashes (i.e. subciliary, scars here heal best) extended laterally beyond the lateral canthus; initially skin only is elevated to leave a cuff of muscle (overlying the tarsus).
  - A variant is to use a subciliary incision, and then raise a skin-only flap over the preseptal orbicularis. This can be used in cases of skin excess but the dissection is rather tedious and may cause scarring of the skin/muscle.
- Excision of a triangular piece of skin/muscle is determined by redraping the flap without tension over the lash line. A rough guide is 3.5 mm; or

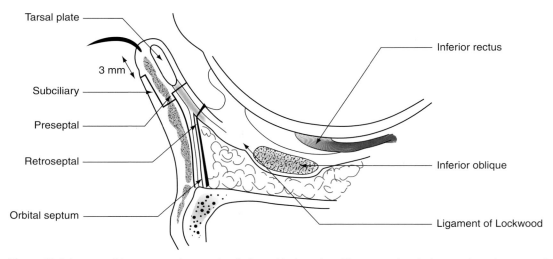

Figure 10.4 Lower eyelid anatomy and approaches for lower blepharoplasty. The transconjunctival approach can be preseptal or retroseptal and avoids an external skin scar.

estimate pre-operatively by marking with the patient's eyes and mouth open.

- Excise fat from each of the three lower lid compartments as above but avoid over-excision which gives a 'hollowed out' appearance.

Fat may be removed via a **transconjunctival approach** (incise above the fornix) if there is no need for skin excision, thus avoiding post-operative lower lid retraction from the scar. After dissection of the plane between conjunctiva and the tarsal plate, taking a **retroseptal** approach preserves the orbital septum.

- This is more suited to those with little or no excess skin, often the younger age group.
- This may be combined with laser resurfacing of the lid skin.
- It is useful as a secondary procedure for patients with inadequately corrected palpebral bags.

Complications

- **Asymmetry**.
- **Excessive scleral show**. Lagophthalmos is usually temporary; treatment with massage and taping, though persistent cases may need skin graft.
- **Ectropion** and lagophthalmos – usually due to over-correction; **store removed skin** in case it is needed later. Do not do a wedge resection even if

there is a positive snap test: do not do a blepharoplasty at all or do it transconjunctivally.

- Blindness due to **retrobulbar haematoma** (~1 in 40 000) – also presents as pain, proptosis, ecchymosis, reduced eye movement, dilated pupil, scotomas and raised intraocular pressure. Emergency treatment includes head elevation, rebreathing bag (to raise CO_2), release of sutures, lateral canthotomy/cantholysis and administer mannitol, acetazolamide, steroids and beta blockers. Emergency exploration; consult ophthalmologist.
  - Other causes are central retinal artery occlusion or optic nerve ischaemia.
- Corneal injury – fluorescein stain for diagnosis. Treat with topical antibiotics and eye patch.
- Muscle injury – levator (leading to ptosis), inferior and superior obliques (leading to diplopia, most cases are due to oedema and resolve).

Treatment of tear trough

This is a difficult area to treat. The problem is mostly certainly multifactorial with soft tissue deficiency/descent being the most significant; other factors include bony depression/deficiency. Others have identified it as a gap in the muscle cover below the infero-medial border of the orbicularis oculi or a tight attachment of the muscle to the bone by retaining ligaments and it may also occur in combination with fat herniation.

- **Tissue fillers and autologous fat** have been used to treat the folds and depressions under the eye; the effect is often temporary.
- Many surgical techniques for the tear trough have been described including:
  - ○ **Repositioning** of bulging lower orbital fat into the area of hollowness e.g. Goldberg's repositioning of subseptal fat into a subperiosteal pocket formed after transconjunctival arcus marginalis release. The septal reset is similar to this (Hamra, Loeb).
  - ○ **Synthetic implants**, particularly for bony deformities.
  - ○ Mid-facelift.

Lower lid laxity

- **Tarsal shortening** (Kuhnt–Szymanowski procedure) – pentagonal excision of posterior lamellae lateral to lateral limbus. This is a good option if there is true tarsal excess.
- **Canthoplasty** – divide commissure and reposition the lower canthal tendon (tarsal strip procedure) and lateral canthus.
- **Canthopexy** (retinacular suspension) – suture suspension to the orbital rim. It is a less invasive procedure compared with canthoplasty, and does not involve disinsertion of lateral canthus, but provides only mild lid tightening and canthal elevation.

VII. Rhinoplasty

Anatomy

See also 'Nasal reconstruction'.

Skin over the upper two-thirds (dorsum and side-walls, upper two zones) is thin, whilst skin over the lower third (lower zone, tip and alar) is thick, sebaceous and more fixed.

Muscles

- Levator labii superioris alaeque nasi – keeps the external nasal valve open.
- Depressor septi nasi – hyperactivity shortens upper lip and reduces tip projection with smiling.

Nasal vault

- Bony vault – paired nasal bones and frontal process of maxilla.
- Upper cartilaginous vault – paired upper lateral cartilages that lie under the bones by 6–8 mm. This overlapping zone is called the **keystone area** – it is the widest part of the dorsum and is important for the dorsal aesthetic line. They join the septum in the midline.
- Lower cartilaginous vault – paired lower lateral cartilages with medial (middle) and lateral crus. The lateral crus overlaps the upper lateral cartilage in three-quarters of cases with the reverse pattern in 11%.

Nasal tip

The projection and support of the tip comes from major and minor tip support mechanism:

- Major: alar cartilages (size, shape, thickness and resilience), their abutment/attachment with piriform aperture, upper lateral cartilage and caudal septum.
- Minor:
  - ○ Domal suspensory ligament.
  - ○ Anterior septal angle.
  - ○ Skin.
  - ○ Nasal spine and caudal septum.
  - ○ Sesamoid cartilage complex extending support of lateral crura to piriform aperture.

Assessment

History

- Previous trauma or surgery.
- Symptoms such as nosebleeds, allergic rhinitis and olfactory disturbances.
- Drug history – aspirin, warfarin, steroids.
- Medical problems e.g. diabetes, hypertension, smokers.

Examination

Photographs are vital.

- **Skin quality and thickness** – specifically telangiectasia (that can get worse). In addition, the thicker the skin, the stronger and more angular the framework required to be visible through the skin envelope.
- **Assess proportions and symmetry** of nose and relationship to thirds of face. Note that

micrognathia will make the nose look bigger and in this case, is best treated by chin augmentation or genioplasty. The nose needs to match the ethnicity of the patient.

- ○ Width of bony base should be 75–80% of the width of the alar base.
- ○ Width of alar base approximates to the intercanthal distance (wider alar may be due to flaring or a truly wide base).
- **Evaluate the nasal lines**.
  - ○ **Nasal deviation** – look at the dorsal line from the middle of the glabellar to the middle of the philtrum (to mentum).
  - ○ 'Aesthetic lines' – two curved lines from medial supraciliary ridges to the tip defining points.
  - ○ Consider the **dorsum** and the presence of any hump, supratip deformity etc.
- **Evaluate the tip:** according to Sheen, the essential landmarks of a refined tip are the lateral projections of the right and left domes, the points of tip differentiation from the dorsum (supratip break), and the columellar/lobular junction (columellar break).
  - ○ Alar rim symmetry – it should resemble a gull wing. On a basilar view the alar rim and tip should approximate to an equilateral triangle with ratio of 1/3 lobule to 2/3 columella. The nostrils are teardrop shaped with apex medial to the base (in Whites).
  - ○ Tip defining points – one each side, forming the lateral corners of a vertical rhombus/diamond (two equilateral triangles) with the supratip break and columellar break forming the upper and lower angles.
  - ○ Tip projection – tip to alar cheek junction. In the 'aesthetic tip', 50–60% of this line is anterior to the upper lip.
  - ○ Tip rotation – columellar/nasolabial angle: males – 90°, females – 100°.
- Examine the septum for deviation and check for collapse of the internal valve and turbinate hypertrophy.

Post-operative

Patient should expect to have a painful swollen nose with black eyes.

- Nasal packs (24 hours).
- Plaster of Paris (1 week).

Complications include:

- Infection, haematoma/epistaxis.
- Under-correction (residual deformity) or over-correction (new deformity).
- Persistent nasal tip oedema (up to 2 years) and numbness that may include the upper teeth.
- Scars (inner canthus, columella), palpable step at lateral maxillary osteotomy site.
- Airway obstruction.

Reasons for secondary rhinoplasty include residual deformity, deviation and valving.

Airway obstruction and rhinoplasty

The relative importance of septal and nasal valvular surgery in correcting airway obstruction in primary and secondary rhinoplasty
Constantian MB. *Plast Reconstr Surg* 1996;**98**:38–54.

Four factors may cause airway obstruction:

- **Septal deviation** (treatment is a septoplasty for more anterior deviations, submucous resection (SMR) is more suited for more posterior problems).
- **Inferior turbinate hypertrophy** (inferior turbinate infracture/crush/diathermy/resection – the last should be approached with caution as chronic exposure to air flow may cause mucosal changes leading eventually to atrophic rhinitis or ozena).
- **External valve problem**.
  - ○ The external valve is formed by the alar rim (lateral crus of the alar cartilage, soft tissue of the alae), membranous septum and the nasal sill. The nasalis dilates this during inspiration. Malposition or over-resection of the alar cartilages may compromise the external valve mechanism; treat by insertion of onlay tip lateral crural grafts to stiffen the lower lateral cartilage or support alar rim with alar batten grafts (10×6 septal or conchal cartilage inserted in a tight pocket in the area of collapse).
- **Internal valve problem**.
  - ○ Narrowing the nose by dorsal resection, osteotomy and in-fracture may render the internal valve too narrow; treat by insertion of **dorsal spreader grafts** between upper lateral cartilage and septum. The spreader grafts maintain the valve whilst also buttressing/straightening up a slightly deviated septum and smoothing the profile. Alar batten grafts may be use for lateral wall supra-alar pinching.

Internal nasal valve

The nose accounts for 50% of upper airway resistance and a major contributor is the internal nasal valve which lies at the angle (usually ~15°) made by the caudal edge of the upper lateral cartilages with the septum. Note that according to Poiseuille's law, air flow increases to the fourth power of the radius and the converse is also true. Treatment options include:

- Lateral traction on the cheeks (**Cottle's manoeuvre**) or sprung devices worn by athletes open up the internal nasal valve and reduce airway resistance.
- Spreader grafts.

Nasal cycle: the inferior turbinate undergoes a 3–4-hourly cycle of congestion and decongestion in 80% of the population. This is a normal phenomenon; persistent congestion due to turbinate hypertrophy may warrant inferior turbinectomy.

Assessment

History: bilateral obstruction that has variable severity suggests a mucosal problem (most common e.g. allergic or viral rhinitis) whilst a more constant/consistent obstruction suggests a fixed i.e. skeletal problem such as septal deviation.

- If Cottle's manoeuvre alleviates the problem then part of the obstruction, at least, is localized to the internal nasal valve.
- Assess alar rim including collapse.
- Examine septum.

Approaches

The **closed approach** i.e. endonasal, has the advantages of no external scar and dissection is limited to the area needed with a precise pocket for graft insertion and fixation; this reduces post-operative oedema. However, the learning curve is significant, and the view (for surgeon and student) is limited. The incision placement depends on the problem that needs correction:

- Intercartilaginous – between the upper lateral cartilage and the lower lateral (alar) cartilages; evert to deliver the alar cartilage.
- Transcartilaginous – through the alar cartilage, this allows access to the alar cartilage.
- Marginal – caudal to alar cartilage (will also need intercartilaginous incision to deliver alar cartilage into wound). A true 'rim' incision is rarely used.

Septal incisions

- **Complete transfixion** – this is usually made as a continuation of the inter- or trans-cartilaginous incisions. It separates the membranous septum (and medial crura) from the caudal septum to free the tip, exposing the nasal spine and depressor septi muscles. The septum is also free for mucoperichondrial flaps to be raised. However, as the attachment of the medial crural footplates to the caudal septum is disrupted, there is a loss of tip support and potential loss of tip projection (which may be a desirable outcome in some cases).
  - ○ Limited partial transfixion – this is indicated if less tip access is required with preservation of the attachments between the caudal septum and medial crural footplate.
  - ○ Partial transfixion incision – the incision begins caudal to the anterior septal angle and

Figure 10.5 Types of incision for rhinoplasty.

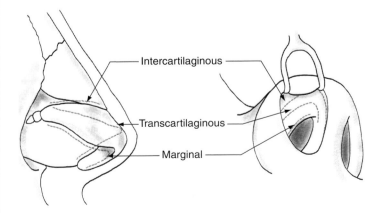

Intercartilaginous

Transcartilaginous

Marginal

continues just short of the medial crural attachments to the caudal septum.

- **Hemitransfixion** (Cottle 1960) – this is a unilateral incision at the junction of the caudal septum and columella. Typically, this is used for procedures in which caudal septum is deviated and needs resection for tip rotation or columellar adjustment.
- **High septal transfixion** (Kamer 1984) – this transcartilaginous incision does not violate the junction of caudal septum and medial crura/membranous septum and so does not alter tip support.

The open approach is useful for tip work and is often the preferred routine approach for patients with cleft nose or needing a secondary rhinoplasty.

Closed versus open rhinoplasty

Greater exposure is afforded by the open approach:

- This makes diagnosis of deforming factors and connections easier.
- Repositioning of cartilaginous framework and application of grafts can be secured under direct vision including dorsal spreader grafts and onlay grafts to the dorsum and tip.
- Allows excellent haemostasis.
- It facilitates teaching.

However, the main disadvantages of the open approach are the transcolumellar scar, longer operative time and prolonged tip oedema that result. There may be delayed healing of the wound. Under certain circumstances, the closed approach may be contraindicated:

- Cantilever graft is needed.
- Excess skin needs to be excised.
- Extreme cephalic malposition of lateral crura which makes alar dissection difficult with a closed approach.
- Cocaine nose.

Alterations in nasal sensibility following open rhinoplasty

Bafaqeeh SA. *Br J Plast Surg* 1998;**51**:508–510.

The nerve supply to the nasal skin is derived from:

- Infratrochlear nerve (V1, branch of nasociliary) – over nasal bones.
- External nasal nerve (V1, terminal branch of anterior ethmoidal) – over upper lateral cartilages, tip and upper columella.

- The nerve emerges between the nasal bones and the upper lateral cartilages and is at risk when elevating lateral nasal skin.
- Infra-orbital nerve (V2) – over lower lateral cartilages and columella.

Following open rhinoplasty, altered sensation at the nasal tip and upper columella was recorded at 3 weeks and had recovered by a year, which may be due to nerve regeneration or recruitment from adjacent areas.

Nasal tip

Tip projection depends on the supporting structures; some have likened the tip to a tripod (Anderson) with each lateral crus forming a leg, and the third leg from the conjoined medial crura. The medial crura are shorter and have additional support by attachments to the septum.

- Upward rotation of the tip occurs if the lateral limbs are shortened or if the central limb is lengthened. With short noses, the aim is to derotate the tip.

The support structures to the tip are often divided into major (alar cartilage configuration and their attachments, particularly the medial cural footplates to the causal septum) and minor.

Increase projection – columellar strut grafts and suture techniques are used before cartilage tip grafts that may be palpable in thinner-skinned patients.

- **Columellar strut grafts**.
  - Floating – able to increase tip projection by 1–2 mm; place it 2–3 mm anterior to the nasal spine and secured in pocket between the medial crura.
  - Fixed grafts are used if > 3 mm projection is needed. Rib cartilage is often used and placed on top of the nasal spine.
- **Suture techniques** can increase projection by 1–2 mm and can help refine/define tip.
  - Medial crural sutures – stabilizes columellar strut and refines nasal tip.
  - Medial crural septal sutures – between the medial cura and septum, cause **rotation** of the nasal tip which increases tip projection and corrects drooping nose e.g. ageing.
  - Interdomal sutures – i.e. dome binding, increases infratip columellar projection and refines tip.

○ Transdomal sutures between medial and lateral parts of the same alar cartilage which allows correction of domal asymmetry and increases tip projection.

- **Tip graft**.
  ○ Infralobular (hexagonal or rhomboid/diamond) (Sheen).
  ○ Onlay graft – provides tip projection and refinement, can be doubled up (or more) (Peak).
  ○ Combinations (Gunter).

Reduce projection – a maximum of 2 mm can be reduced without noticeable columellar bowing or alar flaring.

- Closed approach – transfixion incision to separate alar cartilage from septum and reduce support.
- Open approach – resection of attachment of medial crura to septum to remove support from intercartilaginous ligaments.
  ○ Volume reduction of alar cartilage leaving at least 6–8 mm to prevent external valve collapse.
  ○ To reduce projection further, then transect the lateral crura and overlap them; repeating this with the medial crura can reduce projection further – interrupted strip technique.

Nasal dorsum

- **Dorsal hump reduction** – separate the upper lateral cartilage from the septum and shave down the septum with a blade (this avoids reducing the upper lateral cartilage which may lead to collapse of the internal nasal valve and an irregular dorsum) – if the upper lateral cartilage protrudes it can then be shaved flush. The bony hump is reduced with a downbiting rasp or osteotome. If there is an open roof deformity (gap between septum and bone) then it can be closed with osteotomies.
- **Dorsal augmentation**
  ○ Cartilage grafts – septal, costal cartilage (may need K-wire and suture fixation).
  ○ Alloplastic e.g. silicone, is popular in Asians and despite the theoretical problems with infection risk seems to be well tolerated and this may be due in part to the thicker skin. The use of Alloderm has also been described.

Osteotomies

The bony vault is likened to a pyramid with the paired nasal bones and maxilla, and the shape can be altered with osteotomies (but may lead to upper lateral cartilage collapse). Relative contraindications include:

- Elderly with thin bones.
- Patients who need to wear heavy spectacles.
- Ethnic nose that is particularly flat and broad.

Lateral osteotomies can narrow the side-walls of the dorsum as well as close an open roof deformity and straighten a deviated nasal pyramid. Periosteal dissection should be limited to maximize support to the nasal bones and osteotomy should not be carried above the intercanthal line where the bone becomes thicker.

- **Low–high** osteotomy can be used to mobilize moderately widened nasal bones or a small open roof. The osteotomy starts low (lateral) to the piriform aperture and extends upwards to the intercanthal line ending high (medial) on the dorsum. This tends to narrow the airway slightly.
- **Low–low** osteotomy can be used for wide nasal bones or a large open roof. It begins low and continues low to the dorsal region at the intercanthal line.
- **Double-level** – for excessive lateral wall convexity or lateral nasal wall deformities. A lateral osteotomy is performed along the nasal wall along the nasomaxillary suture and combined with a low–low osteotomy.

Medial osteotomies separate nasal bones from the bony nasal septum and may be used in cases of traumatically narrowed vaults or for patients with widened nasal bones to create a line for a controlled fracture. They should be performed before lateral osteotomies, advancing with a two-tap technique.

Nasal alae

The main support to the alar rim comes from the lateral crural attachments to accessory cartilages (lateral crural complex) and to the piriform aperture, upper lateral cartilage and suspensory ligament of the tip. The posterior 50% of the alar rim is made of fibrofatty tissue and devoid of cartilage. Collapse of the rim, e.g. due to decreased cartilage support, may cause external nasal (valve) obstruction.

- **Non-anatomic alar contour grafts** can be used in selected cases with minimal vestibular lining loss and at least 3 mm of the alar cartilage still remaining; conversely it is not suitable for those with rim retraction second to lining loss, absent alar cartilages or severe alar scarring. A pocket is created above the rim for a 2–6 mm graft, verifying that the rim contour is corrected without the graft being visible.
- Lateral crural strut grafts are placed on the deep surface of the lateral crura and may be used for cases of malpositioned or misshapen lateral crura, as well as alar rim collapse or retraction. These are usually harvested from the septal cartilage (3×4×20 mm) and positioned during an open rhinoplasty in a pocket under the lateral crus and sutured in.

Alar base

The width of the alar base is approximately equal to the intercanthal distance; a wide alar base may be due to a truly wide alar base or excessive alar flare (> 2 mm difference between base and maximum width).

Alar base excision can be used in patients in the latter group – a wedge of tissue is excised (wider skin side and not carried into vestibule, but can pass under the nasal sill) preserving 1–2 mm of the alar base above the groove.

For a wide alar base:

- A wedge excision of the alar base that extends to the vestibule.
- Excision of nasal sill.
- Some have described an 'alar cinch' stitch with a non-resorbable suture on a straight needle, that is passed through a hypodermic needle passed from stab incisions at the alar bases/creases under the soft tissue of the base of the nose.

Septoplasty (SMR)

- A vertical incision is made on the side of the deviation in front of the deformity and subperichondrial dissection carried out over the buckled cartilage.
- The septum is incised to pick up the subperichondrial plane on the other side which is developed and cartilage is excised with a Ballenger swivel knife.

'Typical' open rhinoplasty
Exposure
- Local anaesthesia including nasal block and cocaine pack/spray; shave vibrissae.
- Evert nostril with a double hook and make a curved marginal/rim incision in the nasal mucosa connecting the two sides with a stepped columellar incision at its narrowest part.
- Lift the columellar skin and nasal tip soft tissues off the cartilage framework and then separate the lower lateral cartilages from each other and the septum.
- Dissect the mucosa off the septum and create extramucosal tunnels beneath the upper lateral cartilages; use scissors to separate the upper lateral cartilages from the septal cartilage.

Identify and reduce the bony hump.

- Trim the upper edges of upper lateral and septal cartilages (soft hump) and then use an osteotome to cleanly excise the bony hump (save the bone as it may be needed for radix graft).

Close the 'open roof'.

- Make a stab incision in the inner canthus, and then use a periosteal elevator to dissect a subperiosteal tunnel down the side of the nasomaxillary angle for maxillary osteotomy.
- Introduce a 2 mm osteotomy and create a series of perforations along the proposed osteotomy line; then in-fracture the nasal bones with digital pressure and correct any irregularities by rasping.

Return to the tip (i.e. should be last or nearly the last step).

- Excise a portion of the cephalic edge of the lower lateral cartilages to refine the tip and approximate with 6/0 ethilon.
  - Bulbous tip – excise a wedge or dart.
  - Bifid tip – widely separated medial crura must be plicated in the midline.
  - Hanging tip due to columella lacking adequate skeletal support (e.g. after over-resection of the caudal edge of the septum) – needs a 'T'-shaped cartilage graft e.g. from the septum.

Closure:

- Close mucosa with 5/0 vicryl rapide and skin with 6/0 ethilon.

Post-operative care

- Place jelonet packs in 'trouser' pattern and dorsal plaster of Paris.
  - Remove packs after 24–48 hours.
  - Remove plaster and sutures after 1 week.
- The patient must be instructed to keep relaxed and not to blow nose for 2 weeks.

Secondary rhinoplasty

- **Saddle deformity**.
  - Excessive removal of dorsal bone and cartilage; this needs a cartilage (septal or conchal) graft to fill in the contour defect.
- **Pinched tip deformity**.
  - When the lateral crura have fractured resulting in loss of a dome-like projection, the dome needs to be restored with an onlay cartilage graft.
- **Supra-tip deformity** may be due to several reasons.
  - Inadequate septal dorsal hump reduction (lower the septal hump further).
  - Inadequate correction of a bulbous tip (further tip work and fatty debulking).
  - Over-reduction of the cartilaginous skeleton (dorsal onlay graft).

Rhinophyma

Rhinophyma: review and update
Rohrich RJ. *Plast Reconstr Surg* 2001;**110**:860–870.

Greek: *rhis* is nose; *phyma* is growth.

Rhinophyma is a severe form of acne rosacea and affects up to 10% of the population, more commonly males particularly of Celtic races. It may be related to androgens (higher 5α-reductase activity in acne-prone skin) and there is a familial component in around half of patients.

Contrary to popular opinion, there is no aetiological link with alcohol, although facial flushing following alcohol makes the nose look redder (acne-prone skin may be more vasoreactive to certain stimuli including alcohol and stress).

In its severest form:

- The skin is thickened (dermal hyperplasia), red-purple, pitted, fissured and scarred.
- There is sebaceous hyperplasia, with pustules being a common feature.
- The underlying nasal skeleton remains unaffected.

The nasal tip is affected more than the rest of the nose although other areas may also be affected: mentophyma, otophyma and zygophyma. **Occult basal cell carcinoma** has been reported in up to 10% of rhinophyma.

Freeman classification
Reconstructive rhinoplasty for rhinophyma
Freeman BS. *Plast Reconstr Surg* 1970;**46**:265–270.

- Early vascular.
- Moderate diffuse enlargement.
- Localized 'tumour'.
- Extensive diffuse enlargement.
- Extensive diffuse enlargement plus localized tumour.

Non-surgical treatment:

- Antibiotics: metronidazole, tetracycline.
- Retinoids: tretinoin and isotretinoin – however, as it impairs re-epithelialization, concurrent surgery should be avoided.

Surgical treatment:

- Excision of affected tissue ('sculpting') and healing by secondary intention.
  - Dermabrasion, CO_2 and argon lasers or combined techniques.

VIII. Liposuction

In liposuction, fat is sucked into the openings on the cannula tip and then avulsed as the suction cannula moves back and forth. The fibrous stroma surrounding neurovascular bundles remains relatively intact, preserving blood supply and sensation to the overlying skin.

Classification

- Level – deep vs. superficial (leaving 8–10 mm of subcutaneous tissue vs. 2–4 mm respectively).
- System – syringe vs. machine.
- Assistance – ultrasound, mechanical.
- Infiltration – dry (historical only), wet (100–300 ml per area), superwet (1:1 for aspirate) or tumescent (to skin turgor, ~3 ml per ml aspirate).

The commonest indication is cosmesis – the removal of localized deposits of fat that are not responsive to dieting/exercise. It can also be applied for reduction of fatty tissue in other situations e.g. flap thinning, debulking lipomas, treating gynaecomastia (and selected cases of female breast reduction) as well as treatment for fat necrosis and extravasation injuries. It can also be used to harvest fat for injection.

Assessment

- Establish the patient's expectations and concerns.
- History including weight changes.
- Medical history including anything suggesting a bleeding disorder.

Examination

The body mass index (BMI) should be documented.

- Skin: striae, scars and cellulite. Pinch testing and tissue elasticity.
- The typical appearance of cellulite arises due to the fibrous septae in the superficial fat layer that anchors the skin whilst the fat hypertrophies and the skin loses elasticity with age. Patients with skin laxity may not benefit from liposuction alone.
- Fat distribution.

Procedure

- Pre-operative topographical markings are used to outline areas of proposed fat removal.
- Fluid is infiltrated according to the surgeon's preference.
- Incisions are made in inconspicuous areas agreed with the patient: the areas are 'pretunnelled' before the suction cannulae are used.
- Endpoints include: bloody aspirate, loss of resistance or achieving final contour.

Whilst many may be treated as day cases and can go home with simple oral analgesia, it is suggested that those with large volumes aspirated should be monitored overnight/24 hours with blood tests to check haemoglobin and electrolytes. The use of urinary catheters is not universal.

Patients should expect bruising, numbness and swelling – the latter may take months to settle, meaning that the full benefit may not be evident for up to 6 months. Post-operatively, support garments to extremities are worn for at least 2 weeks – most suggest 6 weeks whilst some say that 3 months is required for the best results.

Complications of liposuction

Toxicity due to local anaesthetics and fat embolism is very rare. Complications are more likely with large volume liposuction although what actually constitutes a 'large volume' is not clearly defined and ranges from 2–5 litres or more depending on the surgeon.

- Infection, bleeding.
- Contour irregularity requiring further liposuction or fat injection. Lax skin.
- Seroma/haematoma.
- Injury to nerves, major blood vessels and overlying skin. The risk of inadvertent entry into the body cavity e.g. bowel perforation is extremely small.
- DVT/PE 0.03% in Whites.
- Death: 1 in 50 000 (compared with 1 in 3000 when combining liposuction with abdominoplasty).

Conventional liposuction includes a blunt tip cannula attached to a vacuum pump (~1 atm), alternatively suction can be generated by a syringe.

- **Ultrasound-assisted liposuction** was pioneered by Zocchi and his technique was outlined in 1992. Ultrasonic waves are converted into mechanical vibration (20 000 cycles/s) at the tip of the titanium cannula causing cavitation 1–2 mm from the tip, which induces fragmentation and melting of fat whilst the collagen network is left intact. The proposed advantages are less bleeding and reduced energy expenditure by the surgeon, whilst the overall volume of fat removed may be increased.
  - However, there is a **risk of burns** (0.07%) at the deep surface of the overlying skin ('tip hits'); it is therefore important to keep the cannula moving but with slower strokes, and a heat-insulating sleeve is needed at the entry site meaning that **larger incisions** are needed. The extra liquefying step before suctioning means that it can take a little longer than conventional liposuction. UAL is a popular choice in the treatment of gynaecomastia.

Ultrasonic assisted liposuction – effect on peripheral nerves

Howard BK. *Plast Reconstr Surg* 1999;**103**:984–989.

Ultrasound-assisted liposuction selectively liquefies fat. Myelin sheaths have a high fat content and so are potentially at risk, however, no adverse sequelae could be demonstrated in a rat sciatic nerve model unless the probe made direct contact with the nerve in which case reversible changes in ultrastructure and conductivity were seen.

Vibration Amplification of Sound Energy at Resonance – VASER

The acronym VASER (Vibration Amplification of Sound Energy at Resonance) is a trade name/term for an ultrasound-assisted system (third generation) of liposuction often referred to as liposelection. The ultrasound energy is pulsed and delivered from specially designed probes with grooves along the sides that are said to allow ultrasound energy to be delivered in a safer manner, supposedly preserving blood vessels, nerves and fibrous tissue more than conventional UAL. Its use is increasing and it is often used for sculpting of body contours, particularly the 'six pack' (Vaser Hi Def$_{TM}$).

Tissue temperatures during ultrasound-assisted lipoplasty
Ablaza VJ. *Plast Reconstr Surg* 1998;**102**:534–542.

Subcutaneous temperature probes were used to measure tissue temperatures during UAL.

- Infiltration of tumescent fluid at room temperature dropped tissue temperature to ~24 °C but this rapidly recovered to ~32 °C; thus tumescent fluid may reduce elevation of tissue temperature during UAL, though it had no effect on core temperature which remained in a narrow range (35.7–36.3 °C).
- During the procedure tissue temperatures remained stable except when treating the thighs, when temperature rose to 41 °C but this did not result in a burn.

Ultrasound-assisted lipoplasty: a clinical study of 250 consecutive patients
Maxwell GP. *Plast Reconstr Surg* 1998;**101**:189–202.

UAL effectively treats fibrous areas such as the male breast whilst also being less physically demanding on the operator. There is very little bruising after UAL but seromas seem to be more frequent. It is generally recommended that aggressive superficial UAL (stay ~10 mm from the dermis) should be avoided.

Body contouring with external ultrasound
Kinney BM. *Plast Reconstr Surg* 1999;**103**:728–729.

External ultrasound used in the presence of tumescent fluid before liposuction with the aim of heating up and cavitation of fat. Constant motion of the ultrasound paddles and application of hydrogel is required to prevent burn injury to the skin (which has been reported).

The use of external ultrasound was introduced by Silberg in 1998. The paper above was a Safety report and concluded that further data was awaited. There was a rash of papers soon after but overall, external UAL is not widely used and evidence of its usefulness is conflicting.

The effect of ultrasound-assisted liposuction and conventional liposuction on the perforator vessels of the abdominal wall
Blondeel PN. *Br J Plast Surg* 2003;**56**:266–271.

The authors used a cadaveric study to explore the theory that ultrasound-assisted liposuction is less traumatic to perforating vessels perfusing an abdominal skin flap than conventional liposuction. The territory of a lower abdominal skin flap was marked out and each half subjected to the following procedures:

- Infiltration of tumescent solution plus UAL vs. control.
- Infiltration of tumescent solution plus UAL vs. infiltration.
- Infiltration of tumescent solution plus UAL vs. infiltration plus conventional liposuction.
- A typical formula of 25 ml of 2% lidocaine, 1 ml of 1:1000 adrenaline in 1 L of crystalloid will give approximately (since volume is 1026 ml) 0.05% lidocaine and 1 in 10^6 adrenaline.

After each experiment the abdominal flap was removed and radio-opaque injection studies were undertaken by injecting the deep inferior epigastric arteries on each side.

This was followed by a human volunteer study, where tumescent solution was infiltrated plus UAL vs. infiltration plus conventional liposuction prior to removing skin and fat as an abdominoplasty procedure. There was **no significant difference** in the degree of vessel disruption between UAL and conventional liposuction.

Tumescent technique

This technique was introduced by Klein in 1986 as a measure to reduce operative pain and bleeding whilst assisting the passage of the cannula as a lubricant of sorts. Most use something that lies between 'superwet' (roughly equivalent to the estimated aspirate) and tumescent.

The 'classic' tumescent formula combines 1 L of normal saline with 50 mL of 1% lidocaine, 1 mL of 1:1000 adrenaline and 2.5 mL of 8.4% sodium bicarbonate. The solution is injected until the tissues are swollen, firm and under pressure ('fountain sign'), with injection into the deep tissues before the superficial. Blanching is seen after 10 minutes but the vasoconstriction is more effective after waiting for another 10 minutes. There are many different formulae in use but for most:

- Blood loss is reduced to 1–2% of aspirate volume compared with > 40% without adrenaline.
- Adrenaline is effective in dilutions of up to 1 in a million (though it takes longer to work).
- Large doses of local anaesthetic are infiltrated but it is absorbed slowly and some is re-aspirated. Bupivacaine provides long-lasting anaesthesia and is sometimes combined with or replaces lidocaine.

At least 70% of the total volume of tumescent fluid remains in the tissues and intravascular space at the end of the procedure, thus it is important to avoid infiltrating large volumes in the elderly or those with congestive heart failure.

Fluid resuscitation after liposuction

Tumescent liposuction. A surgeon's perspective
Pitman GH. *Clin Plast Surg* 1996;**23**:633–641.

- If the volume of tumescent solution infiltrated is greater than twice the aspirated volume, then no fluid resuscitation is required.
- If the volume of the injected tumescent solution is less than twice the aspirate volume, then the deficit is administered.

Safety considerations and fluid resuscitation in liposuction: an analysis of 53 consecutive cases
Trott SA. *Plast Reconstr Surg* 1998;**102**:2220–2229.

The authors state that assuming that 70% of the infiltrated volume is absorbed into the intravascular space, fluid resuscitation in addition to maintenance needs (5–6 ml/kg/hour) is not necessary in aspirations of less than 4 L. Their suggested guidelines for fluid resuscitation after liposuction were:

- Small volume (< 4 L aspirated): resuscitation is provided by maintenance fluid and the subcutaneous wetting solution infiltrated.
- Large volume (≥ 4 L aspirated): fluid administered includes maintenance needs, subcutaneous wetting solution and additional fluid – 0.25 ml of intravenous crystalloid per ml of aspirate removed after 4 L.

A lower volume of resuscitation fluid aimed to prevent fluid overload. The authors state that urine output is a useful indicator of volaemic status.

Antibacterial effects of tumescent liposuction fluid
Craig SB. *Plast Reconstr Surg* 1999;**103**:666–670.

A low incidence of infection is observed after liposuction (< 0.05%). Whilst there is some evidence that lidocaine has bactericidal properties at concentrations of > 0.8%, studies show no in-vitro growth-inhibiting activity at the dilutions used clinically (0.1% lidocaine, 1:1 million adrenaline and 0.012 mEq sodium bicarbonate).

Tumescent technique: the effect of high tissue pressure and dilute epinephrine on absorption of lidocaine
Rubin JP. *Plast Reconstr Surg* 1999;**103**:990–996.

During routine liposuction the 'safe' dose of lidocaine is often exceeded 4–5× (35 mg/kg, peaking at about 12 hours i.e. well after surgery). In this study, 7 mg/kg lidocaine was injected with or without 1:1 million adrenaline into healthy volunteers and serum levels were measured.

- There was a slower rise in serum levels in adrenaline solutions but the peak concentration was the same with or without adrenaline.
- High- or low-pressure injection techniques did not influence absorption.

Although lidocaine has vasodilatory properties, the vasoconstrictive effect of adrenaline is greater.

- Dilution of both lidocaine and adrenaline in the tumescent solution causes **net vasoconstriction** as 1:1 million adrenaline has a biological effect whereas 0.1% lidocaine has little or none (in terms of vasodilation). The reduction in local blood flow to the area inhibits absorption, thus giving high total doses of lidocaine is safe.

IX. Abdominoplasty

Fat anatomy

- The fat above Scarpa's fascia is compact with many fibrous septae.
- The fat below Scarpa's fascia is globular with fewer fibrous septae; its distribution is responsible for the typical sex-related body shapes.

It is usually said that the number of fat cells in adults is fixed and moderate weight gain is accompanied by fat cell hypertrophy – cell hyperplasia usually only occurs in massive weight gain.

Umbilicus

The umbilicus is exactly in the midline in only 17% (Rohrich 2003), lying halfway between the xiphoid and pubis at the level of the superior iliac crest. The shape is extremely variable (outie vs. innie, etc), though many regard the ideal umbilicus to have superior hooding, inferior retraction and relatively shallow and narrow in the vertical axis (resulting in an almost 'T' shape sometimes). Sensation comes from T10 (the whole abdomen is T7–12) with nerves running in the plane between the internal oblique and transversalis abdominis muscles.

Arterial vascular anatomy of the umbilicus
Stokes RB. *Plast Reconstr Surg* 1998;**102**:761–764.

The blood supply comes from several sources including the subdermal plexus and several deep sources – small branches from the deep inferior epigastric arteries, ligamentum teres and the median umbilical ligament. The latter two are smaller vessels constituting a minor source normally but that would be the only source in a bilateral TRAM patient.

Huger's zones (1979) of blood supply to the anterior abdominal skin, can be used as a guide in planning a safe operation:

- Huger zone I – the central zone supplied by the vertical deep epigastric arcade.
- Huger zone II – the lower abdomen is supplied by superior epigastric, external pudendal and circumflex iliac arteries.
- Huger zone III – the lateral zone/flanks supplied by the 6 lateral intercostal arteries and 4 lumbar arteries.

During an abdominoplasty, zone I and II supplies are divided with the flap dependent on zone III. Liposuction in zone III may theoretically interfere with perfusion to the upper skin flap and thus should be used judiciously. Matarasso wrote about the 'safe zones' for liposuction in abdominoplasty.

Matarasso classification

The majority of abdominoplasty procedures carried out are type IV. There is a trend that moves away from the 'traditional' method of wide flap elevation – a central column is raised wide enough to allow rectus plication (thus reducing the elevation in the subcostal region).

Table 10.2 Matarasso classification of patients with reference to treatment of abdominal tissue excess.

Type	Features	Treatment
I	Excess fat only	Liposuction
II	Mild skin excess Infra-umbilical divarication	Mini abdominoplasty, infra-umbilical plication and liposuction
III	Moderate skin excess Divarication above and below	Mini abdominoplasty, plication above and below umbilicus + liposuction
IV	Severe skin excess Severe rectus divarication	Standard abdominoplasty + sheath plication + liposuction

Assessment

The aims of an abdominoplasty are to improve contour whilst minimizing scarring and maintaining a natural umbilicus.

- The patient's complaints and expectations should be elicited. Smoking and use of anticoagulants including herbal remedies is particularly relevant.

Examine the patient for skin excess and for musculoaponeurotic laxity (diastasis of the recti), and also scars. The incision lines and expected scar lines should be discussed with the patient; they can be tailored to their preferred types of underwear/swimwear to a certain extent. Prepare an abdominal binder/pressure garment for the patient to wear immediately postoperatively.

- A **mini-abdominoplasty** removes infra-umbilical skin excess without the need to reposition the umbilicus. A traditional abdominoplasty removes the entire abdominal skin excess, usually to a point above the umbilicus with undermining of the flap to the costal margins.
- Use the **fleur-de-lis technique** for those with vertical skin excess; this is particularly suited to those who have experienced significant weight loss.
- **Reverse abdominoplasty** (Baroudi 1979) has been suggested using a W-shaped inframammary incision.

Typical technique

- Antibiotics, DVT prophylaxis e.g. intermittent compression devices, and urinary catheter.

- A folding table is needed. Ensure that the placement of the hips is correct.
- Subcutaneous infiltration of tumescent solution reduces blood loss.
- Use a lower incision within the pubic hairline 5–7 cm above the anterior vulval commissure and bevel the upper skin flap edge. Most incisions are variations of Regnault or the 'handlebar'. Watch for the lateral cutaneous nerve of the thigh in the lateral part of the incision.
- Raise the abdominal flap as needed. Leaving the flimsy fascia overlying the rectus sheath (fascia of Gallaudet) may help reduce seroma; other strategies including quilting sutures.
- Plicate the rectus sheath if there is any diastasis with two continuous sutures (e.g. looped nylon) – one above and one below the umbilicus to avoid umbilical strangulation. A long umbilicus stalk can be tacked to the abdominal fascia (with needles left attached, and then brought through the new aperture later on). De-fat in the midline below the umbilicus. Others suggest additional paramedian and transverse plication.
  - Plication seems to increase post-operative pain; some inject bupivacaine locally.
- Fold the table and excise the excess tissue. Do not make the skin closure over-tight. The superficial fascial system should be closed separately.
- The use of drains is common, though some have suggested that the use of quilting/'adhesion' sutures obviates this need (Arantes HL. *Aesth Plast Surg* 2010;**34**:102–104) whilst others have suggested that quilting sutures do not reduce the incidence of seromas after abdominoplasty (Ovens L. *Eur J Plast Surg* 2009;**32**:177–180).

Complications

- Early.
  - Umbilical necrosis.
  - Flap necrosis (especially in smokers), wound dehiscence/infection (10%).
  - Haematoma, seroma (up to 24%).
  - Injury to lateral cutaneous nerve (10%).
  - Thromboembolic complications approximately 0.1%. Death, though rare, may result from PE.
- Late.
  - Scarring and altered sensation, revisional surgery may be needed e.g. for dog ears (up to a third).

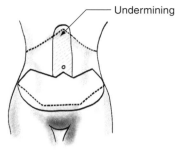
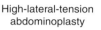
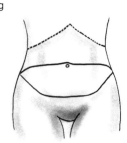

High-lateral-tension abdominoplasty

Traditional abdominoplasty

Figure 10.6 High-lateral-tension abdominoplasty – undermining is restricted to the paramedian area for muscle plication.

Male abdominoplasty patients are more likely to be dissatisfied which may be due in part to less realistic expectations, to their thicker, less elastic skin and having a larger amount of intra-abdominal fat.

High-lateral-tension abdominoplasty

High-lateral-tension abdominoplasty was described by Lockwood in 1995. The technique is based on the belief that epigastric skin excess is primarily horizontal whilst infra-umbilical skin excess is horizontal, thus less skin should be taken centrally and more laterally compared with a traditional abdominoplasty. This results in an oblique lift vector and an element of lift to the anterior and lateral thigh.

Subcostal undermining is minimized; only the central portion is raised to allow rectus sheath plication.

Fleur-de-lis abdominoplasty

The fleur-de-lis (French for 'lily flower') abdominoplasty is an abdominoplasty with a component of vertical skin resection, and is particularly used in patients who have lost large amounts of weight e.g. after bariatric surgery.

Fleur-de-Lis abdominoplasty: a safe alternative to traditional abdominoplasty for the massive weight loss patient

Friedman T. *Plast Reconstr Surg* 2010;**125**:1525–1535.

The rectus plication and resection of the transverse component is performed first, and then towel clips are used to judge the vertical tissue excess which is then removed by excising to just below the xiphisternum. There should be minimal undermining to maximize the number of perforators to the skin flaps. The superficial fascial system is closed and the umbilicus set in the incision line without excising additional skin to reduce widening. The authors reported a minor complication rate of 26.3% and major complication rate of 5.6%.

Fleur-de-lys abdominoplasty. A consecutive case series
Duff C. *Br J Plast Surg* 2003;**56**:557–566.

This is a retrospective review of 68 procedures. The authors emphasize the minimal undermining of skin flaps. Rectus diastasis was corrected as necessary but liposuction was not performed. Two-thirds of patients developed one or more complications postoperatively.

- Early wound dehiscence/infection in nine patients.
- Delayed wound healing in 17 patients.
- Aesthetic complications in 12 patients.

In this study, there was no correlation between:

- Smoking and risk of a complication.
- BMI and wound breakdown in this series.

However, there was a correlation between complications and increasing age, increasing BMI/weight and mass of tissue resected.

Should diastasis recti be corrected?
Nahas FX. *Aesthetic Plast Surg* 1997;**21**:285–289.

The recti muscles maintained their corrected position (2 layer 2'0 nylon repair) as assessed by CT up to 6 months post-operatively in a group of 14 patients.

Pregnancy
Abdominoplasty is generally not advised when the patient plans to become pregnant in the near future. Apart from the effects on the aesthetics, there is concern that the reduced abdominal wall flexibility may pose risks to both the mother (fascial tears, organ compression) and child.

Pregnancy after abdominoplasty
Menz P. *Plast Reconstr Surg* 1996;**98**:377–378.

Pregnancy after abdominoplasty is possible but where midline rectus sheath plication has been performed the pregnancy should be closely monitored, with delivery by an elective Caesarean section.

Pregnancy in the early period after abdominoplasty
Borman H. *Plast Reconstr Surg* 2002;**109**:396–397.

This is another report of a successful pregnancy in a patient who became pregnant 2 months after surgery.

Pregnancy after abdominoplasty
Nahas FX. *Aesth Plast Surg* 2002;**26**:284–286.

A patient had an uneventful pregnancy 2.5 years after abdominoplasty with correction of rectus diastasis. A CT scan after the pregnancy demonstrated that the correction was intact.

General plastic surgery

I. Skin grafts

Classification of skin grafts

Skin grafts can be classified in many ways, for example according to:

- Thickness/composition: split thickness, full thickness, composite (more than one type of tissue).
- Origin: autograft, allograft, xenograft.

Skin graft take

The take of skin grafts is traditionally described as consisting of four phases: adherence, plasmatic imbibition, revascularization and remodelling.

- **Adherence** – fibrin bonds form between the graft and recipient bed leading to adherence, which, at least empirically, seems stronger on fascia and granulation tissue. The relatively weak adherence can be disrupted by shear forces etc. (see Skin graft failure to take). Fibroblasts in a skin graft are derived from circulating monocytes or perivascular mesenchymal cells, and by the third day there is ingrowth of collagen from these fibroblasts (and formation of vascular channels) that strengthens the attachment.
- **Plasmatic imbibition** – the breakdown of intracellular proteoglycans in graft cells leads to more osmotically active subunits, causing absorption of interstitial fluid by osmosis, and thus graft swelling and oedema.

- **Revascularization** – the circulation to a skin graft is restored after 4–7 days with thicker grafts taking longer as might be expected. Two of the mechanisms put forward to explain the restoration of a blood supply include pre-existing blood vessels linking up with graft vessels (inosculation) or ingrowth/formation of new vessels (angiogenesis); they may co-exist. Lymphatic circulation is restored after approximately 1 week.
- **Remodelling/graft maturation** – from day 7 onwards, this includes epidermal hyperplasia (increased mitoses from day 3 onwards) and contracture of the graft bed.
  - **Appendages:** regeneration can occur especially of sweat glands and hair follicles. Hair is usually noticeable after 14 days in well-vascularized full thickness skin grafts (FTSG), however full thickness grafts tolerate ischaemia poorly and may lose appendages.
  - **Re-innervation:** nerves enter existing neurilemmal sheaths (thus more in FTSG). Sensory re-innervation of split skin grafts (SSG) occurs faster (from 3–4 weeks onwards) than FTSG but will probably be less complete. Final sensation may approximate that of adjacent skin unless bed is severely scarred. For example an SSG on the fingertip will have an average two-point discrimination (2 pd) of 5 mm, compared with 3 mm on corresponding area of finger on normal opposite hand. The 2 pd is worse if the recipient bed is scarred; another qualifier is the availability of end organs in the grafts

e.g. Meissner's corpuscles are only found in glabrous skin.

○ Sympathetic innervation of **sweat glands** can be re-established and resultant sweating activity tends to parallel the recipient site (e.g. emotion vs. temperature) rather than the donor site.

○ **Pigmentation:** pigment changes in skin grafts are usually temporary but good colour match can be achieved with carefully selected donor sites. The occurrence of hyperpigmentation can be reduced somewhat by avoiding ultraviolet stimulation of melanocytes by reducing deliberate exposure to sunlight. Hyperpigmented grafts may be treated by dermabrasion.

○ **Contraction.** Although usually undesirable e.g. ectropion from cheek SSGs, some contracture may be beneficial, e.g. SSG grafts on the fingertip contracting to draw sensate skin over the tip.

– Primary contraction is the immediate contraction due to the elastin fibre content of the dermis and thus is greater in FTSG (~40% vs. ~10%).

– Secondary contraction (from day 10 and continues for up to 6 months): the recipient bed, not the skin graft, is the site of contracture. Thicker grafts contract less as dermal elements are said to inhibit myofibroblast contraction. Other factors that decrease graft contracture include a rigid recipient site (e.g. periosteal bed leads to little contracture compared with mobile areas) and greater percentage graft take/less meshing (leaving fewer areas that need to heal by secondary intention).

Skin graft failure to take

● Shear – repeated movement between graft and recipient site. The use of tie-over dressings is common (and many different methods have been described); negative pressure dressings may be useful for graft fixation in more complex situations.

● Haematoma/seroma – increasing the diffusion barrier.

● Infection – e.g. bacterial collagenases. Streptococcal infection (classically group A beta

haemolytic) is regarded as particularly deleterious to skin grafting.

● Unsuitable bed (avascular) e.g. bare bone, cartilage, tendon.

Aftercare

● Avoid ultraviolet exposure to reduce hyperpigmentation.

● Use emollients to moisturize grafts until sebaceous activity returns.

● Use pressure garments if hypertrophic scarring occurs.

● Protection: sensory return begins at 3–4 weeks and can continue to improve for 2 years.

SSG vs. FTSG

Full thickness skin grafts potentially offer a better cosmetic and functional outcome.

● Adnexal structures are better maintained in FTSG and there is a potential for hair transplantation e.g. eyebrows can be reconstructed with strip full thickness grafts of hairy scalp, though it is not the best method.

● There is more (secondary) contraction (of the recipient/wound bed) following SSG, thus making it unsuitable for resurfacing areas such as the face, particularly lower eyelid/upper cheek and the hand, particularly digits.

However:

● SSGs survive better during the phase of plasmic imbibition and can tolerate longer revascularization times, and in general will offer more guaranteed take. This is more relevant in less than optimal recipient sites.

● Harvesting SSG leaves less donor-site morbidity when large areas are needed. Some may argue that a good linear scar e.g. in the groin or post/pre-auricular creases after FTG harvest is very well tolerated. On the other hand, the final appearance will be poorer when an FTSG donor site has to be closed by an SSG (e.g. when harvesting large blocks of FTSG for resurfacing the face).

○ There are many different strategies for dressing the SSG donor site and though the healing times may be similar, other factors such as patient comfort and fewer dressing changes may be significant factors.

II. Other tissue grafts

Bone grafts

(See also wound healing.)

The manner of 'take' of a bone graft (and contributions of osteoconduction, osteoinduction and osteogenesis) depends on the composition of bone.

- Cortical bone tends to form a non-viable scaffold matrix. The osteocytes within lacunae die leaving an intact Haversian canal system and graft take occurs by **osteoconduction** i.e. the bone graft is a scaffold or surface to 'conduct' cells at the recipient bone ends, which migrate, proliferate and carry out their functions. In effect, there is osteoclastic resorption and osteoblastic deposition and eventual replacement of the cortical bone graft. Characteristically there is initially high strength that decreases with bone resorption and is regained after remodelling is complete.
- Cancellous bone consists of morcellized pieces of bone that are readily vascularized by surrounding tissues and the presence of viable osteoblasts in the graft allow **osteogenesis** and contribute to new bone growth. **Osteoinduction** can occur by factors such as bone morphogenetic proteins (BMPs, which are the most widely studied) or other factors that cause undifferentiated mesenchymal cells to differentiate along osteoblastic pathways. Consequently such grafts tend to have initially low tensile strength but this increases as more bone is incorporated.

The most basic requirement for a bone graft to work is for it to be **osteoinductive**; osteoinduction and osteogenesis will theoretically promote faster integration of the graft.

- **Distraction osteogenesis** – just as bone is resorbed when exposed to compressive forces, it is laid down when exposed to tension forces.

Cartilage grafts: due to the low metabolic requirements of cartilage, take of a cartilage graft is generally high as long as it can be vascularized by surrounding tissues. One of the commonest applications is in rhinoplasty. Perichondrium usually needs to be excluded, for example in precise reconstructions, as its chondrogenic potential may distort the graft. Donor options for nasal reconstructions include:

- Septal cartilage – easily harvested, good for structural support but limited in quantity.

- Auricular/conchal cartilage (elastic cartilage) – tends to be curved and relatively thin, thus less useful for support but can be used for the tip and alar. It is more brittle than septal cartilage making it more difficult to carve.
- Costal cartilage – large amounts are available but the potentially poor donor scar limits its wider use. In addition, when it needs to be carved it tends to warp; unilateral carving/scoring often leads to curling (Gibson's principle). Calcification typically occurs after the ages of 50 or so, making it more difficult to carve but less liable to deform.

Fat grafts: Fat is a well-vascularized tissue with high metabolic activity. The number of fat cells in an individual is generally assumed to be stable after the completion of adolescent growth, and subsequent changes in the overall volume of fatty tissue relate to the size of the cells and their overall lipid content, rather than their number. Conversely, fat cells will shrink with overall weight loss and, in fact, may de-differentiate. Fat cells removed by liposuction or other surgical procedures do not regenerate but subsequent weight gain causes redifferentiation of the remaining cells with a resultant increase in volume.

The choice of fluid for fat suspension is somewhat controversial; most commonly, normal saline or Ringer's lactate is used, whilst serum-free culture medium is also available, but it is more expensive. Some groups advocate additives such as heparin, insulin, vitamin E and non-steroidal anabolic hormones. The contribution of lidocaine is also debatable.

Fat cells can be disrupted by the harvesting and refining process, thus care is needed (e.g. Coleman technique) to maximize cell survival. Viable fat cells will survive if they can receive nutrients from the surrounding tissues, thus survival is improved by injecting in small aliquots.

- Host replacement theory – host histiocytes invade the fat graft, take on lipids and eventually replace the adipose tissue of graft.
- Cell survival theory – after revascularization, histiocytes acts as fat scavengers (also removing dead/dying graft cells) but do not replace graft adipose tissue. Healthy living adipocytes in the graft maintain the adipose tissue. This theory is more favoured.

Dermal fat grafts: dermis is included in the graft, adding collagen bulk and may improve take (compared with a block fat graft alone).

Table 11.1 The common types of collagen.

Number	Distribution	Disorders
I	Bone, skin, tendon, ligaments, cornea	Deficient in osteogeneis imperfecta
II	Cartilage, vitreous humour of eye	Deficient in chondrodysplasia
III	Skin, blood vessels, intestines, uterus	Excessive: early wound, early Dupuytren's contracture, hypertrophic scar Deficient: Ehlers–Danlos syndrome
IV	Basal laminae, eye lens	
V	Associated with type I	Found in active stage Dupuytren's contracture

Collagen synthesis

Collagen is a triple helix formed from three α-helical chains. Twenty-five different α-chains have been identified, each encoded by a separate gene. There are at least 16 different types of collagen but 90% of body collagen is type I. In normal skin the ratio of types I:III = 3:1.

- Synthesis from gene translation forms the pro-α-chains, with post-translational hydroxylation of proline and lysine residues (this requires vitamin C and iron).
- Pro-α-chains are assembled into pro-collagen which is then secreted out of the cell in secretory vesicles.
- Cleavage of pro-peptides on α-chains converts pro-collagen into collagen with covalent cross-linking between collagen molecules forming fibrils, followed by aggregation of fibrils into fibres.

III. Local flaps and Z-plasty

Types of local flap

Flaps should be raised to include at least full thickness skin to reduce secondary contraction, whilst taking care to avoid including too much bulk/fat that would impede flap movement; in practice, the flap includes the subdermal plexus along with a little subcutaneous fat.

Reading man   Rhomboid

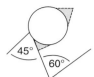 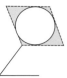

Figure 11.1 Reading man flap (a type of unequal Z-plasty) for closure of circular defects. It sacrifices less healthy tissue (ratio 1:2.5 approximately) than a rhomboid flap.

Flaps that move about a pivot point

- **Rotation flap:** a semicircular flap that rotates about a pivot point through an arc of rotation into an adjacent defect. The donor site either closes directly (buttock rotation flap) or with a skin graft (e.g. scalp rotation flap). Back cuts may be needed.
- **Advancement flap:** a flap that moves forwards without rotation or lateral movement e.g. V–Y, Y–V, Reiger flap on the nasal dorsum, lip advancement techniques. Rectangular advancement flaps usually require excision of Burow's triangles.
- **Transposition flap:** a flap that moves laterally about a pivot point into an adjacent defect e.g. Limberg flap, bilobed flap and Z-plasty. Other examples include a posterior thigh flap for ischial sores. A hatchet flap is probably a combination of rotation and transposition; it can be likened to a rotation with a large back cut.
- **Interpolation:** a flap that moves laterally about a pivot point into a defect which is not immediately adjacent to it e.g. nasolabial island flap to the nasal tip and a deltopectoral flap to the head and neck. Some describe this as an islanded flap.
- **Z-plasty:** technique involving the transposition of two adjacent triangular flaps and at the completion of the transposition the 'Z' has rotated by 90°. All limbs of the 'Z' must be of equal length though the angles (between 30° and 90°) do not have to be the same (this asymmetric variety is sometimes referred to as the skewed Z-plasty). Although it had been described before, the geometry was worked out by Limberg in 1929.

The **actual length gain** is less than the theoretical length gain due to the visco-elastic properties of skin, and the actual gain is proportionately less with shorter limbs. In clinical practice, 60° permits a maximal length gain **whilst still allowing easy transposition of the two triangles.** The tension required to close a

Table 11.2 The effect of the angle of Z-plasty flaps and the theoretical length gains.

Angle of flaps (°)	Theoretical gain in length (%)
30	25
45	50
60	75
90	100

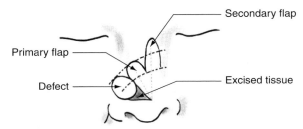

Figure 11.2 Bilobed flap for reconstruction of a nasal defect (Zitelli modification). The smaller angle between defect and adjacent flaps is about 45° which reduces the size of the standing cone. Secondary flap is longer and thinner. It may cause alar rim retraction and should not be used if the rim is less than 10 mm away from the defect.

90°–90° Z-plasty is 10 times that required to close a 30°–30° Z-plasty, though to reduce this tension, the 90°–90° Z-plasty could be divided into four flaps, each with an angle of 45°.

Greater gain in length is achieved by **one large Z-plasty** than by multiple small Z-plasties whose total central limb length is equal. Although length gain is additive, the field of tension exerted by each Z-plasty affects the neighbouring flaps and thereby reduces actual overall length gain and the tissue recruited laterally is equivalent to that of one small Z-plasty alone. However, lateral skin availability may be limited so a single large Z-plasty may not always be practical. In addition, in axillary surgery, the 'unwanted' transposition of hair-bearing skin is reduced with smaller multiple flaps.

Z-plasties are useful to:

- Transpose normal tissue into a critical area, e.g. return a vermilion step into alignment.
- Break up a linear scar and change the direction of a scar.

- Lengthen a scar, e.g. burn scar contracture, lip lengthening with the Tennison cleft repair.
- Treat a web. Some authors emphasise that the problem is multiplanar.

Tip necrosis may be a complication particularly in previously burnt/scarred skin; using wide or rounded tips may help in addition to careful tissue handling, and avoid directly suturing the tip, using glue or steri-strips instead.

Some thoughts on chooosing the Z-plasty: the Z made simple

Hudson DA. *Plast Reconstr Surg* 2000;**106**:665–671.
Multiple Z-plasties:

- **Z-plasties in series:** the central flaps tend to develop a square shape and do not interdigitate easily. This technique may be better applied to a long scar with less lateral tissue available (e.g. correcting volar skin shortage associated with Dupuytren's contracture).
- **Double opposing Z-plasty:** a Z-plasty in reverse follows a Z-plasty; this produces triangular flaps that interdigitate easily.
- **Four-flap Z-plasty:** wide flaps of either 90° or 120° are bisected into two sets of flaps. This produces good length gain, equal to that of two individual 45° or 60° Z-plasties (100% and 150%) but the flaps are easier to transpose as triangles. There are two possible end results depending on which triangle moves the least. It represents two Z-plasties **in parallel** and is better applied to a short scar with a greater amount of lateral tissue available e.g. **deepening a web space.** Adding another triangle of the outside of each side produces a six-flap Z-plasty (described by Mir L. *Plast Reconstr Surg* 1973;**52**:625–628).
- **Five-flap Z-plasty:** a double opposing Z-plasty that incorporates a V–Y advancement and is otherwise known as a 'jumping man flap'. The length gain of 125% is better than a double opposing Z-plasty alone but has less lengthening than a four-flap Z-plasty for a given scar length.
- **'Single' limb Z-plasty:** used to introduce a triangular flap of skin into an area of skin shortage, it breaks up the contracted scar but does not offer the mechanical advantages of the Z-plasty.

465

IV. Pedicled and free flaps

Blood supply of the skin

Cutaneous arteries

The arterial supply of the skin comes from:

- Direct branches of segmental arteries (concentration of direct cutaneous perforators near axial lines and intermuscular septae).
- Perforating branches from nutrient vessels supplying deep tissues especially muscle, i.e. indirect.

Plexuses are formed at different levels:

- Subepidermal.
- Dermal.
- Subdermal.
- Fascial.
- Subfascial.

There are anastomoses between neighbouring cutaneous arteries:

- True anastomoses do not have a change in calibre.
- Choke vessels, which have reduced calibre or are closed under normal circumstances but dilate to restore blood flow to areas of flap ischaemia.

Cutaneous veins

There are oscillating veins (valved or avalvular) in the subdermal plexuses with bidirectional flow between adjacent venous territories with equilibration of flow and pressure.

- Valved channels tend to direct blood away from a venous plexus or towards a central draining vein.
- Interconnecting system of choke veins, tend to be oscillating.

The vascular territories (angiosomes) of the body
Taylor GI. *Br J Plast Surg* 1987;**40**:113–141.

Three-dimensional blocks of tissue supplied by a single artery and its venae comitantes are called angiosomes and venosomes respectively. Adjacent angiosomes are connected by true anastomoses or small calibre choke vessels; flaps can be larger than one angiosome as choke vessels allow perfusion from adjacent angiosomes.

Junctional zones tend to occur within muscles, hence muscle choke vessels dilate to provide collateral circulation to an adjacent angiosome. If one source vessel is small, the adjacent source vessel is usually large – 'law of equilibrium'.

Delay phenomenon

This term is used to describe the practice of elevating part of a flap (and thus dividing part of its vascular supply) for the purpose of expanding the territory prior to further elevation and definitive transfer. The mechanism underlying this is not fully understood.

- Conditions the flap to survive with reduced blood flow (metabolic adaptation to hypoxia).
- Partially sympathectomizes the flap to facilitate opening of choke vessels and angiogenesis.
- Choke vessel hypertrophy and hyperplasia maximal at 48–72 h.
- Vascular reorientation along longitudinal axis of flap.

A newly configured A–V circulation is established within 7 days whilst the maximally augmented blood flow occurs at 2–3 weeks. It is said that delay will be optimal if carried out in stages by elevating flap from base to tip. Tissue expansion is considered a type of delay whilst the delay phenomenon is also exploited in flap prefabrication.

- One method of testing vascularity involves injecting 20 ml 5% fluorescein IV and then observing the pattern of yellow–green fluorescence under UV light (Wood's lamp) in a darkened room.

Skin flaps – Mathes and Nahai classification

Direct cutaneous flaps:

- Axial cutaneous arteries, e.g. groin, scapular area.
- The horizontal cutaneous vessels travel in loose connective tissue rather than on the deep fascia. There is usually soft tissue laxity.

Fasciocutaneous flaps:

- The horizontal cutaneous vessels lie on the deep fascia which is not strictly essential to the flap vascularity. However, it is difficult to separate the vessels off the fascia so it is safest to include the fascial layer in the flap.
- The skin is relatively immobile over deep fascia, e.g. limbs, scalp.
- Cutaneous nerves often travel parallel to vessels; hence, many fasciocutaneous flaps are neurosensory.

Septocutaneous flaps – the perforators come from the subfascial source vessel and course along intermuscular septae, e.g. lateral arm flap ('in-transit perforators').

Musculocutaneous flaps – occasionally perforators arise as indirect branches from muscle branches off the source vessel (gluteal area).

Classification of fasciocutaneous flaps

Mathes and Nahai

- Type A: Direct cutaneous perforator.
- Type B: Septocutaneous perforator.
- Type C: Musculocutaneous perforator.

Cormack and Lamberty

- Type A: Multiple perforators.
- Type B: Solitary perforator.
- Type C: Segmental perforator.

Classification of flaps according to their blood supply

- **Random pattern** flap relies for its vascularity upon the vessels of the dermal and subdermal plexuses of the skin.
- **Axial pattern** flap is vascularized by vessels running longitudinally within it:
  - Direct cutaneous artery.
  - Fasciocutaneous artery.
  - Septocutaneous artery.
  - Muscle perforators.

Blood supply of muscles

Mathes and Nahai classification

A dominant pedicle is defined as a vessel which can perfuse the whole muscle. If there is only one dominant pedicle then this is critical to muscle survival; where more than one vessel is dominant, these are called **major** vessels.

- **Non-dominant or minor** pedicle – vessels that cannot support the whole muscle on their own; may be variable in number.

Muscle flaps need to be raised on dominant pedicles; a portion of the muscle can be based on a minor pedicle but the whole muscle will not survive.

- I – one dominant pedicle, e.g. TFL, gastrocnemius.
- II – dominant pedicle(s) plus minor pedicle(s), e.g. gracilis, soleus. The commonest type of muscle flap.
  - Delaying a type II muscle flap by ligation of a non-dominant vessel may improve survival.
    - A portion of the muscle can be based on a minor pedicle.
- III – two dominant pedicles, e.g. pectoralis minor, serratus, rectus abdominis, temporalis, gluteus maximus. Type III muscles are suited to split design, e.g. pectoralis minor for facial reanimation, with slips to orbit and angle of the mouth.
  - Some surgeons propose ligation of the inferior epigastric pedicle some 10 days before harvesting of a superiorly pedicled TRAM flap.
- IV – segmental supply, e.g. sartorius. Muscle will not survive if too many segmental vessels are divided.
- V – one dominant plus segmental vessels e.g. latissimus dorsi, pectoralis major. Such flaps will survive if the dominant vessel is ligated as long as all/most of the segmental vessels are preserved, e.g. pectoralis major turnover flap for sternal defects. Some have investigated the effects of delaying the latissimus dorsi by ligating the segmental perforator vessels, e.g. prior to harvest for cardiomyoplasty.

Taylor classification of muscle innervation

- I – single nerve, branches within the muscle e.g. latissimus dorsi.
- II – single nerve, branches before entering the muscle e.g. vastus lateralis.
- III – multiple nerves from the same nerve trunk e.g. serratus anterior.
- IV – segmental nerve supply e.g. rectus abdominis.

Free and pedicled flaps and their application

A free flap is a composite block of tissue that is moved from a donor site to a distant recipient site where its circulation is restored by microvascular anastomosis. A pedicled flap keeps its circulation intact during transfer which is thus limited by the vascular axis.

Flap selection

- The aim is to replace like with like: the types and volume of tissue required are determined by the defect.
  - Sensate or insensate.
- Donor site availability.
  - Ease of harvesting including changes of position.
- Recipient vessels available and matching to the length of pedicle needed.

Anaesthesia

- Keep the patient warm and well filled whilst avoiding vasoconstrictors.
- Muscle relaxation.
- Monitor volume status with urine output and haematocrit (0.30–0.35).
- Prevention of pressure sores.

Flap monitoring

Clinical monitoring remains the most commonly used and the most practical.

- Colour.
- Refill.
- Temperature.
- Bleeding on pinprick.

Other methods include:

- Temperature (δ-T, i.e. the difference between the flap temperature and control site temperature).
- Doppler signal – the presence of neighbouring vessels can be misleading; some use implantable Doppler probes.
- Oxygen saturation.
- Transcutaneous oxygen saturation/thermography/ laser Doppler/near infra-red spectrometry.

Monitoring of **buried flaps** e.g. in pharyngeal reconstruction offers another challenge and methods that have been described include:

- Implantable Doppler probes popularized by Swartz (Swartz WM. *Plast Reconstr Surg* 1994;**93**:152).
- Surface Doppler probe (with or without markings on the skin surface) – may be prone to misinterpretation due to interference from other vessels.
- Exteriorized segment of flap e.g. skin, muscle or mucosa (in jejunal flaps), that may be incorporated into the skin closure or divided secondarily. Window technique (Bafitis H. *Plast Reconstr Surg* 1989;**83**:896–897).
- Exteriorized vessel stumps (Yang JC. *Ann Plast Surg* 2007;**59**:378–381).
- Endoscopy (but not contrast swallows) for pharyngeal reconstructions.

Lining of the microanastomosis

- Day 1–3 platelets.

- Day 4–14 pseudointima.
- Day 14 intima.

Causes of free flap failure

- Mechanical: problem with anastomosis or pedicle such as kinking, twisting, stretching or compression e.g. by haematoma or by brachytherapy tubes.
- Hydrostatic.
  - ○ Inadequate perfusion (hypovolaemia, spasm, hypothermia).
  - ○ Inadequate drainage (inadequate vein size, dependency, shunting via a superficial system).
- Thrombosis: traumatized vessels due to surgical dissection or using vessels in a zone of injury.
  - ○ Hypercoagulable states.
  - ○ Reperfusion injury (prolonged ischaemia time).

Maximum warm ischaemia times (maximum cold ischaemia)

- Jejunum less than 2 hours.
- Muscle less than 2 hours (8 hours).
- Bone flaps less than 3 hours (24 hours).
- Skin and fascia 4–6 hours (12 hours).

Antispasmodics

- Papaverine – salt of opium alkaloid that causes smooth muscle relaxation by adrenoceptor blockade.
- Verapamil – calcium channel inhibitor.
- Lidocaine 2% – membrane stabilization by sodium channel blockade, produces potent local vasodilatation.

No reflow phenomenon

This is the failure of a flap to perfuse after anastomosis which has been shown to be technically satisfactory i.e. patent. It is possibly due to endothelial injury or platelet aggregation, after reperfusion injury, blocking off the microcirculation.

Ischaemia–reperfusion injury: a review
Kerrigan CL. *Microsurgery* 1993;**14**:165–175.

Ischaemia – tissue and cellular hypoxia causes build up of products of anaerobic metabolism, e.g. lactate, in proportion to the metabolic activity of the tissue. This causes disturbance to membrane transport systems, resulting in the influx of calcium into the cell, which triggers the production of inflammatory mediators (heparin, kinins, prostaglandins) by tissue mast cells.

Reperfusion – restoration of perfusion provides oxygen for formation of oxygen free radicals by neutrophils – 'respiratory burst' (xanthine oxidase pathways). Further influx of calcium into cells increases the generation of inflammatory mediators.

Cigarette smoking, plastic surgery and microsurgery
Chang LD. *J Reconstr Microsurg* 1996;**12**:467–474.

There is no proven adverse affect on the actual microanastomosis or free tissue transfer although smoking may compromise healing at the flap–recipient interface and at the donor site. Smokers are advised to stop smoking for at least 3 weeks pre- and post-operatively for the vascular effects; stopping smoking will also benefit general cardiorespiratory function, as well as reducing cancer risk.

There is a thrombogenic state due to effects of smoking on:

- Dermal microvasculature.
- Blood constituents.
- Vasoconstrictive prostaglandins – nicotine leads to increased TXA2 and decreased PGI2.

Carbon monoxide causes formation of carboxyhaemoglobin which exacerbates tissue hypoxia and increased platelet adhesiveness. Overall, there are several adverse effects on surgical procedures:

- Those that involve extensive undermining, e.g. facelift surgery, and thus rely upon subdermal and dermal plexuses.
- Where a block of tissue depends upon a single vascular pedicle for survival, e.g. breast reduction, pedicled TRAM flaps.

Smoking one cigarette reduces blood flow velocity to the hand by 42% for up to 1 hour; thus digital replants are at particular risk in smokers.

Muscle flaps

Muscle-only flaps can provide a large surface area and volume coverage, whilst the donor site can still be closed directly. The flap tissue is well vascularized – a quality that is often said to aid in combating infection.

- Some muscle flaps may be split to allow further customization.
- Some may retain motor function for reanimation/restoring motor function.

Fasciocutaneous flaps

These are often used in the extremities (Pontén B. *Br J Plast Surg* 1981;**34**:215–220). Their advantages include providing a thin, pliable, potentially sensate flap with a useful length:breadth ratio (= 3:1). There is relatively little donor morbidity, and the donor site can often be closed directly.

Perforator flaps

The perceived advantages are of less donor site morbidity (due to sparing of muscles) and patient recovery, as well as more versatility in flap design.

Perforator flap terminology:update 2002
Blondeel PN. *Clin Plastic Surg* 2003;**30**:343–346.

Direct and indirect perforator flaps
Hallock GG. *Plast Reconstr Surg* 2003;**111**:855–865.

A perforator flap is a flap of skin/fat supplied by a perforating branch of the source vessel, passing through deep tissues and fascia to supply the flap.

- Indirect perforators: the perforating vessel passes through muscle and fascia before supplying the flap tissue.
  - Muscle/musculocutaneous perforator – perforating vessel passes through muscle before supplying the flap tissue, e.g. DIEP flap, S-GAP flap and most ALT flaps.
  - Septal/septocutaneous perforator – perforating vessel passes along a fascial septum before supplying the flap tissue e.g. the minority of ALT flaps.
- Direct perforators: these are perforators that pass from the source vessel directly through fascia (but not septum) to supply the overlying tissue (most axial pattern fasciocutaneous flaps of the extremities).

Flaps based on nerves

More specifically, these are flaps based on the vascular axis of nerves.

- Sural flap – this is based on the arterioles around the sural nerve that perfuse the nerve and overlying skin island. The short saphenous vein is included.
- Cephalic flap – this is based on the axis of the lateral cutaneous nerve of the arm; it includes the cephalic vein.

Other flaps

- **Bone flaps** – bone is harvested with endosteal and periosteal circulations maintained, and the flap heals in a similar manner to simple fractures at the flap-recipient interfaces and at the wedge osteotomies used to conform the donor bone.

- **Toe and joint transfers** – replace composite functioning tissues e.g. in thumb reconstruction. The transferred tissue has sensory potential; the donor defect can usually be closed primarily. Toe pulp may be transferred independently.
- **Gastrointestinal flaps** e.g. jejunal. Due to the high metabolic rate of the tissue, it is important to keep ischaemic time to a minimum to avoid mucosal sloughing. Caution is required in patients with a history of previous abdominal surgery.
- Other specialized tissues: vascularized nerves and vascularized tendons.

Leeches

Leeches are annelid worms with 'V'-shaped mouth parts. Their three jaws, each with > 100 teeth, form a 'Mercedes Benz symbol' shape. **Hirudin** is secreted in leech saliva which binds activated thrombin, prevents fibrinogen being converted to fibrin, blocks activation of factors V, VIII, XI and vWF and decreases activation of tPA, protein C and plasmin. Hirudin prolongs thrombin dependent coagulation tests, but there is no direct effect on platelets or endothelial cells.

The leech harbours *Aeromonas hydrophila* in its gut, and there is a risk of transmission to the patient which increases with any regurgitation of blood (e.g. traumatic removal including the use of salt water to detach it). Therefore the use of prophylactic antibiotics (third-generation cephalosporins, quinolones e.g. *ciprofloxacin* or trimethoprim-sulfamethoxazole (TMP-SMX)) is advisable. Leeches are meant to be used once only though some authors have described the use of saline to cause regurgitation and allow re-use in the same patient. They can be ordered as required.

V. Individual flaps

Latissimus dorsi

This a type V muscle flap. The dominant pedicle is the thoracodorsal artery which is the continuation of the subscapular artery from the third part of the axillary artery – this passes through the **triangular space** (when viewed from the front: teres minor (some say subscapularis), teres major and long head of triceps) to gain the posterior axilla. The artery and (usually) single vein are ~2 mm diameter.

The muscle arises from a broad origin stretching from the spinous processes from T7 downwards, and then across to the posterior superior iliac crest. It runs superomedially to converge upon the bicipital groove of the humerus and forms the lower border of the posterior axilla. It is innervated by the thoracodorsal nerve (C6,7,8 – posterior cord of brachial plexus) and on contraction, extends and adducts at the shoulder and also medial rotation of the humerus. The best way to test its function is to palpate the lower border during resisted adduction. There does not seem to be any difference in shoulder strength when one muscle has been harvested (Laitung JK. *Br J Plast Surg* 1985;**38**:375–379).

Common uses

- As an islanded flap may be used for chest wall, breast, shoulder, back and neck reconstruction. It can provide a functional muscle flap for proximal upper limb reconstruction.
- As a free flap it is often used for defects of the scalp and lower limb. A larger flap can be raised by also harvesting the serratus anterior ± rib. The blood supply to the inferior fascial portion may be precarious.

Surface markings

Origins and attachments as above. Find the lower border by asking the patient to adduct against resistance and mark the inferior border of the posterior axilla. The vessels enter the deep surface of the upper part of the muscle in the axilla along with the thoracodorsal nerve. A skin paddle, if required, can be transverse (especially for breast reconstruction, with scar hidden in the bra band), or oblique; a skin paddle of up to 8 cm in width allows primary closure.

Technique

The patient is placed in a mid-lateral position with arm abducted to 90°. The border of the skin paddle is incised, bevelling edges outwards; usually the upper border is developed first, then sweeping downwards to avoid inadvertent elevation of serratus anterior which is intimately associated with the deep surface of the muscle from its scapular attachment to the ninth rib. The paravertebral perforators and vertebral attachments need to be divided. During dissection, identify and preserve the long thoracic nerve and serratus vessels, although the branch to serratus anterior may be divided along with the circumflex scapular artery for greater pedicle length.

Other points

- The flap may also be pedicled on the segmental perforators – the reversed latissimus dorsi.
- The flap may be harvested in some cases if the thoracodorsal artery has been divided previously e.g. from prior axillary node dissection. In such cases, the flap is sustained by retrograde flow in the serratus anterior branch.
- Seroma is fairly common and some recommend a quilting technique to reduce its incidence.

Rectus abdominis

The muscle flap is a type III muscle (two dominant pedicles); the tissue in this region may alternatively be harvested as a myocutaneous TRAM or cutaneous DIEP flap.

The rectus muscle is attached superiorly to the fifth–seventh costal cartilages and inferiorly by two heads to the pubic symphysis and upper border of the pubic crest. The pyramidalis muscle arises from the pubic crest and blends with its counterpart at the linea alba 4 cm above its origin. The muscle is embryologically derived from segmental anterior mesodermal somites, thus explaining its segmental innervation T7–12. The muscle has distinctive tendinous intersections to which the anterior rectus sheath is firmly adherent; there is one intersection at the umbilicus, one at the xiphisternum and one in between (occasionally also below). The muscle acts to flex the trunk (first 30–40°), depress the ribs with the pelvis stabilized and raise intra-abdominal pressure.

The arterial supply comes from the superior epigastric (terminal branch of internal thoracic) and deep inferior epigastric (branch of the external iliac) **plus** small segmental branches entering the deep surface from the lower six intercostal arteries (travelling with the accompanying intercostal nerves). The deep inferior epigastric vessels are larger than the superior epigastric vessels (2–4 mm in diameter vs. 1–2 mm) and are 6–8 cm in length on average; there are usually two accompanying venae comitantes (venous valves become incompetent for reverse flow). The flap can be delayed by dividing one set of vessels.

Common uses

Defects requiring muscle (it is between gracilis and latissimus dorsi in size) – functional segments may be raised by preserving the intercostal nerves. This segmental pattern of nerve supply does limit its usefulness in functional muscle transfer though small strips can be used for facial reanimation.

- Lower and upper limb defects as a muscle flap (myocutaneous flap is usually too bulky).
- Breast reconstruction (TRAM pedicled or free, DIEP).
- Perineal/groin reconstruction (inferiorly pedicled).

Surface markings

The DIEA arises 1 cm above the inguinal ligament and enters the muscle on its deep lateral surface midway between the umbilicus and the pelvic crest (i.e. roughly at the level of the arcuate line).

Technique

Vertical paramedian incision can be utilized for raising a rectus muscle flap or a vertical ellipse for VRAM whilst a transverse ellipse is used for a TRAM.

For a TRAM, elevate without fascia to the perforators (largest ones are para-umbilical) on the pedicle side and include these in a strip of anterior rectus sheath (these can be diathermied if a muscle-only flap is needed). For a free TRAM, isolate and divide superior pedicle, then follow inferior pedicle along the lateral side of the flap inferiorly.

Other points

- The muscle contracts after harvesting: on average, it measures ~30 × 10 cm *in situ* but only 20 × 8 cm after raising.
- Caution is advised following previous intra-abdominal surgery, but a typical (low) Caesarean section is not a contraindication for a free TRAM. Obese patients may be unsuitable for a TRAM because of reduced reliability of para-umbilical perforators.
- Mesh repair may be required if the rectus sheath cannot be closed directly.

Radial forearm flap

The radial forearm flap (RFF) is a fasciocutaneous flap (type C), typically used as a free flap but can be pedicled or distally based with reversed flow from the ulnar artery via the palmar arches.

- A 10–12 cm segment of lateral cortex of radius can also be harvested if required.
- The palmaris longus can be included e.g. in lower lip reconstruction as a sling.
- Either the venae comitantes or the superficial veins (usually cephalic) can be used for microanastomosis; some advise against anastomosing both, due to the possible risk of reduced flow leading to thrombosis.

The use of this flap is contraindicated where Allen's test indicates poor perfusion by the ulnar artery (7–12 seconds, 15% do not have complete palmar arches); some have suggested reconstruction of the artery with reversed cephalic or saphenous vein grafting. Note that the ulnar artery may be superficial in ~9% of patients and thus vulnerable during RFF harvesting.

Surface markings

The non-dominant forearm is usually preferred; generally avoid the most distal parts of the forearm over the wrist crease. The radial artery may be palpated at the wrist and traced proximally beneath brachioradialis to the antecubital fossa (a Doppler probe may help). It is useful in flap design to pre-operatively mark out tributaries of the cephalic vein – the cephalic vein often communicates with the venae comitantes near the antecubital fossa and this can drain the whole flap.

Common uses

The RFF is the archetypal 'Chinese flap' (its use in penile reconstruction was described by Chang) and its use for mandibular reconstruction was first described in the English literature by Soutar in 1983. It remains commonly used in head and neck surgery particularly when thin pliable flaps are required e.g. intra-oral, as well as resurfacing of the dorsum of the hand and penile reconstruction. The RFF can also be used as a flow-through flap due to its vascular anatomy.

When used as a reverse distally based flap (best pivot point is about 2–3 cm proximal to the wrist), the communicating channels between venae comitantes allow bypass of venular valves; alternatively, valves may become incompetent.

Technique

The use of an arm tourniquet is common but not universal; some inflate without exsanguination to make the veins more pronounced whilst stopping arterial bleeding. It is more common to begin elevation on the ulnar side and work radially, taking care to preserve paratenon particularly on FCR. On the radial side of FCR the dissection proceeds from superficial to the tendon to a deeper plane to ensure fascial continuity between vessels and skin paddle. The distal artery is temporarily clamped to check hand perfusion with the tourniquet down before transecting it. The flap can then be raised from distal to proximal. Care should be taken to avoid injury to the superficial branches of the radial nerve.

- When harvesting bone, do not dissect beneath the vessels but maintain septocutaneous continuity and a cuff of FPL muscle origin. Stress fracture of the radius may occur in post-menopausal women.
- If the flap is intended to be sensate then either the medial or lateral cutaneous nerves of the forearm can be included.

The donor site is the main perceived disadvantage with this flap; it can be poor in young or obese patients. It is usually closed with a skin graft (non-take is most common over the FCR tendon) but many alternative techniques are described in the literature.

Scapular flap

This is a (fascio)cutaneous flap based upon the horizontal or transverse branch of the circumflex scapular artery from the subscapular artery which emerges through the triangular space. The artery roughly divides the scapula into two halves; the average pedicle length is 4–6 cm with a 1.5–3 mm diameter artery with two large but thin-walled venae comitantes. The flap can be raised without fascia (suprafascial) or with bone from the scapula or in combination with other flaps on the subscapular artery axis such as latissimus dorsi or serratus anterior with or without rib for large composite defects.

The parascapular flap can be harvested on the descending branch of the circumflex scapular artery that courses down the lateral border of the scapula.

Surface markings

A horizontal ellipse drawn over the centre of the scapula, with apices in the posterior axilla at the position of the triangular space and within 2–3 cm of the midline. The maximum dimensions allowing primary closure are ~10 × 20 cm in the average-sized person. A bilateral scapular flap that crosses the midline can be harvested but requires two anastomoses and has been used for total face reconstruction (Angrigiani C. *Plast Reconstr Surg* 1997;**99**:1566–1575).

Common uses

The free scapular flap was first described by Gilbert A (*Plast Reconstr Surg* 1982;**69**:601–604). It is a thin versatile flap that is easy to raise and is often used in limb resurfacing and facial reconstruction, but having to reposition patients adds to the operative time.

Technique

With the patient prone or in mid-lateral position, elevation progresses medial to lateral in a bloodless plane superficial to the deep fascia towards fat-filled triangular space; smaller flaps may be passed anteriorly through this space e.g. for anterior defects.

Deep circumflex iliac artery

The deep circumflex iliac artery (DCIA) flap was first described by Taylor GI (*Plast Reconstr Surg* 1979:**64**:595–604). It is based over the iliac crest and may include some of this bone (up to 7 cm). The pedicle is the deep circumflex iliac artery, a branch from the lateral aspect of the external iliac artery 2 cm above the inguinal ligament that then skirts the inner pelvic rim deep to the fascia overlying iliopsoas muscles. The skin perforators emerge in a row just above the inner lip of the iliac crest, commencing near the ASIS and emerging at 2 cm intervals; the largest perforator is usually the terminal branch and arises 6–8 cm beyond the ASIS. The pedicle length is on average 5–8 cm with large vessels of diameters 1.5–4 mm; the venae comitantes run lateral to the external iliac artery and then cross either in front of (50%) or behind (50%) the artery as they ascend medially to join the external iliac vein. There is an ascending muscular branch from the pedicle 1–2 cm medial to the ASIS which does not contribute to the skin or bone of the flap.

Surface markings

The cutaneous paddle (up to 14 × 27 cm) is centred on the iliac crest with two-thirds of its area lying above the iliac crest. It can be extended medially to the femoral vessels and laterally 8–10 cm away from the ASIS.

Common uses

As an osseocutaneous flap, it is perhaps most suited to the reconstruction of curved bone (though step osteotomies can be used for straightening, the fibular is preferred for straight bone) e.g. using the ipsilateral hip for hemimandible and composite intra-oral defects; the bone can be orientated at right angles to the skin.

Technique

The medial upper part of the flap is usually raised first, along with a segment of the anterior abdominal wall (external oblique/internal oblique/transversus abdominis) to identify and preserve the superficial circumflex iliac vessels. The DCIA is followed laterally maintaining a cuff of iliacus between the vessels and the bone. The inferior border is then raised cutting through TFL and the gluteal muscles as an outer muscle cuff. Since the bone is supplied from its medial cortex, it can be split to harvest this cortex alone while preserving the outer cortex.

- The superficial circumflex vessels may be anastomosed to the ascending muscle vessels as an internal shunt.
- The upper cut edge of abdominal wall muscle is attached to the pelvic side-wall using a strong nylon suture anchored through bone.
- The donor site is relatively inconspicuous but the flap is usually a poor colour match and often bulky.

Free fibula

This flap can be raised as bone only, or combined with skin, muscle or both. It is supplied by the peroneal artery which arises from the posterior tibial artery 2.5 cm below its origin (the popliteal artery divides into anterior and posterior tibial arteries at the level of politeus muscle). The artery is in the posterior compartment along with the posterior tibial artery, running beneath the attachment of flexor hallucis longus posteromedial to the fibula and gives off muscle branches to flexor digitorum longus and tibialis posterior; other muscle branches wind around the fibula to supply peroneus longus and brevis and a nutrient branch is given off to the fibula itself at the junction of the upper and middle third with ascending and descending branches. It terminates as the lateral calcaneal artery and a perforating branch which penetrates the interosseus septum to reach the anterior compartment.

There are usually four septocutaneous perforators running in the intermuscular septum between peroneus longus and soleus around the junction between the upper and middle thirds of the fibula. Sometimes the perforators arise from muscular branches of the peroneal necessitating intermuscular dissection of soleus. In up to 10%, the skin island over the fibula is supplied by a system of vessels separate from the peroneal artery and cannot be harvested together.

Surface markings

Mark out the fibula head and lateral malleolus, and draw the line along the posterior border of the bone which forms the axis of the skin paddle (maximum dimensions 22–25 × 10–14 cm but any more than 8–10 cm wide will require skin grafts) with most perforators at the junction of the upper and middle third.

Mark a line 6–8 cm distal to the fibula head as site of proximal osteotomy (distal to common peroneal nerve but proximal to peroneal vessels; the nerve may be palpable as it travels forwards over the neck of the fibula to divide in the substance of peroneus longus into branches – superficial to peroneal compartment and deep to anterior compartment). Maintain at least 5 cm proximal to the lateral malleolus to avoid disrupting the ankle joint. Ankle weakness may be due to excessive bony resection or detachment of muscles (FHL, FDL and tibialis posterior).

Common uses

The fibula flap offers about 22 cm of straight tubular bone that is good for weight bearing; it is commonly used for mandibular reconstruction and segmental long bone defects. Its use was first described by Taylor GI (*Plast Reconstr Surg* 1975;**55**:533–544). The rich periosteal supply allows the bone to be osteotomized to reconstruct the curve of an angle to angle mandibular defect and to be double-barrelled.

Technique

The skin paddle is raised from both anterior and lateral borders, preserving the intermuscular septum with the septocutaneous perforators which are traced whilst dissecting free the posteromedial surface of the fibula, taking care to maintain the periosteal layer.

The distal osteotomy is usually performed first and the peroneal vessels emerging from the lower border of FHL are ligated. Allow 1–2 cm extra bone than required to fit the defect at either end with flaps of periosteum for wrapping around the fixation. Continue the dissection proximally, freeing the anteriomedial surface whilst preserving the vascular pedicle. A proximal segment of bone can be excised to allow more room for mobilization during the superior dissection.

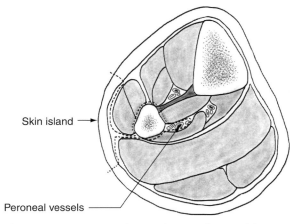

Figure 11.3 Cross-section showing the tissues harvested during an osteocutaneous fibula flap.

Wedge osteotomies can be performed whilst the flap is still attached by its pedicle; some prefer out-fractures with opening osteotomies to the conventional closing osteotomy after excision of a wedge.

Serratus anterior

The serratus anterior is a type III muscle flap – there are two dominant pedicles (lateral thoracic artery to the upper part plus serratus branch of thoracodorsal artery to the lower part). It can also be raised with some skin and rib.

The muscle arises from first to eighth/ninth ribs; the upper half inserts into the deep aspect of the medial edge of the scapula whilst the lower slips insert into the angle. When it contracts it causes protrusion of the scapula and rotates the scapula upwards and outwards. It can be tested by pushing the outstretched hand against a wall – absence or denervation produces characteristic winging.

It is innervated by the **long thoracic nerve** (C5, 6 and 7) which lies anterior to the artery but still deep to the deep fascia; the nerve joins the artery at the level of the sixth rib to enter at the junction of middle and posterior third of the muscle. The upper four muscle slips are innervated by C5, next two by C6 and lowest two by C7 fibres – the lower half thus has an independent nerve and blood supply lending itself to easy splitting.

Common uses

The serratus anterior flap is most often used for coverage of defects of the head and neck and extremities. It may also be used as a functional flap for facial and hand reanimation.

Technique

The incision parallels the eighth rib on the lateral chest side-wall, curving superiorly to the axilla. Identify the anterior border of latissimus dorsi and separate it from the posterior part of the serratus anterior under it; the anterior part is exposed by elevation of the overlying skin. Elevate the lower slips of serratus off their rib origins, tying off intercostal perforators unless underlying bone and/or overlying skin are required.

The pedicle is traced superiorly; tying off the thoracodorsal artery (latissimus dorsi) and the circumflex scapular artery will provide an extremely long pedicle (whole of subscapular artery). The nerve is preserved if an innervated muscle is required – it is possible to separate out a discrete bunch of fascicles to the lower part of the muscle only.

Lateral arm flap

The lateral arm flap is a fasciocutaneous flap (type C) that is easy to make sensate. It can also be raised as a fascia-only flap or with a piece of the humerus as an osseofasciocutaneous flap. It is based upon the posterior radial collateral artery (and its venae comitantes) from the profunda brachii artery (it continues behind the lateral malleolus to anastomose with the radial artery). The skin island is innervated by the **lower lateral cutaneous nerve of the arm**, a branch of the radial nerve which pierces the belly of triceps, whilst the upper cutaneous nerve of the arm is a terminal branch of the axillary nerve. There will be an area of numbness along the lateral forearm as a result of flap harvest. The pedicle has a diameter 1–2 mm with a maximum length 8 cm (requires splitting of the lateral head of triceps).

Common uses

It provides a thin flap suited for soft tissue defects of the dorsal and volar surfaces of the hand, as well as the foot and anterior surface of tibia. It is particularly suited as a covering for tendons because deep surface is fascia. It can also be used for facial or intra-oral defects.

Technique

The skin paddle lies on the axis of a line drawn between deltoid insertion and lateral epicondyle which also marks the position of the lateral intermuscular septum

(anterior to septum are biceps, brachialis, brachioradialis and ECRL whilst posteriorly are lateral (above spiral groove) and medial (below groove) heads of tricep). A narrow sterile tourniquet can be used but is not necessary. The posterior incision is made first and the flap is elevated forwards in the subfascial plane, then it is dissected from the front and the vessel can then be seen in the intermuscular septum. The distal vessel is ligated and the fascial septum progressively detached from bone unless bone is needed. The flap can be cut between perforators to form two paddles when needed.

The pedicle is followed proximally, a process which is made easier by incising the lateral head of triceps, taking care to preserve the radial nerve that lies between brachialis and brachioradialis, and the spiral groove.

The radial nerve gives off the posterior cutaneous nerve of the arm, which runs through the flap but innervates only the skin on the back of the arm but must be taken in the flap. Donor sites of up to 6 cm width will close directly.

Groin flap

The groin flap is a cutaneous/fat flap that can be used either free or pedicled. It is the archetypal axial pattern flap. The pedicle is the superficial circumflex iliac artery from the femoral artery at the medial border of sartorius. The vessels have a narrow diameter, usually about 1 mm, which is similar to the superficial temporal or facial vessels, hence these are often used as recipient vessels. There are paired venae comitantes and by a direct cutaneous vein draining into the saphenous bulb, ~2 mm diameter, which drains the whole flap.

Common uses

It is a versatile flap first described by McGregor IA (*Plast Reconstr Surg* 1972;**49**:41–47) and can be used for a variety of defects such as the head and neck, chest and extremities. It can be de-epithelialized to fill out contour defects of the face.

Flaps of up to 15 × 30 cm can be raised and closed directly leaving an inconspicuous linear donor site scar and is thus often described as being 'dispensible'. However it is not so useful in obese patients though liposuction can subsequently be used to reduce bulkiness. The main 'complaint' levelled at the flap is that the pedicle is small, short and inconsistent – expect anatomical variations.

Technique

The long axis of the flap parallels the inguinal ligament, 2 cm below. The flap is raised from the lateral edge first (in the flank the full-thickness of fat need not be elevated but can be thinned to the dermis at this point) taking care to preserve the lateral cutaneous nerve of the thigh. As sartorius is approached the fascia is included in the flap since this transmits a number of cutaneous perforators at this point. The superficial circumflex iliac vessels are on the underside of the flap and can be traced forwards; preserve the inferior epigastric vein as it runs beneath the medial part of the flap since this has a sizeable tributary from the groin skin.

Gracilis flap

The gracilis is a type II muscle flap with a major pedicle from medial branch of circumflex femoral artery (and venae comitantes) and one or two minor pedicles from branches of superficial femoral artery distal to the origin of the medial circumflex femoral artery. The pedicle is 6–8 cm long and enters the muscle on its deep surface 10 cm from the pubic tubercle.

The muscle arises as a flat sheet from the inferior pubic ramus, narrowing inferiorly to insert into medial side of the subcutaneous surface of the tibia, just below and behind the sartorius insertion. It is innervated by the **obturator nerve** which enters the muscle on its medial side, lying just superior (2 cm) to the vessels. It is an adductor of the hip, flexor of the knee and medially rotates the flexed knee.

Common uses

Primarily it is used as a muscle flap as the skin paddle is generally regarding as being relatively unreliable. It provides well-vascularized muscle (up to 5 × 20 cm) for use at sites where bulk is a disadvantage such as long thin defects following lower extremity trauma and osteomyelitis, as well as for facial and hand reanimation as well as contour restoration in the head and neck.

Since the obturator nerve trifurcates at its entry point to the muscle, the gracilis can be split to provide slips if needed. 10–12 cm of nerve is available.

Technique

The incision runs from the midpoint of the symphysis pubis and ischial tuberosity superiorly to the medial femoral condyle inferiorly, keeping the long saphenous vein anteriorly which crosses the muscle.

The muscle is raised from inferior to superior, ligating the multiple perforators from the gracilis pedicle to the overlying adductor longus. The latter muscle can be retracted to expose the full length of the pedicle right up to its origin.

Rectus femoris myocutaneous flap

The rectus femoris muscle has two heads from the anterior inferior iliac spine and upper part of acetabulum, which unite to contribute to the patellar tendon along with the vastus muscles (some recommend that the latter should be centralized after flap harvest). The pedicle comes from the descending branch of the lateral circumflex femoral artery and enters the flap 8 cm below the inguinal ligament.

This is a useful flap for perineal reconstruction, and it can also be used for defects of the lower abdominal wall and greater trochanter. It has a longer length and arc of rotation than the TFL and the pivot point is at the anterior thigh rather than lateral thigh. Freeing the proximal attachments will increase the arc of rotation further.

The flap can also be raised as a musculocutaneous flap with a skin paddle of 15 × 40 cm, supplied by three-to-four perforators proximally. The skin and muscle components can be split and used to fill separate defects.

Tensor fascia lata flap

The TFL flap is supplied by a transverse branch of the lateral femoral circumflex artery which enters the muscle 6–8 cm below the ASIS. The muscle arises from the ASIS and greater trochanter of the femur and inserts as fascia lata into the iliotibial tract (lateral tibial condyle) and thus helps to maintain lateral knee stability.

A myocutaneous flap can be harvested with a skin paddle reaching up 8 cm above the lateral femoral condyle. It is a suitable option for reconstruction of perineal, ischial and lower abdominal/groin defects; freeing up the proximal attachments can increase arc of rotation. The donor site can be closed directly or skin grafted.

Pectoralis major

This myocutaneous flap was first described by Ariyan S (*Plast Reconstr Surg* 1979:**63**:78–81), and was commonly used in head and neck reconstruction though its use has reduced after the introduction of the RFF and other flaps.

The muscle has sternocostal (upper six ribs) and clavicular heads, which combine to insert into the lateral lip of the bicipital groove of the humerus; the muscle forms the anterior border of the axilla and acts as a powerful adductor and medial rotator of the humerus.

The nerve supply comes from the medial and lateral pectoral nerves. The blood supply comes from the lateral thoracic arteries and pectoral branch of the thoraco-acromial trunk – the latter provides the pedicle that runs medially along a line drawn from the acromion to the xiphisternum after dropping down vertically to meet it.

Technique

The skin paddle is positioned medial to the nipple according to the reconstructive needs; in females it is often better to position the paddle below the nipple. A 'defensive' incision is often used even though the use of the deltopectoral flap has reduced significantly; direct donor site closure is usually possible. The inferior border of the flap is dissected first to define the extent of the muscle to ensure that the skin island is located suitably. The dissection is continued to lift up the muscle, and the pedicle is easily visualized; traditionally a generous cuff is kept around the vessels.

Wei described the 'muscle-free' flap in 1984 with sparing of the clavicular head to reduce donor morbidity. A later 'functional island flap' was said to be comparable to a radial forearm flap but is more suited to larger volume defects and further reduces shoulder dysfunction following radical neck dissection in which trapezius is often denervated.

The Palmer and Bachelor modifications aim to reduce the donor morbidity further:

- The upper portion of the sternocostal head is also left intact.
- The lateral pectoral nerve and as much as possible of the medial nerve are left intact.

The proximal portion of the pectoral branch before it enters the muscle is surrounded by loose areolar tissue and can be dissected off overlying muscle and the islanded flap delivered through a 'button-hole' between the fibres of the clavicular head of the muscle and overlying fascia. This increases the pedicle length by about 4 cm to reach the oral cavity, a greater arc of rotation and less compromise of shoulder function.

Superior gluteal artery flap

This is a type II muscle or myocutaneous flap, and the latter is an option in breast reconstruction when the abdominal flaps are not available. A pedicled perforator flap based on the artery alone (S-GAP perforator flap) is a good option for sacral pressure sores.

The free S-GAP flap is recommended as a sensate flap for autologous breast reconstruction (Blondeel PN. *Br J Plast Surg* 1999;**52**:185–193) and benefits include the inconspicuous donor site with no functional deficit. It provides a skin paddle 25–35 × 9–13 cm with a fat layer of up to 8 cm and flap volume of up to 800 ml. The pedicle length is short at 3 cm but the vessels are a good size with a diameter 2–3 mm, and can be anastomosed to internal mammary vessels or axilla (vein graft may be needed). However, the need to turn the patient during the operation is a disadvantage.

The **gluteus maximus** is a broad, flat sheet of muscle which lies most superficially in the buttock and crosses the gluteal fold at 45°, passing from the gluteal surface of the ilium, the lumbar fascia, the sacrum and the sacrotuberous ligament to the gluteal crest of the femur and the iliotibial tract. It contracts to extend and externally rotate the femur, and acting through the fascia lata it also supports the extended knee. The muscle is supplied by the inferior gluteal nerve only whilst the arterial supply comes from both the superior and inferior gluteal arteries.

The superior gluteal artery arises from the posterior branch of the internal iliac artery whilst the inferior gluteal artery is one of three parietal branches from the anterior branch (the others being the pudendal and obturator arteries).

- The superior gluteal artery emerges from the greater sciatic foramen with the superior gluteal nerve, passing between gluteus medius above and piriformis below, and divides into deep and superficial branches. The latter branch supplies gluteus maximus and the overlying skin.
- The inferior gluteal artery emerges from the pelvis below piriformis, and hence through the lesser sciatic foramen, along with the sciatic nerve.

Surface markings

The superior gluteal artery emerges from the pelvis at a point between the upper third and lower two-thirds of a line connecting the posterior superior iliac spine (PSIS) and greater trochanter, 6 cm below the PSIS and 4 cm lateral to the midline of the sacrum. The flap may be drawn horizontally based upon this to conform to a bikini line.

Technique

Circumcise the skin flap down through the deep fascia. Divide the upper third of gluteus maximus in line with the upper skin incision and identify the superior gluteal pedicle emerging from between gluteus medius and piriformis. The inferior incision can then be completed, elevating the flap from lateral to medial.

Temporoparietal fascial flap

The temporoparietal fascia (TPF) is a large thin fascial sheet which covers the temporal, parietal and occipital areas of the scalp. It is an extension of the SMAS layer, passing from face to scalp, and continues above the temporal line as the galea aponeurosis, densely adherent to overlying skin/fat via connective tissue and separated by loose areolar tissue from the underlying pericranium. The temporalis muscle and temporalis fascia (deep temporal fascia) lie deep to the temporoparietal fascia inferior to the temporal line.

The TPF flap can be used as a free or pedicled flap (the skin or underlying parietal cranial bone can be included). It is a very thin flap with cosmetic donor site unless there is male pattern baldness. It is often used in head and neck reconstruction or upper limb reconstruction as it allows tendon gliding.

It is supplied by large, anatomically consistent vessels with artery size of up to 2 mm (and vein > 2 mm in diameter) from the superficial temporal artery which is the terminal branch of the external carotid artery and can be palpated or identified by Doppler. The artery and vein ascend anterior to the ear with the vein lying superficially and the auriculotemporal nerve supplying sensation to the scalp lying posterior to the pedicle.

The incision is made posterior to the pedicle at the level of the tragus; the pedicle is identified and traced superiorly. A skin paddle of up to 3 cm wide may be closed directly; transient alopecia has been observed. Note that the frontal branch of the facial nerve passes from a point 0.5 cm below the tragus to 1.5 cm superior to the lateral brow.

Omental flap

This is a flap of omentum which is largely a mass of fat attached along the greater curvature of the stomach as far as the first part of the duodenum and loops down and backwards to attach to the transverse colon.

It provides an extensive vascular film to restore moving tissue planes and has been used for certain purposes such as scalp reconstruction and filling in of contour deformities (Romberg's disease). It has been advocated in the past for augmenting lymphatic drainage in lymphoedema. The pedicle is the right gastroepiploic artery (and vein) roughly 3–4 cm in length, which is a terminal division of the gastroduodenal artery. There are many vessels in the attachments that need to be ligated.

It can be harvested by open laparotomy or through endoscopic harvest; its use is relatively contraindicated by previous abdominal surgery.

Anterolateral thigh flap

This is a fasciocutaneous flap based upon myocutaneous or septocutaneous perforators from the descending branch of the lateral circumflex femoral artery. It has become a workhorse flap in head and neck reconstruction in particular including pharyngeal reconstruction as a tubed flap. The surface markings are fairly consistent; a line drawn from ASIS to the lateral border of patella marks the lateral intermuscular septum between vastus lateralis and rectus femoris, and most perforators are seen in the lateral inferior quadrant of a 3 cm circle centred on the midpoint of this line. The pedicle is 7–12 cm long with a 1.5–2.5 mm diameter artery. The TFL is a 'lifeboat' if there are no 'typically' located perforators; otherwise a medial thigh flap can often be raised.

Pre-operative identification of the location of perforators is commonly performed with Doppler ultrasound although some have documented experience with computed tomography angiography (CTA) or magnetic resonance angiography (MRA). A flap is based on these perforators with the medial incision usually made first down to the rectus femoris. Lateral subfascial dissection towards the intermuscular septum allows identification of perforators which are gradually traced back to the origin and may need significant intramuscular dissection.

The flap provides a large skin paddle (which can be sensate) and can be used as a flow-through flap. When suitable perforator configuration/numbers permit, **chimeric type** flaps with multiple skin islands or components e.g. skin and muscle can be harvested. The donor site morbidity is relatively minimal if direct closure is possible; compartment syndrome has been reported after overtight closure (Addison PD. *Ann Plast Surg* 2008;**60**:635–638).

VI. Tissue expansion

Aims:

- Allows replacement of like with like by using local skin for the best match of colour, texture, and hair-bearing quality (if needed) and is potentially sensate.
- The donor site can be closed directly under most circumstances.

History

- Neumann 1957 – expansion of postauricular skin for ear reconstruction with an air-filled subcutaneous implant. However, this did not become popular.
- Radavon 1975 – developed the silicone expander and used it clinically initially in a case of arm flap tissue expansion to cover an adjacent defect (1976), and later breast reconstruction (1982). At the same time, Austad had done similar work in developing an implant independently.
- Austad ED. *Plast Reconstr Surg* 1982;**70**:704–710 – histological evaluation of the changes accompanying tissue expansion in animals.

Histological changes

- Epidermis thickens due to cellular hyperplasia (**the only layer/tissue that thickens**) and there are increased mitoses in the basal layer. Rete ridges are less pronounced.
- Dermis thins despite increased dermal collagen that also realigns – fibrils straighten and become parallel.
  - Rupture of elastin fibres.
  - Appendages unaltered.
- Muscle thins – sarcomeres thin and become compacted. There are increased numbers of mitochondria.
- Adipose tissue atrophies with some permanent loss.
- Nerves – altered conductivity.

Cyclic loading

The mobile microarchitecture of dermal collagen

Gibson T. *Br J Surg* 1965;**52**:764–770.

Application of a load to skin causes it to stretch, and when the load is removed it relaxes back. However, when an excessive load is applied, it stretches without subsequent relaxation.

Creep vs. stretch: a review of the viscoelastic properties of skin

Wilhelmi BJ. *Ann Plast Surg* 1998;**41**:215–219.

Skin is viscoelastic and responds to stretch in a characteristic manner.

- **Mechanical** creep is the elongation of skin under a constant load over time:
  - Collagen fibres stretch out and become parallel.
  - Elastin undergoes microfragmentation.
  - Water/interstitial fluid is displaced.
  - Some mechanical creep occurs during intra-operative tissue expansion and skin suturing under tension.
- **Biological creep** is the generation of **new tissue** secondary to a persistent chronic stretching force i.e. the type of creep seen in pregnancy and conventional tissue expansion.
- **Stress–relaxation** describes the tendency for the resistance of the skin to a stretching force to decrease when held at a given tension over time e.g. skin becomes tight when expanded but by the next visit, it is no longer tight.

Molecular basis for tissue expansion: clinical implications for the surgeon

Takei T. *Plast Reconstr Surg* 1998;**102**:247–258.

Mechanical strain was shown to induce transcription of cellular proto-oncogenes such as *c-fos*, *c-myc* and *c-jun*.

- **Up-regulation of growth factors** such as EGF, TGF-β and PDGF.
- Deformational forces acting on the cell membrane and disruption of integrins **reduce cell–matrix adhesion**.
- Stretch-induced conformational changes of membrane proteins cause **opening of calcium channels** leading to signal transduction and effects on the cytoskeleton (microfilament contraction), transduction pathways such as phospholipase C/protein kinase C.
- The actin cytoskeleton transmits mechanical forces intracellularly resulting in **mitosis** (growth and regeneration) via interaction with protein kinases, second messengers and nuclear proteins.

Stretch and growth: the molecular and physiological influences of tissue expansion

De Filippo RE. *Plast Reconstr Surg* 2002;**109**:2450–2462.

Mechanical stretch leads to activation of signal transduction pathways (via protein kinase C receptors) that increase DNA synthesis and cell proliferation.

Vascular endothelial growth factor expression in expanded tissue: a possible mechanism of angiogenesis in tissue expansion

Lantieri LA. *Plast Reconstr Surg* 1998;**101**:392–398.

Tissue expansion is angiogenic and the expanded skin has increased vascularity and blood flow. The authors looked at human skin samples after expansion and found an increased number of cells expressing VEGF.

Radiotherapy: effects on expanded skin

Goodman C. *Plast Reconstr Surg* 2002;**110**:1080–1083.

This study in rabbits aimed to investigate the effects of external beam radiotherapy upon the skin overlying a tissue expander and its capsule. Half of the expanded area was irradiated 3 weeks after insertion whilst the other half acted as an internal control; three groups received 20 Gy, 25 Gy or 35 Gy in unfractionated doses. The skin was harvested 6 weeks after irradiation and the findings were:

- Dermal thickness and the surrounding capsule remained unchanged.
- Epidermal thickness increased to up to 130% in the highest radiation dose group.

Biomechanical comparison between conventional and rapid expansion of skin

Zeng YJ. *Br J Plast Surg* 2003;**56**:660–666.

The authors compared the biomechanical properties of rapidly expanded skin (daily expansion for 2 weeks) and conventionally expanded skin (weekly for 6 weeks) in a canine model. There was a maintaining time after expansion (1 week, 2 weeks or 4 weeks). The results showed no difference in total area of skin expansion and biomechanical properties (stress–strain, stress–relaxation, tensile strength, creep and stretch–back). Their conclusion was that rapid expansion can be undertaken to provide skin with similar biomechanical properties to conventionally expanded skin whilst a **4-week maintaining time** optimizes the stretch–back ratio.

Indications

Burn scar alopecia

Tissue expansion is an important option in burn scar excision e.g. of the face (including ear) and neck (expanders can be placed in the neck without causing vascular compromise) particularly where the scar is on the scalp and thus causes alopecia. It is common to base rotation or advancement flaps on named arteries such as temporal, occipital, taking care to orientate direction of hair growth. It is possible to expand to double the size of the scalp without separating follicles unduly.

- The expander is placed beneath the galea (scoring at the time of flap mobilization may aid expansion) and the implant is expanded over 6–8 weeks.

Others

- Forehead expansion for nasal reconstruction – critics suggest that this will lead to suboptimal results as the skin flap retracts.
- Expansion of myocutaneous pedicled and free flaps (prefabrication) to increase volume of tissue transported and facilitate donor site closure.

Technique

The defect should be considered in terms of its shape and site, and the type of flap to be used. A significant disadvantage in the use of tissue expanders is the prolonged process needing two operations and multiple visits in between. Using multiple expanders could reduce the overall duration of expansion.

- Expanders should be placed either through an incision which will be later excised or one remote from the scar/defect. Remote radial incisions will tend to be under less tension with expansion and thus need less delay to allow for wound healing compared with circumferential incisions that form the leading edge of the advancing flap; however, using radial incisions usually means adding another scar.
- Make the largest pocket possible and chose the expander base size to fill this pocket.
- The port can be placed internally or externalized (useful in children). A moderate amount of fluid is usually injected for an initial expansion that takes up dead space. Expansion proper is commenced after 1–2 weeks and continues weekly to the limits of patient tolerance (blanching is another clue to the adequacy of fill).
- The capsule can be kept if there is sufficient tissue as it is extremely vascular; incision of the capsule (capsulotomy) adds a slight amount of mobility whilst excision of the capsule (capsulectomy) increases the mobility further, making it thinner

and more compliant but risks compromising the vascularity.

Potential difficulties

- Judging if the skin has been expanded adequately.
  - There are many different formulae that have been used to determine the amount of expanded skin, ranging from the simple, e.g. subtraction of base size from the circumference of the expanded skin, to more complex mathematical formulae. For many practical reasons (leakage from port, stretchback etc.), the actual tissue gained always seems to be less than predicted, thus in practice expanding just a bit more is always a safe practice.
- Using the expanded skin in the most efficient manner.
  - It can be difficult to convert a three-dimensional area of skin into a flap to cover what is usually a flat defect. In most cases, simple rotation or advancement flaps are used. It may be easier to visualize the expanded skin as five sides of a cube (minus the base) that can be split along its sides creating a flap as a chain of three 'squares' with the wings being positioned variably at these links.

Complications

Tissue expansion does have a significant rate of complications:

- Extrusion and wound dehiscence.
- Infection.
- Rupture.
- Migration – less with textured expanders.

Extremity expansion, especially lower limb, associated with more complications including sural nerve neuropraxia. Expansion in **children** and in previously irradiated tissue is also more problematic.

Tissue expansion in children

It is traditionally accepted that there is a higher incidence of complications in children (~20%) and this is often higher in burn scars as the tissue is less malleable.

Risk factors for complications for pediatric tissue expansion

Friedman R. *Plast Reconstr Surg* 1996;**98**:1242–1246.

The authors report on their experience with 180 expanders in children with an overall complication rate of 9%. Internal ports were associated with a higher complication rate (puncture). Overall, more complications were expected for burn scar surgery, soft tissue loss and age <7 years (perceived lack of cooperation).

Tissue expansion in children: a retrospective study of complications

Gibstein L. *Ann Plast Surg* 1997;**38**:358–364.

Indications for the use of tissue expanders in this study included congenital naevus, craniofacial anomalies, aplasia cutis congenita and myelomeningocoele. Overall, 17% had complications and these were not related to gender, site, numbers, indication or use of drains.

Calvarial deformity and remodelling following prolonged scalp expansion in a child

Calobrace MB. *Ann Plast Surg* 1997;**39**:186–189.

Using a scalp expander causes bone resorption and a deformity known as **saucerization**. The authors describe a 5-year-old boy undergoing scalp expansion for burn scar alopecia over 15 months. Burn scar is regarded as being unyielding and so may transmit more pressure to the calvarium. A 3-cm deep depression had been created in the calvarium with bone lipping (deposition) at the margins. The changes were **reversible** and were fully remodelled by 6 months.

Algorithm of hair restoration surgery in children

Kolasinski J. *Plast Reconstr Surg* 2003;**112**:412–422.

The authors reviewed their experience with 57 children with hair loss over the 18-year study period. The aetiology of hair loss included congenital alopecia, trauma including burns and surgical scars, irradiation for CNS neoplasms.

Scalp skin in a child is more pliable and responsive to expansion (but scars also stretch more). There is less subcutaneous fat and the hair is sparser and widely separated.

They used the McCauley classification of hair loss (1990):

- **I.** Single defect.
  - Subtypes A–D depending upon size of defect (25% increments).
- **II.** Segmental defects (2).
- **III.** Multiple defects, multiple islands of intact scalp.
- **IV.** Total scalp loss.

Treatment options:

- Excision with direct closure or scalp flap reconstruction.

- Tissue expansion for cases of extensive hair loss – consider direction of hair growth when moving flap(s).
- Hair transplantation for smaller areas of hair loss, in multifocal hair loss and for thinned hair after radiotherapy.

Tissue expansion in the limbs

Tissue expansion at limb and non-limb sites
Pandya AN. *Br J Plast Surg* 2002;**55**:302–306.

The authors present an 8-year retrospective review. In their practice, expanders are placed via short incisions, radial to direction of expansion; intra-operative expansion with saline and methylene blue is used to close the dead space and is useful at subsequent expansion to confirm correct needle placement in the port.

- Non-limb expansion mainly for breast reconstruction.
- Limb expansion for post-traumatic scarring and other contour deformities.

The commonest complications were infection and exposure of the expander.

- Overall complication rate of 43% in limbs, with **more complications in the lower limb**.
- Overall complication rate 27% in non-limb sites.

Despite the different complication rates, the authors report similar rates of successful outcome at limb and non-limb sites (83% and 86% respectively).

- Exposed or infected expanders were managed by hospitalization, antibiotics and dressings until healed and then further expansion was commenced if possible. Those unresponsive to conservative management had the expander removed after rapid expansion and judicious use of the expanded tissue.

Soft tissue expansion in the lower extremities
Manders EK. *Plast Reconstr Surg* 1988;**81**:208–217.

The vasculature in the leg is of the 'terminal' type with few axial vessels and a poorly formed subdermal plexus.

- Expanders should be at least as long as the defect to be closed and placed **above** muscle fascia.
- Incisions perpendicular to the long axis of the expander are safest.
- Over-expand or expand as long as the patient tolerates it – expansion below the knee is often a

slower process and overall much less successful than in the thigh.

There is a high complication rate including 50% infection rate. An open wound at or distal to the knee is a relative contraindication to the use of expanders.

Is soft tissue expansion in lower limb reconstruction a legitimate option?
Vogelin E. *Br J Plast Surg* 1995;**48**:579–582.

The authors reviewed their series of 34 consecutive cases with indications such as excision of unstable scars and chronic ulcers. The process was ultimately successful in 68% but the local complication rate was high at 44%. The authors suggest the following contraindications to tissue expansion in the lower limb:

- Extensive areas of scarring with compromised skin vascularity.
- Vascular disease.
- Osteomyelitis.

They recommend that these problems should be treated with muscle flaps.

Tissue expansion in the lower limb: complications in a cohort of 100 patients
Casanova D. *Br J Plast Surg* 2001;**54**:310–316.

This was a review of the use of 207 expanders in the lower limb with roughly equal proportions of remote internal ports and external ports – the latter had less leakage but more infections. The complication rate was 15.5% (with expansion abandoned in 5%) commonly sepsis, exposure and damage due to undermining.

Advancement flaps were preferred to transposition flaps. They suggest the following regarding expander selection and placement:

- Avoid bony areas, joints, scars or irradiated skin.
- Place expanders in a longitudinal direction; multiple expanders preferable.
- Use remote radial incisions, then atraumatic blunt dissection above fascia.

The begining of a new era in tissue expansion: self-filling osmotic tissue expander – four-year clinical experience
Ronert MA. *Plast Reconstr Surg* 2004;**114**:1025–1031.

These expanders are made from an osmotically active hydrogel and manufactured to 10% of its final volume. The expander gradually absorbs fluid to achieve final size over 6–8 weeks thus obviating the need for an inflation port, painful injections and regular clinic attendances for expansion. There is some discomfort that abates after the early postoperative period. A round expander is used in the breast whilst a rectangular expander is used in most other situations.

The authors suggest that these may be used for most other tissue expansion indications, particularly breast skin expansion prior to replacement with a silicone implant:

- May be left *in situ* for up to 6 months before replacement.
- Requires healthy skin/muscle coverage and thus unsuitable in previously irradiated areas.

Wound dehiscence occurred in some patients and led to a modification to the expander with a silicone membrane to limit the rate of expansion and improvement of the success rate from 82% to 91%. One criticism of this technique is the lack of control over speed as well as extent of expansion.

Osmotic expanders have been used by some surgeons in paediatric patients particularly burns (Chummun S. *J Burn Care Res* 2009;**30**:744–746) and clefts. Avoiding the need for regular injections is a major advantage but many (Chummun S. *J Plast Reconstr Aesthet Surg* 2010;**63**:2128–2132) suggest caution, given the high complication rate despite 'adequate precautions' and the lack of control over the expansion.

Index